Equine Clinical Immunology

To Nora and Robin.
To my family, friends and mentors who shared their support all the way.

Equine Clinical Immunology

Edited by

M. Julia B. Felippe

MedVet, MSc, PhD, Diplomate ACVIM
Associate Professor of Large Animal Medicine
College of Veterinary Medicine, Cornell University
Ithaca, New York, USA

WILEY Blackwell

This edition first published 2016 © 2016 by John Wiley & Sons, Inc.

Editorial offices: 1606 Golden Aspen Drive, Suites 103 and 104, Ames, Iowa 50010, USA
The Atrium, Southern Gate, Chichester, West Sussex, PO19 8SQ, UK
9600 Garsington Road, Oxford, OX4 2DQ, UK

For details of our global editorial offices, for customer services and for information about how to apply for permission to reuse the copyright material in this book please see our website at www.wiley.com/wiley-blackwell.

Library of Congress Cataloging-in-Publication Data

Equine clinical immunology / [edited by] M. Julia B. Felippe.
   p. cm.
   Includes bibliographical references and index.
   ISBN 978-1-118-55887-4 (cloth)
   1. Horses–Immunology. 2. Horses–Diseases. I. Felippe, M. Julia B. (Maria Julia B.), editor.
   [DNLM: 1. Horse Diseases–immunology. 2. Immune System Diseases–veterinary. 3. Immunotherapy–veterinary. SF 951]
   SF951.E5423 2016
   636.1'0896079–dc23

                                                                              2015019958

A catalogue record for this book is available from the British Library.

Wiley also publishes its books in a variety of electronic formats. Some content that appears in print may not be available in electronic books.

Set in 9.5/12pt MinionPro-Regular by Thomson Digital, Noida
Printed and bound in Singapore by Markono Print Media Pte Ltd

1   2016

Contents

Contributors

Amanda A. Adams, PhD
Department of Veterinary Science
Gluck Equine Research Center
University of Kentucky
Lexington, Kentucky

Michelle H. Barton, DVM, PhD, Diplomate ACVIM
Department of Large Animal Medicine
College of Veterinary Medicine
University of Georgia
Athens, Georgia

Angela I. Bordin, DVM, MS, PhD
Department of Large Animal Clinical Sciences
College of Veterinary Medicine and Biomedical Sciences
Texas A&M University
College Station, Texas

Michela Bullone, DVM, MSc
Département de Sciences Cliniques
Faculté de Médecine Vétérinaire
Université de Montréal
Montréal, Canada

Noah D. Cohen, VMD, MPH, PhD, Diplomate ACVIM
Department of Large Animal Clinical Sciences
College of Veterinary Medicine and Biomedical Sciences
Texas A&M University
College Station, Texas

Lais R.R. Costa, MedVet, MS, PhD, Diplomate ACVIM, Diplomate ABVP
Department of Clinical Sciences
College of Veterinary Medicine
Mississippi State University
Mississippi State, Mississippi

Elizabeth G. Davis, DVM, PhD, Diplomate ACVIM
Department of Clinical Sciences
College of Veterinary Medicine
Kansas State University
Manhattan, Kansas

Catharina De Schauwer, DVM, PhD, Diplomate ECAR
Department of Obstetrics, Reproduction, and Herd Health
Ghent University, Belgium
Merelbeke, Belgium

Thomas J. Divers, DVM, Diplomate ACVIM, Diplomate ACVECC
Department of Clinical Sciences
College of Veterinary Medicine
Cornell University
Ithaca, New York

Sian Durward-Akhurst, BVMS
Department of Veterinary Population Medicine
College of Veterinary Medicine
University of Minnesota
St. Paul, Minnesota

M. Julia B. Felippe, MedVet, MSc, PhD, Diplomate ACVIM
Department of Clinical Sciences
College of Veterinary Medicine
Cornell University
Ithaca, New York

Lisa A. Fortier, DVM, PhD, Diplomate ACVS
Department of Clinical Sciences
College of Veterinary Medicine
Cornell University
Ithaca, New York

Brian C. Gilger, DVM, MS, Diplomate ACVO, Diplomate ABT
Department of Clinical Sciences
College of Veterinary Medicine
North Carolina State University
Raleigh, North Carolina

Kelsey A. Hart, DVM, PhD, Diplomate ACVIM
Department of Large Animal Medicine
College of Veterinary Medicine
University of Georgia
Athens, Georgia

David W. Horohov, PhD
Department of Veterinary Science
Gluck Equine Research Center
University of Kentucky
Lexington, Kentucky

Laszlo L. Hunyadi, DVM, MS, PhD
Veterinary Medical Teaching Hospital
UC-Davis School of Veterinary Medicine
University of California
Davis, California

Jean-Pierre Lavoie, DMV, Diplomate ACVIM
Département de Sciences Cliniques
Faculté de Médecine Vétérinaire
Université de Montréal
Montréal, Canada

Mathilde Leclère, DMV, PhD, Diplomate ACVIM
Département de Sciences Cliniques
Faculté de Médecine Vétérinaire
Université de Montréal
Montréal, Canada

Erin L. McConachie, DVM, Diplomate ACVIM
Department of Large Animal Medicine
College of Veterinary Medicine
University of Georgia
Athens, Georgia

SallyAnne L. Ness, DVM, Diplomate ACVIM
Department of Clinical Sciences
College of Veterinary Medicine
Cornell University
Ithaca, New York

Gillian A. Perkins, DVM, Diplomate ACVIM
Department of Clinical Sciences
College of Veterinary Medicine
Cornell University
Ithaca, New York

**Jeanine Peters-Kennedy, DVM,
Diplomate ACVP, Diplomate ACVD**
Department of Biomedical Sciences
College of Veterinary Medicine
Cornell University
Ithaca, New York

Jamie W. Prutton, BVSc, MRCVS, Diplomate ACVIM
Veterinary Medical Teaching Hospital
UC-Davis School of Veterinary Medicine
University of California
Davis, California

**Nicola Pusterla, DVM, PhD,
Diplomate ACVIM**
Department of Medicine and Epidemiology
UC-Davis School of Veterinary Medicine
University of California,
Davis, California

**Rolfe M. Radcliffe, DVM, Diplomate
ACVS, Diplomate ACVECC**
Department of Clinical Sciences
College of Veterinary Medicine
Cornell University
Ithaca, New York

Rebecca E. Ruby, BVSc, MS
Department of Biomedical Sciences
College of Veterinary Medicine
Cornell University
Ithaca, New York

Nathan M. Slovis, DVM, CHT, Diplomate ACVIM
Hagyard Equine Medical Institute
Lexington, Kentucky

**Tracy Stokol, BVSc, PhD, Diplomate ACVP
(Clinical Pathology)**
Department of Population Medicine and Diagnostic Sciences
College of Veterinary Medicine
Cornell University
Ithaca, New York

Rebecca L. Tallmadge, PhD
Department of Clinical Sciences
College of Veterinary Medicine
Cornell University
Ithaca, New York

**Stephanie J. Valberg, DVM, PhD,
Diplomate ACVIM**
Department of Veterinary Population Medicine
College of Veterinary Medicine
University of Minnesota
St. Paul, Minnesota

Gerlinde R. Van de Walle, DVM, PhD
Baker Institute for Animal Health
College of Veterinary Medicine
Cornell University
Ithaca, New York

Bettina Wagner, DVM, Dr.vet.med. habilitation
Department of Population Medicine and Diagnostic Sciences
College of Veterinary Medicine
Cornell University
Ithaca, New York

Preface

The major motivation for gathering the information in this book was to highlight the field of clinical immunology using accessible and applied approaches for students and practitioners with interest in furthering horse health. The topics covered include developmental immunology, immunodeficiencies, inflammation, hypersensitivity reactions, immune-mediated diseases, oncology, vaccinology, transplantation, and regenerative medicine. These areas cover both routine and advanced equine clinical cases.

Clinical immunology is grounded on the history of infectious disease outbreaks in humans and animals but this is just the beginning. A dysfunctional immune system has been associated with the pathophysiology of tissue damage, poor healing, and cancer, involving one or multiple organs. Organ-specific specialties investigate diseases that one way or another implicate the immune system, and much of the gathered clinical immunology knowledge and principles come from these basic applied studies. Natural immunodeficiencies have taught us about mechanisms of immune response and immunity. In addition, the growing fields of transplantation and regenerative medicine attempt to explore the connection and involvement of the immune system with their success in cell and tissue restoration.

The chances of an effective treatment increase with our ability to diagnose and understand the mechanisms of disease. Working as a large animal internist in a referral hospital, and as a clinical immunologist with emphasis in immunodeficiencies, I am reminded about the broad participation of the immune system in the cause and/or effect of the great majority of diseases. However, it is at the primary care level that clinical immunology offers the most significant contributions to patient care, when the curiosity of a clinician brings questions about the role of the immune system in a clinical context, and allows the early considerate intervention before tissue damage ensues.

Inspiration is the fuel for moving forward and, in the planning of this book, I got mine from my patients and students throughout the years. Some of my patients came with aberrant susceptibility to infections or excessive inflammatory response, and my students were curious about explanations for the cause and approaches for treatment. My inspiration also came from the pioneers in the studies of equine clinical immunology, who identified and characterized the first primary immunodeficiency of the horse, shared their discoveries on developmental immunology of the fetus and foal, described the mechanisms of endotoxemia, and created the critical reagents and diagnostic tools for basic and applied research of the immune system of the horse. Although we have achieved answers to many of our questions, the gaps are still considerable, and much work is ahead of us in order to better define diseases, promote healing and, ultimately, ensure prevention.

I hope this book inspires you in pursuing knowledge and training in clinical immunology.

M. Julia B. Felippe

1

The Immune System

M. Julia B. Felippe

1.1 Definition

The immune system is a network of cells and proteins that interact in tissues and organs to protect the body from infection, and also to promote healing. In general, immunity involves: the generation of inflammation; the removal and destruction of pathogens; the expansion of immune cell population and development of memory, specifically against the antigenic insult; control of inflammation; and tissue repair. The immune mechanisms aim to recognize and attack non-self molecules, although dysregulation can cause immunodeficiencies (e.g., insufficient protective response) or immune-mediated damage of self-molecules (i.e., autoimmune diseases and hypersensitivity reactions).

Classically defined, the immune system promotes immunity through *innate* and *adapted* segments. The innate immune cells and proteins provide immediate response and action against pathogens in a somewhat unspecific manner, while the adapted immune cells require priming with pathogen, cell co-stimulation and activation before function, and development of memory.

Immune cells cross-activate or cross-repress each other through cell-cell interactions, and in response to *cytokines* and *chemokines*, which are secreted proteins that function primarily in autocrine and paracrine manners and, sometimes, endocrine. Ligand-receptor or cytokine-cytokine receptor interactions lead to corresponding cell signaling, transcription and translation for immunostimulatory or immunosuppressive outcomes.

1.2 The organs of the immune system

The organs of the immune system are referred to as *central* (e.g., bone marrow and thymus), where cells are produced and go through initial or complete development; or *peripheral* (e.g., lymph nodes, spleen, and mucosa-associated lymphoid tissues (MALT), also known as bronchus-associated (BALT) and gut-associated (GALT) lymphoid tissues), in which cells complete their development and become activated upon encountering antigen.

Epithelial cells of the skin and mucosa comprise anatomical barriers to pathogens and toxins. Secretions (e.g., lysozymes in saliva and tears, low stomach pH) and clearance mechanisms (e.g., mucociliary system of the respiratory tract) add protection as physiological barriers. In addition, epithelial and endothelial cells can become activated by pathogens and secrete cytokines (e.g., interferon-beta, TNF-alpha), chemokines and selectins/integrins, which attract inflammatory cells. Damage to these structures and mechanisms decreases protection and favors pathogen invasion and replication.

Immune cells circulate through blood and lymph throughout the body, and migrate to tissues and lymphoid tissues, often attracted by chemokines; they can either settle and become resident cells, or constantly recirculate in search of an antigen or a site of inflammation. Cells circulating in the lymphatics re-enter the blood circulation via the thoracic duct and, from the blood, they can be attracted and migrate to tissues via diapedesis. From tissues, they can reach regional lymphoid structures and draining lymph nodes via draining lymphatics. Immune cells and antigens reach the spleen via blood, which works as a filter, with small capillary structures surrounded by organized lymphoid tissues.

Diapedesis is the process of extravasation of leukocytes from the blood stream into tissues. Sentinel cells of the immune system resident at tissue sites (e.g., macrophages, mast cells) detect the presence of pathogens or tissue destruction through their receptors. Cell signaling, transcription and translation follow, and these cells secrete inflammatory cytokines (e.g., tumor necrosis factor-alpha, TNF-alpha; interleukin-1,IL-1; IL-6) and chemokines (e.g., IL-8), which attract other inflammatory cells to the site. They cause fever and vasodilation, and increase capillary permeability, responsible for the clinical signs observed during inflammation (Chapter 18, Table 18.1).

The inflammatory cytokines also induce the expression of *adhesion molecules* called selectins (e.g., E-selectin) and integrins (e.g., vascular cell adhesion molecule-1, VCAM-1) on the luminal surface of local endothelial cells that bind (initially gently, then tightly) to the surface of leukocytes in the blood flow. This process induces the expression of similar adhesion molecules on the leukocyte surfaces (e.g., L-selectin; integrin CD11a-CD18 or LFA-1 lymphocyte-function associate antigen 1). With time, leukocytes roll along the luminal endothelium, then attach tightly to the endothelial cells and, finally, pass through gaps

Equine Clinical Immunology, First Edition. Edited by M. Julia B. Felippe.
© 2016 John Wiley & Sons, Inc. Published 2016 by John Wiley & Sons, Inc.

between them. A similar process is used in the absence of inflammation, when monocytes leave the blood stream into tissues and become resident macrophages, the immune sentinels. Once in the tissue, leukocytes follow the chemokine (e.g., interleukin-8, IL-8; complement component C5a) gradient produced by the macrophages and other inflammatory cells and proteins, and find the site of inflammation.

1.3 The immune cells and soluble molecules

The immune cells originate from myeloid and lymphoid precursors in the bone marrow, and follow stepwise genetically and epigenetically controlled lineage differentiation from hematopoietic stem cells. The bone marrow milieu has cell lineage niches that receive and respond to systemic signals (i.e., hormones, cytokines) with the production of new hematopoietic cells.

1.3.1 Myeloid cells

Myeloid cells comprise neutrophils, monocytes, macrophages, dendritic cells, eosinophils, basophils, mast cells, red cells and thrombocytes. These cells can complete maturation in the bone marrow, although further differentiation upon antigen encounter may happen at peripheral sites (e.g., monocytes differentiating into macrophages). Neutrophils, monocytes, macrophages and dendritic cells are phagocytes. They recognize pathogens, phagocytose and kill them, becoming activated during this process, and secreting cytokines and chemokines to signal other cells and expand the inflammatory response (Chapter 18, Table 18.4).

The recognition of pathogens by phagocytes is based on their *pattern-recognition receptors* (PRR). Signaling PRR include Toll-like receptors (TLRs, e.g., TLR-2, TLR-4, TLR-7 – about 11 described thus far); nucleotide-binding oligomerization receptors (NOD-like receptors – about 20 described thus far); or retinoic-acid inducible protein-1 (RIG-1-like receptors, also known as RLRs) (Figure 1.1; see also Chapter 18, Table 18.3).

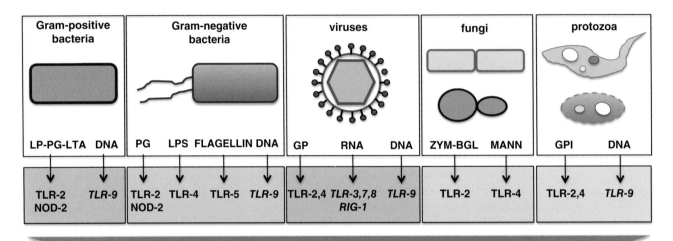

Figure 1.1 The pathogen-associated molecular patterns (PAMPs) and pathogen-pattern receptors (PRRs).
Pathogen small molecular motifs (PAMPs) or extracts (vaccines) can be detected by cell-membrane or intracellular (endosomic) receptors (PRRs) in phagocytes (e.g., macrophages and dendritic cells). PAMP-PRR binding triggers receptor-specific cell signaling events that lead to the production of inflammatory mediators (pro-inflammatory cytokines and type 1 interferons). Bacterial lipopeptide (LP), peptidoglycan (PG), lipoteichoic acid (LTA), lipopolysaccharide (LPS), and flagellin are detected by different cell-membrane toll-like receptors (TLRs) and intracellular nucleotide-binding oligomerization receptors (NOD-like receptors). Viral glycoprotein is detected by TLR-2 and TLR-4. Protozoal-released glycosylphosphatidylinositol (GPI)-anchored proteins are recognized by TLR-2 and TLR-4. Fungal zymogen and beta-glucosidase (BGL) are recognized by TLR-2, and mannose by TLR-4. Viral nucleic acids ribonucleic acid (RNA) is detected by intracellular TLR-3, TLR-7 and TLR-8, and retinoic-acid inducible protein-1 (RIG-1-like receptors); bacterial, viral and protozoal DNA (i.e., unmethylated cytosine-phosphodiester-guanine deoxynucleotide (CpG) motif) is recognized by intracellular TLR-9.

Located on the cell membrane or in the cytosol, they detect extracellular and intracellular pathogens, respectively. Each of these receptors recognizes distinct *pathogen-associated molecular patterns* (PAMPs), for which it has affinity.

In addition, endogenous molecules released by cell damage serve as *danger* alert, also known as *damage-associated molecular patterns* (DAMPs). As signaling receptors, PRR binding to a certain PAMP induces a determined cell-signaling configuration that results in the transcription and translation of a determined type of inflammatory response. Hence, the type of pathogen, defined by its signature molecular pattern, determines the type of immune response that, hopefully, will eliminate it. Early danger signals will recruit inflammatory cells that promptly potentiate this capacity.

Phagocytosis is the process of engulfing particles (endocytosis), including organisms, cells, proteins and other molecules. Phagocytes use different receptors to initiate phagocytosis. Some of them bind directly to the pathogens (e.g., mannose-receptors), while others require opsonization (*coating*) of the organism with immunoglobulin or complement, so they can bind to immunoglobulin or complement receptors on phagocytes. Once the pathogen adheres to the phagocyte surface, the cellular actin-myosin system contracts and expands the cell to engulf the pathogen and form a phagosome, which is rapidly fused with a cytosolic lysosome to form a *phagolysosome*. In the phagolysosome, proteolytic enzymes, oxygen-reactive species (e.g., hydrogen peroxide, hypochlorite, superoxide) and nitrogen-reactive species (e.g., peroxynitrite) produced through oxidative burst activity degrade the pathogens, and waste material is expelled from the cell.

Neutrophils are short-lived cells that arrive very quickly at the site of inflammation and competently phagocytose and kill pathogens, along with macrophages. Phagocytosis is much efficient when the pathogen is opsonized, creating a certain dependence on immunoglobulins and complement for phagocytic function. In addition, for some organisms (e.g., encapsulated bacteria), phagocytosis and killing require opsonization with both immunoglobulin and complement. As the early phase of inflammatory response supported primarily by neutrophils controls infection, macrophages become the predominant anti-inflammatory cells for tissue repair. Nevertheless, persistence of infection leads to chronic inflammation, with imbalanced tissue damage and repair.

Macrophages originate from circulating monocytes but live in tissues. They receive different names, accordingly: histiocytes, microglia, alveolar macrophages, osteoclasts, giant cells. There are pro-inflammatory macrophages (M1 cells) that are involved in the inflammatory response described above, and anti-inflammatory macrophages (M2 cells), which are involved in tissue repair. These cells co-exist during inflammation but their roles are more predominant in one phase or another, and both cell types have important roles. These cells require phenotypic and functional analyses for characterization. For example, exposure to the pro-inflammatory cytokine interferon-gamma

(IFN-gamma) and PAMP lipopolysaccharide (LPS, endotoxin) activate TLR-4 and differentiate macrophages into M1 cells, which subsequently express more pro-inflammatory cytokines (e.g., IL-12, IL-23, TNF-alpha), and promote inflammatory responses by activating lymphocytes and neutrophils. In addition, activation of M1 cells leads to the production of enzymes involved in oxidative burst activity, increasing the risk of tissue damage via oxidative stress. M2 cells, on the other hand, differentiate from exposure to IL-4, and secrete the anti-inflammatory cytokine IL-10. They promote tissue remodeling and decrease inflammation, which can also favor the development of tumors.

Dendritic cells and B cells can also function as phagocytes with lower efficiency for pathogen removal and killing, but with the objective to interact with T lymphocytes. Dendritic cells and Langerhans cells (skin) have the same PRRs for pathogen recognition and mechanisms for phagocytosis. Upon pathogen binding, immature dendritic cells found in tissues become mature cells and migrate to the regional lymph nodes, where they function as antigen presenting cells (APCs). Dendritic cells process killed extracellular pathogens into small peptides that are loaded to molecules called major histocompatibility (MHC) class II. The expression of MHC class II is increased after maturation, and the dendritic cells use their large cell surface area (proportionate to their dendritis) to express high amounts of MHC molecules loaded with foreign peptides.

The foreign peptides presented with MHC class II molecules may be recognized by a CD4$^+$ T cell that has a T cell receptor (TCR) with affinity for the peptides, and become partially activated (Chapter 13, Figure 13.1). Dendritic cells then express co-stimulatory molecules (CD40, CD86), which reinforce T cell activation when they bind to ligands on CD4$^+$ T cells (CD40L, CD28, respectively). In addition, dendritic cells secrete cytokines (e.g., IL-12) that can modulate and activate CD4$^+$ T cells and induce their proliferation. In essence, dendritic cells promote the development and guide the direction of the acquired immunity, based on the nature of its own antigenic stimulus (i.e., the PRR and cell signaling induced by the PAMP encountered). Macrophages are also capable of antigen presentation but perhaps dendritic cells provide greater co-stimulatory support to naïve T cells during their first antigen encounter.

Cell markers used for myeloid cell recognition in immunologic testing for horses include CD11b, CD14, CD172a, CD86, CD250, and MHC class II. Monocytes, macrophages and dendritic cells express these markers in different quantities, according to their stage of development and activation.

Eosinophils, basophils (circulating) and mast cells (tissue residents) are granular cells that participate in cytotoxicity reactions against parasites and allergens. Eosinophils respond to IL-5 for activation and proliferation. Basophils and mast cells express epsilon receptors for IgE, and most IgE is bound to these receptors by its constant region; upon allergen/antigen binding to the variable region of IgE, immediate cell degranulation releases vasoactive amines (e.g., histamine, leukotrienes, heparin, proteolytic enzymes), which cause cytotoxicity, vascular

Immunoglobulin Structure

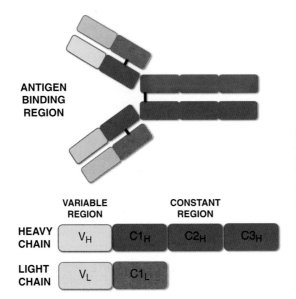

ANTIGEN BINDING REGION

V(D)J genes encode the variable region

| V | D | J |
| V | J |

VARIABLE REGION   **CONSTANT REGION**

HEAVY CHAIN V_H $C1_H$ $C2_H$ $C3_H$

LIGHT CHAIN V_L $C1_L$

Figure 1.2 The immunoglobulin structure. Immunoglobulin has two heavy chains (with variable and constant regions) and two light chains (also with variable and shorter constant regions) that form a 'Y' shaped structure. The heavy and light chain variable regions bind to antigens; and the heavy chain constant region determines the immunoglobulin isotype (IgA, IgE, IgG, or IgM) and promotes specific immune functions. The diversity in the variable region of the immunoglobulin is achieved by DNA recombination during B cell development, precisely of a region of genes named V (variability), D (diversity) and J (joining).

permeability, and the release of cytokines (an important source of IL-4) (see Chapter 4, Figure 4.1 and Chapter 8, Figure 8.2).

Myeoloid cells play an important role in the detection and removal of blood-borne pathogens and particles, and aged erythrocytes and platelets, through the mononuclear phagocyte system and the pulmonary intravascular macrophages. The mononuclear phagocyte system (formerly known as the reticuloendothelial system) comprises monocyte precursors in the bone marrow, circulating monocytes and tissue macrophages. Pulmonary intravascular macrophages are resident cells of the capillary endothelium of lungs, and have a similar morphology to the Kupfer cells of the liver. Together, these cells have the phagocytic, microbicidal, and secretory properties of other phagocytes. It is possible that the detection of and response to immunomodulators (e.g., bacterial extracts, endotoxin) is initiated by the pulmonary intravascular macrophages in the horse.

1.3.2 Lymphoid cells

Lymphoid cells derive from common lymphoid progenitors in the bone marrow and comprise B and T lymphocytes, and natural killer (NK) cells.

B lymphocytes complete their initial development into immature B cells in the bone marrow in the absence of foreign antigens and, subsequently, B cells continue their differentiation and selection after antigen encounter in peripheral tissues. The goal of a B cell during development in the bone marrow is to form a B cell receptor (BCR) that does not recognize self-molecules, but can individually and specifically recognize an infinite number of structures (molecules) present in the vast world of pathogens (antigens). Consequently, a very large number of autoreactive cells or cells that cannot build their BCR are eliminated daily during this process. The BCR is formed by a cell-surface bound IgM molecule and supporting transmembrane molecules (CD19, CD79a, CD79b), which

promote cell signaling and activation of B cells upon antigen binding to the receptor.

The immunoglobulin structure has two heavy chains (with variable and constant regions) and two light chains (also with variable and shorter constant regions) that form a 'Y' shaped structure. The heavy and light chain variable regions (forming the 'V') bind to antigens; and the heavy chain constant region (the 'I') determines the immunoglobulin isotype and promotes specific immune functions (Figure 1.2).

When B cells are developed in the bone marrow, each cell is produced with different variable regions in order to create an arsenal of cells that recognizes the enormous variety of antigens/pathogens to which an individual is exposed in a lifetime. This diversity is achieved thanks to DNA recombination during B cell development, precisely of a region of genes named V (variability), D (diversity) and J (joining). Different gene segments from these regions are trimmed and reunited (recombination) to form diverse exons that, consequently, encode different variable regions of the heavy or light chains of the immunoglobulin. Diversity is additionally obtained by the addition of nucleotides during the recombination process that reunite the DNA segments (junctional diversity, using N and P nucleotides). Diversity also follows in the periphery, with point mutations in the variable region to improve antigen recognition and binding. The constant region of a developing B cell is of IgM isotype. Once a B cell accomplishes its BCR on the cell surface and tests negative for self-recognition, it leaves the bone marrow towards peripheral tissues, in search of its matching foreign antigen. Cell markers used for B cell recognition in horses include B220, CD19, CD20, CD21, CD79a, IgG, and IgM.

T lymphocytes are long-lived cells that originate in the bone marrow from a common lymphoid progenitor, and move to the thymus to complete their differentiation; they also produce a T cell receptor. T cell receptors are heterodimers formed by alpha and beta chains (alpha-beta T cell), or gamma and delta chains (gamma-delta T cells), each with variable and constant regions. The variable regions are put together using the same process for the immunoglobulins in B cells. Alpha and beta TCRs need to be positively selected for their fit to the host MHC class I or class II molecules; if a TCR fails to recognize a MHC molecule, it is eliminated. An alpha-beta T cell that recognizes MHC class I becomes a CD8[+] (cytotoxic) T cell (CTL); an alpha-beta T cell that recognizes MHC class II becomes a CD4[+] (helper) T cell. A CD3 molecule for transmembrane signaling accompanies alpha-beta TCRs. T cells that recognize self-peptides (autoreactive) are eliminated in the thymus and are not released in the circulation. Cell markers used for alpha-beta T cell recognition in horses include CD3, CD4, and CD8.

Gamma-delta T cells also develop in the thymus and have diverse TCR, but are not restricted to recognition of peptides bound to MHC molecules (i.e., they can also bind to whole molecules), and they perhaps offer complementary mechanisms to detect antigen in the early stages of infection, likewise innate immune cells. They circulate in blood and tissues, and express a variety of cytokines (IFN-gamma, TNF-alpha, IL-17, IL-4) that signal inflammation upon activation. Gamma-delta T cells have not been thoroughly described in the horse and, if present, they represent a small population.

Regulatory CD4[+] T cells (Tregs) can develop in the thymus or in the periphery (induced Tregs), and comprise a small percentage of the circulating T cells. Tregs are heterogeneous cell populations that suppress the activation and proliferation of effector T cells; they play an important role in preventing tissue damage and autoimmunity, and provide peripheral immunotolerance. Their suppressive mechanism is not completely known, but involves the anti-inflammatory cytokines IL-10 and TGF-beta. Subpopulations of Tregs have been described in the horse. Cell markers used for Tregs include CD4, CD25, FoxP3, and IL-10; however, these markers are not exclusive to Tregs, and are also present in CD4[+] effector T cells.

The MHC class I and MHC class II molecules are polymorphic, and are encoded by different genes among individuals; these are the molecules evaluated before transplantation procedures for tissue compatibility, as they can function as foreign antigens in the recipient, and induce immune response and rejection. MHC class II is expressed primarily in APCs, but is also constitutively expressed in equine lymphocytes, and conditionally expressed in some activated cells (e.g., endothelial cells).

MHC class II molecules are loaded with processed peptides (between 18 and 20 amino acids) after phagocytosis and killing of extracellular organisms (Figure 1.3). The peptide presented in the context of the MHC class II molecule can be recognized by a TCR on CD4[+] T cells with specific affinity for it (Figure 1.4). MCH class I molecules are expressed in almost all nucleated cells of the body; they are also polymorphic, and are implicated in transplantation. MHC class I molecules are loaded with endogenously processed self- or non-self (e.g., tumoral, viral) peptides (between 8 and 10 amino acids) (Figure 1.3). The peptide presented in the context of the MHC class I molecule can be recognized by a TCR on CD8[+] T cells with specific affinity for it (Figure 1.4).

The CD8[+] (cytotoxic) T cells (CTLs) are activated by antigen presentation via MHC class I on APCs (cross-presentation), the co-stimulation from molecules expressed on activated CD4[+] T cells, and their secreted IFN-gamma. In the periphery, activated CTLs search for infected cells that express processed pathogen peptides in the context of MHC class I molecules. CD8[+] T cells kill infected target cells using elements that alter cell permeability (e.g., perforins, granzymes).

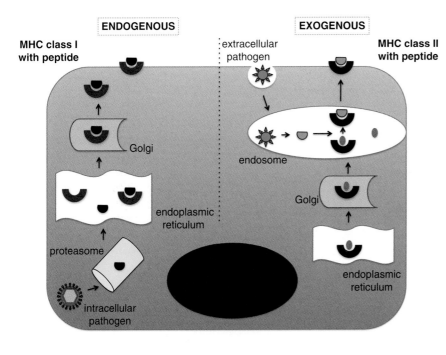

Figure 1.3 Pathways for peptide processing and loading in major histocompatibility complex (MHC) molecules.
(*left*): Endogenous pathway for peptide processing. An intracellular pathogen (e.g., virus) is processed through the proteasome and broken into small peptides (8–10 amino acids), which are loaded into a MHC class I molecule in the endoplasmic reticulum. The complex is moved through the Golgi apparatus and expressed on the cell surface. Some viruses and tumoral cells can interfere in many points of this pathway to prevent antigen presentation to CD8 cytotoxic T cells (CTLs).
(*right*): Exogenous pathway for peptide processing. An extracellular pathogen is endocytosed and broken by lysozymes into small peptides (18–20 amino acids), which are loaded in the MHC class II molecule in the endosome and expressed on the cell surface for presentation to CD4 T cells.

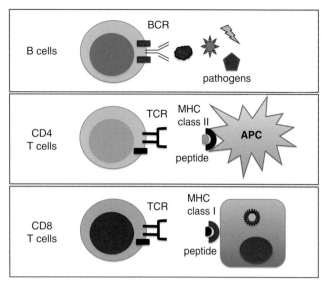

Figure 1.4 Antigen recognition by lymphocytes.
B and T cells recognize and bind specifically to antigens through their receptors, B cell receptor (BCR) and T cell receptor (TCR), respectively. The variable region of the BCR directly binds *unprocessed* antigen. On the other hand, the variable region of the TCR binds to *processed*, small peptides presented in the context of major histocompatibility (MHC) molecules. CD4 T cells recognize peptides presented by MHC class II molecules, and CD8 T cells recognize peptides presented by MHC class I molecules. Binding to antigen is the first signal for activation, and co-stimulation (with cytokines and interaction of co-stimulatory cell surface molecules) is required for full activation.

Natural killer (NK) cells are large granular cells, which also develop from common lymphoid precursors in the bone marrow but do not go through thymic maturation and do not express TCR or BCR. Hence, they are considered innate immune cells. NK cells kill target cells that do not express MHC class I, using granzymes and perforins that destroy cell membranes. Tumoral cells and virus-infected cells can downregulate the expression of MHC class I in order to escape $CD8^+$ T cell cytotoxicity. Without the expression of MHC class I, the target cells cannot inhibit the killer-cell immunoglobulin-like receptor (KIR), and cannot prevent the activation of NK cells (Figure 1.5). In addition, an NK cell can be activated when its Fc gamma RIII receptor (CD16, its classic marker) binds IgG attached to target cells expressing non-self antigens, a cell-destruction mechanism known as antibody-dependent cell-mediated cytotoxicity (ADCC). NK cells can become activated by lectins, and subsequently secrete inflammatory cytokines IL-2, IFN-gamma, and TNF-alpha.

1.3.3 Complement system

The complement system consists of circulating glycoproteins (C1 to C9) produced in the liver in response to inflammation. These pro-proteins are inactive until pathways induce sequential proteases that trigger the protein activation cascade:
- *classical* (antigen is bound by IgG or IgM molecules, and the C1-complex becomes activated when it binds to the antibodies);

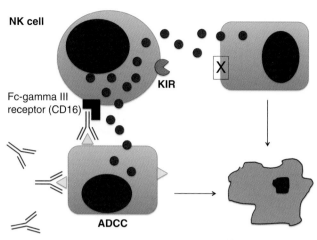

Figure 1.5 Natural killer (NK) cells kill infected cells.
NK cells recognize infected cells when they do not express MHC class I, a mechanism used by viral and tumoral cells to escape cytotoxic T cell (CTL) immunity. Without the expression of MHC class I (demonstrated by X), the target cells cannot inhibit the activation of the killer-cell immunoglobulin-like receptor (KIR). Subsequently, NK cells release granzymes and perforins (red circles) that destroy cell membranes of the target cells. In addition, an NK cell can be activated when its Fc gamma RIII receptor (CD16, its classic marker) binds IgG attached to target cells expressing non-self antigens, a cell-destruction mechanism known as antibody-dependent cell-mediated cytotoxicity (ADCC).

- *lectin* (antigen is bound by mannose-binding lectin and ficolins, and C4 becomes activated); or
- *alternative* (spontaneous complement C3 activation).

The ultimate outcome is the formation of the membrane attack complex (MAC) that creates pores on the cell surface of cells, with consequent lysis. After activation, opsonic, chemoattractant, anaphylactic and cytotoxic fragments are produced. Complement glycoproteins are regulated by circulating or membrane-bound (e.g., CD59) complement control proteins, which prevent activation of early or late complement cascade events.

Phagocytic activity is facilitated by complement, which opsonizes foreign structures, and binds to complement receptors on phagocytes.

1.4 B and T cell activation in lymphoid tissues

Upon phagocytosis of antigen in tissues, dendritic cells migrate to regional lymph nodes to interact with $CD4^+$ helper T cells (Figure 1.6A). Dendritic cells present processed antigen peptide via MHC class II that binds to the TCR, and conclude $CD4^+$ helper T activation with co-stimulatory molecules CD40 (binds to CD40L in lymphocytes) and CD86 (binds to CD28 in lymphocytes), and cytokines (Figure 1.6B). This is the time that determines the fate of $CD4^+$ helper T cells. Cytokine IL-12 secreted by APCs induces Th1 cells, whereas IL-23 induces Th17 cells, and IL-4 is necessary for Th2 differentiation (although its origin is not well determined) (see Chapter 13, Figure 13.2 and

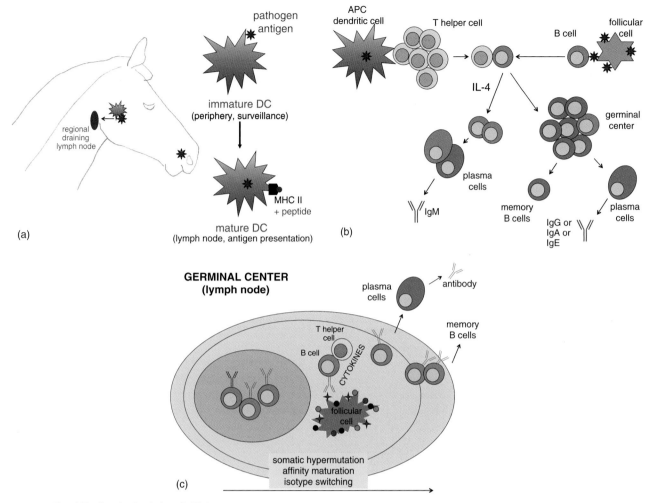

Figure 1.6 B and T cell activation in lymphoid tissues.

(a) Immature dendritic cells in peripheral tissues encounter, phagocytose and process antigen (e.g., respiratory pathogen, intranasal vaccine) and migrate to regional (draining) lymph nodes, where they become mature.

(b) In the paracortical region, they interact with naïve CD4 T cells, which become activated (helper cells) and proliferate. Also in the paracortical region, naïve IgM⁺ B cells encounter their matching unprocessed antigen on the surface of follicular cells, which initiates cell activation. Nevertheless, B cells require interaction with CD4 helper T cells in order to get second signals for full activation and, subsequent, proliferation. Some of the proliferating B cells, in the presence of IL-4 secreted by Th2 cells, quickly differentiate into plasma cells and secrete IgM. The rest of the activated B cells migrate to the cortical region and form germinal centers.

(c) Germinal centers contain highly proliferative B cells that undergo point mutation (somatic hypermutation) in their variable region to increase affinity and avidity for the triggering antigens. The new variable region needs to be tested again with binding to antigen (provided by follicular cells) and another round of interaction with CD4 T cells (affinity maturation). After approval, B cells keep their variable region, but change their constant region through isotype switching into IgA, IgE or IgG. Finally, at this point, some B cells become plasma cells (which secret antibodies) or long-lived memory cells.

Chapter 25, Figure 25.2). The many types of CD4⁺ helper T cells express the same cell markers, and can only be defined by the cytokines they secrete. Among many other types of helper T cells, Th1 cells secrete IFN-gamma, Th2 cells secrete IL-4, IL-5, IL-9, IL-13, and Th17 cells secrete IL-17.

After immature B cells leave the bone marrow, they also circulate in lymphoid tissues to encounter antigens. Whole (unprocessed) antigens reach the lymph nodes through lymph, the spleen through the blood, and the MALT through M cells in the mucosal epithelium. Antigens are often opsonized by local complement or immunoglobulins, which allows them to bind to

the surface of follicular dendritic cells. These cells are not hematopoietic, and do not process antigens, but serve as a *buffet* of antigens to B cells in search of a match for their BCRs (opsonized antigens bind to Fc receptors and complement receptors on the surface of follicular cells, exposing the antigen to B cells).

When the BCR binds to antigens, it triggers the first signal for activation of B cells. However, a second signal is necessary, and it comes from the activated CD4⁺ helper T cells. Both B cells and CD4⁺ T cells are activated by the same triggering antigen (organism), but BCRs (cell surface immunoglobulin) can bind to unprocessed antigen (i.e., directly to the pathogen), whereas TCR can only bind to processed antigens (i.e., peptides presented via MHC class II molecule).

B cells interact with CD4$^+$ helper T cells in the same manner in which APCs interact with them, namely, via MHC class II molecule presenting a processed peptide. After the BCR binds to and internalizes the antigen, it is processed into small peptides, which are presented to CD4$^+$ helper T cells via MHC class II. Co-stimulation with CD40-CD40L and CD86-CD28 molecules reinforce the interaction (hence, B cells are also APCS).

Once a B cell receives both signals (antigen binding and CD4$^+$ helper T cell co-simulation), it proliferates for clonal expansion. Some of the clonal cells, in the presence of IL-4 secreted by CD4$^+$ helper T cells (Th2 cells), differentiate immediately into plasma cells and secrete IgM, which is the same immunoglobulin expressed on the cell surface during bone marrow development. IgM, therefore, is the predominant immunoglobulin produced in a primary response or immunization. Part of the proliferating B cells form germinal centers, in which further B differentiation and proliferation occurs.

In the germinal centers, rapidly proliferating B cells (also known as centrocytes) develop point mutations (somatic hypermutation) in the immunoglobulin variable region (known as the complementarity determining region) to increase affinity and avidity for the triggering antigen (Figure 1.6C). Once the immunoglobulin changes its variable region, it needs to be re-tested against the antigen (provided by follicular dendritic cells) to check for improvement or deterioration of binding. If there is improvement, B cells interact again with CD4$^+$ helper T

cells to receive survival signals, and this process is called affinity maturation. At this point, no more changes happen in the variable region of the cell surface immunoglobulin (BCR), and the B cell proceeds to switch the immunoglobulin isotype from IgM into IgG, IgA or IgE. The cells then differentiate into plasma cells and secrete antibodies, or differentiate into memory cells that can be activated by antigens in a subsequent exposure. The immunoglobulin isotype is determined by the cytokine milieu created by the interacting T cells.

1.4.1 Immunoglobulins

There are five major isotypes of immunoglobulins (IgM, IgG, can, IgE and IgD). These isotypes are distinguished by their heavy chain constant regions encoded by the genes mu, gamma, alpha, epsilon and delta, respectively. Each immunoglobulin isotype promotes distinct functions for neutralization, complement fixation and opsonization, and mucosal protection (Figures 1.7A and 1.7B). The combination of isotypes provides a functional strategy for removal of pathogens, and lack of specific isotypes may facilitate certain pathogen establishment and disease. For example:

1 IgG, IgA and IgM directly neutralize bacteria, viruses and toxins, preventing them to bind to cell surface ligands for invasion or dysfunction.
2 IgG and IgA opsonize organisms for phagocytosis.
3 IgG and IgM activate complement component C1q.
4 IgG participates in ADCC.
5 IgE degranulates mast cells.

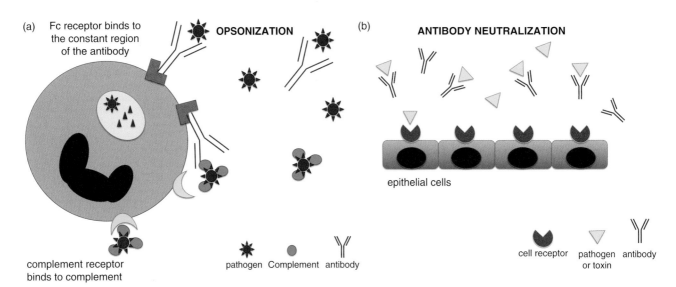

Figure 1.7 Opsonization and neutralization.
(a) Antibodies and complement opsonize (directly coat) antigens (e.g., pathogens, toxins). Neutrophils, macrophages and dendritic cells have antibody receptors on the cell surface (Fc-gamma and Fc-alpha receptors) that bind to the constant region of IgG and IgA antibodies, while their variable region binds to the antigen. These cells also have complement receptor. Once attached to these receptors, efficiency of phagocytosis is increased and, consequently, reactive oxygen and nitrogen species are produced for the destruction of pathogens. In other words, opsonization is essential for effective pathogen clearance. For encapsulated bacteria, opsonization with both immunoglobulin and complement is required for effective phagocytosis and killing.
(b) Antibody-binding prevents pathogens or toxins to attach to cell surface receptors (neutralization effect).

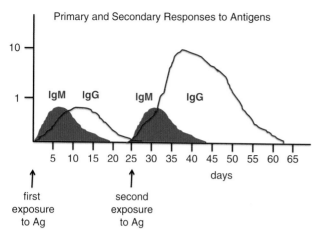

Figure 1.8 Primary and secondary immune responses.
Serum antigen-specific antibody concentrations serve to illustrate primary and secondary immune responses. First exposure to antigens induces initial population expansion and activation, with production of antibodies and memory cells. In a primary response, serum antigen-specific IgM concentration rises within a few days, and soon decays. Serum antigen-specific IgG concentration also rises, but requires a few more days to reach its peak, then levels decay. Upon a second encounter, a larger population of cells (memory cells) can recognize the antigen and respond quickly with antibody production. In a secondary response, again antigen-specific IgM rises quickly, but is now accompanied by IgG (faster response), which reaches much greater levels.

Therefore, the most significant impact in humoral protection is provided by IgG. However, other immunoglobulin isotypes broaden and reinforce immunity. Immunoglobulin isotype concentrations vary according to age, breed, and type of immune stimulation (type of pathogen, type of vaccine and adjuvant). Such differences may have implications for the quality and duration of protection, but overlapping of functions through the different immunoglobulin isotypes provides robust immunity.

In the horse, the immunoglobulin repertoire includes IgM, IgA, IgE, IgD, and seven different IgG isotypes, defined by different amino acid sequences in the heavy chain constant region. The most abundant of these are IgG_1 (formerly known as IgGa), $IgG_{3/5}$ (IgGT), and $IgG_{4/7}$ (IgGb), while IgG_2 and IgG_6 (IgGc) are found in smaller concentrations (their specific functions are unknown). IgG is present in blood, tissues and colostrum, and produced in large amounts in secondary responses (Figure 1.8). Colostral IgG is actively transported across the intestinal epithelium via the neonatal Fc receptor (FcRn). IgM molecules form pentamers, and are very efficient in activating complement.

IgM is the prevalent isotype in primary immune responses. IgA is produced in the lymph nodes and spleen in a monomeric form, and in the lamina propria of the MALTs in a dimeric form. In the latter, IgA binds to a receptor on the basolateral surface of the epithelial cells, and the receptor-IgA complex is taken up by endocytosis, moves toward the apical surface, and is finally secreted in the lumen. IgE is encountered in the blood and in tissues (e.g., skin, mucosa) already associated with mast cells, and is involved in allergic reactions.

Phagocytic activity is largely facilitated by immunoglobulin, which opsonizes foreign structures, and binds to immunoglobulin Fc receptors on phagocytes. In the absence of antigen-specific immunoglobulins, phagocytosis is largely inefficient; phagocytes may be present in large numbers, but cannot control infection by pathogen removal and killing – a scenario often observed in foals with low circulating IgG levels.

1.5 When the immune response goes wrong

Homeostasis is widely dependent on a protective and balanced response of the immune system, which involves redundant inflammatory and regulatory mechanisms. Occasionally, the immune system reacts to a non-self structure or a danger signal inadequately, either by not responding to it (immuno-suppression or tolerance), or by over-reacting to it (auto-immunity). In these conditions, selective activation or suppression of specific responses becomes necessary.

Autoimmunity is an immune response against self-molecules involving B lymphocytes (antibodies) and/or T lymphocytes (CD4$^+$ helper or CD8$^+$ cytotoxic cells). Auto-reactive B and T cells are common to all individuals, but they may or not have an adverse effect in the body tissues with clinical manifestation. B and T cells are controlled by mechanisms of central and peripheral tolerance. However, immune dysfunction involving antigen-presentation and co-stimulation, genetic defects, and environmental factors may lead to autoimmunity.

The failure of the anti-idiotype control mechanism of antibody production may facilitate the circulation of autoantibodies: (an antibody is considered a new molecule (antigen) because of its variable region, and additional antibodies are developed against that variable region). In addition, molecular mimicry of microbes and self-epitopes may result in immune responses that overcome immunological tolerance and lead to tissue injury. Exposure of self-antigens present in systems that are not normally visited by lymphocytes (e.g., breakdown of the blood-brain-barrier or blood-ocular-barrier), or the development of new epitopes on self-proteins (e.g., infection with viruses, exotoxin damage of cell membranes, penicillin hapten binding to red cell membrane, or exposure to chemicals), can lead to the production of autoantibodies. In some cases, autoimmunity is associated with aging and immune system malfunction, or the effect of sexual hormones. The mechanisms that induce tissue injury are the ones described in hypersensitivity reactions.

Hypersensitivity reactions are inflammatory and damaging immune responses. The classification of hypersensitivity reactions is based on the type of cells and immune mediators that promote tissue injury:

(a) *Type I hypersensitivity reactions* (e.g., urticaria, insect-bite hypersensitivity, and food allergy) are mediated by antigen-specific IgE, mast cells, basophils and their mediators (see Chapter 4, Figure 4.1 and Chapter 5, Figure 5.2).

Table 1.1 Classification system of hypersensitivity reactions according to Gell and Coombs.

Type	Names	Definition	Examples
Type I	Immediate hypersensitivity	Mediated by IgE attached to mast cells in tissues or circulating basophils; reaction in minutes to hours; requires prior antigen sensitization	Anaphylaxis, Insect hypersensitivity, Food allergy
Type II	Antibody-dependent	IgG or IgM antibodies bind directly to cell membranes and cause tissue destruction via neutrophil chemotaxis and complement deposition; reaction in a few days	Immune-mediated hemolytic anemia, Immune-mediated thrombocytopenia, Pemphigus, Vasculitis, Glomerulonephritis
Type III	Antibody-antigen immune-complex	IgG or IgM form complexes with antigens, which deposit on cell membranes and cause tissue destruction via neutrophil chemotaxis and complement deposition; reaction in a few days	Purpura hemorrhagica, Vasculitis, Glomerulonephritis Serum sickness, Arthus reaction
Type IV	Delayed hypersensitivity, Antibody-independent	Mediated by CD4 T cells that activate macrophages, causing tissue damage or granulomas; delayed reaction in 2 to 3 days	Contact dermatitis Tuberculin test

prepared by Dr. Rolfe M. Radcliffe, Cornell University.

(b) *Type II hypersensitivity reactions* (e.g., immune-mediated hemolytic anemia or thrombocytopenia, pemphigus foliaceus, vasculitis, glomerulonephritis, drug hypersensitivity) involve auto-antibodies IgM or IgG against self cell-surface or extracellular matrix antigens. The antibodies function as opsonins, activating neutrophils and complement.

(c) *Type III hypersensitivity reactions* (e.g., purpura hemorrhagica, vasculitis, glomerulonephritis, serum sickness, Arthus reaction) are promoted by the random deposition of antigen-antibody immune-complexes in capillary vessels, with subsequent activation of neutrophils and complement (Chapter 8, Figure 8.2).

(d) *Type IV hypersensitivity reactions* (e.g., granulomas, tuberculin test, contact dermatitis) are mediated by sensitized CD4[+] T cells (Th1) and CD8[+] T cells (direct cytotoxic effect), which secrete inflammatory cytokine IFN-gamma that induces infiltration and activation of macrophages (Table 1.1; and see Chapter 13, Figure 13.3).

Immunodeficiencies are rare disorders of the immune system that result in failure to build protection against pathogens, leading to recurrent fevers and infections (Table 1.1; and see Chapter 21). These conditions may be transient or lasting, primary (genetic, inherited) or secondary (viral infections, immunosuppressive therapy, stress, endocrine disorders, nutritional deficiencies), and affect one or more arms of the immune system (humoral, cellular, and/or phagocytic systems). Described immunodeficiencies in the horse can be diagnosed using immunologic or genetic testing.

References

Abbas, A.K., Lichtman, A.H.H. and Pillai, S. (2014). *Cellular and Molecular Immunology*, eighth edition. Elsevier Saunders.

Parham, P. (2014). *The Immune System*, 4th Edition. Garland Science.

2 The Immune System of the Young Horse

Rebecca L. Tallmadge

2.1 Definition

Neonates have the formidable task of rapidly expanding their immune system while generating appropriate immune responses to pathogens and environmental antigens. It is important to appreciate the nuances of the neonatal immune system in order to distinguish age-related developmental programs from deficiencies of the immune system. Previously, neonates were not considered to be immunocompetent. However, studies of horse, human, and mouse neonates have revealed that neonates are capable of generating protective immune responses to certain pathogens or types of vaccines.

2.2 Equine immune system development

2.2.1 The immune system of the fetus

In the course of equine gestation, a great portion of the development of the immune system occurs during fetal life (Figure 2.1). The lymphoid population of the thymus is under development by approximately 80 days of gestation, circulating lymphocytes are observed by 120 days of gestation, and secondary lymphoid tissues (particularly the spleen) are populated soon afterwards (Mackenzie, 1975; Perryman, 1980). Primary germinal centers are evident in day 200 fetal spleen, pre-suckle neonatal spleen and mesenteric lymph node, with foci of IgM$^+$ cells among CD3$^+$, CD4$^+$, or CD8$^+$ T cells (Perryman, 1980; Tallmadge, 2009).

Based on molecular data, B cell differentiation reaches the mature B cell stage and immunoglobulin isotype switching is active during mid-gestation. Fetal liver, bone marrow, and spleen tissues, at approximately 100 days of gestation, express transcripts for all B cell genes tested (CD20, CD21, CD22, CD27, CD40, CD45/B220, CD79A, CD79B, and immunoglobulin recombination genes RAG-2 and TdT), indicating successful B lymphopoiesis (Tallmadge, 2009). At 100 days of gestation, mRNA expression of not only IGHM and the lambda light chain (IGLC) can be detected in the bone marrow, but also IGHD, IGHG1, IGH3, IGHG5, IGHG6, IGHG7, and IGHA isotypes indicating immunoglobulin isotype- switching capacity during development. Immunoglobulin gene expression is similar in pre-suckle neonatal bone marrow, although expression of the IGHG4 gene is active in pre-suckle neonatal spleen.

The wide repertoire of immunoglobulin antigen specificity is derived from usage of different immunoglobulin heavy chain variable (V), diversity (D), and joining (J) gene segments, and diversity in immunoglobulin sequence content through addition of non-templated nucleotides or somatic hypermutation. Limitations in fetal immunoglobulin gene segment usage and sequence diversity have been reported in humans and mice (Lawler, 1987; Jeong, 1988; Raaphorst, 1992). However, in the equine fetus, the complement of immunoglobulin heavy chain variable, diversity, and joining gene segments used and CDR3H lengths are comparable to those of neonatal, foal, and adult horse immunoglobulin sequences (Tallmadge, 2013). Unexpectedly, the diversity of immunoglobulin sequence content (i.e., the variation between immunoglobulin transcripts and germline sequences) significantly increases between 100 days of gestation and birth, as do the lengths of non-templated nucleotide insertions (Tallmadge, 2013).

Prior to 200 days of gestation, both IgM and IgG proteins are evident in fetal serum (Perryman, 1980). Antigenic responses during fetal life have been identified histologically and by antigen-specific antibody production, including antigen-specific IgG isotype switching (Martin, 1973; Mackenzie, 1975; Morgan, 1975). At birth, foals have low, but detectable, amounts of serum IgM and IgG, and high titers of pre-suckle antibodies to *Neospora hughesi* have been detected in foals born to naturally infected mares (Rouse, 1971; Jeffcott, 1974; Perryman, 1980; Tallmadge, 2009; Pusterla, 2011).

Together, these findings indicate that the fetal humoral immune system repertoire undergoes expansion and limited diversity in an antigen-independent manner during gestation, and can respond to pathogens when they are present, with production of small levels of antibodies of different isotypes.

2.2.2 Passive transfer of immunity to the neonate

The epitheliochorial placenta of the horse prevents the transfer of maternal antibodies to the fetus *in utero*; thus, foals are born with small, non-protective amounts of endogenous serum IgM and IgG (Perryman, 1980; Tallmadge, 2009). Generation of

Equine Clinical Immunology, First Edition. Edited by M. Julia B. Felippe.
© 2016 John Wiley & Sons, Inc. Published 2016 by John Wiley & Sons, Inc.

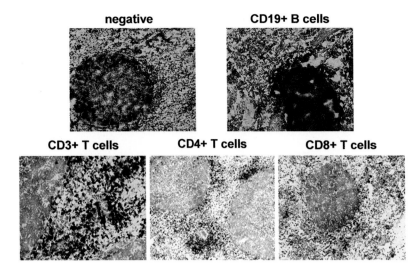

Figure 2.1 Peripheral lymphoid tissue in the equine neonate.

Immunohistochemical staining of microsections from spleen collected from a healthy foal at one day old. The distribution of B cells (CD19) and T cells (CD3, CD4 and CD8) was tested using monoclonal antibodies against the cell markers and 3-amino-9-ethylcarbazole, AEC; positive cells are red. Note the abundance of B and T cells, and the organization of germinal centers (Julia Felippe, Cornell University).

primary immune responses requires approximately 10–15 days, and perhaps 3–4 months for protective levels, leaving the foal vulnerable to pathogens in this window. The dam's colostrum provides passive transfer of antibodies, which requires good quality and adequate, timely suckling to achieve its efficiency (Figure 2.2).

Colostrum provides a plethora of soluble factors for the neonatal foal, including innate immune proteins such as complement components (i.e., C3, serum amyloid A), cytokines (i.e., tumor necrosis factor alpha (TNF-alpha), IL-6), lysozyme, ferritin, and antibodies that are absorbed by the foal (Jeffcott, 1974; Zou, 1998; McDonald, 2001; Gardner, 2007; Burton, 2009; Secor, 2012; Numata, 2013). In mammalian species, colostrum also contains maternal lymphocytes, neutrophils, macrophages, and epithelial cells (Le Jan, 1996). In the horse, colostrum CD4$^+$ and CD8$^+$ T lymphocytes have been shown to be responsive to

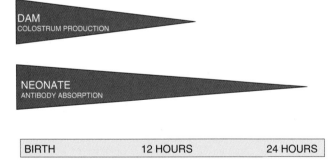

Figure 2.2 Time line for production of and absorption of IgG from colostrum.

Mares start producing colostrum a couple of weeks before foaling, and cease production by 12 hours after foaling. Foals should ingest colostrum within hours after birth, as peak absorption of antibodies through the intestinal epithelium occurs by eight hours after foaling and decreases gradually in the subsequent hours. By 24 hours, absorption is minimal and inefficient. Therefore, foal serum IgG concentrations should be greater than 800 mg/dL (ideally >1000 mg/dL) by 12–14 hours after birth in normal conditions.

mitogens *in vitro*, and produce inflammatory cytokines IL-17 and IFN-gamma (Perkins, 2014).

Maternal IgG isotypes and small amounts of IgM, IgA, and IgE antibodies are absorbed in the small intestine from colostrum in the first 24 hours of life (Table 2.1; Jeffcott, 1974; Jeffcott, 1975; Kohn, 1989; Sheoran, 2000; Wagner, 2006). Impressively, absorption of colostrum can protect SCID foals that inherently lack T and B lymphocytes for up to four months of life against certain organisms (Poppie, 1976). Antigen-specific antibody transfer via colostrum has been demonstrated for *Clostridium perfringens, Clostridium difficile, Pseudomonas aeruginosa, Streptococcus equi, Rhodococcus equi, Actinobacillus spp.*, equine arteritis virus, West Nile Virus, *Theileria equi, Neospora hughesi, Strongylus vulgaris*, among others (Jeffcott, 1974; Ueda, 1982; Galan, 1986; Prescott, 1996; Hullinger, 1998; Sternberg, 2001; Wilkins, 2006; Kumar, 2008; Pusterla, 2011; Kaur, 2013; Artiushin, 2013; Nielsen, 2014).

Colostrum-derived antibodies should confer protection not only after foaling, but for the first three months of life, when endogenous antibody production in normal foals reaches levels close to protection (e.g., >500 mg/dL).

2.2.3 The immune system of the neonate
2.2.3.1 Innate immune system

A functional innate immune system comprised of pre-existing or rapidly induced defenses is critical for newborn foals, particularly while antigen-specific immune responses require exposure and time for development after birth. Competence of the innate immune system has been measured in the foal by function of phagocytes, activation markers, expression of cytokines, and phagocytosis and killing capacity. In addition, other cells of the innate immune system have been tested in the neonate and young foal; accordingly, lymphokine-activated killing cell activity has been documented to be present at birth (Flaminio, 2000).

Intrinsic phagocytic and oxidative burst activities are present in neonatal phagocytes at birth, and foal neutrophils express

Table 2.1 Immunoglobulin concentrations in adult horses, colostrum, and neonatal foals.

Immunoglobulin	Original designation	Adult serum	% Adult serum	Colostrum	Pre-suckle foal serum	Post-suckle foal serum	Half-life (days)	Complement fixation
IgM	IgM	103		86–123	16–32	34–54	5	yes
IgG$_1$	IgGa	340	15.2	8200	3–5.4	1000	17.6	yes
IgG$_2$								no
IgG$_3$	IgG(T)	363–400	16.8	4400	ND	480	21	yes
IgG$_5$	IgG(T)							no
IgG$_4$	IgGb	1114–1960	65.1	18,300	ND, 8	2900	32	yes
IgG$_7$	IgGb							yes
IgG$_6$	IgGc	20	0.7	30	ND	ND		no
Total IgG		1913		8000–46,000	5–7.5	300–4600		
IgA	IgA	40–225		900–957	ND	40–58	3.4	poor

Ig concentration units are mg/dL; ND – not detectable.
Data compiled from Perryman, 1980; Siegel, 1980; Kohn, 1989; Lavoie, 1989; Flaminio, 1999, 2000; Sheoran, 2000; Lewis, 2008; Secor, 2012; and Tallmadge, 2009.

more integrin molecule CD18 during their initial three weeks of life when compared to adult horses, providing efficient diapedesis and cell-to-cell interactions (Wichtel, 1991; Gröndahl, 1999; Flaminio, 2000). Nevertheless, phagocytosis and bacterial killing are dependent on the synergistic opsonization of the pathogen by circulating complement and antibodies (Gardner, 2007). Prior to colostrum ingestion, foal serum has significantly less chemotactic and opsonic factors, compared to foal serum after ingestion of colostrum or adult serum. Accordingly, administration of adult plasma to one week old foals significantly increases opsonic capacity, particularly in the presence of sepsis (Bernoco, 1987; Gröndahl, 1999; Gardner, 2007; McTaggart, 2005). Opsonic capacity in foals becomes comparable to that of adults by 3–4 weeks of life, and there is an age-dependent increase in complement concentration in serum (Gröndahl, 2001; Gardner, 2007).

Serum amyloid A (SAA), an acute phase protein produced in the liver and also present in colostrum (SAA3), induces chemotaxis, cell degranulation, opsonization, phagocytosis, and pathogen killing (Badolato, 1994, 2000). SAA3 peak levels are detected on the second day of life in foals, and indicate colostrum transfer (Stoneham, 2001). SAA levels increase dramatically in foals with septicemia or focal infection, and are higher in foals with bacterial infections than in those with non-bacterial infections (Stoneham, 2001; Hulten, 2002; Gardner, 2007).

Toll-like receptors (TLRs) are key components of the innate immune system, because they recognize conserved structural pathogen-associated molecular patterns (PAMPs) and initiate signaling cascades upon ligand binding to activate immune cells. TLR-8 recognizes single-stranded RNAs and has a role in the innate antiviral immune response. Foal neutrophils of all ages express TLR-8 mRNA constitutively, and stimulation of the TLR-8 signaling pathway with a synthetic agonist (R848) induces mRNA expression of pro-inflammatory cytokines IL-6 and IL-8 (Harrington, 2012). TLR-9 detects bacterial DNA, which is distinguished by unmethylated CpG motifs (Hemmi,

2000). TLR-9 signaling promotes functional activity of neutrophils including enhanced neutrophil phagocytic activity; induction of IL-6, IL-8, and TNF-alpha; increased production of reactive oxygen species; and delay in apoptosis (Weighardt, 2000; Hayashi, 2003; Jozsef, 2004).

Neutrophils from newborn and two-month-old foals express levels of TLR-9 mRNA comparable to those of adult horse neutrophils, and stimulation of foal and adult neutrophils with CpG induces IFN-gamma, IL-8, and IL-12p35 mRNA expression, whereas TNF-alpha mRNA is decreased (Liu, 2009). Neutrophil *in vitro* stimulation with a CpG-agonist or *R. equi* induces degranulation at two days old (Bordin, 2012). Foal dendritic cells and macrophages express TLR-9 mRNA levels comparable to adult horse cells (Flaminio, 2007). Foal neutrophils express high levels of cytokine mRNA (IFN-gamma, TNF-alpha, IL-4, IL-6, IL-8, IL-10, IL-12p35, IL-12p40, IL-17, IL-23p19) in response to *in vitro R. equi* stimulation, which most likely stimulates TLR-2 and TLR-4 (Nerren, 2009; Bordin, 2012; Kaur, 2013).

These examples illustrate that the neonatal foal's innate immune system is able to recognize and respond to pathogens by way of phagocytosis, degranulation, cytokine modulation, and killing in early life. Nevertheless, these mechanisms are highly dependent on opsonization with colostrum-derived IgG, followed by endogenously-produced IgG.

2.2.3.2 Adaptive immune system

Although much of the lymphoid tissue develops during gestation, the foal adaptive immune system is naïve to environmental organisms at birth. The exposure to an abundant and diverse population of pathogens in early life induces a massive expansion of antigen-specific lymphocyte populations, reflected by a 2–3 times increase in the number of circulating lymphocytes and an increase in mass of secondary lymphoid tissues (Flaminio, 2000). Also, there is an increase in the circulation of cells through the gut and the appearance of gut-homing T cells, which are likely driven by antigen. The postnatal immune system development includes an increase in size of the total lymphocyte compartment and the establishment of primed cells (Banks, 1999).

Circulating B and T lymphocyte populations expand in a linear fashion over the first five months of life, plateauing at a number greater than that of adult horses for a few months, before dropping toward adult horse reference values (Flaminio, 1999; Smith, 2002). The lymphocyte population expansion reflects exposure to a multitude of environmental antigens and pathogens, with lymphocyte activation and proliferation. Indeed, increasing total lymphocyte counts and subpopulations (CD4$^+$ and CD8$^+$ T cells, and B cells) in the young foal is a desirable sign of an active immune system (Figure 2.3). Foal peripheral blood lymphocytes proliferate in response to mitogen stimulation, with lower levels in the first few weeks of life, then reaching adult horse levels by four weeks old (Flaminio, 2000). In secondary lymphoid tissues, increase in density and follicular organization of B and T zones are obvious in the first three months of life (Tallmadge, 2009).

Several aspects of neonatal antigen presenting cells (APCs, dendritic cells and macrophages) exhibit age-dependent changes over the first three months of life. Reduced MHC class II expression in foals less than three months old may limit the capacity to present processed extracellular antigens to T cells (Barbis, 1994; Flaminio, 2000; Smith, 2002; Flaminio, 2007). Foal APCs do not alter cytokine mRNA expression in response to CpG agonist (CpG-ODN 2135) stimulation up to three months of life, although this CpG agonist can induce proliferation of foal leukocytes at two days old (Flaminio, 2007). Despite the fact that the co-stimulatory marker CD86 is present on foal APCs at adult-like levels from birth, fewer numbers of mature dendritic cells with the CD14$^-$CD1b$^+$CD86$^+$ phenotype are detected in foals (Flaminio, 2007; Merant, 2009). It is possible that foal APCs, like human neonates, require multiple stimuli (e.g., more than one TLR stimulation or a certain threshold of cytokine milieu) for competent activation.

While the thymus, spleen, and some systemic lymph nodes develop their structure during fetal life, foals do not present organized lymphoid tissue in the lungs at birth. T lymphocytes and plasma cells are virtually absent in lung tissues in the first week of life, and bronchus-associated lymphoid tissue (BALT) is only observed by 12 weeks old (Banks, 1999). Consequently, there is an increase in leukocyte populations in the bronchoalveolar lavage fluid (BALF) with age (Blunden and Gower, 1999; Flaminio, 2000). However, for the first three months, the foal has a small leukocyte population in BALF (Figure 2.3). CD4$^+$ T cell distribution equivalent to that found in adult horse BALF is reached by three weeks old, and CD8$^+$ T cell numbers near adult horse levels by ten weeks old (Balson, 1997). Very few B lymphocytes or plasma cells are identified in BALF until eight weeks (Blunden and Gower, 1999; Flaminio, 2000). BALF lymphocytes from foals younger than six weeks old have lower MHC class II expression than that observed in adult horse BALF

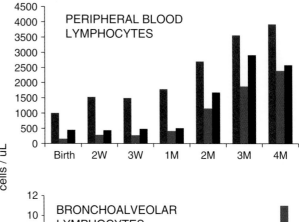

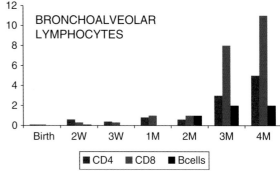

Figure 2.3 Dynamic changes of foal lymphocyte subpopulation distributions.
The number of total CD4 and CD8 T cells, and B cells, progressively increases in the first months of life in peripheral blood (likely reflecting lymph node activity) and bronchoalveolar lavage fluid. In the latter, note the paucity of lymphocytes during the first two months of life (adapted from Flaminio, 1999, 2000). "W" indicates weeks and "M" indicates months.

lymphocytes, consistent with peripheral blood lymphocytes (Balson, 1997). Few alveolar macrophages are recovered in BALF up to two weeks of life but, by the third week, greater than 70% of cells recovered are alveolar macrophages, and this level is sustained (Zink, 1984; Liu, 1987).

IgG isotypes are detected in foal nasal washes after passive transfer via colostrum, but IgA is not detected in the airway until 28 days old (Sheoran, 2000). Thus, it is suggested that fewer lymphocytes in the lung and lack of mucosal IgA may predispose young foals to respiratory tract disease. In the gut, the immunoglobulins present in colostrum and milk offer significant passive mucosal protection, particularly IgA, which offers effective neutralization and opsonization of pathogens and toxins. The development of intestinal tract lymphoid tissue is intense after birth, and Payer's patches and mesenteric lymph nodes become grossly obvious beyond the first three weeks of life. Although the foal is likely born with most resources for the mucosal immune system, it is only after exposure to organisms (i.e., normal flora PAMPs) that the expansion of the lymphocyte population occurs. Therefore, exposure to pathogenic organisms before this necessary priming would cause disease in the foal and, in addition, elements that may affect the proliferation of resident bacteria may affect or delay protective immune response.

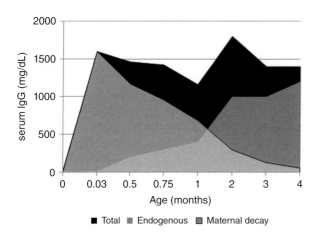

Figure 2.4 Serum immunoglobulin profile of young foals. The total serum IgG profile is comprised of increasing endogenous production and decay of colostrum-derived (half-life 28–32 days) antibodies. A nadir in total IgG is observed between the first 1–2 months of life (adapted from Jeffcott, 1974; Holmes, 1991; and Flaminio, 2000).

Endogenous immunoglobulin production occurs already during fetal life, although serum IgM and IgG levels are low and not protective at birth; appreciable endogenous serum IgM and IgG levels are attained by 2–3 months of life, irrespective of colostrum ingestion (Jeffcott, 1975; Lavoie, 1989; Flaminio, 1999; Flaminio, 2000; Tallmadge, 2009). If passive transfer successfully occurs, a nadir of serum IgM and IgG levels occurs between 1–3 months old, due to the decay of colostrum-derived antibodies, although the half-life of each isotype differs (Figure 2.4; Table 2.1) (Flaminio, 1999; Flaminio, 2000; Sheoran, 2000). Measurable concentrations of endogenous antibody has been observed around two weeks old in newborn foals deprived of colostrum, with robust synthesis observed by 28–42 days in newborn foals given bovine colostrum in place of suckling their dams (Jeffcott, 1974; Lavoie, 1989; Holmes, 1991).

One important aspect of this dynamic phase of circulating colostrum-derived antibodies and endogenously-produced antibodies is the need for humoral protection, not only at birth but also in the initial few months of life. Therefore, what is considered to be standard adequate transfer of antibodies through colostrum at birth (e.g., at least 800 mg/dL), questionably, in theory, provides humoral protection in the second and third months of life, when considering an IgG half-life of approximately 30 days, and a minimal circulating level of 500 mg/dL. Therefore, levels greater than 1000–1200 mg/dL would be more certain of protection in the first few months of life. Indeed, adequate transfer of immunoglobulins occurs naturally at levels much higher than 800 mg/dL (>1200 mg/dL), and varies among breeds (Flaminio, 2000). A quantitative assay, such as the turbidimetric or radial immunodiffusion assay, provides the actual blood immunoglobulin concentration achieved after passive transfer, which could be used for clinical planning and monitoring of foals at risk of developing infections.

IgG$_{4-7}$ (IgGb) is the most abundant IgG isotype in adult serum and colostrum and, functionally, it is able to bind complement and mediate respiratory burst in phagocytes, yet delayed endogenous production has been reported in foals (Sheoran, 2000; Holznagel, 2003; Lewis, 2008). Other studies have revealed IgG$_{4-7}$ expression at earlier time points: IgG$_{4-7}$ mRNA expression is present in pre-suckle neonatal spleen, young foal peripheral blood and spleen; IgG$_{4-7}$ proteins are present in pre-suckle serum and young foal lymphoid tissues; and serum IgG$_{4-7}$ is produced in foals younger than one month when challenged with *Rhodococcus equi* (Jacks, 2007a; Tallmadge, 2009).

Most IgE bound to the surface of neonatal basophils is of maternal origin (Wagner, 2006). Endogenous production of IgE appears to be delayed until six months old, with robust serum IgE levels by 9–11 months, despite the decay of colostrum-derived IgE by four months (Marti, 2009). The effect of this window of absent/low IgE expression on immune responses to parasites and allergies is not understood.

Some studies suggest that passively transferred antibodies have a suppressive effect on the foal's endogenous immunoglobulin production. This assertion stems from observations of accelerated onset of immunoglobulin production in colostrum-deprived foals and vaccine studies (Jeffcott, 1974; Van Oirschot, 1991; Wilson, 2001). It has been suggested that colostrum-derived antibodies could interfere, either by clearing antigen and thereby precluding the foal's detection and response, or by inhibition of B cell activation by Fc-gamma-receptor mediated signals (Siegrist, 2003). However, there are many examples which indicate that foals are able to generate antigen-specific immune responses in early life, despite circulating colostrum-derived antibodies, perhaps with different magnitude (Chong, 1992; Jacks, 2007a; Ryan, 2010).

Foal peripheral blood mononuclear cells (PBMCs) exhibit active cytokine production in the first month of life, including TNF-alpha, IL-1beta, IL-2, IL-4, IL-6, IL-8, IL-10, IL-12p35, IL-15, and IL-18. Expression of IFN-gamma, IL-1alpha, and TGF-beta1 mRNA increases with age over the first month of life (Boyd, 2003; Merant, 2009). Small numbers of PBMCs expressing IFN-gamma, IL-4, and IL-10 protein can be detected after stimulation from birth on (Wagner, 2010). The proportion of IFN-gamma and IL-10 producing-cells increases over the first six weeks of life then stabilizes; IFN-gamma expression reaches adult levels by three months old (Breathnach, 2006; Wagner, 2010).

Experimental infection and vaccine challenges have revealed the ability of young foals to generate antigen-specific humoral and cell-mediated immune responses. Three day old foals generated vaccine-specific IgG responses, and three week old foals generated *R. equi*-specific cytotoxic T lymphocyte (CTL) response (Ryan, 2010; Harris, 2011). Therefore, foals are immunocompetent, but may require a specific immunogenic context to generate the desired immune response. Nevertheless, memory response has not been yet characterized in the foal.

2.3 Unique susceptibilities and disorders of young horses

2.3.1 Failure of passive transfer of immunoglobulins

Colostrum preparation initiates a couple of weeks pre-foaling, and is active in the first 12 hours post-foaling. The equine neonate has a small window of time for absorption of immunoglobulins from ingested colostrum, which peaks around eight hours post-foaling, and lasts with limitations up to 24 hours. Therefore, the earlier a foal nurses, the more efficient and faster is this process. Equine colostrum is rich primarily in $IgG_{4/7}$, with small amounts of other IgG isotypes, IgM, IgA and IgE (Table 2.1) (Sheoran, 2000; Holznagel, 2003). As indicated previously, the colostrum-derived IgG is essential for humoral protection of foals, with vital neutralization and opsonization properties. Nevertheless, it is the combination of immunologic strategies that provide the best protection against pathogens in any phase of life.

Failure of passive transfer (FPT) of immunoglobulins may occur if the foal does not suckle adequate amounts of colostrum soon after birth, or if foals cannot absorb immunoglobulin efficiently through the intestinal epithelium (e.g., in the case of ischemic hypoxia), or if the colostrum does not contain adequate amounts of immunoglobulin (e.g., mares with systemic disease late in gestation, pre-partum loss of colostrum due to placentitis). Consequently, foals remain hypogammaglobulinemic and, thus, susceptible to infection by environmental pathogens and sepsis (McGuire, 1975; Robinson, 1993; Raidal, 1996). FPT is classically defined by serum IgG concentration less than 800 mg/dL by 24 hours old, and foals with serum IgG between 400 and 800 mg/dL are considered to have partial FPT.

Based on a serum IgG concentration below 400 mg/dL, retrospective surveys estimate the incidence of failure of passive transfer to be between 10–18% of foals (Baldwin, 1991; Clabough, 1991; Stoneham, 1991; LeBlanc, 1992; Raidal, 1996; Tyler-McGowan, 1997; Erhard, 2001). One study found that failure of passive transfer was most prevalent in foals born to dams older than 15 years, foals that ingested colostrum with specific gravity less than 1.06, and foals born in wet, cold environments (LeBlanc, 1992).

Evaluation of foal serum or blood IgG concentration at 12–14 hours post-suckling will reveal whether FPT is possible, and allows remediation with colostrum supplementation (when less than 24 hours after birth) or, with more certainty, intravenous plasma transfusion (after 24 hours).

Foals with FPT of immunoglobulins often present with pulmonary or gastrointestinal infections or sepsis within the first month of life. In addition, foals that did not have FPT at birth, as classically defined, but had marginal transfer of immunoglobulins through colostrum (around 800 mg/dL), may not have adequate humoral protection during the transition period when colostrum-derived antibodies decay and endogenously-produced antibodies rise, at around 2–3 months of life. These foals tend to present recurrent fevers and pneumonia into the first 4–5 months of life, or until endogenous serum IgG concentration reaches protective levels (500–800 mg/dL). They require antibiotic therapy during this period to treat infections.

2.3.2 Septicemia

Septicemia in foals less than one week old is a life-threatening systemic condition that may arise from respiratory, oral, and umbilical routes, including intrauterine placentitis (Koterba, 1984; Morris, 1987). Failure of passive transfer may predispose foals to sepsis, although foals with adequate passive transfer may also become septic, and foals may be born septic when there is intrauterine infection (Robinson, 1993; Raidal, 1996).

Sepsis involves an excessive and systemic inflammatory response during infection, and foals respond effectively with neutrophilia and a left shift, unless they present with prematurity or immaturity. Nevertheless, a transient neutropenia may be accompanied by decreased phagocytic function and oxidative burst activity in the acute phase (Hotchkiss, 2003; Gardner, 2007).

In addition, studies of cytokine expression in PBMC of septic foals have reported decreased gene expression of TNF-alpha, TGF-beta, and IL-4; increased expression of TLR4; and comparable levels of IFN-gamma, IL-beta, IL-6, IL-8, and IL-10, compared with healthy foals (Pusterla, 2006; Gold, 2007; Burton, 2009; Castagnetti, 2012). Though cytokine analyses of blood from septic foals have been contradictory to date, perhaps reflecting immune response to different types of infectious organisms or transient immunosuppression, expression of some cytokines could serve as survival predictors (Pusterla, 2006). Although some septic foals are blood culture-negative, Gram-negative bacteria have been implicated as causative agents in the majority of cases, including *Actinobacillus equuli*, *Escherichia coli*, undifferentiated coliforms, *Pseudomonas* spp., and *Arcanobacterium pyogenes* (Brewer and Koterba, 1988; Robinson, 1993).

Opsonins are important for phagocytosis and bacterial killing, and so are highly consumed during bacterial infection and/or sepsis. Hence, intravenous plasma transfusion is used not only for prophylaxis, but also for treatment of sepsis in neonates, along with broad-spectrum antibiotic, fluid and anti-inflammatory therapies (McTaggart, 2005).

2.3.3 *Rhodococcus equi* infection

Rhodococcus equi is a common cause of pneumonia in foals younger than six months old, in contrast to adult horses, which are largely unaffected by *R. equi* infection. The susceptibility to disease exclusively in young animals suggests specific and physiologic age-dependent development of the immune system that favors the pathogen virulence (Prescott, 1987). *R. equi* is a facultative intracellular bacterium that can survive in the soil and is detected in the feces of herbivorous animals; hence, *R. equi* can become endemic on breeding farms. The virulence of *R. equi* is dependent on the presence of a plasmid-encoding virulence-associated protein A (VapA), which allows survival and replication in certain host cells, including macrophages (Jain, 2003). Retrospective epidemiologic analysis suggests that foals are infected during the first days or weeks of life, when their immune system is naïve and expanding (Horowitz, 2001).

Neutrophils from foals on the first day of life, stimulated with *R. equi in vitro*, significantly increase the mRNA expression of IFN-gamma, TNF-alpha, IL-6, IL-8, IL-12p35, and IL-23p19 cytokines when compared with control cells (Nerren, 2009). Neutrophils from three day old foals can phagocytose and kill *R. equi*, and this ability has a >90% improvement in the presence of *R. equi*-specific antibodies (Zink, 1985; Hietala, 1987; Martens, 1988). Opsonization inhibits the extracellular growth of *R. equi*, emphasizing the importance of *R. equi*-specific antibodies on the mucosal surface at the time of infection (Dawson, 2011). In the equine neonate, therefore, *in vivo* neutrophil function against *R. equi* requires the presence of *R. equi*-specific antibodies, likely absorbed through colostrum or transferred through plasma transfusion.

Providing *R. equi*-specific neutralizing antibodies via hyperimmune plasma to neonatal foals prior to experimental *R. equi* exposure protected foals from terminal disease (Martens, 1989). Similarly, providing hyperimmune plasma to neonatal foals decreased the incidence of *R. equi* pneumonia on a farm endemic for *R. equi*, and provided more protection than nursing colostrum from dams vaccinated with *R. equi* during pregnancy (Madigan, 1991). However, other field trials of hyperimmune plasma did not find significant increase in foal protection over control foals, perhaps indicating the need for improving

administration protocols, such as defining optimal dose, timing, and plasma quality variables (Giguere, 2002; Perkins, 2002).

R. equi infects and proliferates in host APCs, such as alveolar macrophages. Therefore, alveolar macrophages are permissible to *R. equi*, and somewhat facilitate the seeding of infection in the lungs. It seems that specific macrophage activation, dependent on inflammatory cytokines IFN-gamma and TNF-alpha, is necessary for *R. equi* killing in macrophages (Darrah, 2000). Nevertheless, upon *in vitro R. equi* infection, foal monocyte-derived macrophages and dendritic cells express CD40 and CD86 co-stimulatory markers at levels equivalent to adult horse APCs, and increase IL-12p35 and IL-12p40 mRNA expression over adult horse levels, suggesting detection of and activation upon *R. equi* encounter (Flaminio, 2009).

Between the first 5–9 weeks of life, healthy foals produce *R. equi*-specific IgM and IgG in concentrations equivalent to that found in adult horses (Takai, 1986). Experimental infection of one week old foals revealed production of *R. equi*-specific IgG$_1$ (IgGa) and IgG$_{4-7}$ (IgGb) at significantly greater serum concentrations than that of *R. equi* infected adults 15 days post-infection (Jacks, 2007a). Notably, bronchial lymph node cells from these foals also expressed significantly more IFN-gamma mRNA than control foals or infected adult horse cells when stimulated *in vitro* with soluble *R. equi* antigens (Jacks, 2007a). In fact, higher *R. equi* doses have been shown to induce higher concentrations of serum IgM and IgG$_{3-5}$ (IgGT) than low doses of *R. equi* in one week old foals (Jacks, 2010). Hence, it is uncertain why the young foal is still susceptible to disease.

The respiratory tract and gut are the main routes of entry for virulent *R. equi*, so development of mucosal immunity, in addition to a systemic response, is of importance. Mucosal IgA is a component of the respiratory tract immune barrier, yet endogenous IgA is not detected on the nasal mucosal surfaces in foals less than one month old (Sheoran, 2000). Further, it has been determined that serum antibodies detect a different VapA epitope than IgA antibodies in tracheal washes (Taouji, 2002). Production of mucosal antibodies varies with the route of exposure to *R. equi*; experimentally, IgM and IgA were only detected in lung washes from foals infected intra-tracheally (Takai, 1987). This lack of mucosal IgA may represent another facet of vulnerability in young foals to *R. equi* infection.

Following experimental intrabronchial infection at one week old, foals exhibit VapA-specific recall lymphoproliferative responses and IFN-gamma mRNA equivalent to adult horses, indicative of a Th1 response (Jacks, 2007b). Cytotoxic T lymphocytes able to lyse *R. equi* infected cells are detectable in foals at six weeks old, although vaccination can induce CTL at three weeks old (Patton, 2005; Harris, 2011).

Research has clearly demonstrated that foals have functional innate antibacterial defenses and can mount *R. equi*-specific humoral and cell-mediated responses. However, given the very early exposure, environmental abundance of *R. equi*, and the pathogen virulence, preventing infection remains a considerable task in endemic farms.

2.4 Vaccinology teaches about neonatal immunity

Foal vaccination has been an area of active research with strides of progress in recent years. However, refinement of optimal formulation and thorough assessment of protection is ongoing. An alternative approach is to vaccinate mares before foaling, in an effort to maximize antigen-specific antibody transfer to the neonate. This approach has seen success for some pathogens and environmental conditions, although the quality of colostrum-derived antibodies and efficiency of transfer to/absorption by foals is variable, and individuals within a herd may still not be protected (Madigan, 1991; Becu, 1997).

The paradox of neonatal vaccination is the need of immediate protection early in life with long-term memory, the perceived limitations of the immune system of the neonate, and the theory of maternal antibody interference. It is recommended to delay vaccination against influenza until after six or 12 months of life, in order to avoid maternal antibody interference (Wilson, 2001). However, given a half-life of 30 days for IgG, it is likely that colostrum-derived antibodies reach low levels around 2–3 months old. In addition, pathogen-specific cellular immunity is not efficiently transferred by colostrum and, consequently, foals would be susceptible to disease between the decay of colostrum-derived antibodies and vaccine-induced immunity. Therefore, further studies are needed to better define vaccination strategies in foals.

Protecting foals against *R. equi* infection and disease (which occurs early in life) has been the subject of much research and, despite impressive gains, *R. equi* remains a leading cause of foal pneumonia. A variety of vaccine formulations and routes of administration have been investigated, including DNA and peptide vaccines, and oral route. Impressively, oral vaccination of foals at two, seven, and 14 days of life provided protection against virulent *R. equi* challenge at three weeks old and stimulated *R. equi*-specific antibodies (Hooper-McGrevy, 2005). Further studies with the same vaccination strategy revealed that three week old foals are able to generate *R. equi*-specific CTLs and produce IFN-gamma mRNA equivalent to adult horse levels (Harris, 2011). Primary DNA vaccination of 8–15 day old foals, followed by DNA and protein boosters, induced VapA-specific antibodies in serum and BALF in a subset of foals (Lopez, 2003). It is likely that management practices, availability of good quality hyperimmune plasma, enhanced innate immunity, and environmental considerations are essential to limit *R. equi* infection, in addition to a vaccination program.

Despite nearly 70 years of studies, EHV-1 and EHV-4 vaccines are still being improved (Patel and Heldens, 2005). Foals represent a particular challenge for EHV vaccination, because they are likely to be exposed by their dams early in life and are considered to be a reservoir in EHV-1 transmission. Thus, vaccine strategies must consider both early exposure and optimal timing for stimulating long-term protective immune responses. Intramuscular vaccination of foals in the first 1–2 months of life with a mutant EHV-1 strain lacking glycoprotein E induced production of serum neutralizing EHV-1 antibodies and decreased viral load following challenge infection (Tsujimura, 2009). This vaccine candidate is being evaluated further, particularly for measures of mucosal immunity and CTL induction.

Intra-rectal vaccination of 4–6 month old foals against *Lawsonia intracellularis* induced serum immunoglobulin response in the majority of foals after one dose, and nearly all foals after boosting (Pusterla, 2010). A further study, including intra-rectal experimental challenge, demonstrated complete protection against proliferative enteropathy following vaccination (Pusterla, 2012).

Intra-muscular vaccination of three and six month old foals with a model antigen keyhole limpet hemocyanin (KLH), induced KLH-specific IgG response after the first vaccination (Sturgill, 2010). Foals vaccinated at one month generated KLH-specific IgG after a booster dose, but not after the primary vaccination (Sturgill, 2010). In the presence of colostrum-derived antibodies, vaccination at four and eight weeks did not induce detectable circulating KLH-specific IgG, although a robust response was observed after a dose at 26 weeks (Sturgill, 2010).

The immune response to live-attenuated *Mycobacterium bovis* bacillus Calmette-Guérin (BCG) has been tested in human, bovine and equine neonates and adults, with measurable antibody and cell-mediated responses. BCG, an antigen that is closely related to *R. equi*, has been shown to induce antibody responses in equine neonates and foals, with age-dependent differences in the quantity and quality of IgG subtypes. The effect of BCG in the production of IFN-gamma, IL-4, and IL-10 was partially investigated in this study, with no effect on whole blood cytokine production in any age group, but significant effect in delayed-type hypersensitivity reaction in neonates and foals (Sturgill, 2014).

Collectively, these studies suggest that vaccination of neonates can induce measurable immune responses, although effective administration strategies (product, adjuvant, route, boosters), and correlates of protection, need still to be defined.

References

Artiushin, S., Timoney, J.F., Fettinger, M., Fallon, L. and Rathgeber, R. (2013). Immunisation of mares with binding domains of toxins A and B of *Clostridium difficile elicits* serum and colostral antibodies that block toxin binding. *Equine Veterinary Journal* **45**, 476–480.

Badolato, R., Wang, J.M., Murphy, W.J., Lloyd, A.R., Michiel, D.F., Bausserman, L.L., Kelvin, D.J. and Oppenheim, J.J. (1994). Serum amyloid A is a chemoattractant: induction of migration, adhesion and tissue infiltration of monocytes and polymorphonuclear leukocytes. *The Journal of Experimental Medicine* **180**, 203–209.

Badolato, R., Wang, J.M., Stornello, S.L., Ponzi, A.N., Duse, M. and Musso, T. (2000). Serum amyloid A is an activator of PMN antimicrobial functions: induction of degranulation, phagocytosis and enhancement of anti-Candida activity. *Journal of Leukocyte Biology* **67**, 381–386.

Baldwin, J.L., W.L. Cooper, D.K. Vanderwall and H.N. Erb (1991). Prevalence (treatment days) and severity of illness in hypogamma-globulinemic and normogammaglobulinemic foals. *Journal of the American Veterinary Medical Association* **198**, 423–428.

Balson G.A., Smith, G.D. and Yager, J.A. (1997). Immunophenotypic analysis of foal bronchoalveolar lavage lymphocytes. *Veterinary Microbiology* **56**, 237–246.

Banks, E.M., Kyriakidou, M., Little, S. and Hamblin, A.S. (1999). Epithelial lymphocyte and macrophage distribution in the adult and fetal equine lung. *Journal of Comparative Pathology* **120**(1), 1–13.

Barbis, D.P., Bainbridge, D., Crump, A.L., Zhang, C.H. and Antczak, D.F. (1994). Variation in expression of MHC class II antigens on horse lymphocytes determined by MHC haplotype. *Veterinary Immunology and Immunopathology* **42**, 103–114.

Becht, J.L. and Semrad, S.D. (1985). Hematology, blood typing and immunology of the neonatal foal. *The Veterinary Clinics of North America: Equine Practice* **1**, 91–116.

Becu, T., Polledo, G. and Gaskin, J.M. (1997). Immunoprophylaxis of Rhodococcus equi pneumonia in foals. *Veterinary Microbiology* **56**, 193–204.

Bernoco, M., Liu, I.K., Wuest-Ehlert, C.J., Miller, M.E. and Bowers, J. (1987). Chemotactic and phagocytic function of peripheral blood polymorphonuclear leucocytes in newborn foals. *Journal of Reproduction and Fertility Supplement* **35**, 599–605.

Blunden, A.S. and Gower, S.M. (1999). A histological and immuno-histochemical study of the humoral immune system of the lungs in young Thoroughbred horses. *Journal of Comparative Pathology* **120**, 347–356.

Bordin, A.I., Liu, M., Nerren, J.R., Buntain, S.L., Brake, C.N., Kogut, M.H. and Cohen, N.D. (2012). Neutrophil function of neonatal foals is enhanced in vitro by CpG oligodeoxynucleotide stimulation. *Veterinary Immunology and Immunopathology* **145**, 290–297.

Boyd, N.K., Cohen, N.D., Lim, W.S., Martens, R.J., Chaffin, M.K. and Ball, J.M. (2003). Temporal changes in cytokine expression of foals during the first month of life. *Veterinary Immunology and Immunopathology* **92**, 75–85.

Breathnach, C.C., Sturgill-Wright, T., Stiltner, J.L., Adams, A.A., Lunn, D.P. and Horohov, D.W. (2006). Foals are interferon gamma-deficient at birth. *Veterinary Immunology and Immunopathology* **112**, 199–209.

Brewer, B.D. and Koterba, A.M. (1988). Development of a scoring system for the early diagnosis of equine neonatal sepsis. *Equine Veterinary Journal* **20**, 18–22.

Burton, A.B., Wagner, B., Erb, H.N. and Ainsworth, D.M. (2009). Serum interleukin-6 (IL-6) and IL-10 concentrations in normal and septic neonatal foals. *Veterinary Immunology and Immunopathology* **132**, 122–128.

Castagnetti, C., Mariella, J., Pirrone, A., Cinotti, S., Mari, G. and Peli, A. (2012). Expression of interleukin-1beta, interleukin-8 and interferon-gamma in blood samples obtained from healthy and sick neonatal foals. *American Journal of Veterinary Research* **73**, 1418–1427.

Chong, Y.C. and Duffus, W.P. (1992). Immune responses of specific pathogen free foals to EHV-1 infection. *Veterinary Microbiology* **32**, 215–228.

Clabough, D.L., Levine, J.F., Grant, G.L. and Conboy, H.S. (1991). Factors associated with failure of passive transfer of colostral antibodies in Standardbred foals. *Journal of Veterinary Internal Medicine* **5**, 335–340.

Darrah, P.A., Hondalus, M.K., Chen, Q., Ischiropoulos, H. and Mosser, D.M. (2000). Cooperation between reactive oxygen species and nitrogen intermediates in killing of Rhodococcus equi by activated macrophages. *Infection and Immunity* **68**(6), 3587–3593.

Dawson, D.R., Nydam, D.V., Price, C.T., Graham, J.E., Cynamon, M.H., Divers, T.J. and Felippe, M.J. (2011). Effects of opsonization of Rhodococcus equi on bacterial viability and phagocyte activation. *American Journal of Veterinary Research* **72**, 1465–1475.

Erhard, M.H., Luft, C., Remler, H.P. and Stangassinger, M. (2001). Assessment of colostral transfer and systemic availability of immu-noglobulin G in new-born foals using a newly developed enzyme-linked immunosorbent assay (ELISA) system. *Journal of Animal Physiology and Animal Nutrition* **85**, 164–173.

Flaminio, M.J., Rush, B.R., Cox, J.H. and Moore, W.E. (1998). CD4$^+$ and CD8$^+$ T-lymphocytopenia in a filly with *Pneumocystis carinii* pneumonia. *Australian Veterinary Journal* **76**, 399–402.

Flaminio, M.J., Rush, B.R. and Shuman, W. (1999). Peripheral blood lymphocyte subpopulations and immunoglobulin concentrations in healthy foals and foals with *Rhodococcus equi* pneumonia. *Journal of Veterinary Internal Medicine* **13**, 206–212.

Flaminio, M.J., Rush, B.R., Davis, E.G., Hennessy, K., Shuman, W. and Wilkerson, M.J. (2000). Characterization of peripheral blood and pulmonary leukocyte function in healthy foals. *Veterinary Immunology and Immunopathology* **73**, 267–285.

Flaminio, M.J., Borges, A.S., Nydam, D.V., Horohov, D.W., Hecker, R. and Matychak, M.B. (2007). The effect of CpG-ODN on antigen presenting cells of the foal. *Journal of Immune Based Therapies and Vaccines* **5**, 1.

Flaminio, M.J., Nydam, D.V., Marquis, H., Matychak, M.B. and Giguère, S. (2009). Foal monocyte-derived dendritic cells become activated upon Rhodococcus equi infection. *Clinical and Vaccine Immunology* **16**, 176–183.

Galan, J.E., Timoney, J.F. and Lengemann, F.W. (1986). Passive transfer of mucosal antibody to *Streptococcus equi* in the foal. *Infection and Immunity* **54**, 202–206.

Gardner, R.B., Nydam, D.V., Luna, J.A., Bicalho, M.L., Matychak, M.B. and Flaminio, M.J. (2007). Serum opsonization capacity, phagocyto-sis and oxidative burst activity in neonatal foals in the intensive care unit. *Journal of Veterinary Internal Medicine* **21**, 797–805.

Giguère, S., Gaskin, J.M., Miller, C. and Bowman, J.L. (2002). Evaluation of a commercially available hyperimmune plasma product for pre-vention of naturally acquired pneumonia caused by *Rhodococcus equi* in foals. *Journal of the American Veterinary Medical Association* **220**, 59–63.

Gold, J.R., Perkins, G.A., Erb, H.N. and Ainsworth, D.M. (2007). Cytokine profiles of peripheral blood mononuclear cells isolated from septic and healthy neonatal foals. *Journal of Veterinary Internal Medicine* **21**, 482–488.

Gröndahl, G., Johannisson, A., Demmers, S. and Jensen Waern, M. (1999). Influence of age and plasma treatment on neutrophil phago-cytosis and CD18 expression in foals. *Veterinary Microbiology* **65**, 241–254.

Gröndahl G., Sternberg, S., Jensen-Waern, M. and Johannisson, A. (2001). Opsonic capacity of foal serum for the two neonatal patho-gens *Escherichia coli* and *Actinobacillus equuli*. *Equine Veterinary Journal* **33**, 670–675.

Harrington, J.R., Wilkerson, C.P., Brake, C.N. and Cohen, N.D. (2012). Effects of age and R848 stimulation on expression of Toll-like receptor 8 mRNA by foal neutrophils. *Veterinary Immunology and Immunopathology* **150**, 10–18.

Harris, S.P., Hines, M.T., Mealey, R.H., Alperin, D.C. and Hines, S.A. (2011). Early development of cytotoxic T lymphocytes in neonatal foals following oral inoculation with *Rhodococcus equi*. *Veterinary Immunology and Immunopathology* **141**, 312–316.

Hayashi F., Means, T.K. and Luster, A.D. (2003). Toll-like receptors stimulate human neutrophil function. *Blood* **102**(7), 2660–2669.

Hemmi, H., Takeuchi, O., Kawai, T., Kaisho, T., Sato, S., Sanjo, H., Matsumoto, M., Hoshino, K., Wagner, H., Takeda, K. and Akira, S. (2000). A Toll-like receptor recognizes bacterial DNA. *Nature* **408** (6813), 740–745.

Hietala, S.K. and Ardans, A.A. (1987). Neutrophil phagocytic and serum opsonic response of the foal to *Corynebacterium equi*. *Veterinary Immunology and Immunopathology* **14**, 279–294.

Holmes, M.A. and Lunn, D.P. (1991). A study of bovine and equine immunoglobulin levels in pony foals fed bovine colostrum. *Equine Veterinary Journal* **23**, 116–118.

Holznagel, D.L., Hussey, S., Mihalyi, J.E., Wilson, W.D. and Lunn, D.P. (2003). Onset of immunoglobulin production in foals. *Equine Veterinary Journal* **35**, 620–622.

Hooper-McGrevy, K.E., Wilkie, B.N. and Prescott, J.F. (2005). Virulence-associated protein-specific serum immunoglobulin G-isotype expression in young foals protected against *Rhodococcus equi* pneumonia by oral immunization with virulent *R. equi*. *Vaccine* **23**, 5760–5767.

Horowitz, M.L., Cohen, N.D., Takai, S., Becu, T., Chaffin, M.K., Chu, K.K., Magdesian, K.G. and Martens, R.J. (2001). Application of Sartwell's model (lognormal distribution of incubation periods) to age at onset and age at death of foals with *Rhodococcus equi* pneumonia as evidence of perinatal infection. *Journal of Veterinary Internal Medicine* **15**, 171–175.

Hotchkiss, R.S. and Karl, I.E., (2003). The pathophysiology and treatment of sepsis. *The New England Journal of Medicine* **348**, 138–150.

Hullinger, P.J., Wilson, W.D., Rossitto, P.V., Patton, J.F., Thurmond, M.C. and MacLachlan, N.J. (1998). Passive transfer, rate of decay and protein specificity of antibodies against equine arteritis virus in horses from a Standardbred herd with high seroprevalence. *Journal of the American Veterinary Medical Association* **213**, 839–842.

Hulten, C. and Demmers, S. (2002). Serum amyloid A (SAA) as an aid in the management of infectious disease in the foal: comparison with total leucocyte count, neutrophil count and fibrinogen. *Equine Veterinary Journal* **34**, 693–698.

Jacks, S., Giguère, S., Crawford, P.C. and Castleman, W.L. (2007a). Experimental infection of neonatal foals with *Rhodococcus equi* triggers adult-like gamma interferon induction. *Clinical and Vaccine Immunology* **14**, 669–677.

Jacks, S., Giguère, S. and Prescott, J.F. (2007b). *In vivo* expression of and cell-mediated immune responses to the plasmid-encoded virulence-associated proteins of *Rhodococcus equi* in foals. *Clinical and Vaccine Immunology* **14**, 369–374.

Jacks, S. and Giguère, S. (2010). Effects of inoculum size on cell-mediated and humoral immune responses of foals experimentally infected with *Rhodococcus equi*: a pilot study. *Veterinary Immunology and Immunopathology* **133**, 282–286.

Jain, S., Bloom, B.R. and Hondalus, M.K. (2003). Deletion of vapA encoding Virulence Associated Protein A attenuates the intracellular actinomycete *Rhodococcus equi*. *Molecular Microbiology* **50**, 115–128.

Jeffcott, L.B. (1974). Studies on passive immunity in the foal. 1. Gamma-globulin and antibody variations associated with the maternal transfer of immunity and the onset of active immunity. *Journal of Comparative Pathology* **84**, 93–101.

Jeffcott, L. B. (1975). The transfer of passive immunity to the foal and its relation to immune status after birth. *Journal of Reproduction and Fertility Supplement* (23) 727–733.

Jeffcott, L.B. and Jeffcott, T.J. (1974). Studies on passive immunity in the foal. III. The characterization and significance of neonatal proteinuria. *Journal of Comparative Pathology* **84**, 455–465.

Jeong, H.D. and Teale, J.M. (1988). Comparison of the fetal and adult functional B cell repertoires by analysis of VH gene family expression. *Journal of Experimental Medicine* **168**, 589–603.

Jozsef, L., Khreiss, T. and Filep, J.G. (2004). CpG motifs in bacterial DNA delay apoptosis of neutrophil granulocytes. *FASEB Journal* **18** (14), 1776–1778.

Kaur, N., Townsend, H., Lohman, K., Marques, F. and Singh, B. (2013). Analyses of lipid rafts, Toll-like receptors 2 and 4 and cytokines in foals vaccinated with Virulence Associated Protein A/CpG oligonucleotide vaccine against Rhodococcus equi. *Veterinary Immunology and Immunopathology* **156**(3–4) 182–189.

Kohn, C.W., Knight, D., Hueston, W., Jacobs, R. and Reed, S.M. (1989). Colostral and serum IgG, IgA and IgM concentrations in Standardbred mares and their foals at parturition. *Journal of the American Veterinary Medical Association* **195**, 64–68.

Koterba, A.M., Brewer, B.D. and Tarplee, F.A. (1984). Clinical and clinicopathological characteristics of the septicaemic neonatal foal: review of 38 cases. *Equine Veterinary Journal* **16**, 376–382.

Kumar, S., Kumar, R., Gupta, A.K. and Dwivedi, S.K. (2008). Passive transfer of Theileria equi antibodies to neonate foals of immune tolerant mares. *Veterinary Parasitology* **151**, 80–85.

Lavoie, J.P., Spensley, M.S., Smith, B.P. and Mihalyi, J. (1989). Absorption of bovine colostral immunoglobulins G and M in newborn foals. *American Journal of Veterinary Research* **50**, 1598–1603.

Lawler, A.M., Lin, P.S. and Gearhart, P.J. (1987). Adult B-cell repertoire is biased toward two heavy-chain variable-region genes that rearrange frequently in fetal pre-B cells. *Proceedings of the National Academy of Sciences of the United States of America* **84**, 2454–2458.

LeBlanc, M.M., Tran, T., Baldwin, J.L. and Pritchard, E.L. (1992). Factors that influence passive transfer of immunoglobulins in foals. *Journal of the American Veterinary Medical Association* **200**, 179–183.

Le Jan, C. (1996). Cellular components of mammary secretions and neonatal immunity: a review. *Veterinary Research* **27**, 403–417.

Lewis, M.J., Wagner, B. and Woof J.M. (2008). The different effector function capabilities of the seven equine IgG subclasses have implications for vaccine strategies. *Molecular Immunology* **45**, 818–827.

Liu, I.K., Walsh, E.M., Bernoco, M. and Cheung, A.T. (1987). Bronchoalveolar lavage in the newborn foal. *Journal of Reproduction and Fertility Supplement* **35**, 587–592.

Liu, M., Liu, T., Bordin, A., Nerren, J. and Cohen, N. (2009). Activation of foal neutrophils at different ages by CpG oligodeoxynucleotides and *Rhodococcus equi*. *Cytokine* **48**, 280–289.

Lopez, A.M., Hines, M.T., Palmer, G.H., Knowles, D.P., Alperin, D.C. and Hines, S.A. (2003). Analysis of anamnestic immune responses in adult horses and priming in neonates induced by a DNA vaccine expressing the vapA gene of *Rhodococcus equi*. *Vaccine* **21**, 3815–3825.

Mackenzie, C. D. (1975). Histological development of the thymic and intestinal lymphoid tissue of the horse. *Journal of the South African Veterinary Association* **46**, 47–55.

McTaggart, C., Penhale, J., and Raidala, S.L. (2005). Effect of plasma transfusion on neutrophil function in healthy and septic foals. *Australian Veterinary Journal* **83**(8), 499–505.

Madigan, J.E., Hietala, S. and Muller, N. (1991). Protection against naturally acquired *Rhodococcus equi* pneumonia in foals by administration of hyperimmune plasma. *Journal of Reproduction and Fertility Supplement* **44**, 571–578.

Martens, J.G., Martens, R.J. and Renshaw, H.W. (1988). *Rhodococcus (Corynebacterium) equi*: bactericidal capacity of neutrophils from neonatal and adult horses. *American Journal of Veterinary Research* **49**, 295–299.

Martens, R.J., Martens, J.G., Fiske, R.A. and Hietala, S.K. (1989). *Rhodococcus equi* foal pneumonia: protective effects of immune plasma in experimentally infected foals. *Equine Veterinary Journal* **21**, 249–255.

Marti, E., Ehrensperger, F., Burger, D., Ousey, J., Day, M.J. and Wilson, A.D. (2009). Maternal transfer of IgE and subsequent development of IgE responses in the horse (*Equus callabus*). *Veterinary Immunology and Immunopathology* **127**, 203–211.

Martin, B.R. and Larson, K.A. (1973). Immune response of equine fetus to coliphage T2. *American Journal of Veterinary Research* **34**, 1363–1364.

McDonald, T.L., Larson, M.A., Mack, D.R. and Weber, A. (2001). Elevated extrahepatic expression and secretion of mammary-associated serum amyloid A 3 (M-SAA3) into colostrum. *Veterinary Immunology and Immunopathology* **83**, 203–211.

McGuire, T.C., Poppie, M.J. and Banks, K.L. (1975). Hypogammaglobulinemia predisposing to infection in foals. *Journal of the American Veterinary Medical Association* **166**, 71–75.

Merant, C., Breathnach, C.C., Kohler, K., Rashid, C., Van Meter, P. and Horohov, D.W. (2009). Young foal and adult horse monocyte-derived dendritic cells differ by their degree of phenotypic maturity. *Veterinary Immunology and Immunopathology* **131**, 1–8.

Morgan, D.O., Bryans, J.T. and Mock, R.E. (1975). Immunoglobulins produced by the antigenized equine fetus. *Journal of Reproduction and Fertility Supplement* **23**, 735–738.

Morris, D.D. and Whitlock, R.H. (1987). Therapy of suspected septicemia in neonatal foals using plasma-containing antibodies to core lipopolysaccharide (LPS). *Journal of Veterinary Internal Medicine* **1**, 175–182.

Nerren, J.R., Martens, R.J., Payne, S., Murrell, J., Butler, J.L. and Cohen, N.D. (2009). Age-related changes in cytokine expression by neutrophils of foals stimulated with virulent Rhodococcus equi in vitro. *Veterinary Immunology and Immunopathology* **127**, 212–219.

Nielsen, M.K., Vidyashankar, A.N., Gravatte, H.S., Bellaw, J., Lyons, E.T., Andersen, U.V. (2014). Development of Strongylus vulgaris-specific serum antibodies in naturally infected foals. *Veterinary Parasitology* **200**(3–4) 265–270.

Patel, J.R. and Heldens, J. (2005). Equine herpesviruses 1 (EHV-1) and 4 (EHV-4)– epidemiology, disease and immunoprophylaxis: a brief review. *Veterinary Journal* **170**, 14–23.

Patton, K.M., McGuire, T.C., Hines, M.T., Mealey, R.H. and Hines, S.A. (2005). *Rhodococcus equi*-specific cytotoxic T lymphocytes in immune horses and development in asymptomatic foals. *Infection and Immunity* **73**, 2083–2093.

Perkins, G.A., Yeager, A., Erb, H.N., Nydam, D.V., Divers, T.J. and Bowman, J.L. (2002). Survival of foals with experimentally induced *Rhodococcus equi* infection given either hyperimmune plasma containing *R. equi* antibody or normal equine plasma. *Veterinary Therapeutics: Research in Applied Veterinary Medicine* **3**, 334–346.

Perkins, G.A., Goodman, L.B., Freer, H., Babasyan, S. and Wagner, B. (2014). Maternal T-lymphocytes in equine colostrum express a primarily inflammatory phenotype. *Veterinary Immunology and Immunopathology*, **161**(3–4), 141–150.

Perryman, L.E. and McGuire, T.C. (1980). Evaluation for immune system failures in horses and ponies. *Journal of the American Veterinary Medical Association* **176**, 1374–1377.

Perryman, L.E., McGuire, T.C. and Torbeck, R.L. (1980). Ontogeny of lymphocyte function in the equine fetus. *American Journal of Veterinary Research* **41**, 1197–1200.

Prescott, J.F. (1987). Epidemiology of *Rhodococcus equi* infection in horses. *Veterinary Microbiology* **14**, 211–214.

Prescott, J.F., Johnson, J.A. and Markham, R.J. (1980). Experimental studies on the pathogenesis of *Corynebacterium equi* infection in foals. *Canadian Journal of Comparative Medicine* **44**, 280–288.

Prescott, J.F., Fernandez, A.S., Nicholson, V.M., Patterson, M.C., Yager, J.A., Viel, L. and Perkins, G. (1996). Use of a virulence-associated protein based enzyme-linked immunosorbent assay for *Rhodococcus equi* serology in horses. *Equine Veterinary Journal* **28**, 344–349.

Pusterla, N., Magdesian, K.G., Mapes, S. and Leutenegger, C.M. (2006). Expression of molecular markers in blood of neonatal foals with sepsis. *American Journal of Veterinary Research* **67**, 1045–1049.

Pusterla, N., Jackson, R., Mapes, S.M., Noland, J., Stenbom, R.M. and Gebhart, C. (2010). *Lawsonia intracellularis*: humoral immune response and fecal shedding in weanling foals following intra-rectal administration of frozen-thawed or lyophilized avirulent live vaccine. *Veterinary Journal* **186**, 110–112.

Pusterla, N., Conrad, P.A., Packham, A.E., Mapes, S.M., Finno, C.J., Gardner, I.A., Barr, B.C., Ferraro, G.L. and Wilson, W.D. (2011). Endogenous transplacental transmission of *Neospora hughesi* in naturally infected horses. *The Journal of Parasitology* **97**, 281–285.

Pusterla, N., Vannucci, F.A., Mapes, S.M., Nogradi, N., Collier, J.R., Hill, J.A., Difrancesco, M., White, A.M., Akana, N.K., Simonek, G. and Gebhart, C.J. (2012). Efficacy of an avirulent live vaccine against *Lawsonia intracellularis* in the prevention of proliferative enteropathy in experimentally infected weanling foals. *American Journal of Veterinary Research* **73**, 741–746.

Raaphorst, F.M., Timmers, E., Kenter, M.J., Van Tol, M.J., Vossen, J.M. and Schuurman, R.K. (1992). Restricted utilization of germ-line VH3 genes and short diverse third complementarity-determining regions (CDR3) in human fetal B lymphocyte immunoglobulin heavy chain rearrangements. *European Journal of Immunology* **22**, 247–251.

Raidal, S.L. (1996). The incidence and consequences of failure of passive transfer of immunity on a thoroughbred breeding farm. *Australian Veterinary Journal* **73**, 201–206.

Robinson, J.A., Allen, G.K., Green, E.M., Fales, W.H., Loch, W.E. and Wilkerson, C.G. (1993). A prospective study of septicaemia in colostrum-deprived foals. *Equine Veterinary Journal* **25**, 214–219.

Rouse, B.T. (1971). The immunoglobulins of adult equine and foal sera: a quantitative study. *The British Veterinary Journal* **127**, 45–52.

Ryan, C. and Giguère, S. (2010). Equine neonates have attenuated humoral and cell-mediated immune responses to a killed adjuvanted vaccine compared to adult horses. *Clinical and Vaccine Immunology* **17**, 1896–1902.

Secor, E.J., Matychak, M.B. and Felippe, M.J. (2012). Transfer of tumour necrosis factor-alpha via colostrum to foals. *The Veterinary Record* **170**, 51.

Sheoran, A.S., Timoney, J.F., Holmes, M.A., Karzenski, S.S. and Crisman, M.V. (2000). Immunoglobulin isotypes in sera and nasal mucosal secretions and their neonatal transfer and distribution in horses. *American Journal of Veterinary Research* **61**, 1099–1105.

Siegel, R.C. and Cathou, R.E. (1980). Conformation of Immunoglobulin M. III. Structural requirements of antigen for complement fixation by equine IgM. *Journal of Immunology* **125**, 1910–1915.

Siegrist, C.A. (2003). Mechanisms by which maternal antibodies influence infant vaccine responses: review of hypotheses and definition of main determinants. *Vaccine* **21**(24), 3406–3412.

Smith, R. 3rd, Chaffin, M.K., Cohen, N.D. and Martens, R.J. (2002). Age-related changes in lymphocyte subsets of quarter horse foals. *American Journal of Veterinary Research* **63**, 531–537.

Sternberg, S. (2001). Specific immune response of mares and their newborn foals to Actinobacillus spp. present in the oral cavity. *Acta Veterinaria Scandinavica* **42**, 237–242.

Stoneham, S.J., Digby, N.J. and Ricketts, S.W. (1991). Failure of passive transfer of colostral immunity in the foal: incidence and the effect of stud management and plasma transfusions. *The Veterinary Record* **128**, 416–419.

Stoneham, S.J., Palmer, L., Cash, R. and Rossdale, P.D. (2001). Measurement of serum amyloid A in the neonatal foal using a latex agglutination immunoturbidimetric assay: determination of the normal range, variation with age and response to disease. *Equine Veterinary Journal* **33**, 599–603.

Sturgill, T.L. and Horohov, D.W. (2010). Vaccination Response of Young Foals to Keyhole Limpet Hemocyanin: Evidence of Effective Priming in the Presence of Maternal Antibodies. *Journal of Equine Veterinary Science* **30**, 359–364.

Sturgill, T.L., Giguere, S., Berghaus, L.J., Hurley, D.J. and Hondalus, M.K. (2014). Comparison of antibody and cell-mediated immune responses of foals and adult horses after vaccination with live *Mycobaterium bovis* BCG. *Vaccine* **32**, 1362–1367.

Takai, S., Kawazu, S. and Tsubaki, S. (1986). Immunoglobulin and specific antibody responses to *Rhodococcus (Corynebacterium) equi* infection in foals as measured by enzyme-linked immunosorbent assay. *Journal of clinical Microbiology* **23**, 943–947.

Takai, S., Kawazu, S. and Tsubaki, S. (1987). Humoral immune response of foals to experimental infection with *Rhodococcus equi*. *Veterinary Microbiology* **14**, 321–327.

Tallmadge, R.L., McLaughlin, K., Secor, E., Ruano, D., Matychak, M.B. and Flaminio, M.J. (2009). Expression of essential B cell genes and immunoglobulin isotypes suggests active development and gene recombination during equine gestation. *Developmental and Comparative Immunology* **33**, 1027–1038.

Tallmadge, R.L., Tseng, C.T., King, R.A. and Felippe, M.J. (2013). Developmental progression of equine immunoglobulin heavy chain variable region diversity. *Developmental and Comparative Immunology* **41**, 33–43.

Taouji, S., Breard, E., Peyret-Lacombe, A., Pronost, S., Fortier, G. and Collobert-Laugier, C. (2002). Serum and mucosal antibodies of infected foals recognized two distinct epitopes of VapA of Rhodococcus equi. *FEMS Immunology and Medical Microbiology* **34**, 299–306.

Tsujimura, K., Shiose, T., Yamanaka, T., Nemoto, M., Kondo, T. and Matsumura, T. (2009). Equine herpesvirus type 1 mutant defective in glycoprotein E gene as candidate vaccine strain. *The Journal of Veterinary Medical Science* **71**, 1439–1448.

Tyler-McGowan, C.M., Hodgson, J.L. and Hodgson, D.R. (1997). Failure of passive transfer in foals: incidence and outcome on four studs in New South Wales. *Australian Veterinary Journal* **75**, 56–59.

Ueda, Y., Sanai, Y. and Homma, J.Y. (1982). Enzyme-linked immunosorbent assay for detection of antibody to *Pseudomonas aeruginosa* and measurement of antibody titer in horse serum. *American Journal of Veterinary Research* **43**, 55–60.

Van Oirschot, J.T., Bruin, G., de Boer-Luytze, E. and Smolders, G. (1991). Maternal antibodies against equine influenza virus in foals and their interference with vaccination. Zentralblatt fur Veterinarmedizin. Reihe B. *Journal of Veterinary Medicine Series B* **38**, 391–396.

Wagner, B., Flaminio, J.B., Hillegas, J., Leibold, W., Erb, H.N. and Antczak, D.F. (2006). Occurrence of IgE in foals: evidence for transfer of maternal IgE by the colostrum and late onset of endogenous IgE production in the horse. *Veterinary Immunology and Immunopathology* **110**, 269–278.

Wagner, B., Burton, A. and Ainsworth, D. (2010). Interferon-gamma, interleukin-4 and interleukin-10 production by T helper cells reveals intact Th1 and regulatory TR1 cell activation and a delay of the Th2 cell response in equine neonates and foals. *Veterinary Research* **41**, 47.

Weighardt, H., Feterowski, C., Veit, M., Rump, M., Wagner, H. and Holzmann, B. (2000). Increased resistance against acute polymicrobial sepsis in mice challenged with immunostimulatory CpG oligodeoxynucleotides is related to an enhanced innate effector cell response. *Journal of Immunology* **165**(8), 4537–4543.

Wichtel, M.G., Anderson, K.L., Johnson, T.V., Nathan, U. and Smith, L. (1991). Influence of age on neutrophil function in foals. *Equine Veterinary Journal* **23**, 466–469.

Wilkins, P.A., Glaser, A.L. and McDonnell, S.M. (2006). Passive transfer of naturally acquired specific immunity against West Nile Virus to foals in a semi-feral pony herd. *Journal of Veterinary Internal Medicine* **20**, 1045–1047.

Wilson, W.D., Mihalyi, J.E., Hussey, S. and Lunn, D.P. (2001). Passive transfer of maternal immunoglobulin isotype antibodies against tetanus and influenza and their effect on the response of foals to vaccination. *Equine Veterinary Journal* **33**, 644–650.

Zink, M.C. and Johnson, J.A. (1984). Cellular constituents of clinically normal foal bronchoalveolar lavage fluid during postnatal maturation. *American Journal of Veterinary Research* **45**, 893–897.

Zink, M.C., Yager, J.A., Prescott, J.F. and Wilkie, B.N. (1985). In vitro phagocytosis and killing of Corynebacterium equi by alveolar macrophages of foals. *American Journal of Veterinary Research* **46**, 2171–2174.

Zou, S., Brady, H.A. and Hurley, W.L. (1998). Protective factors in mammary gland secretions during the periparturient period in the mare. *Journal of Equine Veterinary Science* **18**, 184–188.

3 The Immune System of the Older Horse

Amanda A. Adams and David W. Horohov

3.1 Definition

Improvements in health care and advancements in science and medicine over the past century have extended the average lifespan of humans and companion animals, including horses. We now have the dilemma of having a horse population with increased longevity, facing the potential for age-associated diseases. Thus, a better understanding of the mechanisms leading to a decline in physiologic function with age is important for providing optimal care for old horses. The process of aging is an ubiquitous and complex phenomenon; while there is no universal definition of aging, it is expected that the effectiveness of several physiological systems becomes compromised. One of the most recognized consequences of aging is a decline in the functionality of the immune system.

When does a horse become *old*? The term *old* has a broad meaning of *lived for many years*, or *not young*. Some refer to the old as being *geriatric* or *aged*, which implies there are health problems occurring with the process of aging. However, there is considerable variation in the aging process, and there is no set chronological age at which an individual is considered old. This difficulty is due to the fact that chronological age does not equal biological age.

Chronological age is simply an individual's age in years, whereas biological age refers to one's age at the cellular level (Lloyd, 2014). These two concepts of age are often not equal. Some horses remain physically active and healthy well into their twenties, while others become biologically old or geriatric by their mid-to-late teens. These individual differences are due to a variety of factors, including genetics, environment, and management practices. For the purposes of this chapter we will refer to the aged horse as being "old" rather than "geriatric". With regard to chronological age for an old horse, we will use ≥20 years of age, as this is a typical cut-off used in studies comparing physiological responses of old horses to young horses.

Population information regarding the aged horses is limited. In 2003, Brosnahan and Paradis surveyed horse owners and reported that they perceived their horses as being old at approximately 22 years of age. Data from a retrospective study showed that in 1989, only 2% of equine referral cases at a university veterinary hospital were over 20 years of age, but this had increased to 12.5% by 1999 and to almost 20% by 2003

(Brosnahan, 2003b). However, in 2005, a survey of the horse population in the United States reported only 7.6% of the total population to be over 20 years of age (USDA, 2006). It has been estimated that 29% of the equine population in the United Kingdom is 15 years or older (Ireland, 2011a, 2011b).

3.2 Clinical conditions associated with aging

There are several clinical conditions that are acknowledged as being more prevalent in the older horse. While these conditions may be present in younger horses, their frequency and severity often increases with age. In a survey conducted in 2005, owners considered ≈ 43% of old horses (≥ 20 years old) to present health disorders, compared with ≈ 33% in the six to ten year old age group (Cole, 2005). The most frequently reported problems in horses ≥ 20 years fall into the category of gastrointestinal, musculoskeletal and respiratory systems (Brosnahan, 2003a, 2003b).

In a more recent survey, Australian horse owners were most concerned with weight loss, arthritis, lameness, and dental problems in caring for old horses (McGowan, 2010). The most commonly cited clinical conditions of the old horse include: pituitary pars intermedia dysfunction (PPID) (McFarlane, 2011); colic (Brosnahan, 2003, 2003); dental abnormalities (Graham, 2002); glaucoma (Chandler, 2003); decline in cardiac output (McKeever, 2010); respiratory dysfunction (Deaton, 2004); osteoarthritis (Brama, 1999); decline in reproductive function of the mare (Madill, 2002); neoplasia, including intestinal lipomas, melanomas, and squamous cell carcinomas (Brosnahan, 2003a, 2003b); and increased risk for bacterial and viral infections (Allen, 2008; Adams, 2011). In terms of these latter conditions, an overall decline in immune function most likely contributes to the increased susceptibility to infections.

3.3 Immunosenescence and vaccination

It has been appreciated for many years that the immune system undergoes gradual deterioration with age, referred to as

Equine Clinical Immunology, First Edition. Edited by M. Julia B. Felippe.
© 2016 John Wiley & Sons, Inc. Published 2016 by John Wiley & Sons, Inc.

immunosenescence (Walford, 1969). The classic definition of immunosenescence is an age-related, unidirectional decline in immune function. However, recent studies indicate that this process is more complex, where nearly every component of the immune system undergoes age-associated changes, leading to both diminished and enhanced (*inflamm-aging*) (Franceschi, 2000a) characteristics. The two terms "immunosenescence" and "inflamm-aging" may sound contradictory; however, they are intertwined.

Immunosenescence is the biological aging process associated with a progressive decline in overall systemic immunity and increased prevalence of cancer, autoimmune and chronic diseases, poor responses to vaccination, and increased susceptibility to common infectious organisms. Both innate and adaptive arms of the immune system are affected by immunosenescence, including a wide range of cell types:

1 Hematopoietic stem cells, lymphoid progenitors in the bone marrow, and thymic stroma (Linton, 2004).

2 Macrophages, dendritic cells and neutrophils of the innate response (Plackett, 2004).

3 B cells and T cells (Globerson, 2000; Colonna-Romano, 2008).

While few studies have investigated the effect of aging on the innate immune system of the horse, innate immunity appears to remain intact in the aged horse. A study by Horohov and colleagues (1999) demonstrated that aged horses (mean age 25 years) had lymphokine-activated killer cell activity equivalent to that of younger animals (mean age 7.5 years) (Horohov, 1999). Circulating monocyte and granulocyte counts in young and aged horses are also reported to be similar (Guirnalda, 2001). These findings are in concordance with those of human studies that similarly showed little effect of aging on innate immune function (Franceschi, 2000b).

Horses, like other species, experience thymic involution (Perryman, 1988). Studies have looked at age-associated changes in lymphocyte populations ($\geq$ 20 years) and found that old horse exhibit a decline in the total lymphocyte count, as well as lymphocyte subset cell counts ($CD5^+$, $CD4^+$ and $CD8^+$ T cells, and B cells) (McFarlane, 2001; Horohov, 2002). While there were no significant differences in the immunoglobulin (Ig) isotypes in aged horses, compared to younger controls, there was a trend towards a higher concentration of IgA and IgG (McFarlane, 2001).

Among the immunological changes seen in aged humans and experimental animals, T cells are most frequently found to be responsible for defects in humoral and cell-mediated immunity (Miller, 1996; Pawelec, 2002; Effros, 2003a). Moreover, dysfunctional T cells have been associated with increased morbidity and mortality in the elderly (Goodwin, 1995). The most noted changes in T cell populations of the elderly are decreased frequencies of naïve T cells (Globerson, 1995), expanded pools of dysfunctional memory T cells (Effros, 2003b; Goronzy, 2005), shrinkage of the T cell repertoire, and decreased T cell proliferative responses *in vitro* (Naylor, 2005). In fact, decreased T cell proliferation is a hallmark characteristic of immunosenescence

in many species, including humans (Pawelec, 2002); primates (Messaoudi, 2006); mice (Douziech, 2002); cats (Campbell, 2004); dogs (HogenEsch, 2004); and horses (Fermaglich, 2002, Horohov, 2002, Adams, 2008).

Proliferation of T cells or clonal expansion is essential for maintaining function of the adaptive immune system (Effros, 2003a). During development, T cells generate receptors with diversity that allows recognition of all possible antigens they may encounter over the lifespan (Janeway, 2005). Once generated, a lymphocyte's receptor specificity does not change. Following exposure to their specific antigen, the lymphocytes divide and mature into effector cells that are involved in clearance of the antigen. Once antigen clearance occurs, most of the cells die by apoptosis, leaving a small number of memory cells with the same antigen receptor specificity (Gupta, 2005). Re-exposure to the antigen results in a repeat of the process of activation and proliferation, though at a more rapid rate because of the presence of memory cells. Thus, proliferation is important process in generating sufficient numbers of T cells to fight an infection (Weng, 1998; Miller, 2000).

The mechanisms responsible for decreased proliferation are not completely known. In one study of aged horse immunosenescence, T cell proliferation remained depressed after supplementation with recombinant interleukin (IL)-2, suggesting that decreased proliferation cannot be solely attributed to decreased expression of IL-2 (Horohov, 2002). Telomere-driven replicative exhaustion has been proposed as a mechanism leading to immunosenescence of both T and B lymphocytes (Goronzy, 2006). Telomeres are specialized protein structures that cap and protect the ends of chromosomes to maintain the stability and integrity of the DNA. Telomeres shorten with each cycle of cell division, and sufficient telomere loss acts as a molecular clock that triggers cell senescence (Lord, 2002). Indeed, leukocyte telomere length (LTL) is an emerging marker of biological age (O'Donovan, 2011).

Progressive telomere shortening with age in humans has been demonstrated in many studies, and this age-associated loss of telomeres has been observed in different types of leukocytes (Goronzy, 2006). In fact, this age-associated loss of telomeres also occurs in equine peripheral blood mononuclear cells, and has been correlated with decreased proliferation potential and other immunosenescent characteristics (Katepalli, 2008).

These age-related changes in immune function likely contribute to reduced responsiveness to vaccination and infectious agents (Walford, 1969; Effros, 2003a; Pawelec, 2005). Several studies have examined the immune responses to equine influenza vaccination in order to evaluate the secondary or anamnestic immune responses of aged horses. These studies have shown that old horses have a reduced humoral immune response to inactivated influenza virus vaccines, compared with younger horses (Goto, 1993; Horohov, 1999; Muirhead, 2008).

Another study investigated the antibody response to rabies vaccination, which was used as a measure of a primary immune response, when an animal is exposed to an antigen for the first time. This was possible because the study was performed on Prince Edward Island, which is rabies-free, so most horses there are not vaccinated against rabies (Muirhead, 2008). This primary response involves the process of recruiting naïve lymphocytes, which become activated, proliferate and create memory T and B cells. These memory cells will play a role in providing protection from subsequent challenges by the same antigen. Interestingly, the results of this study demonstrated that aged horses mounted an anti-rabies virus antibody response that was similar to younger horses. However, the aged horses did not maintain an adequate antibody titer following a single dose of rabies vaccine, compared with the younger horses.

Since alternative vaccination approaches may prove more efficacious in aged horses, a study measuring both antibody and cell-mediated immune responses of aged horses to a canarypox recombinant virus vector expressing the haemagglutinin antigen of influenza (Recombitek® Influenza) was undertaken (Adams, 2011). The vaccine was effective at inducing both antibody and cell-mediated immune responses to equine influenza in young naïve horses. While the old horses had prior evidence of pre-existing immunity to influenza, their antibody responses were enhanced only slightly by the vaccine. The old horses' cell-mediated immune responses post-vaccination were present, but were not statistically significant over time.

Only one study has investigated the efficacy of a canarypox-vectored influenza vaccine in aged horses. Adams and colleagues (2011) demonstrated that aged horses remain susceptible to infection with equine influenza virus, despite the presence of circulating antibodies. The vaccine did not induce significant cell-mediated immune responses for protection from clinical disease in these aged horses.

Taken together, these studies showed that, while aged horses have pre-existing humoral immune responses, these levels may not be sufficient enough to sustain protection in the face of an infectious challenge. Therefore, periodic vaccination is important, in order to maintain a protective level of immunity by preserving memory responses.

3.3.1 Inflamm-aging

A lifetime of exposure to various antigens can have an impact on immunosenescence and can contribute to the process of *inflamm-aging*, or chronic, low-grade pro-inflammatory state, via the mechanism of *clonal exhaustion* (Franceschi, 2000b, 2014). While this exact association has yet to be identified for the aged horse, the process of inflamm-aging has been well characterized in humans.

Inflammation is a complex combination of molecular and cellular interactions directed to return physiological homeostasis (Vasto, 2007). Unlike acute inflammation, chronic inflammation is not resolved within minutes or hours, and involves various processes, including cytokine production, tissue injury and healing over a long period (Vasto, 2007). An imbalance between pro- and anti-inflammatory cytokines contributes to the process of age-associated chronic inflammation.

The production of pro-inflammatory cytokines IL-6 beta (IL-6b), IL-1 and tumor necrosis factor alpha (TNF-alpha), by monocytes and macrophages, responds to a variety of stimuli, including mitogens, bacteria, viruses, tissue damage, and cytokines themselves (Dinarello, 1998; Van Snick, 1990; Baud, 2001; Bruunsgaard, 2003). One cytokine in particular – interferon-gamma (IFN-gamma) – has been known as a chief mediator of innate, as well as adaptive immunity, and plays a central role in the process of inflamm-aging. IFN-gamma, produced by activated T cells, stimulates macrophages to produce a number of inflammatory cytokines (Schroder, 2004). The production of IFN-gamma is itself induced by other cytokines (IL-12 and IL-18) secreted by dendritic cells, macrophages and NK cells. This network of cells and cytokines can result in amplification and chronicity of the inflammatory response, such as in inflamm-aging.

Serum levels of inflammatory cytokines IL-6b (Harris, 1999; Roubenoff, 2003) and TNF-alpha (Bruunsgaard, 2003) are significantly elevated in the elderly, while the anti-inflammatory cytokine IL-10 (Saurwein-Teissl, 2000) is decreased. Furthermore, it has been shown *in vitro* that, as T cells undergo replicative senescence, the production of pro-inflammatory cytokines IFN-gamma and TNF-alpha increases (Effros, 2003a). *In vitro* studies of mononuclear cells from aged humans have shown increased IL-1b, IL-6, IFN-gamma and TNF-alpha production (Fagiolo, 1993). These inflamm-aging cytokine profiles measured *in vitro* likely reflect dysfunctional activity of senescent cells *in vivo*.

Elevated levels of these inflammatory cytokines, in particular TNF-alpha and IL-6b, have been associated with morbidity and predict mortality in the elderly (Bruunsgaard, 2003; Krabbe, 2004). Moreover, chronic inflammation is a characteristic of the pathological processes of age-related diseases, such as: atherosclerosis (Ross, 1999); osteoarthritis (Goldring, 2007); Alzheimer's (Akiyama, 2000); Parkinson's (Dobbs, 1999); osteoporosis (Pacifici, 1999); and type 2 diabetes (Paolisso, 1999). It remains controversial whether inflammatory mediators have a causal relationship, simply contribute and/or aggravate the pathologies of these age-related diseases, or are simply the consequence of age-related diseases (Franceschi, 2000b, 2007; Bruunsgaard, 2003; Krabbe, 2004).

Studies have shown evidence of inflamm-aging in aged horses that may contribute to the development of age-associated conditions similar to those found in humans. More specifically, it has been shown that old horses have significantly higher levels of inflammatory cytokines (IL-1b, IL-15, IL-18 and TNF-alpha) in peripheral whole blood, compared with younger horses (Adams, 2008). Adams and colleagues (2008) also found that old horses, in contrast to young ones, have increased inflammatory cytokine TNF-alpha and IFN-gamma production from peripheral blood mononuclear cells, and the frequency of these cells in circulation is increased. Obese old horses have even higher frequencies of lymphocytes and monocytes producing inflammatory cytokines (TNF-alpha and IFN-gamma) compared to old thin horses (Adams, 2009). Increased adiposity or obesity may contribute to the inflamm-aging process, because reduction of body weight and adiposity in these old horses significantly reduced lymphocyte and monocyte expression of TNF-alpha and IFN-gamma, and serum levels of TNF-alpha (Adams, 2009).

This age-related dysregulation of pro-inflammatory cytokine production has not only been shown to occur in the peripheral blood samples but, recently, also in the lung. The frequency of IFN-gamma producing lymphocytes in bronchoalveolar lavage fluid (BALF) cells and peripheral blood mononuclear cells (PBMCs) from old horses was found significantly increased, compared with those in young horses (Hansen, 2013). This age-associated increase of pro-inflammatory cytokine production may be a co-factor for the pathogenesis of equine airway diseases.

When old horses were subjected to an influenza challenge, they showed an exacerbated increased production of pro-inflammatory cytokines post-infection, which is consistent with the concept of inflamm-aging (Franceschi, 2000a; Adams, 2011). Moreover, it has been shown that horses with pituitary pars intermedia dysfunction have increased expression of IL-8 (McFarlane, 2008). This chronic inflammatory activity is proposed as a promoter of biological aging in general. Older horses with high levels of inflammatory activity may be at increased risk for accelerated leukocyte telomere shortening, and those with short telomeres may suffer the consequences of increased risk for diseases with an inflammatory etiology (Katepalli, 2008). Thus, it is critical to further characterize and understand the cause of inflamm-aging in old horses.

3.4 Nutrition in enhancing immunity in the old horse

Nutritional immunology is a new field of study, in which nutrition is used as a modifiable factor in impacting immune function, particularly to delay or reverse immunosenescence and to improve resistance to infections. Nutritional interventions are practical, cost-effective approaches to mitigating age-related breakdown in immune function. Natural dietary compounds found in a variety of plants, roots, fruits, vegetables, nuts and seeds are promising candidates for helping to combat the effects of an aging immune system, with a broad biological activity: anti-oxidative; anti-inflammatory; detoxification; regulation of signaling pathway; modulation of enzyme activities; and improvement of immune responses to vaccines (Pae, 2012).

Since old horses have increased levels of inflammation and long-term use of non-steroidal anti-inflammatory drugs (NSAIDs), nutritional interventions are studied to counteract the inflamm-aging process. Flavonoid and polyphenolic compounds from blueberries, red grapes, turmeric, and green or black tea were tested *in vitro* side-by-side with NSAIDs for inflammatory cytokine production from isolated leukocytes

---

Take home message

Immunosenescence is the biological aging process associated with a progressive decline in overall systemic immunity and increased prevalence of cancer, autoimmune and chronic diseases, poor responses to vaccination, and increased susceptibility to common infectious organisms. Therefore, both decreased specific immunity and chronic inflammation are part of immunosenescence.

A lifetime of exposure to various antigens with the activation of inflammatory cells and production of inflammatory mediators (cytokines) can contribute to the process of *inflamm-aging*, also known as a chronic, low-grade pro-inflammatory state. Old horses have significantly higher levels of inflammatory cytokines (IL-1b, IL-15, IL-18 and TNF-alpha) in peripheral whole blood, compared with younger horses, and obesity and endocrine disorders (pituitary pars intermedia dysfunction, PPID) exacerbate this condition.

Horses aged 20 years or over show a decline in the total lymphocyte count, lymphocyte subpopulation cell counts (CD4[+] and CD8[+] T cells and B cells). Changes in immune function of the aged horse likely contribute to reduced responsiveness to vaccination and infectious agents. Aged horses, despite pre-existing humoral immune responses, do not produce or sustain antibody production after vaccination at the same level of younger horses.

Dysfunctional T cells have been associated with increased morbidity and mortality in the elderly. The most common changes in T cell populations of the elderly are decreased frequencies of naïve T cells, expanded pools of dysfunctional memory T cells, shrinkage of the T cell repertoire, and decreased T cell proliferative responses *in vitro*. T cells are most frequently found to be responsible for defects in both humoral and cell-mediated immunity.

---

from aged horses (Siard, 2013). At varying doses, each of the compounds and NSAIDs (curcuminoids, hydroxyperostilbene, pterostilbene, quercetin, resveratrol, flunixin meglumine and phenylbutazone) significantly reduced inflammation. Interestingly, curcuminoids appear to have the potential to outperform NSAIDs (Siard, 2013).

Few studies have been conducted to better understand the effect of nutrition on modulating or improving immune responses of the aged horse. Petersson and colleagues (2010) conducted a study to examine the effect of vitamin E supplementation on immune function and response to vaccination in older horses. Vitamin E is a very effective chain-breaking, lipid-soluble antioxidant, present in the membrane of all cells and particularly enriched in immune cells. Vitamin E supplementation in the elderly has been shown to enhance immune response, which is possibly associated with increased resistance against oxidative damage and several pathogens (Pae, 2012). In the study conducted by Petersson and colleagues (2010), aged horses were supplemented daily with 15 times the Nutrient Requirements of Horses (2007) for 16 weeks, and immune responses measured throughout. The results of this study showed that Vitamin E supplementation improved the bacteria-killing ability of monocytes and neutrophils. Furthermore, humoral immune responses were enhanced, based on increased subtypes of IgG concentrations in response to vaccination, when vitamin E was supplemented.

Prebiotics and probiotics, or generally categorized as *functional foods*, are increasingly being recognized as effective, immune-modulating nutritional factors. These functional foods are thought to modulate the immune system at the mucosal surfaces throughout the gastrointestinal tract. In fact, several studies have shown that supplementation with either of these functional foods can enhance both the innate and adaptive arms of the immune system in the elderly (Pae, 2012). Studies have been conducted (Adams, 2015) involving aged horses fed commercially available senior diet, with or without a proprietary prebiotic yeast, for 86 days, and administered an influenza vaccine on day 42, followed by measurements of immune response throughout the study. Preliminary results of this study showed that old horses supplemented with the prebiotic yeast had reduced levels of inflammation and enhanced humoral immune responses after vaccination, compared with horses not receiving the supplement. More studies are warranted to identify effective and optimal conditions for various nutritional intervention regimens that can improve the immune function of the aged horse.

3.5   Conclusion

Given the growing number of older horses worldwide, we are now facing new challenges with the paradox of an old horse population with increased longevity and the potential of increased age-associated diseases. Immune responses decrease with aging, likely contributing to the increased incidence of different chronic diseases with an inflammatory component referred to as inflamm-aging. Thus, a better understanding of the mechanisms contributing to age-associated immune dysfunction may at least in part help explain the aging process and will allow us to provide optimal care of the older horse.

References

Adams, A.A., Breathnach, C.C., Katepalli, M.P., Kohler, K. and Horohov, D.W. (2008). Advanced age in horses affects divisional history of T cells and inflammatory cytokine production. *Mechanisms of Ageing and Development* **129**(11), 656–664.

Adams, A.A., Katepalli, M.P., Kohler, K., Reedy, S.E., Stilz, J.P., Vick, M.M., Fitzgerald, B.P., Lawrence, L.M. and Horohov, D.W. (2009). Effect of body condition, body weight and adiposity on inflammatory cytokine responses in old horses. *Veterinary Immunology and Immunopathology* **127**(3–4) 286–294.

Adams, A.A., Sturgill, T.L., Breathnach, C.C., Chambers, T.M., Siger, L., Minke, J.M. and Horohov, D.W. (2011). Humoral and cell-mediated immune responses of old horses following recombinant canarypox virus vaccination and subsequent challenge infection. *Veterinary Immunology and Immunopathology* **139**(2–4) 128–140.

Adams, A.A. Vineyard, K.R. Gordon, M.E. Reedy, S. Siard, M.H. and Horohov, D.W. (2015). The effect of n-3 polyunsaturated fatty acids (DHA) and prebiotic supplementation on inflammatory cytokine production and immune responses to vaccination in old horses. *Journal of Equine Veterinary Science.* Abstracts. **35** (407–408).

Akiyama, H., Barger, S., Barnum, S., Bradt, B., Bauer, J., Cole, G.M., Cooper, N.R., Eikelenboom, P., Emmerling, M., Fiebich, B.L., Finch, C.E., Frautschy, S., Griffin, W.S., Hampel, H., Hull, M., Landreth, G., Lue, L., Mrak, R., Mackenzie, I.R., McGeer, P.L., O'Banion, M.K., Pachter, J., Pasinetti, G., Plata-Salaman, C., Rogers, J., Rydel, R., Shen, Y., Streit, W., Strohmeyer, R., Tooyoma, I., Van Muiswinkel, F.L., Veerhuis, R., Walker, D., Webster, S., Wegrzyniak, B., Wenk, G. and Wyss-Coray, T. (2000). Inflammation and Alzheimer's disease. *Neurobiology of Aging* **21**(3), 383–421.

Allen, G.P. (2008). Risk factors for development of neurologic disease after experimental exposure to equine herpesvirus-1 in horses. *American Journal of Veterinary Research* **69**(12), 1595–1600.

Baud, V. and Karin, M. (2001). Signal transduction by tumor necrosis factor and its relatives. *Trends in Cell Biology* **11**(9), 372–377.

Brama, P.A., TeKoppele, J.M., Bank, R.A., van Weeren, P.R. and Barneveld, A. (1999). Influence of site and age on biochemical characteristics of the collagen network of equine articular cartilage. *American Journal of Veterinary Research* **60**(3), 341–345.

Brosnahan, M.M. and Paradis, M.R. (2003a). Assessment of clinical characteristics, management practices, and activities of geriatric horses. *Journal of the American Veterinary Medical Association* **223**(1), 99–103.

Brosnahan, M.M. and Paradis, M.R. (2003b). Demographic and clinical characteristics of geriatric horses: 467 cases (1989–1999). *Journal of the American Veterinary Medical Association* **223**(1), 93–98.

Bruunsgaard, H. and Pedersen, B.K. (2003). Age-related inflammatory cytokines and disease. *Immunology and Allergy Clinics of North America* **23**(1), 15–39.

Campbell, D.J., Rawlings, J.M., Heaton, P.R., Blount, D.G., Pritchard, D.I., Strain, J.J. and Hannigan, B.M. (2004). Insulin-like growth factor-I (IGF-I) and its association with lymphocyte homeostasis in the ageing cat. *Mechanisms of Ageing and Development* **125**(7), 497–505.

Chandler, K.J., Billson, F.M., and Mellor, D.J. (2003). Ophthalmic lesions in 83 geriatric horses and ponies. *The Veterinary Record* **153**(11), 319–322.

Cole, F.L., Hodgson, D.R., Reid, S.W. and Mellor, D.J. (2005). Owner-reported equine health disorders: results of an Australia-wide postal survey. *Australian Veterinary Journal* **83**(8), 490–495.

Colonna-Romano, G., Bulati, M., Aquino, A., Vitello, S., Lio, D., Candore, G. and Caruso, C. (2008). B cell immunosenescence in the elderly and in centenarians. *Rejuvenation Research* **11**(2), 433–439.

Deaton, C.M., Marlin, D.J., Smith, N.C., Harris, P.A., Roberts, C.A., Schroter, R.C. and Kelly, F.J. (2004). Pulmonary epithelial lining fluid and plasma ascorbic acid concentrations in horses affected by recurrent airway obstruction. *American Journal of Veterinary Research* **65**(1), 80–87.

Dinarello, C.A. (1998). Interleukin-1, interleukin-1 receptors and interleukin-1 receptor antagonist. *International Reviews of Immunology* **16**(5–6), 457–499.

Dobbs, R.J., Charlett, A., Purkiss, A.G., Dobbs, S.M., Weller, C. and Peterson, D.W. (1999). Association of circulating TNF-alpha and IL-6 with ageing and parkinsonism. *Acta Neurologica Scandinavica* **100** (1), 34–41.

Douziech, N., Seres, I., Larbi, A., Szikszay, E., Roy, P.M., Arcand, M., Dupuis, G. and Fulop, T. Jr. (2002). Modulation of human lymphocyte proliferative response with aging. *Experimental Gerontology* **37**(2–3), 369–387.

Effros, R.B. (2003b). Replicative senescence: the final stage of memory T cell differentiation? *Current HIV Research* **1**(2), 153–165.

Effros, R.B., Dagarag, M. and Valenzuela, H.F. (2003a). In vitro senescence of immune cells. *Experimental Gerontology* **38**(11–12), 1243–1249.

Fagiolo, U., Cossarizza, A., Scala, E., Fanales-Belasio, E., Ortolani, C., Cozzi, E., Monti, D., Franceschi, C. and Paganelli, R. (1993). Increased cytokine production in mononuclear cells of healthy elderly people. *European Journal of Immunology* **23**(9), 2375–2378.

Fermaglich, D.H. and Horohov, D.W. (2002). The effect of aging on immune responses. The Veterinary Clinics of North America. *Equine Practice* **18**(3), 621–630, ix.

Franceschi, C. and Campisi, J. (2014). Chronic inflammation (inflammaging) and its potential contribution to age-associated diseases. *The Journals of Gerontology. Series A Biological Sciences and Medical Sciences* 69 Suppl 1, S4–9.

Franceschi, C., Bonafe, M., Valensin, S., Olivieri, F., De Luca, M., Ottaviani, E. and De Benedictis, G. (2000a). Inflamm-aging. An evolutionary perspective on immunosenescence. *Annals of the New York Academy of Sciences* **908**, 244–254.

Franceschi, C., Bonafe, M. and Valensin, S. (2000b). Human immunosenescence: the prevailing of innate immunity, the failing of clonotypic immunity, and the filling of immunological space. *Vaccine* **18**(16), 1717–1720.

Franceschi, C., Capri, M., Monti, D., Giunta, S., Olivieri, F., Sevini, F., Panourgia, M.P., Invidia, L., Celani, L., Scurti, M., Cevenini, E., Castellani, G.C. and Salvioli, S. (2007). Inflammaging and anti-inflammaging: a systemic perspective on aging and longevity emerged from studies in humans. *Mechanisms of Ageing and Development* **128**(1), 92–105.

Globerson, A. (1995). T lymphocytes and aging. *International Archives of Allergy and Immunology* **107**(4), 491–497.

Globerson, A. and Effros, R.B. (2000). Ageing of lymphocytes and lymphocytes in the aged. *Immunology Today* **21**(10), 515–521.

Goldring, M.B. and Goldring, S.R. (2007). Osteoarthritis. *Journal of Cellular Physiology* **213**(3), 626–634.

Goodwin, J.S. (1995). Decreased immunity and increased morbidity in the elderly. *Nutrition Reviews* **53**(4 Pt 2), S41–44; discussion S44–46.

Goronzy, J.J. and Weyand, C.M. (2005). T cell development and receptor diversity during aging. *Current Opinion in Immunology* **17**(5), 468–475.

Goronzy, J.J., Fujii, H. and Weyand, C.M. (2006). Telomeres, immune aging and autoimmunity. *Experimental Gerontology* **41**(3), 246–251.

Goto, H., Yamamoto, Y., Ohta, C., Shirahata, T., Higuchi, T. and Ohishi, H. (1993). Antibody responses of Japanese horses to influenza viruses in the past few years. *The Journal of Veterinary Medical Science* **55**(1), 33–37.

Graham, B.P. (2002). Dental care in the older horse. The Veterinary Clinics of North America. *Equine Practice* **18**(3), 509–522.

Guirnalda, P.D., Malinowski, K., Roegner, V. and Horohov, D.W. (2001). Effects of age and recombinant equine somatotropin (eST) administration on immune function in female horses. *Journal of Animal Science* **79**(10), 2651–2658.

Gupta, S., Su, H., Bi, R., Agrawal, S. and Gollapudi, S. (2005). Life and death of lymphocytes: a role in immunesenescence. *Immunity & Ageing* **2**, 12.

Hansen, S., Sun, L., Baptiste, K.E., Fjeldborg, J. and Horohov, D.W. (2013). Age-related changes in intracellular expression of IFN-gamma and TNF-alpha in equine lymphocytes measured in bronchoalveolar lavage and peripheral blood. *Developmental and Comparative Immunology* **39**(3), 228–233.

Harris, T.B., Ferrucci, L., Tracy, R.P., Corti, M.C., Wacholder, S., Ettinger, W.H., Jr. Heimovitz, H., Cohen, H.J. and Wallace, R. (1999). Associations of elevated interleukin-6 and C-reactive protein levels with mortality in the elderly. *The American Journal of Medicine* **106**(5), 506–512.

HogenEsch, H., Thompson, S., Dunham, A., Ceddia, M. and Hayek, M. (2004). Effect of age on immune parameters and the immune response of dogs to vaccines: a cross-sectional study. *Veterinary Immunology and Immunopathology* **97**(1–2), 77–85.

Horohov, D.W., Dimock, A., Guirnalda, P., Folsom, R.W., McKeever, K.H. and Malinowski, K. (1999). Effect of exercise on the immune response of young and old horses. *American Journal of Veterinary Research* **60**(5), 643–647.

Horohov, D.W., Kydd, J.H. and Hannant, D. (2002). The effect of aging on T cell responses in the horse. *Developmental and Comparative Immunology* **26**(1), 121–128.

Ireland, J.L., Clegg, P.D., McGowan, C.M., McKane, S.A. and Pinchbeck, G.L. (2011a). A cross-sectional study of geriatric horses in the United Kingdom. Part 2: Health care and disease. *Equine Veterinary Journal* **43**(1), 37–44.

Ireland, J.L., Clegg, P.D., McGowan, C.M., Platt, L. and Pinchbeck, G.L. (2011b). Factors associated with mortality of geriatric horses in the United Kingdom. *Preventive Veterinary Medicine* **101**(3–4), 204–218.

Katepalli, M.P., Adams, A.A., Lear, T.L. and Horohov, D.W. (2008). The effect of age and telomere length on immune function in the horse. *Developmental and Comparative Immunology* **32**(12), 1409–1415.

Krabbe, K.S., Pedersen, M. and Bruunsgaard, H. (2004). Inflammatory mediators in the elderly. *Experimental Gerontology* **39**(5), 687–699.

Linton, P.J. and Dorshkind, K. (2004). Age-related changes in lymphocyte development and function. *Nature Immunology* **5**(2), 133–139.

Lloyd, R.S., Oliver, J.L., Faigenbaum, A.D., Myer, G.D. and De Ste Croix, M.B. (2014). Chronological Age vs. Biological Maturation: Implications for Exercise Programming in Youth. *Journal of Strength and Conditioning Research* **28**(5), 1454–1464.

Lord, J.M., Akbar, A.N. and Kipling, D. (2002). Telomere-based therapy for immunosenescence. *Trends in Immunology* **23**(4), 175–176.

Madill, S. (2002). Reproductive considerations: mare and stallion. The Veterinary Clinics of North America. *Equine Practice* **18**(3), 591–619.

McFarlane, D. (2011). Equine pituitary pars intermedia dysfunction. The Veterinary Clinics of North America. *Equine Practice* **27**(1), 93–113.

McFarlane, D. and Holbrook, T.C. (2008). Cytokine dysregulation in aged horses and horses with pituitary pars intermedia dysfunction. *Journal of Veterinary Internal Medicine* **22**(2), 436–442.

McFarlane, D., Sellon, D.C. and Gibbs, S.A. (2001). Age-related quantitative alterations in lymphocyte subsets and immunoglobulin isotypes in healthy horses. *American Journal of Veterinary Research* **62**(9), 1413–1417.

McGowan, T.W., Pinchbeck, G., Phillips, C.J., Perkins, N., Hodgson, D.R. and McGowan, C.M. (2010). A survey of aged horses in Queensland, Australia. Part 2: Clinical signs and owners' perceptions of health and welfare. *Australian Veterinary Journal* **88**(12), 465–471.

McKeever, K.H., Eaton, T.L., Geiser, S., Kearns, C.F. and Lehnhard, R.A. (2010). Age related decreases in thermoregulation and cardiovascular function in horses. *Equine Veterinary Journal Suppl* (**38**) 220–227.

Messaoudi, I., Warner, J., Fischer, M., Park, B., Hill, B., Mattison, J., Lane, M.A., Roth, G.S., Ingram, D.K., Picker, L.J., Douek, D.C., Mori, M. and Nikolich-Zugich, J. (2006). Delay of T cell senescence by caloric restriction in aged long-lived nonhuman primates. *Proceedings of the National Academy of Sciences of the United States of America* **103**(51), 19448–19453.

Miller, R.A. (1996). The aging immune system: primer and prospectus. *Science* **273**(5271), 70–74.

Miller, R.A. (2000). Effect of aging on T lymphocyte activation. *Vaccine* **18**(16), 1654–1660.

Muirhead, T.L., McClure, J.T., Wichtel, J.J., Stryhn, H., Frederick Markham, R.J., McFarlane, D. and Lunn, D.P. (2008). The effect of age on serum antibody titers after rabies and influenza vaccination in healthy horses. *Journal of Veterinary Internal Medicine* **22**(3), 654–661.

Naylor, K., Li, G., Vallejo, A.N., Lee, W.W., Koetz, K., Bryl, E., Witkowski, J., Fulbright, J., Weyand, C.M. and Goronzy, J.J. (2005). The influence of age on T cell generation and TCR diversity. *Journal of Immunology* **174**(11), 7446–7452.

O'Donovan, A., Pantell, M.S., Puterman, E., Dhabhar, F.S., Blackburn, E.H., Yaffe, K., Cawthon, R.M., Opresko, P.L., Hsueh, W.C., Satterfield, S., Newman, A.B., Ayonayon, H.N., Rubin, S.M., Harris, T.B. and Epel, E.S. (2011). Cumulative inflammatory load is associated with short leukocyte telomere length in the Health, Aging and Body Composition Study. *PLoS One* **6**(5), e19687.

Pacifici, R. (1999). Aging and cytokine production. *Calcified Tissue International* **65**(5), 345–351.

Pae, M., Meydani, S.N. and Wu, D. (2012). The role of nutrition in enhancing immunity in aging. *Aging and Disease* **3**(1), 91–129.

Paolisso, G., Tagliamonte, M.R., Rizzo, M.R. and Giugliano, D. (1999). Advancing age and insulin resistance: new facts about an ancient history. *European Journal of Clinical Investigation* **29**(9), 758–769.

Pawelec, G., Akbar, A., Caruso, C., Solana, R., Grubeck-Loebenstein, B. and Wikby, A. (2005). Human immunosenescence: is it infectious? *Immunological Reviews* **205**, 257–268.

Pawelec, G., Barnett, Y., Forsey, R., Frasca, D., Globerson, A., McLeod, J., Caruso, C., Franceschi, C., Fulop, T., Gupta, S., Mariani, E., Mocchegiani, E. and Solana, R. (2002). T cells and aging, January 2002 update. *Frontiers in Bioscience* **7**, d1056–1183.

Perryman, L.E., Wyatt, C.R., Magnuson, N.S. and Mason, P.H. (1988). T lymphocyte development and maturation in horses. *Animal Genetics* **19**(4), 343–348.

Petersson, K.H., Burr, D.B., Gomez-Chiarri, M. and Petersson-Wolfe, C.S. (2010). The influence of vitamin E on immune function and response to vaccination in older horses. *Journal of Animal Science* **88**(9), 2950–2958.

Plackett, T.P., Boehmer, E.D., Faunce, D.E. and Kovacs, E.J. (2004). Aging and innate immune cells. *Journal of Leukocyte Biology* **76**(2), 291–299.

Ross, R. (1999). Atherosclerosis is an inflammatory disease. *American Heart Journal* **138**(5 Pt 2) S419–420.

Roubenoff, R. (2003). Catabolism of aging: is it an inflammatory process? *Current Opinion in Clinical Nutrition and Metabolic Care* **6**(3), 295–299.

Saurwein-Teissl, M., Blasko, I., Zisterer, K., Neuman B., Lang, B. and Grubeck-Loebenstein, B. (2000). An imbalance between pro- and anti-inflammatory cytokines, a characteristic feature of old age. *Cytokine* **12**(7), 1160–1161.

Schroder, K., Hertzog, P.J., Ravasi, T. and Hume, D.A. (2004). Interferon-gamma: an overview of signals, mechanisms and functions. *Journal of Leukocyte Biology* **75**(2), 163–189.

Siard, M. H., McMurry, K. E., Horohov, D. W., & Adams, A. A. (2013). Effects of polyphenolic bioactive compounds (pterostilbene, resveratrol, curcuminoids, quercetin, and hydroxypterostilbene) on pro-inflammatory cytokine production in vitro. *Journal of Equine Veterinary Science*. Abstracts. **33**(321–399). pg. 343.

Suberville, S., Bellocq, A., Peguillet, I., Lantz, O., Stordeur, P., Fouqueray, B. and Baud, L. (2001). Transforming growth factor-beta inhibits interleukin-10 synthesis by human monocytic cells. *European Cytokine Network* **12**(1), 141–146.

USDA. 2006. Equine 2005, Part I: Baseline Reference of Equine Health and Management, 2005 USDA:APHIS:VS, CEAH. Fort Collins, CO #N451-1006.

Van Snick, J. (1990). Interleukin-6: an overview. *Annual Review of Immunology* **8**, 253–278.

Vasto, S., Candore, G., Balistreri, C.R., Caruso, M., Colonna-Romano, G., Grimaldi, M.P., Listi, F., Nuzzo, D., Lio, D. and Caruso, C. (2007). Inflammatory networks in ageing, age-related diseases and longevity. *Mechanisms of Ageing and Development* **128**(1), 83–91.

Walford, R.L. (1969). *The Immunologic Theory of Aging*. København: Munksgaard.

Weng, Z. and DeLisi, C. (1998). Toward a predictive understanding of molecular recognition. *Immunological Reviews* **163**, 251–266.

4 Anaphylaxis

Rolfe M. Radcliffe

4.1 Definition

Hypersensitivity responses arise from the adaptive immune system, and they may yield both protective and pathologic outcomes (Gershwin, 1978; Wells, 1981; Day, 2011). Prior antigen exposure is required to stimulate specific IgE synthesis and, upon subsequent antigen exposure, the release of inflammatory and vasoactive mediators leads to local and systemic effects (Lunn, 2004; Tizzard, 2013).

Type I hypersensitivity reactions are mediated by antigen-specific IgE on the surface of mast cells, basophils and eosinophils, in response to certain insect bites/stings, drugs or vaccines, and food (Swiderski, 1995; Lunn, 2004; Tizzard, 2013). They are considered immediate reactions, because they arise within seconds or minutes after antigen exposure and binding to IgE. When such immediate hypersensitivity reactions are systemic and life-threatening, they are known as allergic anaphylaxis or anaphylactic shock (Sampson, 2006; Day, 2011). *Anaphylactoid* events are clinically similar reactions, because they involve mast cell degranulation; they are not IgE-mediated, but are triggered by other immune mechanisms (Lieberman, 2006). The traditional Gell and Coombs classification of hypersensitivity reactions has been slightly modified over the years (Gell, 1963; Descotes, 2001; Rajan, 2003; Uzzaman, 2012).

4.2 Signalment and clinical signs

Mild, moderate or severe clinical signs of allergic reaction may occur, depending upon: the dose and route of antigen challenge; the type, quantity and site of mediator release; the activation process of the antigen; the organ system involvement; and the individual inflammatory response of the patient (Eyre, 1973; Swiderski, 1995; Lunn, 2004; Tizzard, 2013).

The more rapid the onset of clinical signs, the more likely a severe anaphylactic event is impending. Urticaria and rhinitis usually occur in mild cases, while angioedema, diarrhea and abdominal pain characterize moderate disease, and respiratory distress, hypotension, and collapse present with severe reactions. The quantity and persistence of antigen exposure will influence the clinical signs. In addition, those drugs that require metabolic processing may delay the onset of clinical signs. The route of antigen exposure will also affect the subsequent type of reaction: inhalation is often associated with upper respiratory tract inflammation, bronchoconstriction and conjunctivitis; topical exposure with urticaria, erythema, pain, and pruritis; and exposure via the parenteral and oral routes with various systemic signs (Swiderski, 1995).

Most type I hypersensitivity reactions provoke local allergic responses within the tissues where antigen contact occurs (Day, 2011). Examples of such diseases include atopic dermatitis and insect bite hypersensitivity affecting the skin, food allergies of the intestinal system, and allergic rhinitis of the respiratory tract. In some cases, systemic reactions follow activation and degranulation of circulating basophils or widespread tissue mast cells, with life-threatening anaphylaxis. Primary systemic anaphylaxis in horses includes hypersensitivity to various drugs, vaccines, and blood products, and severe intestinal anaphylaxis (Wilson, 1992; Jones, 2004; Divers, 2008a).

The shock organs of the horse are considered the respiratory tract and intestine. Therefore, many of the clinical signs of systemic anaphylaxis relate to these organs, including tachypnea, coughing, pulmonary emphysema, dyspnea or respiratory distress; sweating; colic; and diarrhea (Swiderski, 1995; Day, 2011; Tizzard, 2013). Other consequences in severe cases include subcutaneous edema, laminitis, purpura hemorrhagica, hemolytic anemia, and hemorrhagic enterocolitis (Eyre, 1973; Hanna, 1982; Swiderski, 1995; Jones, 2004; Tizzard, 2013).

The most concerning signs of systemic anaphylactic reactions are *dyspnea* and *hypotension*, because they represent asphyxia (secondary to increased bronchial smooth muscle tone, increased mucosal secretion, laryngeal edema, pulmonary edema) and vasculogenic shock (secondary to vasodilation, increased vascular permeability, reduced venous return, cardiac arrhythmias, myocardial ischemia) (Swiderski, 1995). Hypotension may vary from mild cardiovascular changes to severe shock states, depending upon the degree of mediator-induced vasodilation and altered capillary permeability, reduced venous return, cardiac arrhythmias, and myocardial ischemia. Pale mucous membranes, poor peripheral pulses, and cold extremities are common clinical signs associated with cardiovascular collapse.

Equine Clinical Immunology, First Edition. Edited by M. Julia B. Felippe.
© 2016 John Wiley & Sons, Inc. Published 2016 by John Wiley & Sons, Inc.

The prevalence of anaphylactic reactions is unknown in horses. Blood transfusion reactions were reported in seven out of 44 (16%) procedures in adult horses in one study (Hurcombe, 2007), varying from local urticaria to anaphylactic shock. Allergic drug reactions are reported in approximately 6–10% of adverse drug reactions in animals, with penicillin the most common medication implicated (Davis, 1984; Dowling, 2004). In human patients, the prevalence of anaphylactic reactions is estimated at 1.6% (Wood, 2013).

Biphasic or multiphasic anaphylactic episodes, characterized by recurrence of symptoms following an acute episode of anaphylaxis, are possible, usually within eight hours after resolution of the primary event (Lieberman, 2006). Protracted anaphylaxis, with unremitting symptoms that persist for several days despite treatment, is also possible (Simons, 2013).

4.3 Immunologic mechanisms and etiologic associations

Anaphylactic events are acute, generalized reactions, mediated via IgE and antigen binding, and secondary release of mast cell and basophil mediators (Lieberman, 2006). All hypersensitivity reactions consist of two phases: antigen sensitization and subsequent re-exposure, leading to mast cell degranulation (Day, 2011; Tizzard, 2013).

4.3.1 Phase 1: antigen sensitization
Many of the antigens involved in type 1 hypersensitivity reactions are presented to the body at the mucosal and cutaneous surfaces, and use similar principles of sensitization (Day, 2011). Assume that a horse ingests a novel antigen that reaches the intestines. In the gut-associated lymphoid tissues, antigen presenting cells (i.e., dendritic cells) detect, process and present the novel antigen to T helper lymphocytes that, subsequently, activate antigen-specific B cells for clonal proliferation (Figure 4.1). Secretion of high levels of antigen-specific IgE follows, and these bind to specialized receptors on circulating basophils and tissue mast cells. Many of these IgE-coated mast cells will be located beneath the epithelial surface, where the antigen originally presented. The horse is now sensitized.

4.3.2 Phase 2: hypersensitivity response
When this sensitized horse re-encounters the same antigen, a hypersensitivity response may develop. Upon penetration of the

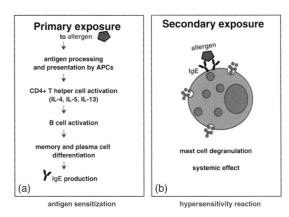

Figure 4.1 Type I hypersensitivity (anaphylactic) reaction.
(a) First exposure: antigen sensitization. Antigen presenting cells (APCs) translate a message of foreign invasion by delivering antigen or allergen (Ag) to regional lymphoid tissues, where T lymphocyte helper 2 (Th2) cells induce B cell differentiation and production of IgE. Antigen-specific IgE subsequently bind to the epsilon receptor on circulating basophils and tissue mast cells, and the horse is now considered *sensitized*.
(b) Second exposure: hypersensitivity response. When the horse reencounters the same antigen or allergen (Ag), a hypersensitivity response develops. The basophils or mast cells already have IgE bound to their epsilon receptors; upon cross-linking of two antibodies with the antigen, the basophil or mast cell is activated and releases granules with inflammatory and vasoactive mediators.

mucosal or skin barrier, the antigen-specific IgE that coats mast cells bind to the antigen, and cross-linking of two of these IgE initiates activation of mast cells, which are abundant in these tissues (Day, 2011; Tizzard, 2013; Figures 4.1 and 4.2). Activated mast cells release a great variety of inflammatory and vasoactive mediators to remove antigens but, in some individuals, they trigger an immediate allergic reaction (Lunn, 2004).

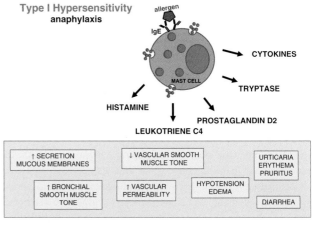

Figure 4.2 Hypersensitivity reaction.
Upon cross-linking of two IgE with the antigen, activation of a basophil or mast cell promotes the release of a variety of inflammatory and vasoactive mediators, creating the classic physiologic changes and clinical signs of hypersensitivity.

A large variety of chemical mediators are involved in anaphylactic reactions and, through their combined effects, they are responsible for increasing vascular permeability, constricting smooth muscle, dilating blood vessels, attracting leukocytes, altering platelet function, and activating the coagulation and complement pathways, among other actions (Hanna, 1982; Swiderski, 1995). Because of this diversity of mediator release during anaphylaxis, it is not surprising that those medications directed at one mediator have limited efficacy. Although mast cells and basophils largely initiate the reaction, macrophages, eosinophils, neutrophils and platelets expand and sustain the inflammatory cascade.

Histamine is the classic mediator described in anaphylaxis. In addition, many other chemical mediators, including tryptase, leucotrienes, prostaglandins, neutral proteases, proteoglycans and chemokines, are involved (Swiderski, 1995; Lieberman, 2006; Simons, 2013). Histamine and serotonin are thought to be the primary mediators of anaphylactic reactions in horses (Tizzard, 2013). Acting via both H_1 and H_2 receptors, histamine causes vasodilation and increased vascular permeability, ultimately leading to systemic hypotension. Histamine acts directly on the heart to increase chronotropy and intropy, thereby expanding cardiac oxygen demand. At the same time, it induces contraction of the respiratory bronchial and gastrointestinal smooth muscles.

Other inflammatory mediators released by mast cells include: neutral proteases and proteases that cause tissue destruction; cytokines such as IL-4, IL-5, IL-13, and tumor-necrosis factor-alpha; proteoglycans; and products of arachidonic acid metabolism (Lunn, 2004; Lieberman, 2006). Nitrous oxide has also been implicated in anaphylactic reactions, and likely contributes toward development of shock via promoting systemic vasodilation and vascular permeability (Lieberman, 2006).

In addition to IgE-mediated activation, other *immune* mechanisms of anaphylaxis not classified under hypersensitivity type 1 have been reported, and these are referred to as *anaphylactoid* reactions (Simons, 2013). Despite dissimilar triggering mechanisms, the clinical signs and outcomes are the same for anaphylaxis and anaphylactoid reactions, because both conditions elicit degranulation and release of anaphylatoxins by mast cells or basophils. Examples of anaphylactoid reactions include: complement system activation, usually following the use of various drugs and blood products; IgG-mediated allergic reactions associated with specific drugs and high molecular weight dextran therapy; and abnormalities of arachidonic acid metabolism associated with aspirin or other non-steroidal anti-inflammatory drug therapy (Lieberman, 2006; Tizzard, 2013).

Whole blood and blood products (e.g., plasma), antibiotics (e.g., penicillin, cephalosporins, sulfonamides, quinolones, vancomycin), anthelmintics, vitamins and minerals (vitamins B and K, selenium, iron, copper), muscle relaxants, general and inhalant anesthetics, or inadvertent injection of other products (e.g., milk) have all been implicated in triggering reactions in horses, many via complement system activation, which does not require

previous antigen exposure and host sensitization with production of IgE (Wilson, 1992; Swiderski, 1995; Divers, 2008a; Alcott, 2010). Vaccine-induced hypersensitivity reactions, including anaphylactic shock, may be related to IgE responses to non-target antigens (e.g., adjuvants) (Gershwin, 2012).

Non-immunologic and non-allergic mechanisms may directly induce mast and basophil cell degranulation into surrounding tissues (Lieberman, 2006; Simons, 2013). Various drugs (e.g., opioids and radiocontrast agents), physical sources (e.g., temperature extremes, sunlight and exercise), electrical and osmotic disturbances may incite direct mediator release (Swiderski, 1995). When the trigger of an anaphylactic event cannot be identified, the condition is termed *idiopathic anaphylaxis* (Simons, 2013).

4.4 Diagnostics

The diagnosis of anaphylaxis is largely based upon the history and clinical presentation of the disease, and laboratory tests are available to confirm diagnosis (Lieberman, 2005; Vadas, 2013; Vitte, 2013; Simons, 2006, 2013).

Anaphylaxis is an immediate allergic reaction having the risk of death (Greenberger, 2012). A *rule of twos* states that reactions begin from two minutes to two hours following injection, infusion, ingestion, contact or inhalation. The sudden onset of respiratory distress, hypotension, rapid development of urticaria and collapse are considered the cardinal signs of systemic anaphylaxis.

Often, more than one body system is affected, including the cutaneous, respiratory, gastrointestinal, cardiovascular or central nervous systems. In humans, 80–90% of patients report signs referable to the skin, followed by the respiratory tract (60%), cardiovascular, gastrointestinal, and central nervous systems, occurring in approximately 35%, 30% and 15% of patients, respectively (Lieberman, 2006; Simons, 2013). Cutaneous signs may be absent with the presence of shock or severe respiratory obstruction (Lieberman, 2005).

The medical history should explore exposure to antigens and agents prior to, and a review of the sequence of events leading up to the reaction. Questions should be asked about the following:
1 Medications (drugs, vaccines, blood products).
2 Diet and recent changes in diet, including pasture.
3 Evidence of insect biting with cutaneous signs (e.g., urticaria, pruritus, and angioedema).

In human medicine, specific clinical criteria have been established to provide emergency health personnel with a simple, rapid method for making a diagnosis of anaphylaxis (Sampson, 2006). According to these recommendations, anaphylaxis is highly likely when any one of the following three criteria are fulfilled:
1 Acute onset of illness with involvement of the skin and/or mucosa, together with either respiratory distress or reduced blood pressure (or symptoms of end-organ dysfunction);
2 Two or more of the following problems occurring rapidly after exposure to a *likely* allergen: skin/mucosal tissue involvement,

respiratory compromise, reduced blood pressure (or associated signs), or persistent gastrointestinal symptoms.

3 Reduced blood pressure after exposure to a *known* allergen.

Laboratory tests may also be useful to confirm a diagnosis of anaphylaxis (Vadas, 2013; Vitte, 2013), although treatment should not be delayed when anaphylaxis is suspected (Simons, 2013). *Serum tryptase levels* are considered the gold standard testing for anaphylaxis in humans (Vitte, 2013), and are preferred to plasma histamine testing because tryptase remains elevated longer than histamine – approximately six hours and one hour, respectively (Lieberman, 2006). However, tryptase concentrations were not elevated in 36% of acute anaphylaxis events, and inconsistently increased during food-induced anaphylactic episodes in humans (Sala-Cunill, 2013; Vitte, 2013). In addition, *platelet-activating factor*, an immerging biomarker of interest in human anaphylaxis, may correlate better with disease severity than either tryptase or histamine (Vadas, 2013).

4.5 Treatment

Several different classes of medications (including physiological antagonists, selective inhibitors, and broad-spectrum anti-inflammatory drugs) have applications for the treatment of hypersensitivity reactions in horses, depending upon the clinical presentation (Eyre, 1976, 1982).

Not all anaphylactic reactions require emergency treatment. Mild forms of anaphylaxis, for example, restricted to urticaria and/or small increases in respiratory rate, may be monitored or treated with antihistamines (Divers, 2008a). Glucocorticoid therapy may be indicated in pruritic conditions such as insect hypersensitivity; these reactions are best managed with a combination of insect control and corticosteroids.

4.5.1 Emergency treatment

In severe cases, though, early recognition of clinical signs and immediate emergency steps are critical for patient survival (Lunn, 2004). Clinicians must recognize that anaphylaxis is rapidly progressive, and that symptoms may become life-threatening quickly unless early emergency treatments are initiated (Lieberman, 2005). Therefore, upon diagnosis or suspicion of an anaphylactic event, the following immediate steps are warranted:

1 Stop exposure to the trigger if possible (i.e., discontinue intravenous administration of the therapeutic drug or agent).

2 Rapid assessment of the patient status:
   (a) airway, breathing, circulation, level of consciousness;
   (b) secure airway and check vital parameters (heart and respiratory rates, blood pressure);
   (c) perform tracheotomy for respiratory distress (Schaer, 2008);

3 Administer epinephrine (Divers, 2008a; Gaughan, 2008).

4 Administer oxygen (Schaer, 2008).

5 Administer intravenous crystalloid and/or colloid fluids (Divers, 2008b).

4.5.1.1 Epinephrine

Epinephrine is the foundation of therapy for anaphylaxis, and it should be administered immediately upon recognition of symptoms, even when there is doubt, and simultaneously during patient assessment (Lieberman, 2005). In fact, delay in epinephrine therapy has been related to increased likelihood of biphasic and protracted anaphylaxis and mortality in humans (Simons, 2013). The great benefits provided by epinephrine therapy are bronchodilation and increased cardiac output, based on its inotropic, chronotropic, and peripheral vasoconstriction effects. Consequently, epinephrine alleviates life-threatening airway obstruction, hypotension and shock (Simons, 2013).

The intramuscular (IM) route of epinephrine injection is preferred in human patients for treatment of anaphylaxis and may be repeated every 5–15 minutes for a total of 3–5 doses when needed (Lieberman, 2005, 2006). The IM method has a considerably wider margin of safety in humans in comparison to intravenous (IV) administration and, in addition, more rapid absorption occurs following IM, compared with subcutaneous (SC) injections (Sampson, 2006; Simons, 2013).

For patients lacking improvement following IM injection, or in shock and exhibiting cardiovascular collapse, IV injection should be considered (Lieberman, 2006; Sampson, 2006). In humans, epinephrine is often diluted in various IV preparations that can be titrated to effect, and the safest and most effective strategy may be continuous low-dose epinephrine infusion (Sampson, 2006). Anxiety, pallor, palpitations and tremors may occur following IV dosing in humans, but are uncommon with IM injection. In addition, serious side effects of epinephrine administration in humans may include potentially lethal tachyarrythmias, myocardial ischemia, hypertension and/or pulmonary edema, particularly when it is not diluted appropriately for intravenous use (Simons, 2013). Cardiac monitoring, via auscultation and electrocardiogram (ECG), is indicated when possible, as many of the medications selected for hypersensitivity therapy (including epinephrine) potentiate arrhythmias (Swiderski, 1995).

The dosage of epinephrine (1: 1000 dilution) recommended for anaphylaxis or cardiopulmonary resuscitation in foals is 0.01 to 0.02 mg/kg (0.5 to 1 ml/50 kg foal), given slowly intravenously (Palmer, 2007). A high dose regimen (0.1 mg/kg) has also been reported for resuscitation, but secondary side effects are likely to decrease survival. In the adult horse, the dose of epinephrine in severe anaphylaxis is 0.01 mg/kg given slowly intravenously (3–6 mls/450 kg horse), although twice this dose may be given IM (approximately 10 mls/450 kg horse) when dyspnea or hypotension are mild, and higher doses via the intratracheal route (20 mls/450 kg horse), when IV access is not possible (Swiderski, 1995; Divers, 2008a; Gaughan, 2008).

Sublingual injection of epinephrine has also been reported as an alternative to IV, and inhaled epinephrine may be performed for cases manifesting laryngeal edema (Lieberman, 2005). Epinephrine may also be given via the intracardiac route during collapse and unresponsiveness. Intravenous administration of

<table>
<tr><td>

Take home message

Upon diagnosis or suspicion of an anaphylactic event:
1 Stop exposure to the triggering agent (drugs, fluids, surface contact);
2 At any point, if clinical signs are concerning, administer epinephrine
   1: 1000 dilution I.M. or I.V slowly at 0.01 to 0.02 mg/kg every 5 to
   15 min.
   o *Foal*: 0.5 to 1 ml/50 kg foal.
   o *Adult horse*: 5 to 10 ml/450 kg horse.
3 Rapidly assess patient:
   o Airway patency, difficulty/noisy breathing, pulse, level of
     consciousness.
   o Secure airway (tracheotomy if needed) and check vital
     parameters (heart and respiratory rates, blood pressure).
4 Administer oxygen
5 Administer bolus fluid therapy
6 Consider nebulization with beta-2 agonists
7 Consider anti-histamine treatment
8 Consider glucocorticosteroid to prevent biphasic reactions

</td></tr>
</table>

the 1: 1000 dilution of epinephrine has been performed safely in horses into large vessels such as the jugular vein, although it may be prudent to dilute the drug for injection into smaller vessels to lessen local vasoconstriction (T. Divers, personal communication, 2013).

4.5.1.2 Oxygen

High-flow supplemental oxygen therapy is indicated during systemic anaphylaxis in order to help improve tissue oxygenation. After epinephrine, oxygen is considered one of the most important treatments in anaphylaxis management (Lieberman, 2005). The recommended flow rate is approximately 5–10 L/min for foals, and 10–15 L/min for adult horses, directly into the nasal passage. The use of two intranasal lines compared with one increases the fraction of inspired oxygen (FiO_2) from approximately 30% to 40% (Schaer, 2008).

Intratracheal oxygen administration may also be considered, and will provide a higher FiO_2 compared with intranasal placement, although remaining below 50%. However, coughing is common when providing oxygen via the tracheal route, and it may be difficult for long periods of time. Oxygen should be delivered through sterile saline for humidification purposes, to prevent airway desiccation. Development of a respiratory acidosis secondary to reduced ventilation, and increased partial pressure carbon dioxide ($PaCO_2$), may develop with prolonged oxygen administration. Oxygen toxicity is unlikely to occur at an $FiO_2 < 60\%$ and, therefore, is not a concern during extended supplemental oxygen therapy.

4.5.1.3 Fluid therapy

Horses that remain hypotensive following epinephrine treatment should receive fluid therapy (Divers, 2008b). Crystalloid and colloid fluids are both useful in helping to restore intravascular fluid volume, cardiac output and aerobic metabolism. Careful dosage and monitoring are critical to evaluate for worsening of tissue edema that accompanies anaphylaxis, particularly of upper airways, lungs and neural tissues.

A crystalloid fluid challenge can be started for foals at 50–80 ml/kg (2.5–4 L/50 kg foal) divided into separate bolus doses, and for adult horses at 10–20 ml/kg/hr (5–10 L/450 kg horse). Reassessment of the patient's volume status is important before additional boluses are administered. The goal is to recover normal central venous pressure (CVP, 7–12 cm H_2O in adult horses) or mean arterial blood pressure (MAP > 60–70 mm Hg), and to ensure vital organ perfusion. A large IV catheter diameter (10 or 12 gauge for an adult horse) allows more rapid provision of fluids during shock (Reddick, 2011).

Hypertonic (7.2%) saline solution (HSS) is also an excellent choice for fluid therapy in adult horses exhibiting shock at 2–4 ml/kg (1–2 L/450 kg horse), simultaneously with crystalloid fluids. As a general rule, approximately 10 L of crystalloid fluids should be provided overtime for each liter of HSS, in order to help restore the fluid shift from the interstitial and intracellular fluid compartments into the intravascular space. Because of concerns of hypernatremia, hypertonic saline should be administered cautiously to foals (Divers, 2008b).

Colloid fluids, combined with crystalloid fluids, can be used to restore and maintain intravascular fluid volume. However, because of complications of acute renal failure, coagulopathies, and increased mortality (during severe sepsis and other critical conditions), they are currently being questioned in the human medical field (Reinhart, 2012). In horses, these complications have not been noted, and hydroxyethyl starch is still used at 2–10 ml/kg/day (1–5 L/450 kg adult horse). The administration of equine plasma, human albumin and dextrans are likely contraindicated during management of anaphylaxis in horses, because of concerns about inducing subsequent anaphylactic events with these products.

4.5.2 Additional treatments

In systemic anaphylactic reactions, after performing the emergency treatments, additional therapy may be considered in patient management. Alternatively, with localized reactions, some of the medications described below may be all that is required for therapy. Vasopressors, bronchodilators, furosemide, antihistamines and corticosteroids may provide important advantages during treatment for anaphylaxis, depending on the clinical problem.

4.5.2.1 Vasopressors

Vasopressors should be considered for horses with persistent hypotension refractory to epinephrine and volume replacement (Divers, 2008b). Dobutamine, dopamine, norepinephrine and vasopressin are all considered valuable drugs for maintaining blood pressure in horses, and should be titrated to maintain a mean arterial blood pressure greater than 60–70 mm Hg. Cardiac monitoring via ECG is recommended, as arrhythmias may develop with these medications.

Dobutamine solution (50 mg diluted in 500 mls of 5% dextrose solution; 100 µg/ml) may be administered at a dose of 5–10 µg/kg/min over 10–20 minutes for an adult horse. Dopamine may be titrated as a continuous infusion at a dose of 1–20 µg/kg/min, depending on the desired clinical effect. At lower doses (3–7 µg/kg/min), dopamine increases glomerular filtration rate and renal blood flow. A positive inotropic effect occurs on the myocardium from 5–10 µg/kg/min, while vasoconstriction predominates above 10 µg/kg/min.

Norepinephrine (0.1–1.5 µg/kg/min), through potent vasoconstrictor effects, increases peripheral vascular resistance and MAP.

Vasopressin may be useful for shock non-responsive to other vasopressor medications, because it produces peripheral vasoconstriction via a different receptor mechanism (Hiruta, 2005). Vasopressin may be administered to adult horses and foals as a continuous infusion for refractory hypotension (0.01–0.04 µg/kg/min), or as a single dose for cardiovascular collapse (0.3–0.6 µg/kg).

4.5.2.2 Bronchodilators

With patients exhibiting bronchospasm resistant to repeated doses of epinephrine, inhalatory therapy with a β_2-agonist (e.g., albuterol) should be considered. Albuterol may be provided every 3–4 hours via an inhaler (720 µg for an adult horse, or eight puffs at 90 µg/puff), or nebulization of a 0.5% solution (approximately 2–5 mls diluted in sterile saline). For horses presenting with severe respiratory distress (i.e., severe laryngeal edema), nasotracheal intubation or placement of a tracheotomy may be necessary to secure the airway prior to epinephrine treatment (Gaughan, 2008; Schaer, 2008).

4.5.2.3 Furosemide

In patients with pulmonary edema due to anaphylaxis, treatment with furosemide (1 mg/kg IV) is indicated, and repeated doses can be used to induce adequate diuresis.

4.5.2.4 Antihistamines

Antihistamines are useful to help control the hypersensitivity clinical signs – especially urticarial and pruritus – and, in humans, a combination of both H_1 and H_2 antagonists are considered more effective for tempering such cutaneous manifestations, compared to an H_1 antagonist alone (Lieberman, 2006; Sampson, 2006). Slow intravenous administration of antihistamines is recommended to avoid the adverse effects of excitement and hypotension. If the cardiovascular status of the horse is stable, doxylamine succinate (0.5 mg/kg slowly IV or IM), pyrilamine maleate (1.0 mg/kg slowly IV, IM or SQ), tripelennamine hydrochloride (1 mg/kg IM; not IV), or hydroxyzine hydrochloride (1–1.5 mg/kg PO) may be administered every 6–12 hours for the relief of clinical signs (Gaughan, 2008). Antihistamines enhance the effects of epinephrine on vascular resistance and, therefore, should be used separately.

4.5.2.5 Glucocorticoids

Systemic corticosteroids, although not useful in the acute response, are indicated to halt progressive inflammation (Swiderski, 1995; Lunn, 2004). Corticosteroids may also prevent recurrence of anaphylaxis, and late-phase or protracted reactions (Sampson, 2006).

Dexamethasone (0.2 to 0.5 mg/kg IV) has been reported for the treatment of rapidly progressing edema (Gaughan, 2008).

Prednisolone sodium succinate (0.25 to 10 mg/kg IV), a rapid-acting corticosteroid, is preferred for systemic reactions, while prednisolone (0.4 to 1.6 mg/kg PO SID) may be useful for managing persistent urticaria.

4.6 Prevention

Several preventative measures may be considered for horses that have a history of anaphylaxis. Importantly, a complete and thorough history is helpful in order to understand the event and establish a diagnosis.

Avoidance of specific food allergens is generally effective in preventing food-triggered anaphylaxis. Similarly, avoidance of relevant stinging insects, using body nets or blankets, insect repellents and overnight barn housing, is effective for animals with a history of insect bite hypersensitivity. Other preventative measures include skin or allergen-specific IgE testing to help investigate sensitivity to various agents, and provocative challenge or desensitization procedures.

For animals with a suspected drug reaction, future therapy should be directed using medications that do not share immunologic or biochemical similarity (Lieberman, 2006). Because parenteral compared to oral administration typically produces a more severe reaction, oral treatment is preferred whenever possible.

When administering an agent of unknown sensitivity to a horse with a history of anaphylaxis, it may be prudent to monitor the animal for a period of 20–30 minutes following injection. Such action will enable early and effective treatment in the event of a serious anaphylactic reaction. In horses requiring treatment with medications associated with previous reactions, pretreatment with flunixin meglumine and antihistamines or corticosteroids and antihistamines may be warranted (Lieberman, 2006; Divers, personal communication, 2013).

Hypersensitivity reactions associated with transfusion of blood products may be minimized through cross-match testing, even though reactions may still occur despite donor and recipient compatibility (Hurcombe, 2007).

Several types of adverse reactions to procaine penicillin G have been recognized, including anaphylaxis, penicillin toxicity, acute pulmonary embolism, and procaine toxicity (Nielsen, 1988; Dowling, 2004). These authors suggest that procaine toxicity may be the most likely cause in their case series, and suggest that clinicians avoid repeated injection sites, administer the drug slowly, and provide proper storage of procaine penicillin G in order to help reduce such adverse reactions in horses.

4.7 Prognosis and clinical outcomes

The prognosis for horses suffering an anaphylactic or anaphylactoid reaction will depend on the type and severity of the event, the speed of disease onset and recognition, the response to treatment, and developing complications. Local reactions are usually not life-threatening, and the prognosis will largely reflect response to treatment. However, systemic reactions, particularly those characterized by cardiovascular collapse or respiratory distress, carry a considerable risk of death (Swiderski, 1995). When the recognition of a systemic reaction or subsequent emergency treatment is delayed, the risk of death increases.

Risk factors reported in humans for anaphylactic reactions include atopy, sex, age, route, constancy of drug administration, time since previous reaction, economic status, and season of the year (Kemp, 1995; Lieberman, 2006). Adverse drug reactions in humans have been associated with females, specific lymphocyte antigen types, and individuals with other allergies or severe illness (Swiderski, 1995). In addition, genetic alterations in basophil and mast cell function, increased IgE synthesis, and hyper-responsive target organs may all play a role in the likelihood of developing anaphylactic reactions in people, although the importance of these mechanisms is not known in the horse.

References

Alcott, C.J. and Wong, D.M. (2010). Anaphylaxis and systemic inflammatory response syndrome induced by inadvertent intravenous administration of mare's milk in a neonatal foal. *Journal Veterinary Emergency Critical Care* **20**(6), 616–622.

Davis, L.E. (1984). Hypersensitivity reactions induced by antimicrobial drugs. *Journal of American Veterinary Medical Association* **185**(10), 1131–1136.

Day M.J. and Schultz, R.D. (2011). Hypersensitivity mechanisms. In: *Veterinary Immunology: Principles and Practice*, pp. 120–130. London, Manson Publishing Ltd.

Descotes, J., and Choquet-Kastylevsky, G. (2001). Gell and Coombs' classification: is it still valid? *Toxicology* **158**(1), 43–49.

Divers, T.J. (2008a). Adverse drug reactions. In: Orsini. J.A. and Divers, T.J. (eds). *Equine Emergencies: Treatment and Procedures*, 3rd edition, pp. 781–785. St. Louis, Elsevier, Inc.

Divers, T.J. (2008b). Shock and systemic inflammatory response syndrome. In: Orsini. J.A. and Divers, T.J. (eds). *Equine Emergencies: Treatment and Procedures*, 3rd edition, pp. 544–552. St. Louis, Elsevier, Inc.

Dowling, P.M. (2004). Antimicrobial therapy. In: Reed, S.M., Bayly, W.M. and Sellon, D.C. (eds). *Equine Internal Medicine*, 2nd edition, pp. 186–220. St. Louis, Elsevier, Inc.

Eyre, P. and Lewis, A.J. (1973). Acute systemic anaphylaxis in the horse. *British Journal of Pharmacology* **48**(3), 426–437.

Eyre, P. (1976). Preliminary studies of pharmacological antagonism of anaphylaxis in the horse. *Canadian Journal of Comparative Medicine* **40**(2), 149–152.

Eyre, P., Hanna, C.J., Wells, P.W. and McBeath, D.G. (1982). Equine immunology 3: immunopharmacology – anti-inflammatory and antihypersensitivity drugs. *Equine Veterinary Journal* **14**(4), 277–281.

Gaughan, E.M., Hanson, R.R. and Divers, T.J. (2008). Integumentary system: burns and acute swellings. In: Orsini. J.A. and Divers, T.J. (eds). *Equine Emergencies: Treatment and Procedures*, 3rd edition, pp. 219–236. St. Louis, Elsevier, Inc.

Gell, P.G.H., and Coombs, R.R.A. (eds, 1963). *Clinical Aspects of Immunology*, 1st edition. Oxford, England, Blackwell.

Gershwin, L.J. (1978). The phylogenetic development of anaphylactic activity and homocytotropic antibodies. *Developmental and Comparative Immunology* **2**(4), 595–615.

Gershwin, L.J., Netherwood, K.A., Norris, M.S., Behrens, N.E. and Shao, M.X. (2012). Equine IgE responses to non-viral vaccine components. *Vaccine* **30**(52), 7615–7620.

Greenberger, P.A. and Ditto, A.M. (2012). Anaphylaxis. *Allergy and Asthma Proceedings* **33**(Suppl 1), S80–S83.

Hanna, C.J., Eyre, P., Wells, P.W. and McBeath, D.G. (1982). Equine immunology 2: immunopharmacology – biochemical basis of hypersensitivity. *Equine Veterinary Journal* **14**(1), 16–24.

Hiruta, A., Mitsuhata, H., Hiruta, M., Horikawa, Y., Takeuchi, H., Kawakami, T., Saitoh, J. and Seo, N. (2005). Vasopressin may be useful in the treatment of systemic anaphylaxis in rabbits. *Shock* **24** (3), 264–269.

Hurcombe, S.D., Mudge, M.C. and Hinchcliff, K.W. (2007). Clinical and clinicopathologic variables in adult horses receiving blood transfusions: 31 cases (1999–2005). *Journal of American Veterinary Medical Association* **231**(2), 267–274.

Jones, S.L. (2004). Inflammatory diseases of the gastrointestinal tract causing diarrhea. In: Reed, S.M., Bayly, W.M. and Sellon, D.C. (eds). *Equine Internal Medicine*, 2nd edition, pp. 884–913. St. Louis, Elsevier, Inc.

Kemp, S.F., Lockey, R.F., Wolf, B.L. and Lieberman, P. (1995). Anaphylaxis: a review of 266 cases. *Archives of Internal Medicine* **155**(16), 1749–1754.

Lieberman, P., Kempm S.F., Oppenheimerm J., Langm D.M., Bernstein, I.L. and Nicklas, R.A. (2005). The diagnosis and management of anaphylaxis: an updated practice parameter. *Journal of Allergy and Clinical Immunology* **115**(3 Suppl. 2), S483–S523.

Lieberman, P. (2006). Anaphylaxis. *Medical Clinics of North America* **90** (1), 77–95.

Lunn D.P. and Horohov, D.W. (2004). Hypersensitivity and autoimmunity. In: Reed, S.M., Bayly, W.M. and Sellon, D.C. (eds). *Equine Internal Medicine*, 2nd edition, pp. 29–36. St. Louis, Elsevier, Inc.

Nielsen, I.L., Jacobs, K.A., Huntington, P.J., Chapman, C.B. and Lloyd, K.C. (1988). Adverse reaction to procaine penicillin G in horses. *Australian Veterinary Journal* **65**(6), 181–185.

Palmer, J.E. (2007). Neonatal foal resuscitation. *Veterinary Clinics of North America: Equine Practice* **23**(1), 159–182.

Rajan, T.V. (2003). The Gell-Coombs classification of hypersensitivity reactions: a re-interpretation. *Trends in Immunology* **24**(7), 376–379.

Reddick, A.D., Ronald, J. and Morrison, W.G. (2011). Intravenous fluid resuscitation: was Poiseuille right? *Emergency Medicine Journal* **28** (3), 201–202.

Reinhart, K., Perner, A., Sprung, C.L., Jaeschke, R., Schortgen, F., Johan Groeneveld, A.B., Beale, R. and Hartog, C.S. (2012). Consensus statement of the ESICM task force on colloid volume therapy in critically ill patients. *Intensive Care Med* **38**(3), 368–383.

Sala-Cunill, A., Cardona, V., Labrador-Horrillo, M., Luengo, O., Esteso, O., Garriga, T., Vicario, M. and Guilarte, M. (2013). Usefulness and limitations of sequential serum tryptase for the diagnosis of anaphylaxis in 102 patients. *International Archives of Allergy Immunology* **160**(2), 192–199.

Sampson, H.A., Muñoz-Furlong, A., Campbell, R.L., Adkinson, N.F. Jr. Bock, S.A., Branum, A., Brown, S.G.A., Camargo, C.A. Jr. Cydulka, R., Galli, S.J., Gidudu, J., Gruchalla, R.S., Harlor, A.D. Jr. Hepner, D.L., Lewis, L.M., Lieberman, P.L., Metcalfe, D.D., O'Connor, R., Muraro, A., Rudman, A., Schmitt, C., Scherrer, D,. Simons, F.E., Thomas, S., Wood, J.P. and Decker, W.W. (2006). Second symposium on the definition and management of anaphylaxis: summary report-second national institute of allergy and infectious disease/food allergy and anaphylaxis network symposium. *Journal of Allergy and Clinical Immunology* **117**(2), 391–397.

Schaer, B.D. and Orsini, J.A. (2008). *Respiratory system: diagnostic and therapeutic procedures. In Equine Emergencies: Treatment and Procedures*, 3rd edition, edited by James A Orsini and Thomas J Divers, pp. 435–446. St. Louis, Elsevier, Inc.

Simons, F.E.R. (2006). Anaphylaxis, killer allergy: long-term management in the community. *Journal of Allergy and Clinical Immunology* **117**(2), 367–377.

Simons, F.E.R. (2013). Anaphylaxis: the acute episode and beyond. *British Medical Journal* **346**, f602.

Swiderski, C. (1995). Hypersensitivity. In: Kobluk, C.N., Ames, T.R. and Geor, R.J. (eds). *The Horse: Diseases and Clinical Management*, pp. 1065–1072. Philadelphia, W.B. Saunders Company.

Tizzard, I.R. (2013). *Type I Hypersensitivity. In: Veterinary Immunology*, 9th edition, pp. 326–345. St. Louis, Elsevier, Inc.

Uzzaman, A., and Cho, S.H. (2012). Classification of hypersensitivity reactions. *Allergy and Asthma Proceedings* **33**(Suppl. 1), S96–S99.

Vadas, P., Perelman, B. and Liss, G. (2013). Platelet-activating factor, histamine and tryptase levels in human anaphylaxis. *Journal of Allergy and Clinical Immunology* **131**(1), 144–149.

Vitte, J. and Bongrand, P. (2013). Serum tryptase determinations in patients with acute allergic reactions (letter to the editor). *Journal of Allergy and Clinical Immunology* **131**(6), 1714–1715.

Wells, P.W., McBeath, D.G., Eyre, P. and Hanna, C.J. (1981). Equine immunology: an introductory review. *Equine Veterinary Journal* **13** (4), 218–222.

Wilson, W.D. and Spensley, M.S. (1992). Preventative medicine programs. In: Robinson, N.E. (ed). *Current Therapy in Equine Medicine*, 23rd edition, pp. 35–50. Philadelphia, W.B. Saunders Company.

Wood, R.A., Camargo, C.A. Jr. Lieberman, P., Sampson, H.A., Schwartz, L.B., Zitt, M., Collins, C., Tringale, M., Wilkinson, M., Boyle, J. and Simons, F.E.R. (2013). Anaphylaxis in America: the prevalence and characteristics of anaphylaxis in the United States. *Journal of Allergy and Clinical Immunology* **133**(2), 461–467.

5 Allergy

Bettina Wagner

5.1 Definition

Horses naturally develop allergic diseases. An allergic reaction is an overreaction of the immune system of some individuals to a normally harmless substance – an allergen – which does not induce any disease or inflammatory reaction in most individuals. Immunoglobulin E (IgE)-mediated allergies are also known as *type I hypersensitivities*. They are characterized by their immediate onset after exposure to allergen, and by immunological mechanisms that involve the production of allergen-specific IgE, binding of IgE to tissue mast cells via high-affinity IgE receptors (a process that is called *mast cell sensitization*), and the release of inflammatory mediators from these sensitized mast cells after exposure to allergen. IgE-mediated allergies of the horse include *Culicoides* hypersensitivity and urticaria (hives). Various other conditions or diseases that have been assumed to be type I allergies, but for which an IgE-mediated pathogenesis has not yet been confirmed, will also be discussed briefly.

5.2 *Culicoides* hypersensitivity

Culicoides hypersensitivity is a seasonal, recurrent allergic dermatitis in horses. It is the most common allergic skin disease of horses, and the first equine disease suspected to be mediated by IgE (Matthews, 1983). *Culicoides* hypersensitivity is known by different names, such as summer eczema, summer seasonal recurrent dermatitis, atopic dermatitis, sweet itch, insect bite hypersensitivity, Kasen or Queensland itch.

5.2.1 Signalment and clinical signs

Culicoides hypersensitivity is characterized by pruritus, alopecia and excoriations, occurring during the summer months, in response to salivary allergens from *Culicoides* midges. Different parts of the body can be affected. Many horses show lesions at the mane, neck and tail. Others are mainly affected on the face, ears and intermandibular space, as well as the chest and belly. Horses can show lesions on just one, a few, or all of these locations (Figure 5.1). Affected horses will rub on any available structure, and can be seen dragging their bellies on the

ground. Secondary bacterial infections of the skin often occur, particularly if the affected areas are not cleaned or treated.

The disease has been frequently described in Icelandic horses (Halldordsottir, 1991; Lange, 2005; Björnsdóttir, 2006), but occurs in most horse breeds, including Thoroughbred, Arabian, Warmblood, Draft, Quarter Horse, Friesian, and different pony breeds. The onset of clinical disease is frequently observed around 3–4 years of age. However, it has also been observed in younger horses, or can first occur when horses are much older. The disease has been found in most countries all over the world and where *Culicoides* midges occur (Braverman, 1988; Larsen, 1988; Greiner, 1990; Anderson, 1993; Littlewood, 1998; Steinman, 2003; van Grevenhof, 2007). In regions that are free of Culicoides midges, including Iceland, New Zealand and Antarctica, the disease does not exist. The prevalence of *Culicoides* hypersensitivity ranges from 3% in Great Britain (McCaig, 1973), to 38% in Germany (Lange, 2005), and 60% in Queensland, Australia (Riek, 1953).

The large variation in prevalence in different countries can be explained by many different factors that influence the disease (Schaffartzik, 2012). Prevalence of *Culicoides* hypersensitivity is influenced by exposure to the midges and, therefore, it varies depending on the environment. Horses that are exclusively kept outside have a much higher chance of being bitten by *Culicoides* midges than do stabled horses. Consequently, disease prevalence varies with climate and, seemingly, between different horse breeds. Because of their different housing styles, pleasure horses are typically more frequently affected with *Culicoides* hypersensitivity than racing or competition horses. Other factors that influence clinical disease are genetic predisposition and the age of the individual horse, including the time that horses first get exposed to *Culicoides*.

This phenomenon was first observed in Icelandic horses. In Iceland, *Culicoides* midges do not occur and the allergy does not exist. Clinical signs only developed after export of the horses from Iceland into *Culicoides*-endemic countries (Larsen, 1988). Epidemiological studies confirmed that between 26–72% of the Icelandic horses exported to Europe developed the disease, while only 7–27% of Icelandic horses born in Europe became affected with *Culicoides* hypersensitivity (Halldordsottir, 1991; Lange, 2005; Björnsdóttir, 2006; Brostrom, 1987).

Equine Clinical Immunology, First Edition. Edited by M. Julia B. Felippe.
© 2016 John Wiley & Sons, Inc. Published 2016 by John Wiley & Sons, Inc.

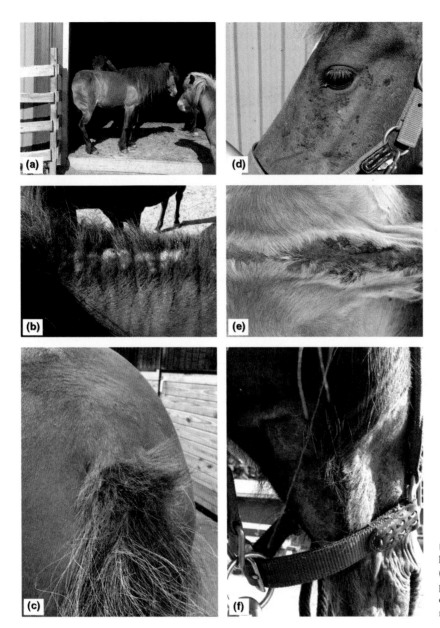

Figure 5.1 Clinical signs in horses with *Culicoides* hypersensitivity.
(**a**) Affected horses frequently scratch several body parts on available surface areas. Skin lesions can be observed at different body locations such as: (**b**) mane; (**c**) tail; (**d**) face; (**e**) belly; or (**f**) chin.

5.2.2 Immunologic mechanisms and etiologic associations

More than 20 years ago, different research groups first described the occurrence of immediate skin reactions after intradermal injection of *Culicoides* extracts (Braverman, 1988; Larsen, 1988; Greiner, 1990; Halldordsottir, 1991). Based on these observations, IgE-mediated allergic mechanisms were implicated in the pathogenesis of *Culicoides* hypersensitivity. Today, the IgE-mediated allergic etiology of *Culicoides* hypersensitivity has been confirmed by transferring the allergic reaction from affected to healthy horses via IgE obtained from allergic horses – a so-called *Prausnitz-Küstner reaction*. After IgE transfer, clinically healthy recipient horses were challenged with *Culicoides* extract. The recipients developed immediate skin reactions at the sites of the IgE transfer from affected donors,

but not at the transfer sites of IgE from healthy donors (Wagner, 2006).

The two major players in the pathogenesis of the *Culicoides* hypersensitivity are IgE and *Culicoides* allergens, required in hypersensitivity type I. Overall, the immune mechanisms of IgE-mediated allergies in horses are considered to be similar to those in humans (Schaffartzik, 2012). The immune pathogenesis of the disease includes the development of allergen-specific IgE, mast cell sensitization, degranulation, and release of inflammatory mediators in the affected skin tissues. During the first summer of exposure, horses are bitten by *Culicoides* and, typically, develop IgE antibodies to different salivary allergens injected by the midges during their blood meals.

IgE production by allergen-specific B cells is initiated in local lymphatic tissues, such as regional lymph nodes, and requires a complex interaction of immune cells, including dendritic cells, CD4 helper T cells (Th cells) and B cells. Once produced, circulating IgE antibodies rapidly bind to high-affinity IgE receptors on surfaces of tissue mast cells – a process called *sensitization*. Mast cell sensitization is a long-lasting process that does not cause any clinical signs in the absence of allergen. After second exposure – typically the second summer of exposure to *Culicoides* – the allergens can now stimulate sensitized tissue mast cells by cross-linking of the receptor-bound IgE on mast cell surfaces. Mast cell stimulation by allergen results in the immediate release of preformed inflammatory mediator histamine from the cells, as well as new production and secretion of additional inflammatory mediators (leukotrienes, prostaglandins) and cytokines (interleukin-4 (IL-4), IL-5, IL-13). Mast cell degranulation initiates an immediate inflammatory reaction in the skin.

Frequent midge bites during the summer rapidly lead to itchiness and the clinical signs of *Culicoides* hypersensitivity. Repeated allergen exposure further supports the production of allergen-specific IgE and mast cell sensitization, causing the allergic condition to continue in the following summer (Figure 5.2). Nevertheless, the detailed immune pathogenesis of *Culicoides* hypersensitivity, the exact cellular immune mechanisms involved and why some horses develop the allergic disease, while other horses in the same environment remain unaffected, are only partially understood. *Culicoides* hypersensitivity is a multi-factorial disease. The development of clinical allergy depends on several parameters, including genetic predisposition, environmental exposure, and the immune status of the individual horse.

Mast cell sensitization always precedes the development of allergy and clinical signs of *Culicoides* hypersensitivity. However, mast cell sensitization with allergen-specific IgE does not always lead to clinical allergy. Many clinically healthy horses are sensitized to *Culicoides* allergens and, despite having similar exposure to *Culicoides* as their allergic herd mates, are able to balance their immune reactions without overreacting and becoming allergic (Wagner, 2009a).

What distinguishes the immune reaction of an allergic from a non-allergic horse? The currently favored hypothesis is that the onset of *Culicoides* hypersensitivity results from immune imbalance characterized by increased numbers of allergen-specific Th2 cells, in combination with reduced immune regulatory mechanisms in affected horses, such as reduced numbers or function of allergen-specific regulatory T cells (Tregs). The decreased regulatory immune functions in allergic horses are supported by experimental results showing that the regulatory cytokines IL-10 and transforming growth factor-β1 (TGF-β1) can reduce IL-4 production in Th2 cells from allergic horses *in vitro* (Hamza, 2008). Stimulation of peripheral blood cells with *Culicoides* extracts also revealed lower numbers of regulatory T cells in allergic horses than in clinically healthy ones (Hamza, 2011). The decreased ability of some horses to regulate immune reactions to *Culicoides* allergens may further increase allergen-specific effector cell responses, such as enhanced Th2 cell immunity and *Culicoides*-specific IgE production, resulting in the development of clinical allergy.

Cellular immune mechanisms involved in *Culicoides* hypersensitivity have been mainly investigated in Icelandic horses. Increased numbers of Th cells and enhanced IL-13 messenger RNA (mRNA) expression were observed in tissues of local skin lesions from allergic horses (Heimann, 2011). Icelandic horses with clinical allergy had increased *Culicoides*-specific Th2 cell responses, compared with clinically healthy horses. Furthermore, exported allergic horses from Iceland had higher allergen-specific Th2 cell numbers than allergic Icelandic horses born in continental Europe (Hamza, 2008). These findings suggest that the increased allergy prevalence in exported Icelandic horses could be influenced by the delayed first exposure to *Culicoides*.

The immune responses of neonatal and young foals differ in many aspects from adult horse immunity (Wagner, 2010). Most horses that are exposed to *Culicoides* early in life likely have

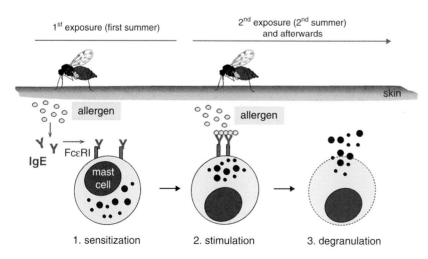

Figure 5.2 Sensitization of skin mast cells and inflammatory mediator release in response to *Culicoides* allergens. During the first summer of exposure, horses get bitten by *Culicoides* midges and develop IgE antibodies to different salivary antigens (allergens):
(**1**) IgE antibodies bind to high-affinity IgE receptors (FcεRI) on the surface of tissue mast cells. This process is called *sensitization*.
(**2**) After second exposure to *Culicoides*, or any following exposure, the allergens can now stimulate sensitized tissue mast cells by cross-linking of receptor-bound IgE on the mast cell surface.
(**3**) Mast cell stimulation by allergen results in the immediate release of inflammatory mediators, initiates an immediate inflammatory reaction in the skin, and leads the clinical signs of *Culicoides* hypersensitivity.

more balanced immune mechanisms, which prevent the development of clinical allergy when older. Young foals have significantly diminished Th2 cell responses, compared with adult horses (Wagner, 2010), and do not produce IgE for several months during the first year of life (Wagner, 2009a). These differences in the foal's immune response might favor the development of *Culicoides*-specific regulatory immune mechanisms when foals are exposed to *Culicoides* allergens early in life. Further investigations of the immune mechanisms leading to development of, or prevention from, clinical disease will allow us to better understand, manage and prevent *Culicoides* hypersensitivity in horses.

5.2.3 Diagnostics

Various techniques are available to detect soluble allergen-specific IgE or the sensitization of mast cells or basophils with allergen-specific IgE (Wagner, 2009b). These tests are called *allergy tests*, although they try to identify the causing allergen(s) for the clinical condition. Allergy testing includes intradermal testing against multiple potential allergens or serological assays – most commonly enzyme-linked immunosorbent assays (ELISAs) – based on a variety of allergens. The goal is to identify the causing allergen in order to develop a management plan toward allergen avoidance and hyposensitization.

Intradermal allergy testing with various environmental allergens has been used to determine allergic responses in horses for over 20 years (Matthews, 1983; Larsen, 1988; Anderson, 1993). Intradermal testing aims to mimic the allergic reaction at the injection site of each causing allergen. Following the injection of a small dose of soluble allergen or anti-IgE into the skin, inflammatory mediators are released from local skin mast cells. A positive immediate skin reaction is characterized by the formation of a wheal developing after 15–30 minutes at the injection site (Wagner, 2006). Horses with clinical signs of *Culicoides* hypersensitivity or urticaria react more frequently to intradermal injection of allergen extracts than do clinically healthy horses (Larsen, 1988; Lorch, 2001). However, allergic horses tend to show multiple positive reactions to intradermal testing, and many allergens are unlikely to be causing the allergic disease (Figure 5.3). Therefore, identifying the allergens that truly induce the patient's allergic disease can be challenging.

Intradermal allergy testing detects sensitization of skin mast cells with allergen-specific IgE, which is required to develop clinical allergy. As discussed above, sensitization of mast cells or basophils with allergen-specific IgE does not necessarily mean that the horse is allergic to that testing allergen. Several clinically healthy horses showed positive skin reaction or *in vitro* sensitization assays to several allergens, including *Culicoides* extract, and never showed any signs of disease (Lorch, 2001; Kolm-Stark, 2002; Lebis, 2002; Wagner, 2008). This further supports that sensitization is a prerequisite, but not always an equivalent, of clinical allergy, and should not be used to diagnose an allergic condition without considering clinical signs.

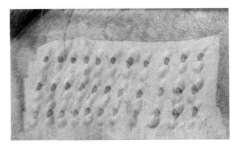

Figure 5.3 Interdermal testing at the lateral neck of an allergic horse 20 minutes after injection.
Two controls and 63 allergen extracts were injected into the skin of the horse. The black marker dots indicate the location of the injection sites. Injections were performed above and below each marker dot. The upper left injection (on top of the first marker dot) is saline (negative control) causing a small wheal induced by the volume of the injection. The second upper left injection (on top of the second marker dot) is histamine (positive control) causing a larger wheal due to local inflammation. All remaining allergen injections are judged relative to these two controls. This horse had positive reactions to multiple allergen extracts.

Serological allergy testing aims to measure soluble allergen-specific IgE antibodies, and to detect the humoral immune response to a particular allergen, by using either an anti-IgE antibody or the human Fc-epsilon RI-alpha chain for IgE detection. The tests are performed by three basic steps:

1 Various allergen preparations are coated to the solid phase of the assay, most frequently an ELISA plate.
2 Patient serum is then added to the testing plate, and serum IgE antibodies bind to respective allergens.
3 An anti-equine IgE reagent is used to detect patient IgE bound to the plate. Despite a straightforward principle, serological allergy tests have a poor performance due to numerous positive reactions, many of which are likely false positive.

One general weakness of the current allergen-specific assays is that they often use crude allergen preparations, which result in binding of many proteins other than the allergen itself to the solid phase of the assay. Consequently, there is a decreased concentration of the allergen available for the assay, and the risk of serum antibody binding to the non-specific proteins (Eder, 2000; Morgan, 2007). Overall, this approach causes false positive reactions that cannot be distinguished from true allergen specific reactivity. Although the principle of allergen-specific IgE detection sounds convincing, in reality, most binding to the crude allergen preparation is due to serum IgG antibodies. IgG antibodies develop to multiple environmental proteins, including allergens; in addition, their serum concentrations are much higher than that of allergen-specific IgE. Consequently, most of the allergen preparation within the serological allergy test is detected by IgGs, and just a small amount of the allergen is available for IgE binding (Morgan, 2007; Langner, 2008).

The specificity of the anti-IgE reagent is the most crucial parameter for the accurate performance of serological allergy tests. A variety of reagents detecting equine IgE have been used for these assays, including polyclonal anti-IgE reagents (Halliwell, 1993; Eder, 2000), monoclonal anti-IgE antibodies (Morgan, 2007; Langner, 2008), and the human Fc-epsilon RI-alpha chain (Frey, 2008). Thus far, convincing specificity against equine IgE has only been reported for monoclonal anti-equine IgE antibodies (Wagner, 2003). There is currently no reported evidence that the human Fc-epsilon RI-alpha chain, which is used in one of the commercial assays, does bind to equine IgE. Therefore, serological allergy tests result in multiple positive reactions, many of which are likely to be false positive, based on the low specificity of some anti-IgE reagents and the poor quality of many allergen preparations. Overall, most authors conclude that serological allergen testing in horses performs poorly, is unreliable, and cannot be recommended using the currently available assays (Eder, 2000; Morgan, 2007; Langner, 2008; Frey, 2008).

5.2.4 Treatment and prevention

Treatment of IgE-mediated allergy in horses is mostly symptomatic. Today, no scientifically proven treatments exist that reliably cure allergy or address the causing mechanisms of the disease to revert the allergic overreaction. Systemic treatments to reduce severe clinical signs include injections of steroids and/or anti-histamines.

The most effective preventive action for allergic horses is allergen avoidance. For *Culicoides* hypersensitivity, this can be achieved by managing the turn-out of affected horses, and by keeping them inside during dusk and dawn. Additional preventive measures include fly control with fly sprays, fly masks, and whole body blankets while horses are outside, plus fans within stalls or sheds. Rough fence or surface areas where affected horses would rub and further damage the affected skin regions should be removed. Instead, providing smooth surfaces or non-damaging brushes for them to rub can help to reduce the severity of clinical signs, secondary infections, and the horse's discomfort.

Supportive care to reduce itchiness, minimize bacterial infection, and improve the healing process of the affected skin areas is work-intensive. However, if it is performed on a regular basis, together with allergen avoidance, severe discomfort of horses affected by *Culicoides* hypersensitivity can be avoided, and the disease may even become non-symptomatic.

Some authors have favored hyposensitization to cure the allergic condition, but this therapy still lacks sufficient experimental proof in horses. A successful hyposensitization approach goes hand in hand with a proper diagnostic of the causing allergen(s). As discussed above, this is also a task that is still difficult to accomplish for most horses, given the current performance of equine allergy tests.

5.2.5 Prognosis and clinical outcomes

IgE-mediated allergies, such as *Culicoides* hypersensitivity and urticaria, usually have no cure and will develop every summer, or whenever the horse is exposed to the causing allergen(s). They can become more severe over time in some horses, but clinical outcome rather depends on allergen pressure and environmental conditions in a given year. If a horse is moved out of the environment with allergen exposure into an allergen-free environment, clinical signs can completely disappear. If this horse is moved back into an area with allergen exposure, clinical allergy can develop again with similar severity, as previously observed. In some cases, allergy may not occur again if the horse has not been exposed to the allergen for extended periods of time, usually several years.

5.3 Urticaria

Urticaria, or hives, is characterized by typical lesions that affect large areas of the skin (Figure 5.4). Lesions can be round, or can have multiple shapes, including linear stripes, or donut-like or papular appearance. In horses, urticaria is not usually associated with pruritus, but it can be in some cases. Severe urticaria may show ventral edema. Food allergens, insect bite, and exposure to environmental allergens have been associated with the development of urticaria. In addition, acute urticaria can occur in response to drug or vaccine administration, or blood transfusion. In recurrent cases, rational diagnostic approaches to identify the inducing allergen(s) can be challenging, and effective causal treatments are often lacking.

Although an IgE-mediated etiology has not yet been directly shown, the similarity to clinical signs with urticaria in humans, and the sudden onset of the lesions, provide support for type I hypersensitivity mechanisms in the pathogenesis of the disease (Lorch, 2001; Jose-Cunilleras, 2001; Rüfenacht, 2005).

Histopathological findings include dermal edema with eosinophilic and/or lymphocytic perivascular cellular infiltrates in the affected areas. Increased numbers of mast cells, eosinophils and macrophages are found in skin lesions from affected horses, compared with normal skin, by immunohistochemistry.

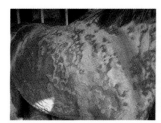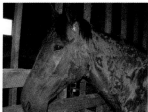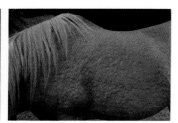

Figure 5.4 Horses with urticaria (hives).

Immunological or mechanistic studies on urticaria in horses are missing.

For horses with urticaria, allergen avoidance can be challenging, because the unknown causing allergen(s).

5.4 Recurrent airway obstruction

Recurrent airway obstruction (RAO) or heaves has been suspected to be mediated by IgE and hypersensitivity type I. However, the involvement of IgE in the pathogenesis remains controversial. RAO is considered to be initiated by a hyperreactive response of the lower respiratory tract to inhaled moulds and organic dusts (Derksen, 1988; McGorum, 1993; Pirie, 2003). The disease is characterized by mucus production, neutrophil accumulation in the airway, bronchial hyperreactivity, and bronchospasm. Inhalation of mold and fungal antigens induces the inflammatory airway response in susceptible horses within six hours after exposure (Gerber, 2004). Nevertheless, the involvement of IgE-mediated mechanisms in the pathogenesis of RAO remains unclear (Marti, 2008).

The support for a role of IgE in RAO was provided in studies that detected increased *Aspergillus*-specific IgE antibodies in bronchoalveolar lavage fluid of affected horses, using a polyclonal anti-IgE reagent (Halliwell, 1993; Schmallenbach, 1998). Nevertheless, these initial findings could not be confirmed in more recently performed studies. It became evident that environmental and genetic factors influence the IgE response to mold allergens (Eder, 2001; Curik, 2003), and a comparison of mold-, mite- or *Aspergillus*-specific IgE responses from horses living in different environments did not result in any differences between RAO-affected and control horses. The authors concluded that IgE serology is not a useful tool for the diagnosis of RAO, or for the determination of antigens causing the disease (Eder, 2000; Tahon, 2009).

Skin testing with mold and fungal allergens in horses with RAO revealed reactions to *Aspergillus fumigatus* and other mold antigens at four hours and/or 24 hours after injection. The authors concluded that the reactivity might, rather, reflect a cell-mediated delayed type hypersensitivity response (Jose-Cunilleras, 2001; Wong, 2005; Tahon, 2009). Overall, evidence for an increase in IgE-mediated immediate skin reactions in RAO-affected horses could not be supported by these studies, and evidence for a causal role of IgE in the pathogenesis of RAO is still missing.

References

Anderson, G.S., Belton, P., and Kleider, N. (1993). Hypersensitivity of horses in British Columbia to extracts of native and exotic species of *Culicoides* (Diptera: Ceratopogonidae). *Journal of Medical Entomology* **30**, 657–663.

Björnsdóttir, S., Sigvaldadóttir, J., Broström, H., Langvad, B. and Sigurdsson, A. (2006). Summer eczema in exported Icelandic horses: influence of environmental and genetic factors. *Acta Veterinary Scandinavica* **48**, 3.

Braverman, Y. (1988). Preferred landing sites of *Culicoides* species (Diptera: Ceratopogonidae) on a horse in Israel and its relevance to summer seasonal recurrent dermatitis (sweet itch). *Equine Veterinary Journal* **20**, 426–429.

Brostrom, H., Larsson, A. and Troedsson, M. (1987). Allergic dermatitis (sweet itch) of Icelandic horses in Sweden: an epidemiological study. *Equine Veterinary Journal* **19**, 229–236.

Curik, I., Fraser, D., Eder, C., Achmann, R., Swinburne, J., Binns, M., Crameri, R., Brem, G., Sölkner, J. and Marti, E. (2003). Association between MHC gene region and variation of serum IgE levels against specific mould allergens in the horse. *Genetic Selection Evolution* **35**, 117–190.

Derksen, F.J., Robinson, N.E., Scott, J.S. and Stick, J.A. (1988). Aerosolized Micropolyspora faeni antigen as a cause of pulmonary dysfunction in ponies with recurrent airway obstruction (heaves). *American Journal of Veterinary Research* **49**, 933–938.

Eder, C., Crameri, R., Mayer, C., Eicher, R., Straub, R., Gerber, H., Lazary, S. and Marti, E. (2000). Allergen-specific IgE levels against crude mould and storage mite extracts and recombinant mould allergens in sera from horses affected with chronic bronchitis. *Veterinary Immunology and Immunopathology* **73**, 241–253.

Eder, C., Curik, I., Brem, G., Crameri, R., Bodo, I., Habe, F., Lazary, S., Sölkner, J. and Marti, E. (2001). Influence of environmental and genetic factors on allergen-specific immunoglobulin E levels in sera from Lipizzan horses. *Equine Veterinary Journal* **33**, 714–720.

Frey, R., Bergvall, K. and Egenvall, A. (2008). Allergen-specific IgE in Icelandic horses with insect bite hypersensitivity and healthy controls, assessed by FcεRIα-based serology. *Veterinary Immunology and Immunopathology* **126**, 102–109.

Gerber, V., Lindberg, A., Berney, C. and Robinson, N.E. (2004). Airway mucus in recurrent airway obstruction – short-term response to environmental challenge. *Journal Veterinary Internal Medicine* **18**, 92–97.

Greiner, E.C., Fadok, V.A. and Rabin, E.B. (1990). Equine *Culicoides* hypersensitivity in Florida: biting midges aspirated from horses. *Journal of Medical Entomology* **4**, 375–381.

Halldordsottir, S. and Larsen, H.J. (1991). An epidemiological study of summer eczema in Icelandic horses in Norway. *Equine Veterinary Journal* **23**, 296–299.

Halliwell, R.E., McGorum, B.C., Irving, P. and Dixon, P.M. (1993). Local and systemic antibody production in horses affected with chronic obstructive pulmonary disease. *Veterinary Immunology and Immunopathology* **38**, 201–215.

Hamza, E., Wagner, B., Jungi, T.W., Mirkovitch, J. and Marti, E. (2008). Reduced incidence of insect-bite hypersensitivity in Icelandic horses is associated with a down-regulation of interleukin-4 by interleukin-10 and transforming growth factor-β1. *Veterinary Immunology and Immunopathology* **122**, 65–75.

Hamza, E., Steinbach, F. and Marti, E. (2011). CD4+CD25+ T cells expressing FoxP3 in Icelandic horses affected with insect bite hypersensitivity. *Veterinary Immunology and Immunopathology* **148**, 139–144.

Heimann, M., Janda, J., Sigurdardottir, O.G., Svansson, V., Klukowska, J., von Tscharner, C., Doherr, M., Broström, H., Andersson, L.S., Einarsson, S., Marti, E. and Torsteinsdottir, S. (2011). Skin-infiltrating T cells and cytokine expression in Icelandic horses affected with insect bite hypersensitivity: a possible role for regulatory T-cells. *Veterinary Immunology and Immunopathology* **140**, 63–74.

Jose-Cunilleras, E., Kohn, C.W., Hillier, A., Saville, W.J.A. and Lorch, G. (2001). Intradermal testing in healthy horses and horses with chronic obstructive pulmonary disease, recurrent urticaria, or allergic dermatitis, *Journal of the American Veterinary Medical Association* **219**, 1115–1121.

Kolm-Stark, G. and Wagner, R. (2002). Intradermal skin testing in Icelandic horses in Austria. *Equine Veterinary Journal* **34**, 405–410.

Lange, S., Hamann, H., Deegen, E., Ohnesorge, B. and Distl, O. (2005). Investigation of the prevalence of summer eczema in Icelandic horses in northern Germany. *Berliner Munchener Tierarztliche Wochenschrift* **118**, 481–489.

Langner, K.F., Darpel, K.E., Drolet, B.S., Fischer, A., Hampel, S., Heselhaus, J.E., Mellor, P.S., Mertens, P.P. and Leibold, W. (2008). Comparison of cellular and humoral immunoassays for the assessment of summer eczema in horses. *Veterinary Immunology and Immunopathology* **122**, 126–137.

Larsen, H.J., Bakke, S.H. and Mehl, R. (1988). Intradermal challenge of Icelandic horses in Norway and Iceland with extracts of *Culicoides* spp. *Acta Veterinary Scandinavica* **29**, 311–314.

Lebis, C., Bourdeau, P. and Marzin-Keller, F. (2002). Intradermal skin tests in equine dermatology: a study of 83 horses. *Equine Veterinary Journal* **34**, 666–671.

Littlewood, J.D. (1998). Incidence of recurrent seasonal pruritus ('sweet itch') in British and German Shire horses. *Veterinary Research* **142**, 66–67.

Lorch, G., Hillier, A., Kwochka, K.W., Saville, W.A. and LeRoy, B.E. (2001). Results of intradermal tests in horses without atopy and horses with atopic dermatitis or recurrent urticaria. *American Journal of Veterinary Research* **62**, 1051–1059.

Marti, E., Gerber, V., Wilson, A. D., Lavoie, J. P., Horohov, D., Crameri, R., Lunn, D. P., Antczak, D., Bjornsdottir, S., Bjornsdottir, T. S., Cunningham, F., Derer, M., Frey, R., Hamza, E., Horin, P., Heimann, M., Kolm-Stark, G., Olafsdottir, G., Ramery, E., Russell, C., Schaffartzik, A., Svansson, V., Torsteinsdottir, S. and Wagner, B. (2008). Report of the 3rd Havemeyer Workshop on Allergic Diseases of the Horse, Iceland, June 2007. *Veterinary Immunology and Immunopathology* **126**, 351–361.

Matthews, A.G., Imlah, P. and McPherson, E.A. (1983). A reagin-like antibody in horse serum: 1. Occurrence and some biological properties. *Veterinary Research Communications* **6**, 13–23.

McCaig, J. (1973). A survey to establish the incidence of sweet itch in ponies in the United Kingdom. *Veterinary Records* **93**, 444–446.

McGorum, B.C., Dixon, P.M. and Halliwell, R.E. (1993). Evaluation of intradermal mould antigen testing in the diagnosis of equine chronic obstructive pulmonary disease. *Equine Veterinary Journal* **25**, 257–258.

Morgan, E.E., Miller, W.H. and Wagner, B. (2007). A comparison of intradermal testing and detection of allergen-specific immunoglobulin E in serum by enzyme-linked immunosorbent assay in horses affected with skin hypersensitivity. *Veterinary Immunology and Immunopathology* **120**, 160–167.

Pirie, R.S., Dixon, P.M. and McGorum, B.C. (2003). Endotoxin contamination contributes to the pulmonary inflammatory and functional response to Aspergillus fumigatus extract inhalation in heaves horses. *Clinical and Experimental Allergy* **33**, 1289–1296.

Riek, R.F. (1953). Studies on allergic dermatitis (Queensland Itch) of the horse I. Description, distribution, symptoms and pathology. *Australian Veterinary Journal* **29**, 177–184.

Rüfenacht, S., Marti, E., von Tscharner, C., Doherr, M.G., Forster, U., Welle, M. and Roosje, P.J. (2005). Immunoglobulin E-bearing cells and mast cells in skin biopsies of horses with urticaria. *Veterinary Dermatology* **16**, 94–101.

Schaffartzik, A., Hamza, E., Janda, J., Crameri, R., Marti, E. and Rhyner, C. (2012). Equine insect bite hypersensitivity: What do we know? *Veterinary Immunology and Immunopathology* **147**, 113–126.

Schmallenbach, K.H., Rahman, I., Sasse, H.H., Dixon, P.M., Halliwell, R.E., McGorum, B.C., Crameri, R. and Miller, H.R. (1998) Studies on pulmonary and systemic *Aspergillus fumigatus*-specific IgE and IgG antibodies in horses affected with chronic obstructive pulmonary disease (COPD). *Veterinary Immunology and Immunopathology* **66**, 245–256.

Steinman, A., Peer, G. and Klemen, E. (2003). Epidemiological study of *Culicoides* hypersensitivity in horses in Israel. *Veterinary Record* **152**, 748–751.

Tahon, L., Baselgia, S., Gerber, V., Doherr, M.G., Straub, R., Robinson, N.E. and Marti, E. (2009). *In vitro* allergy tests compared to intradermal testing in horses with recurrent airway obstruction. *Veterinary Immunology and Immunopathology* **127**, 85–93.

Van Grevenhof, E.M., Ducro, B., Heuven, H.C. and Bijma, P. (2007). Identification of environmental factors affecting the prevalence of insect bite hypersensitivity in Shetland ponies and Friesian horses in The Netherlands. *Equine Veterinary Journal* **39**, 69–73.

Wagner, B. (2009b). IgE in horses: Occurrence in health and disease. *Veterinary Immunology and Immunopathology* **132**, 21–30.

Wagner, B., Radbruch, A., Rohwer, J. and Leibold, W. (2003). Monoclonal anti-equine IgE antibodies with specificity for different epitopes on the immunoglobulin heavy chain of native IgE. *Veterinary Immunology and Immunopathology* **92**, 45–60.

Wagner, B., Miller, W.H., Morgan, E.E., Hillegas, J.M., Erb, H.N., Leibold, W. and Antczak, D.F. (2006). IgE and IgG antibodies in skin allergy of the horse. *Veterinary Research* **37**, 813–825.

Wagner, B., Childs, B.A. and Erb, H.N. (2008). A histamine release assay to identify sensitization to *Culicoides* allergens in horses with skin hypersensitivity. *Veterinary Immunology and Immunopathology* **126**, 302–308.

Wagner, B., Miller, W.H., Erb, H.N., Lunn, D.P. and Antczak, D.F. (2009a). Sensitization of skin mast cells with IgE antibodies to *Culicoides* allergens occurs frequently in clinically healthy horses. *Veterinary Immunology and Immunopathology* **132**, 53–61.

Wagner, B., Burton, A. and Ainsworth, D.M. (2010). Interferon-gamma, interleukin-4 and interleukin-10 production by T helper cells reveals intact Th1 and regulatory TR1 cell activation and a delay of the Th2 cell response in equine neonates and foals. *Veterinary Research* **41**, 47.

Wong, D.M., Buechner-Maxwell, V.A., Manning, T.O. and Ward, D.L. (2005). Comparison of results for intradermal testing between clinically normal horses and horses affected with recurrent airway obstruction. *American Journal of Veterinary Research* **66**, 1348–1355.

6 Immune-Mediated Cytopenias

Thomas J. Divers

6.1 Definition

Immune-mediated anemia, thrombocytopenia, and neutropenia are sporadic diseases in the horse. The immune disease process may result in decreased production of bone marrow-derived cells or, more commonly, enhanced peripheral destruction of the cells. In many of the immune-mediated cytopenia disorders, only one cell line is affected while, in other disorders (e.g., leukemia), two or all three of the cell lineages may be affected simultaneously. The immune process may be the result of primary causes (i.e., autoimmune disorders that are often idiopathic, or secondary to infectious agents, drugs or neoplasia).

Newborn foals may develop alloimmune cytopenias from colostrum-derived antibodies, while isoimmune reactions may occur from blood transfusions. The immune reaction causing the cytopenia is most often considered a cytotoxic type II antibody-mediated response. Diagnosis of immune-mediated cytopenias should include a thorough history and clinical examination, complete blood cell count, and immunological testing when needed. The primary treatments for immune-mediated anemia, thrombocytopenia, or neutropenia include removal of any offending drug or infectious agent, immunosuppressive therapy when indicated, and supportive care such as transfusions, if indicated.

6.2 Immune-mediated hemolytic anemia

6.2.1 Signalment and clinical signs

The signalment and clinical signs often provide a major clue in the diagnosis and cause of the immune-mediated hemolytic anemia (IMHA). Clinical signs of immune-mediated hemolytic anemia are variable, depending upon the severity and speed of onset of the anemia, and the presence of secondary systemic disease or organ system failure, such as disseminated intravascular coagulation or renal failure. Horses and foals with severe IMHA will appear weak, with marked tachycardia and tachypnea, resulting from hypoxia. Icterus is generally noticeable if the immune-mediated anemia has been ongoing for one day or more (Figure 6.1). If the hemolysis is intravascular, which is common in many equine IMHA disorders, the serum and urine may be of a light or dark red color (hemoglobinuria) (Figure 6.2).

Neurologic signs due to bilirubin toxicity (kernicterus) may occur in foals with neonatal isoerythrolysis (NI) when the hemolysis is severe and bilirubin concentration is more than 20 mg/dl. In horses with immune-mediated anemia caused by neoplastic diseases, weight loss, anorexia, fever, or other signs directly attributable to the anatomical location of the neoplastic disease are common signs. Evans syndrome is a rare hematological disease, commonly defined as Coombs-positive hemolytic anemia and immune-mediated thrombocytopenia (Väänänen, 2013).

Foals affected with NI are very young foals usually born to multiparous mares, and the disease is most common in mules. Hemolysis effects may become clinically apparent within hours to a few days after birth. Clinical signs include: depression; weakness; lethargy; tachycardia; tachypnea; icteric or pale mucous membranes; moderate to severe anemia; normal total protein; decreased venous oxygen concentration and saturation; metabolic acidosis due to poor tissue oxygenation; hyperbilirubinemia; hemoglobinemia; and hemoglobinuria. In severe cases, pigmentary nephropathy, azotemia, tissue inflammation due to hypoxia (central nervous system, gastro-intestinal tract, liver), fever and seizures may occur. In addition, kernicterus or bilirubin encephalopathy may lead to severe depression, opisthotonus, rigidity, convulsions and death, due to the deposition of unconjugated bilirubin and necrosis of cerebral gray matter.

6.2.2 Immunologic mechanisms and etiologic associations

Immune-mediated anemia is a result of antibody-mediated destruction of red blood cells (RBCs), either in the bone marrow or peripherally. Peripheral destruction of RBCs due to binding of antibodies to the red blood cell surface (hypersensitivity type II) is the most common cause of cell loss in equine IMHA.

These antibodies may be produced as a primary autoimmune disorder (autoantibodies or isoantibodies) after blood product transfusion or idiopathic causes, or may be absorbed from colostrum (alloantibodies). Production of autoantibodies can be secondary to: lymphoma; hemangiosarcoma; bacterial antigens (*Streptococcus* spp., *Clostridium perfringens*, *Rhodococcus equi*);

Equine Clinical Immunology, First Edition. Edited by M. Julia B. Felippe.
© 2016 John Wiley & Sons, Inc. Published 2016 by John Wiley & Sons, Inc.

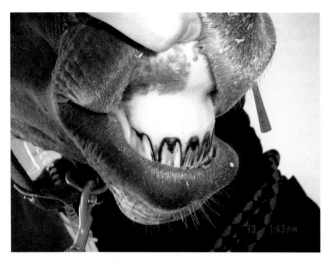

Figure 6.1 Immune-mediated hemolytic anemia.
Adult horse with penicillin induced hemolytic anemia; azathioprine and corticosteroids were required to control the intravascular hemolysis (Thomas Divers, Cornell University).

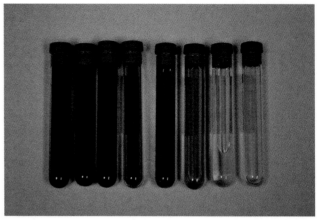

Figure 6.2 Isoimmune hemolytic anemia.
Change in urine discoloration (hemoglobinuria, urine collected in blood tubes) over two days in a mule foal with isoimmune hemolytic anemia (following plasma transfusion) (Sally Ness, Cornell University).

parasitic (uncommonly, *Theleria equi or Babesia* caballi); viral (equine infectious anemia); or drug administration.

Drug-induced immunocytopenia may occur from one or more mechanisms, and there is generally no relationship between the dose of the drug and the reaction (Salama, 2009). Penicillin may be an exception, as there is evidence of dose-related immune hemolytic anemia. Some drugs, such as penicillin, may act as haptens binding to cell surface, or as neoantigens, which result from the interaction of the drug with cell membranes, causing the production of drug-dependent antibodies.

In horses, IgG appears to be the most common primary antibody associated with immunocytopenias, although IgM may be the predominant causative antibody in some cases (Wilkerson, 2000). When complement is activated along with antibody (IgG or IgM) binding, the red cell destruction (hemolysis) happens intravascularly, resulting in discolored serum and urine (hemoglobinuria). In extravascular hemolysis, the latter clinical signs are not obvious, because the antibody (often IgG)-bound red cells are removed via phagocytosis when the antibody binds to the Fc receptor on phagocytes (Salama, 2009). The spleen is thought to be the major site of RBC removal in immune-mediated anemia, through the reticuloendothelial (mononuclear phagocyte) system.

Immune-mediated anemia may be caused by either warm agglutinating antibody, which binds to the red cell antigen at normal or higher body temperature, or by cold agglutinating antibody, which binds to the antigen below normal body temperature. Although not well documented in horses, warm agglutinating antibodies are thought to be mostly associated with IgG, while cold agglutinating antibodies are likely IgM.

In aplastic anemia, the bone marrow is the site of red cell precursor destruction. Aplastic anemia may result from immune-mediated causes or myelophthisic causes (e.g.,

infiltration with neoplasia; in this case, all three hematopoietic cell lines are affected, causing pancytopenia). Drug-induced aplastic anemia/pancytopenia and bone marrow infiltration with lymphosarcoma are the most common causes of aplastic anemia reported in horses (Angel, 1991; Kelton, 2008; Lavoie, 1987).

Red cell aplasia has been reported in horses receiving injections of the first-generation human erythropoietin (Epogen®). Administration of the human product can develop cross-reacting autoantibodies against native equine erythropoietin, and can result in a life-threatening erythroid hypoplasia (Piercy, 1998).

In NI, colostrum-derived alloantibodies directed against the incompatible antigens on the red cell of the affected foal are produced by the dam, because:

(a) the mare was exposed to fetus blood during parturition in a previous pregnancy;

(b) this fetus inherited antigenic blood factors from the sire that are not common to that dam's;

(c) the mare produced antibodies against these factors; and

(d) the affected foal expresses the same incompatible blood factors of the sensitizing fetus (from a previous pregnancy); or

(e) the possibility of NI in a first pregnancy when the mare had received blood transfusion of an incompatible blood type that is the same of the affected foal. The most important blood groups associated with NI are A and Q. The antigens Aa and Qa are responsible for more than 90% of the NI.

6.2.3 Diagnostics

Anemia due to immune-mediated causes tends to be profound, and progresses relatively fast. Historical information, including drug administration, should be considered along with laboratory testing. The initial goal for diagnostics in suspected immune-mediated anemia should be to determine whether the disorder

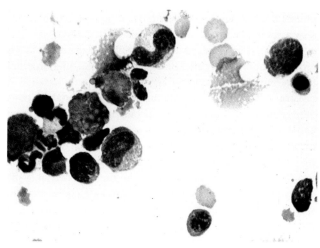

Figure 6.3 Red cell aplasia.
Photograph of bone marrow sample from a horse with red cell aplasia, following multiple injections of human erythropoietin (Thomas Divers, Cornell University).

involves decreased production of red blood cells in the bone marrow, or intravascular/extravascular hemolysis.

When there is no evidence of a regenerative process (increased RBC mean corpuscular volume (MCV), and red cell distribution width (RDW)) of the erythroid cell line, a problem with decreased marrow production (aplastic anemia) should be suspected. In addition, there is no discolored plasma or discolored urine with bone marrow origin anemia, and MCV is low and RDW normal. Pure red cell aplasia (Figure 6.3) is rare, and it is generally associated with the administration of human erythropoietin.

If the IMHA is caused by increased peripheral RBC destruction, MCV and RDW will often be increased, due to the release of larger than normal RBCs from the bone marrow. Although horses with regenerative anemia do not exhibit reticulocytosis on normal Wright's stain, reticulocytosis can be detected with certain automated hematology machines. In intravascular destruction, the plasma may be pink, or at least jaundiced, and urine may be discolored, due to hemoglobinuria.

Another commonly used diagnostic test to confirm IMHA is the direct Coombs' antiglobulin test, which detects antibody attached to the RBC surface. A whole blood sample is collected from the patient, and the RBCs are initially washed to remove the patient's own plasma, then incubated with the Coombs' reagent (anti-horse IgG, IgM and complement C3). A positive Coombs' reaction is shown by the agglutination of RBCs, as the Coombs' reagent (antibodies) bind to the red cell surface autoantibodies and cause cross-linkage of multiple RBCs. In some cases, autoagglutination can be observed, even in the absence of the Coombs' reagent (Owens, 2008). Cold agglutinating antibody is frequently autoagglutinating at 4 °C.

The use of flow cytometry to detect the percentage of antibody-coated red cells can be helpful in the diagnosis

and, in some cases, monitoring the response to therapy (Wilkerson, 2000). Osmotic fragility testing of RBCs can be used as an additional aid in the diagnosis of IMHA, although infectious and toxic causes of hemolytic anemia will also result in increased fragility when RBCs are placed in hypotonic saline solutions.

6.2.4 Treatment

The overall treatments for IMHA include removal of any offending drug, immunosuppressive therapy when indicated, and supportive care, such as blood transfusions, when needed. For drug-induced (secondary) IMHA, the duration of time to recovery following removal of the offending drug is variable.

Immunosuppressive treatments may be indicated when anemia is progressive and/or life-threatening. The two most commonly used immunosuppressive drugs for IMHA are corticosteroids and azathioprine.

Corticosteroids work by controlling both the cell- and antibody-mediated immune responses. Corticosteroid treatment is most effective for warm agglutinin reactions (Michel, 2011). Dexamethasone is generally the preferred corticosteroid in horses, based upon field response reports, although there are no controlled studies comparing different corticosteroids. Starting doses of dexamethasone are generally 0.05–0.1 mg/kg SID, IV or IM. Doses at 0.2 mg/kg may be required in some cases. Duration of treatment depends on the severity of cases and insulting cause but, in general, takes two weeks with tapering doses. The persistence of IgG should be taken into account when tailoring the treatment to the patient's clinical signs. The regular half-life of IgG is 28–32 days. Therefore, in refractory cases, the treatment should be kept for a longer period of time (perhaps a month) before reducing the dose significantly, in order to allow removal of autoimmune IgG while preventing the production of additional antibodies.

For horses that do not respond to corticosteroids or cannot be given high doses of the drug due to metabolic disease, pituitary pars intermedia dysfunction, or risk of laminitis, azathioprine is an alternative treatment (Messer, 1991). Azathioprine is a purine analogue and acts as a prodrug for mercaptopurine, inhibiting an enzyme that is required for the synthesis of DNA. The recommended dose is 3.0 mg/kg SID PO (White, 2005). Duration of treatment is generally one week at this dose if there is a good response, followed by a tapering dose or interval during the following days or weeks, with continued monitoring for evidence of clinical relapse. Combination with dexamethasone (when possible) has also been successful in difficult cases. Although azathioprine is an immunosuppressive drug, and could cause bone marrow suppression, adverse effects in the horse have been rarely reported, even when it is used for several weeks (White, 2005).

Horses with IMHA due to extravascular phagocytosis that do not respond to corticosteroids and azathioprine could be treated by splenectomy, although it is important to rule out lymphoma prior to recommending the procedure.

Supportive care for IMHA includes transfusion of whole blood or packed red cells when required, to maintain adequate global delivery of oxygen to tissues. The need for transfusion can be determined by clinical findings, along with measurement of decreased hematocrit, increased blood lactate, and decreased venous oxygen concentration and saturation. Deciding upon a choice of RBC donor can be challenging, since autoagglutination of RBCs may already exist in the IMHA patient, making cross-matching more difficult to interpret. Mean post-transfusion survival of allogenic RBCs cross-matched compatible is reported to be 39 days in the recipient (Mudge, 2012).

For foals with NI, washed RBCs of the mare, or choosing a gelding of the same breed, are good donor selections when a cross-match is not feasible. Since NI cases are frequently due to transfer of antibodies against red cell surface Aa or Qa, having a pre-selected donor horse negative for Aa and Qa antigen and antibody is desirable, but difficult to find. Additional antigens, such as Pa, Dg, Ka or Qb, may occasionally be the causative antigen in NI (Boyle, 2005). Immunosuppressive therapy is not indicated for the treatment of NI, because of the short presence of maternally-derived antibodies against red cells, and the side-effects of general immunosuppression in foals.

Fluid therapy with an isotonic crystalloid may also be required if the patient is hypovolemic or hypotensive. Although crystalloid therapy will lower the HCT, it does not decrease the total number of RBCs. Without a blood transfusion, crystalloid therapy could be harmful when the HCT is less than 8%, as the viscosity of blood may become so low that it cannot maintain adequate capillary pressure.

Complications from IMHA include renal failure and laminitis. Foals with NI receiving multiple transfusions may develop liver disease, possibly related to iron overload (Boyle, 2005). NI foals also appear to be susceptible to sepsis, possibly associated with immunosuppression from the hemolytic disease, the transfusion, or both. Dogs with IMHA are reported to be pro-thrombotic with increased release of tissue factor (Kidd, 2013), but publication evidence for this in horses could not be found.

6.2.5 Prevention

Except for NI, prevention of tumor-, infection- and drug-associated anemia is difficult, due to the sporadic incidence of IMHA. There is usually no direct relationship between the given dose of a drug and the reaction. Memory cells and antibodies against drugs may persist for years, and previously affected horses should not receive the drug associated with the disorder.

If the foal has NI, or is determined to be at risk of NI, it should not be permitted to nurse the mare for 36 hours, the colostrum should be discarded, and another method of transfer of immunoglobulins (e.g., safe source of banked colostrum orally or plasma transfusion intravenously) instituted. Also, do not use colostrum from mares that have previously received blood transfusions, or from mares that have previous history of NI in their foals. Meanwhile, the foal is muzzled and fed milk replacer or another mare's milk, using a bottle or nasogastric intubation. To ensure adequate levels of antibodies, the foal's serum should be tested for immunoglobulin G levels.

Colostrum can be mixed with a drop of the foal's whole blood on a slide immediately after birth (and before nursing) in order to determine the presence of agglutination. If confirmation is necessary, a jaudince foal agglutination test uses serial dilutions of the dam's colostrum with saline (1 ml of 1 : 2, 1 : 4, 1 : 8, 1 : 16, and 1 : 32 dilutions; 1 ml saline is used as a negative control) mixed with one drop of the foal's whole blood. The mare's blood may also be tested in the same conditions as a negative control, and the presence of agglutination in the red cells may be observed after centrifugation for 2–3 minutes at a medium speed and inversion of the tubes. Minor cross-matching at the time of foaling tests for the presence of antibodies against the blood factors in colostrum or mare's serum. A positive Coombs' test is not specific for NI, but suggests blood group incompatibility.

The risk of NI can also be anticipated and avoided using blood factor assay, which tests for the presence or absence of factors Aa and Qa on the red cells of the dam and sire any time before breeding. If the dam does not have factors Aa or Qa, she is at risk of producing NI-causing antibodies, and she needs to be tested for antibodies before foaling. If the dam is positive for one of the blood groups, there is no risk for that specific blood group. If the sire is negative for both blood groups, there is minimal risk for the disease. In addition, the mare' serum can be cross-matched with the sire's red cells. A negative reaction indicates no risk for the foal, while a positive reaction indicates a 50% risk of NI, and a cross-matching test should be done at foaling or colostrum withheld.

Hemolytic assays test for antibodies against the blood factors in the mare serum within 30 days before foaling. Different dilutions of the serum from the mare are mixed with red cells expressing Aa or Qa or Ca (other factors may be tested in some laboratories). If antibodies are present in the mare's serum, they bind to the red cells (antigen-antibody complex) and, after adding rabbit complement, red cell lysis is induced. Cell lysis intensity is determined from 0–4, and the last dilution of serum that promoted cell lysis is identified. Serum dilutions above 1 : 16 for Aa and Qa that cause hemolysis *in vitro* may produce NI. Antibodies to Aa and Qa factors detected at 1 : 2 serum dilutions require re-test before foaling. Antibodies against Ca factor do not cause NI, but can cause false positive reactions.

6.3 Immune-mediated thrombocytopenia

6.3.1 Signalment and clinical signs

The most common clinical signs are epistaxis, and petechial and ecchymotic hemorrhages of the mucus membranes (Figure 6.4 and Figure 6.5). Less commonly, swollen joints (hemarthrosis), large subcutaneous swellings (hematomas) or internal bleeding can be present. These clinical signs may not be observed in many of the cases, unless platelet counts are below 30,000 platelets/mcL.

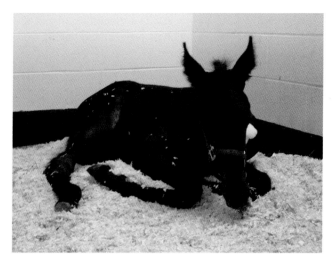

Figure 6.4 Immune-mediated thrombocytopenia.
Epistaxis in a two month old Standardbred foal with IMT after administration of trimethoprim sulfa for five days. Corticosteroids and azathioprine were used in the initial treatment, since the platelet count was <10,000 platelets/μl (Theresa Ollivett and Thomas Divers, Cornell University).

Neurologic signs (due to bleeding into the central nervous system) become more likely when platelet counts decrease to below 10,000 platelets/mcL (Bansal, 2014).

Fever is usually only present if there is an infectious disease. Treatment with trimethoprim-sulfa within the past 5–14 days would be supportive of a drug-induced immune thrombocytopenia. Concurrent neoplasia should be considered as a cause of IMT if drug-associated and infectious causes can be ruled out, and weight loss, anorexia, fever, or other signs attributable to neoplastic disorders are present.

Another disorder is neonatal alloimmune thrombocytopenia (NAIT) in horse and mule foals that ingest colostrum with alloantibody against platelet surface antigens (Perkins, 2005). Similarly to NI, the dam produces antibodies against paternally inherited, incompatible surface molecules on the foal platelets, and most foals affected do *not* have concomitant NI. Alloimmune thrombocytopenia will often develop in subsequent foals from the same mare, even when sired by a different stallion. Affected foals have petechiations or ecchymotic hemorrhages of mucus membranes, hematoma at the site of venipuncture, hematomas, hemoarthrosis, and hyphema and, in addition, dermatitis around the eyes, mouth, and sometimes over the elbow region (Figure 6.6).

Although the platelet counts in the affected foals are sometimes less than 2,000/mcL, life-threatening bleeding is rare. Megakaryocytic hyperplasia is an expected response to the platelet destruction in the periphery, but thrombocytopenia develops despite platelet production, because the binding of maternally-derived antibodies to platelets decreases platelet survival time to a few hours.

Horses with *Anaplasma phygocytophilia* infection often have platelet counts less than 60,000/mcL, but clinical findings

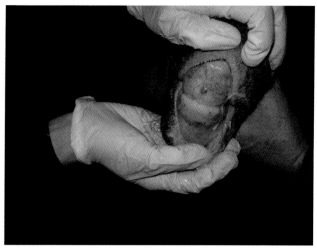

Figure 6.5 Alloimmune thrombocytopenia.
Ecchymosis on the oral mucosa of a foal with alloimune thrombocytopenia (Thomas Divers, Cornell University).

associated with the thrombocytopenia are rare. Evans syndrome, a rare hematological disease defined as Coombs'-positive hemolytic anemia and immune-mediated thrombocytopenia, was reported in a mare with less than 14,000 platelets/mcL and a PCV of 9.5%; the mare died from cerebral hemorrhage (Väänänen, 2013).

6.3.2 Immunologic mechanisms and etiologic associations

Immune-mediated thrombocytopenia is most often caused by hypersensitivity type II, with the binding of autoantibodies to platelet surface and consequent peripheral destruction in the spleen by the reticuloendothelial system. Alternatively, there may be impaired platelet production, due to autoantibodies targeting megakaryocytes in the bone marrow (Khan, 2010).

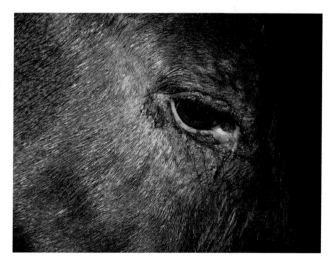

Figure 6.6 Alloimmune thrombocytopenia.
Dermatitis that is often develops concurrently with alloimmune thrombocytopenia in foals (Thomas Divers, Cornell University).

The immune-mediated thrombocytopenia may be classified as *primary*, when there is no underlying cause, or *secondary*, when associated with drug therapy, infectious diseases or known immunologic disorders. Drug-induced thrombocytopenia is most common in horses and foals that have been treated with trimethoprim-sulfa within five days prior to the onset of clinical signs. Although common in humans, heparin administration does not appear to be a common cause of drug-induced thrombocytopenia in horses.

Excessive removal of platelets my also occur, associated with absorption of antibody-antigen complexes onto their surfaces, often referred to as *innocent bystander* cause; platelets express Fc receptors that can bind to the constant region of antibodies. This may occur with bacterial (*Anaplasma phagocytophilium*), or viral infections (EIA), or immune reactions from vaccines.

Specific alloantigens associated with equine NAIT have not been proven, although several platelet membrane glycoproteins with polymorphism are known to occur, and may serve as potential alloantigens (Boudreaux, 2013).

Production of autoantibodies against platelets can be secondary to: lymphoma; hemangiosarcoma; bacterial antigens (*Streptococcus* spp, *Clostridium perfringens*, *Rhodococcus equi*); parasitic (uncommonly *Theleria equi* or *Babesia* caballi); viral (equine infectious anemia); or drug administration (trimethoprim-sulfa).

6.3.3 Diagnostics

There are no highly accurate diagnostic tests to confirm IMT. When the immune-mediated mechanism causes peripheral destruction of platelets, production in the bone marrow is pronounced, resulting in increased mean platelet volume (MPV) and positive reticular staining with New Methylene Blue, which detects RNA in megakaryocytes. Megakaryocytes may also be seen on peripheral blood smears, suggesting enhanced regeneration, and these findings can help support a diagnosis of IMT.

Coagulation profile often reveals prolonged bleeding time, abnormal clot retraction, slightly prolonged activated coagulation, elevated fibrinolytic degradating products (FDP), and normal prothrombin time (PT) and activated partial thromboplastin time (APTT).

Flow cytometry can be used to detect the percentage of antibody-covered platelets although, if the platelet count is extremely low, the interpretation becomes more difficult (McGurrin, 2004). In addition, platelets have Fc receptors that can bind the assay reagents (antibodies), and control samples are essential to interpretation of results.

Pseudothrombocytopenia is very common in blood samples collected in ethylenediaminetetraacetic acid (EDTA) anticoagulant tubes from healthy horse samples. A manual platelet count or test in citrate anticoagulant tubes can rule out thrombocytopenia, in addition to absence of clinical signs or other platelet blood indices.

Important differential diagnosis for ITP include: is excessive consumption of platelets due to disseminated intravascular coagulation (which can be assessed on clinical signs, and also coagulopathy laboratory findings), equine infectious anemia virus, and myelophthisic disease.

6.3.4 Treatment

The decision to treat IMT should be based more on evidence of clinical bleeding than on platelet count alone. Immunosuppressive treatments may be indicated when thrombocytopenia is progressive and/or life threatening. Horses with extremely low platelet counts (e.g., <10,000 mcL) might best be treated even without evidence of hemorrhage, since extremely low platelet counts have been associated with life-threatening intradural bleeding in other species. The two most commonly used immunosuppressive drugs are corticosteroids and azathioprine, and treatment recommendations follow similar guidelines for IMHA (described above).

The use of corticosteroids is the mainstay of first line therapy, and dexamethasone is generally the preferred type, based upon field response reports. Corticosteroids act through inhibition phagocytosis and antibody synthesis, improve platelet production and, possibly, increase microvascular stability. The average time for response to successful corticosteroid treatment is reported in humans to be 1–3 days. A similar response time has been seen in horses with doses of dexamethasone of 0.1 mg/kg SID IV. Doses as high as 0.2 mg/kg have been required in severe cases. Despite the risk of bleeding, intravenous injection of corticosteroids with a 20 gauge needle is preferred, and the vein compressed after drug administration for two minutes. Treatment is generally continued until the platelet count returns to normal, at which time corticosteroid treatment is slowly tapered. The duration of treatment should take into consideration the severity and half-life of IgG, as described for IMHA.

For horses that either do not respond to corticosteroids, or cannot be given high doses of the drug, azathioprine is an alternative treatment (Humber, 1991; Hardefeldt, 2010). The recommended dose is 0.3 mg/kg SID PO. Duration of treatment is generally one week at this dose. If there is a good response, a tapering dose and/or interval is planned during the following days or weeks, with continued monitoring for evidence of relapse of the immune-mediated disease. If IMT is life-threatening, platelet count is less than 10,000/mcL, or serious bleeding is noted, azathioprine and corticosteroids could be used simultaneously until the platelet counts have risen above 40,000/mcL, or when clinical bleeding is resolved.

Other therapies that have been used to treat refractory IMT include vincristine and plasma exchange. Administration of plasma products or concentrated immunoglobulin (IgG) may result in non-specific blockade of the Fc receptor of phagocytes of the reticuloendothelial system, and prevent platelet removal.

Whole blood transfusions or platelet-rich plasma can be administered, but rarely causes a dramatic increase in platelet count. Platelet transfusions are not recommended unless the platelet count is below 20,000/mcL and there is evidence of clinical bleeding. Thromboelastography measurement of maximum amplitude could be used to determine strength of clot if additional information is required regarding the need for transfusion. Centrifuged platelet-rich plasma at $150 \times g$ would be ideal for transfusion but, in practice, collection of citrated blood in plastic bags, followed by allowing the RBCs to settle, and then removing the plasma (which will contain most of the platelets), is an option for platelet transfusion (Dunkel, 2013). Glass bottles cannot be used for blood collection intended for platelet transfusion, because the glass activates platelets. If the transfusion cannot be immediately administered, then plasma should be stored at room temperature and not refrigerated, as this will have a negative effect on platelet function. Platelet survival after transfusion might be 4–5 days (Dunkel, 2013).

Take home message

Immune-mediated cytopenias are a result of antibody-mediated cell destruction, either centrally (in the bone marrow) or peripherally. The initial goal for diagnostics is to determine whether the disorder is central or peripheral.

These antibodies may be produced as a primary autoimmune disorder (autoantibodies or isoantibodies) after blood product transfusion, drug treatment, infections, tumors, or idiopathic causes, or they may be absorbed from colostrum (alloantibodies).

Cell destruction occurs upon binding of the autoantibody or alloantibody to the surface of targeted cells, and activation of complement (hypersensitivity type II).

In bone marrow origin anemia, MCV is low and RDW normal. In immune-mediated hemolytic anemia, peripheral red cell destruction causes increases in both MCV and RDW (release of larger than normal red cells from the bone marrow and/or reticulocytosis when detected by automated equipment), discolored serum and urine (when intravascular hemolysis), positive Coombs' test, and positive detection of antibodies attached to the surface of red cells using flow cytometry.

In intravascular red cell destruction, activation of complement leads to rapid cell lysis. Therefore, the serum and plasma may be pink, or at least jaundiced, and urine may be discolored red due to hemoglobinuria. In extravascular hemolysis, cells are primarily removed by the reticulo-endothelial (mononuclear phagocyte) system, and serum and urine discoloration will not be detected.

In immune-mediated thrombocytopenia, coagulation profile often reveals prolonged bleeding time, abnormal clot retraction, slightly prolonged activated coagulation, elevated fibrinolytic degradating products (FDP), and normal prothrombin time (PT) and activated partial thromboplastin time (APTT).

Treatment for immune-mediated cytopenias is based on clinical and treatment history, and include: removing the insulting element (e.g., discontinue drug, treat infection), when possible; using immunosuppressive therapy; promoting blood product transfusions when life-threatening disorders occur; and providing supportive care.

6.3.5 Prevention

Prevention of drug-associated thrombocytopenia is difficult, due to its sporadic incidence. There is usually no direct relationship between the given dose of drug and the reaction. Antibodies against these drugs may persist for years, and previously-affected horses should not receive the drug associated with the disorder.

6.4 Immune-mediated neutropenia

6.4.1 Signalment and clinical signs

Immune-mediated neutropenia may be seen concurrently with immune disorders that also cause thrombocytopenia or anemia. Neutropenia is relatively common in foals with NIMT, and is sometimes seen with NI. Neutropenia increases the risk of infection, fevers and sepsis, and other clinical signs depend upon the body site involved.

6.4.2 Immunologic mechanisms and etiologic associations

Immune-mediated neutropenia may occur from similar hypersensitivity type II mechanisms, as previously described for IMHA and IMT, and it includes alloimmune and autoimmune (primary) responses against circulating neutrophils or neutrophil precursors in the bone marrow, or secondary immune reaction associated with drug administration, infectious disease or neoplasia.

Autoantibodies may be directed against membrane antigens of neutrophils located on the IgG Fc receptor, causing their peripheral destruction. Alloimmune neonatal neutropenia has also been described in a foal with NI (Wong, 2012), and in foals with alloimmune thrombocytopenia (Perkins, 2005).

6.4.3 Diagnostics

The tentative diagnosis of immune-mediated neutropenia is made by finding a persistent mature neutropenia in the absence of bacterial, viral, toxic or drug-related causes. Anti-neutrophil equine antibodies can be detected by either agglutination test or by flow cytometry, although the interpretation may be difficult, due to the low number of neutrophils in the sample (Davis, 2003). In addition, neutrophils have Fc receptors that can bind the assay reagents (antibodies), and control samples are essential to interpretation of results.

Response to immunosuppressive therapy could also support the diagnosis. Differential diagnosis for severe neutropenia in neonatal foals should include perinatal equine herpesvirus-1 (EHV-1) infection, prematurity and severe sepsis.

6.4.4 Treatment and prevention

Neonatal alloimmune neutropenia generally improves within the first three weeks of life, when the maternally-derived antibodies decline. Treatment is generally conservative, with early antimicrobial treatment. Granulocyte colony-stimulating factor (G-CSF, 3–10 µg/kg IV or SQ, SID, with tapering doses) can be administered to increase production and release of neutrophils from the bone marrow, and this may help to prevent secondary infections. If the immune-mediated neutropenia is believed to be secondary immune-mediated disease or autoimmune, but not alloimmune processes, then corticosteroids might be indicated. Corticosteroid administration in IMN is controversial, and may not be as effective as it is in IMHA and IMT.

References

Angel, K.L., Spano, J.S., Schumacher, J. and Kwapien, R.P. (1991). Myelophthisic pancytopenia in a pony mare. *Journal of the American Veterinary Medical Association* **198**(6), 1039–1042.

Bansal, D., Rajendran, A. and Singhi, S. (2014). Newly diagnosed immune thrombocytopenia: update on diagnosis and management. *Indian Journal of Pediatrics* **81**(10), 1033–1041.

Boudreaux, M.K. and Humphries, D.M. (2013). Identification of potential platelet alloantigens in the Equidae family by comparison of gene sequences encoding major platelet membrane glycoproteins. *Veterinary Clinical Pathology* **42**(4), 437–442.

Boyle, A.G., Magdesian, K.G. and Ruby, R.E. (2005). Neonatal isoerythrolysis in horse foals and a mule foal: 18 cases (1988–2003). *Journal of the American Veterinary Medical Association* **227**(8), 1276–1283.

Davis, E.G., Rush, B., Bain, F., Clark-Price, S. and Wilkerson, M.J. (2003). Neonatal neutropenia in an Arabian foal. *Equine Veterinary Journal* **35**(5), 517–520.

Dunkel, B. (2013). Platelet transfusion in thrombocytopenic horses. *Equine Veterinary Education* **25**(7), 359–362.

Hardefeldt, L.Y., Schambow, R. and Peek, S.F. (2010). Successful treatment of presumptive immune mediated thrombocytopenia and dermatitis with azathioprine in a pregnant mare. *Equine Veterinary Education* **22**(10), 495–500.

Humber, K.A., Beech, J., Cudd, T.A., Palmer, J.E., Gardner, S.Y. and Sommer, M.M. (1991). Azathioprine for treatment of immune-mediated thrombocytopenia in two horses. *Journal of the American Veterinary Medical Association* **199**(5), 591–594.

Kelton, D.R., Holbrook, T.C., Gilliam, L.L., Rizzi, T.E., Brosnahan, M.M. and Confer, A.W. (2008). Bone marrow necrosis and myelophthisis: manifestation of T-cell lymphoma in a horse. *Veterinary Clinical Pathology* **37**(4), 403–408.

Khan, M. and Mikhael, J. (2010). A review of immune thrombocytopenic purpura: focus on the novel thrombopoietin agonists. *Journal of Blood Medicine* **1**, 21–31.

Kidd, L. and Mackman, N. (2013). Prothrombotic mechanisms and anticoagulant therapy in dogs with immune-mediated hemolytic anemia. *Journal of Veterinary Emergency and Critical Care* **23**(2), 3–13.

Lavoie, J.P., Morris, D.D., Zink, J.G., Lloyd, K. and Divers, T.J. (1987). Pancytopenia caused by bone marrow aplasia in a horse. *Journal of the American Veterinary Medical Association* **191**(11), 1462–1464.

McGurrin, M.K., Arroyo, L.G. and Bienzle, D. (2004). Flow cytometric detection of platelet-bound antibody in three horses with immune-mediated thrombocytopenia. *Journal of the American Veterinary Medical Association* **224**(1), 83–87.

Messer, N.T., IV and Arnold, K. (1991). Immune-mediated hemolytic anemia in a horse. *Journal of the American Veterinary Medical Association* **198**(8), 1415–1416.

Michel, M. (2011). Classification and therapeutic approaches in auto-immune hemolytic anemia: an update. *Expert Review of Hematology* **4**(6), 607–618.

Mudge, M.C., Walker, N.J., Borjesson, D.L., Librach, F., Johns, J.L. and Owens, S.D. (2012). Post-transfusion survival of biotin-labeled allogeneic RBCs in adult horses. *Veterinary Clinical Pathology* **41**(1), 56–62.

Owens, S.D., Snipes, J., Magdesian, K.G. and Christopher, M.M. (2008). Evaluation of a rapid agglutination method for detection of equine red cell surface antigens (Ca and Aa) as part of pretransfusion testing. *Veterinary Clinical Pathology* **37**(1), 49–56.

Perkins, G.A., Miller, W.H., Divers, T.J., Clark, C.K., Belgrave, R.L. and Sellon, D.C. (2005). Ulcerative dermatitis, thrombocytopenia, and neutropenia in neonatal foals. *Journal of Veterinary Internal Medicine* **19**(2), 211–216.

Piercy, R.J., Swardson, C.J. and Hinchcliff, K.W. (1998). Erythroid hypoplasia and anemia following administration of recombinant human erythropoietin in two horses. *Journal of the American Veterinary Medical Association* **212**(2), 244–247.

Salama, A. (2009). Drug-induced immune hemolytic anemia. *Expert Opinion on Drug Safety* **8**(1), 73–79.

Väänänen, L., Sihvo, H.K. and Hewetson, M. (2013). Cerebral haemorrhage in a pregnant Standardbred mare with Evan's syndrome. *Equine Veterinary Education* **25**(7), 353–358.

White, S., Maxwell, L.K., Szabo, N.J., Hawkins, J.L. and Kollias-Baker, C. (2005). Pharmacokinetics of azathioprine following single-dose intravenous and oral administration and effects of azathioprine following chronic oral administration in horses. *American Journal of Veterinary Research* **66**(9), 1578–1583.

Wilkerson, M.J., Davis, E., Shuman, W., Harkin, K., Cox, J. and Rush, B. (2000). Isotype-specific antibodies in horses and dogs with immune-mediated hemolytic anemia. *Journal of Veterinary Internal Medicine* **14**(2), 190–196.

Wong, D.M., Alcott, C.J., Clark, S.K., Jones, D.E., Fisher, P.G. and Sponseller, B.A. (2012). Alloimmune neonatal neutropenia and neonatal isoerythrolysis in a Thoroughbred colt. *Journal of Veterinary Diagnostic Investigation* **24**(1), 219–226.

7 Bullous Diseases of the Skin and Mucosa

Jeanine Peters-Kennedy and Rebecca E. Ruby

7.1 Definition

The diseases covered within this chapter include the bullous diseases of the skin and mucous membranes, caused by immune-mediated destruction of a particular component of the epidermis or basement membrane zone, which are characterized by vesicle and bullae formation. The diseases discussed include bullous pemphigoid, cutaneous drug reactions, discoid lupus erythematosus, systemic lupus erythematosus, erythema multiforme and the pemphigus complex, which is comprised of pemphigus foliaceous, pemphigus vulgaris and paraneoplastic pemphigus.

The initiating factors, diagnosis and prognosis of these diseases are varied, and accurate diagnosis will ensure the best management approach and prognosis (Table 7.1). Vesicles can form with a variety of non-immune-mediated diseases in horses, including contact dermatitis, viral infection, photosensitivity, vasculitis, thermal burns, urticarial and various hypersensitivities (Hargis, 2001). As with any clinical presentation, a full clinical history will assist in narrowing the differential diagnosis list.

7.2 Immune-mediated bullous dermatoses

Immune-mediated bullous dermatoses of horses are rare. They can be divided into *primary or autoimmune*, when the lesions are caused by autoantibodies or activated lymphocytes that develop against self-antigens; or *secondary*, when tissue destruction results from an immune response that is directed against nonself-antigens (e.g., drugs, pathogens).

Both vesicles and bullae are intraepidermal or subepidermal sharply demarcated elevated lesions that are filled with clear fluid. Vesicles are up to 1 cm in diameter, and bullae have a diameter greater than 1 cm. Bullae and vesicles are thin, fragile and often transient structures that are prone to rupture, leading to secondary lesions of ulceration and crusts, the most common presentation seen by veterinarians. The dermatologic signs are clinically nonspecific, and cytological and histological evaluations are required for a diagnosis.

7.2.1 Immunologic mechanisms and etiologic associations

The pathomechanisms of autoimmune skin diseases in horses are not well understood. They develop spontaneously, and precipitating factors may not be detected. Autoimmune disease may result from a normal immune response to an abnormal antigen, or can result from an abnormal immune response to a normal antigen. The second category is thought to be the most significant from the perspective of clinical disease. In addition, autoimmune diseases may result from an aberrant response to a single specific antigen, or may be due to a general defect in the regulation of B or T cell functions. Autoimmunity has been associated with a variety of factors, such as: hidden antigens; antigens generated by molecular changes; molecular mimicry; receptor editing; alterations in antigen processing; failure of regulatory control; viral-induced; and microchimers (Tizzard, 2009).

Causes of bullae and vesicle formation include viral diseases that cause ballooning degeneration and immune-mediated dermatoses, characterized by acantholysis, hydropic degeneration, apoptosis/necrosis of basal keratinocytes or subepidermal clefting. They also may occur in dermatitis caused by irritants.

7.2.2 Diagnostics
7.2.2.1 Skin samples
The diagnosis of immune-mediated dermatoses requires demonstration of specific histopathologic features and, ideally, the presence of autoantibodies, immune-complexes or specific cell mediators involved in the immunologic injury. In general, when taking skin samples, it is most useful to obtain fully developed primary lesions with intact vesicles or bullae. Punch biopsies are often satisfactory for most inflammatory and immune-mediated dermatoses, and may be used with small vesicular lesions. However, if the lesion to be biopsied is a bullae or ulcer, wedge biopsy by scalpel excision is preferred.

Multiple biopsy specimens (ideally, 3–5) should always be taken because diagnostic changes can be focal. Secondary lesions, such as crusts, can be diagnostic, especially in cases of pemphigus. Crusts are essentially old pustules, and they may contain acantholytic keratinocytes diagnostic for pemphigus. In the case of ulcerated lesions, biopsy samples should be taken at the edge, with some intact epidermis. Immunopathologic testing

Equine Clinical Immunology, First Edition. Edited by M. Julia B. Felippe.
© 2016 John Wiley & Sons, Inc. Published 2016 by John Wiley & Sons, Inc.

Table 7.1 Summary of the major immune-mediated diseases of horses.

Disease	Site of damage	Mechanism/site of immune targeting	Prognosis
Pemphigus foliaceus	Stratum corneum/granulosum	Desmoglein 1*	Variable, depending on age
Pemphigus vulgaris	Suprabasilar	Desmoglein 3*	Grave
Bullous pemphigoid	Dermal-epidermal junction	Collagen XVII	Poor
Cutaneous drug reaction	Variable	Unknown	Good if drug identified and withdrawn
Erythema multiforme	Keratinocyte	Cell-mediated immunity	Variable based on severity
Systemic lupus erythematosus	Basal keratinocytes/basement membrane zone	Multifactorial	Variable, depending on body systems involved
Discoid lupus erythematosus	Basal keratinocytes/basement membrane zone	Multifactorial	Good with treatment

*major antigen in human, pathogenesis not completely understood in horses.

on tissue specimens may require biopsy samples to be fresh, frozen or in a special fixative, and it is recommended to consult with the veterinary immunopathology laboratory before obtaining and submitting samples for these tests.

When submitting skin biopsy samples, it is best to request evaluation by a veterinary pathologist with an interest or specialization in dermatopathology, or a veterinary dermatologist trained in dermatopathology. Submission of a full clinical history, detailed description of the skin lesions and digital photographs, will aid in the interpretation of the biopsy. If the patient is on immunosuppressive therapy then, when possible, there should be a withdrawal period of at least three weeks for oral and topical corticosteroids, and six weeks for injectable corticosteroids.

7.2.2.2 Immunotesting

Direct immunofluorescence shows the presence of immune complexes in the skin biopsy taken from the patient using fresh biopsy samples. Common locations of immune complex deposition include the dermo-epidermal junction and dermal blood vessels. Typically, a laboratory uses a panel of antibodies that includes IgG, IgA, IgM, and complement. In human medicine, the nature of the immune deposits, the site of deposits, the pattern of deposition, and a semi-quantitative grading of strength of fluorescence, are reported. Based on this interpretation, the biopsy is categorized as vasculitis, bullous disease or lupus. In horses, a linear deposition of immunoglobulin at the dermal-epidermal junction is consistent with an autoimmune disease, but more specific patterns are not well recognized. Consensus in human and veterinary medicine is that an immunofluorescence test is inadequate for interpretation without concurrent histopathologic evaluation.

Indirect immunofluorescence measures the presence of antigen-specific antibodies (autoantibodies) in the patient's serum. This method uses a standardized normal skin biopsy prepared with a salt-split technique, which is bathed in the patient's serum. The pattern of fluorescence corresponds with the level of immunoglobulin deposition. The salt-split preparation widens the epidermal-dermal junction and allows for clear interpretation of whether immunoglobulin is present on the dermal or epidermal component of the basement membrane.

Immunohistochemistry for IgG, IgA and IgM may be performed on formalin fixed skin biopsies, and this is typically done following evaluation of the hematoxylin and eosin staining. This method requires minimal processing, and may show antibody deposition in various locations of the dermis.

7.2.2.3 Classification

Autoimmune dermatoses are classified on the basis of the specific autoallergen being targeted. Specific identification requires techniques such as immunoprecipitation, immunoblotting, and antigen-specific enzyme-linked immunosorbent assay (ELISA). These types of testing are only offered in veterinary immunologic research laboratories. Other tests for immune-mediated and autoimmune skin disease include direct immunofluorescence and immunohistochemistry for detection of autoantibodies, immunoglobulins, and complement within biopsy specimens; and indirect immunofluorescence on serum for the detection of circulating autoantibodies. The later has a high rate of false negatives (Scott, 2011). In addition, these tests may be positive in normal horses. Intercellular and basement membrane zone deposition of immunoglobulins and complement components can occasionally be detected in inflammatory dermatoses (Scott, 2011).

In general, these tests are not warranted for the work-up of most cases. Histopathology and clinical presentation are generally sufficiently diagnostic (Scott, 2011). It should be understood that different diseases, or variants of disease, can have similar histopathologic and/or clinical characteristics and, therefore, may be lumped together.

7.2.3 Treatment and prognosis

In general, drugs with potent immunosuppressive and immunomodulatory effects are used for the treatment of immune-mediated and autoimmune bullous diseases of the skin and mucous membranes of horses.

Glucocorticoids are the most common class of drugs used as immunosuppressant agents to treat immune-mediated bullous skin diseases in horses. Glucocorticoids have a profound and broad effect on immunologic and inflammatory activity, but vary in their relative potency. Optimal therapeutic doses have not been scientifically established for any equine dermatoses. In addition, glucocorticoids can be used alone, or in combination with other therapies, for all of the conditions discussed in this chapter.

In horses, prednisolone or dexamethasone are the most common choices. Immunosuppressive doses of prednisolone in horses are 2–4 mg/kg every 24 hours (Scott, 2011). Immunosuppressive doses of dexamethasone are 0.1–0.2 mg/kg SID PO or IV, and higher doses have been described (Scott, 2011). A therapeutic dose should be given until signs of remission are observed, and then tapered to the lowest possible therapeutic dose. Side-effects from glucocorticoids include: polyphagia; polydipsia/polyuria; behavioral changes; and hypothalamic-pituitary-adrenal (HPA)-axis suppression. Adverse side-effects include: laminitis; gastrointestinal ulceration; diarrhea; hepatopathy; diabetes; hyperlipidemia; hypothyroidism; decreased protein synthesis; delayed wound healing; and secondary infections due to immune suppression (Papich, 2007; Scott, 2011).

Azathioprine is a thioprine immunosuppressive drug that is metabolized to 6-mercaptopurine (6-MP), which interferes with purine metabolism and DNA synthesis in lymphocytes (Papich, 2007). Azathioprine primarily affects rapidly proliferating cells, with its greatest effect on cell-mediated immunity and T-lymphocyte dependent antibody synthesis (Papich, 2007). Azathioprine is usually used in conjunction with systemic corticosteroids for patients that either do not respond to corticosteroids alone, or for a steroid sparing effect in patients with severe corticosteroid side effects. Azathioprine may be beneficial for the treatment of horses with pemphigus foliaceous, pemphigus vulgaris, bullous pemphigoid, and discoid and systemic lupus erythematosus. It may take 3–6 weeks to see clinical improvement (Scott, 2011).

The dosage of azathioprine for horses is 2–3 mg/kg SID PO until clinical response is achieved, and then continued every other day for 30–60 days, with slow tapering to the lowest possible therapeutic dose. Corticosteroids should also be tapered to the lowest possible therapeutic dose, and can be used on alternate days when azathioprine is not given.

Azathioprine treatment potential side effects include: bone marrow suppression (anemia, leukopenia, thrombocytopenia); hypersensitivity reactions; hepatotoxicity; pancreatitis; skin rashes; and alopecia. Significant toxicity in humans and companion animals are possible, but adverse reactions have not been reported in horses (Papich, 2007; Scott, 2011). However, it is recommended to monitor patients initially every two weeks, with complete blood count and serum biochemistry panels. Maintenance monitoring every 4–12 months is recommended, depending on the patient's clinical history.

Pentoxifylline is a methylxanthine derivative that is primarily used as a hemorheological agent, by decreasing blood viscosity and blood flow through narrow vessels, and decreasing platelet aggregation (Liska, 2006). As a phosphodiesterase inhibitor, it suppresses the synthesis of leukotrienes and many inflammatory cytokines, such as interleukin-1 (IL-1), IL-6, and tumor necrosis factor alpha (TNF-alpha), and may inhibit lymphocyte activation (Papich, 2007). Although most reports are anecdotal, pentoxifylline may be beneficial for the use of pemphigus foliaceous in the horse, dosed at 10 mg/kg BID PO. Clinical improvement may not be noted for 4–8 weeks. Side-effects are generally minimal, and include transient sweating, behavior change and conjunctivitis (Scott, 2011).

Chrysotherapy is the use of gold (gold sodium thiomalate, aurothioglucose) as a therapeutic agent. It is generally only considered after failure with corticosteroids and azathioprine. Gold inhibits the epidermal enzymes that may be responsible for blister formation in pemphigus (Scott, 2011). Gold compounds are reported to modulate many phases of immune and inflammatory responses, but the exact mechanism is unknown. Gold reduces the release of inflammatory mediators such as lysosomal enzymes, histamine, and prostaglandin; inactivates complement components; interferes with immunoglobulin synthesizes; inhibits T cell proliferation; suppresses IL-2 and IL-2 receptor synthesis; and inhibits IL-5 mediated eosinophil survival (Scott, 2011). In human patients, reported side-effects include skin eruptions, oral reactions, proteinuria, and bone marrow depression. However, side-effects have not been reported in horses (Scott, 2011).

During the induction phase, hemograms and urinalyses should be performed weekly, and monthly thereafter (Scott, 2011). Gold compounds should not be used in pregnant animals, animals with blood dyscrasias, hepatic or renal disease (Scott, 2011). Aurothioglucose (unavailable in the USA) and gold sodium thiomalate have been reported to be effective in the treatment of equine pemphigus foliaceous (Scott, 2011). Injections should be delayed for four weeks following the discontinuation of azathioprine. Horses are given 1 mg/kg IM weekly until remission occurs (Scott, 2011). Sixteen weeks of therapy may be necessary to see clinical improvement. After remission, the dose is given every two weeks for one month, and then monthly thereafter. Some patients may go into complete remission.

7.3 Pemphigus complex

The pemphigus complex is a group of uncommon-to-rare diseases, characterized by the presence of autoantibodies that target molecules (i.e., desmogleins, desmocollins, desmoplakin, envoplakin, periplakin, plakoglobin, pemphaxin, cholinergic receptors) needed for keratinocyte cell-to-cell adhesion. The resulting destruction leads to loss of keratinocyte adhesion, called acantholysis. Autoantibodies can be produced against various components of the desmosome, and the classification of pemphigus depends on the level where intraepidermal splitting occurs.

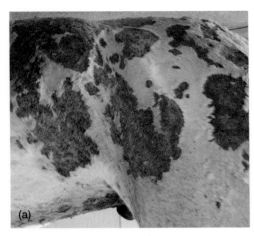 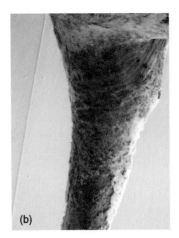 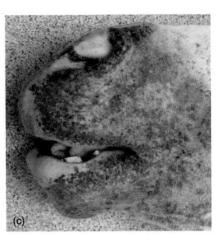

Figure 7.1 Pemphigus foliaceous: Horse with widespread annular alopecia and thick crusts over the **(a)** trunk, **(b)** limb and **(c)** muzzle (Courtesy of Bhupinder Bawa, BVSc, MVSc, PhD, DACVP).

The severity and location of the clinical lesions are related to which components of the desmosome are targeted by autoantibodies. In humans, mucosal dominant pemphigus vulgaris has autoantibodies against desmoglein III. Humans with pemphigus foliaceous have autoantibodies against desmoglein I (Dsg-1). In cases where pemphigus vulgaris progresses to more cutaneous involvement, antidesmoglein I antibodies are produced. The reason for this is unknown, but it may be due to *epitope spreading*, when an immune response to a primary antigen causes tissue damage and exposes self-antigens that then become targeted. Injection of these human autoantibodies into neonatal mice reproduces cutaneous lesions in the patient, and highlights the complexity of lesion distribution.

7.3.1 Pemphigus foliaceus

Pemphigus foliaceus (PF), an intraepidermal vesiculo-pustular disease, is uncommon-to-rare, but is the most common form of pemphigus and the most common autoimmune skin disease of horses. It has also been recognized in humans, dogs, cats, goats and llamas. Autoantibodies are directed against components of desmosomes in the stratified squamous epithelium –notably the stratum corneum or stratum granulosum – which leads to loss of intercellular cohesion (acantholysis) and vesicle/bullae formation within the epidermis.

7.3.1.1 Signalment and clinical signs

There is no breed, age or sex predilection for PF. The condition has been reported in horses ranging from two months to 25 years. PF has also been reported to occur during pregnancy and, in one case, resolved after the mare aborted (Zabel, 2005). In human patients, a link between certain MHC class II alleles and ethnic groups of pemphigus patients exists, suggesting a genetic influence (Grando, 2012). Genetic factors also appear to be important in dogs (Scott, 2011).

Clinical signs may be preceded by stress, drug administration, systemic disease, or hypersensitivity (urticaria). The earliest clinical sign is edema of the ventral abdomen and distal extremities (Vandenabeel, 2004; Zabel, 2005; Scott, 2011). Skin lesions commonly begin on the face, legs, or ventrum. Coronary bands, prepuce and mammary glands may be affected in some cases. Frequently, lesions become generalized within 1–3 months.

The most consistent and prominent lesions in horses with PF are crusts (see Figures 7.1a, b, and c). Lesions begin as vesicles, bullae or pustules, but these are fragile and often very transient lesions that quickly progress to crusts, annular erosions, epidermal collarettes, annular areas of alopecia, and variable degrees of oozing, matted hair coat, and scaling. The disease often involves the mucocutaneous junctions, but the mucous membranes are less often involved. Pruritus and pain are variable, but have been reported in up to 50% of cases of PF. Skin lesions may wax and wane.

Systemic signs, such as fever, depression, lethargy, anorexia, weight loss, nonregenerative anemia, neutrophilia, hypoalbuminemia, hyperglobulinemia, hyperfibrinogenemia and increased levels of alkaline phosphatase, have all been reported. (Vandenabeel, 2004; Zabel, 2005; Scott, 2011).

7.3.1.2 Immunologic mechanisms and etiologic associations

The major antigen involved in PF in humans is Dsg-1 (Freedberg, 2003). Desmogleins are glycoproteins of the cadherin family that allow the formation of desmosomes via a Ca^{2+} dependent homophilic interaction (Miragliotta, 2006). Desmosomes are cell-cell adhesion systems that contribute to the mechanical integrity of the epidermis by linking to keratin intermediate filaments and connecting the cytoskeleton of adjacent keratinocytes. Dsg-1 is thought to be a minor antigen in dogs, and desmocollin 1 may be an important PF antigen in the dog; however, more studies are warranted (Olivry, 2006a, 2009). The exact antigen in the horse has not been identified. Dsg-1 has been identified in the muzzle of a healthy horse using immunohistochemistry and immunoblotting (Miragliotta, 2006).

In horses, a range of conditions has been proposed to initiate autoantibody formation, including insect hypersensitivity, seasonal atopic dermatitis, and ultraviolet light, particularly in PF that recur or intensify on a seasonal warm weather basis. Equine PF has been reported in a group of horses that had *Culicoides* hypersensitivity for 1–3 years (Scott, 2011). Stress and systemic disease may also be triggers. Drugs such as penicillin, trimethoprim/sulfamethoxazole, vaccines, dewormers, and various supplements have been associated with PF (Vandenabeele, 2004; Zabel, 2005; Scott, 2011; Miller, 2013).

In human patients, an endemic form of PF called fogo selvagem (Portuguese: wild fire) has been correlated with exposure to black fly bites (Freedberg, 2003; Scott, 2011). Interestingly, foods containing thiols, isothiocyanates, phenols and tannins – similar to the molecular components of some of the more common drug triggers – have been implicated in cases of human PF (Brenner, 1998). It is thought that the drugs and their metabolites can bind to the cell membrane as haptens, causing inadequate cell-cell adhesion or changing the conformation of the cell-surface antigens and, consequently, leading to antibody production and acantholysis (Vandenabeele, 2004).

7.3.1.3 Diagnostics

Definitive diagnosis of PF is based on history, physical examination, cytology, and skin biopsy. Cytology often reveals variable numbers of non-degenerate neutrophils and/or eosinophils with acantholytic keratinocytes (Figure 7.2a). An acantholytic keratinocyte is an epidermal or follicular epithelial cell that has lost its intercellular attachments. These cells are rounded, and have normal to hypereosinophilic cytoplasm with hematoxylin and eosin stain. Histopathologic features of PF include subcorneal to intragranular vesicle and pustular formation that may span multiple follicles (Figure 7.2b).

Pustules contain predominantly non-degenerate neutrophils, with variable numbers of eosinophils, and individual to rafts of acantholytic keratinocytes. Similar pustules may occur in the follicular outer root sheath. In cases in which pustules are difficult to demonstrate clinically, biopsy of crusts may also demonstrate large numbers of acantholytic keratinocytes. Dermal infiltrates are generally mild and are composed of variable perivascular infiltrates of lymphocytes, neutrophils and eosinophils.

Differential diagnoses of PF in horses include diseases characterized by scaling and crusting, including: dermatophytosis; dermatophilosis; bacterial folliculitis; sarcoidosis; multisystemic eosinophilic epitheliotropic disease; seborrhea; cutaneous adverse drug reaction; and epitheliotropic lymphoma (Miller, 2013). Dermatophytosis due to *Trichophyton equinum* can produce both clinical signs of PF and histopathologic evidence of acantholysis, and should be ruled out with cytology, fungal culture, and/or special histochemical stains on biopsy specimens (Scott, 1994; Miller, 2013).

7.3.1.4 Treatment and prognosis

Treatment options for PF are described as for bullous dermatoses, and include corticosteroids, azathioprine, pentoxifylline, or gold sodium thiomalate. Spontaneous remission of PF is rare, but has been reported (Scott, 2011). Prognosis appears to be associated with age, with horses under one year old having a better prognosis, and those over five years old a less favorable prognosis (Zabel, 2005). PF may be worse and more difficult to control in hot, humid environments (Miller, 2013). Many horses require lifelong treatment, while a portion can be weaned off of treatment. Up to 50% of horses relapse months to years later. Those with multiple rapid relapses may be more difficult to control, with subsequent recurrences (Miller, 2013). Reasons for euthanasia include laminitis associated with corticosteroid administration, and the need for long-term medication in some cases.

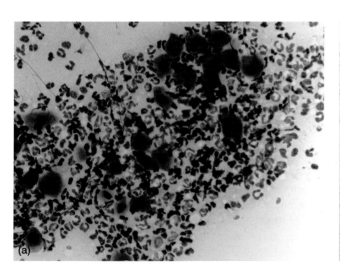
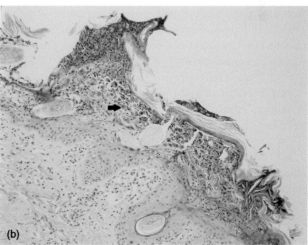

Figure 7.2 Pemphigus foliaceus: (**a**) Cytology shows numerous nondegenerate neutrophils and moderate numbers of acantholytic keratinocytes; magnification 400× (courtesy of William Miller, VMD, DACVD, Cornell University, Ithaca, NY).
(**b**) Photomicrograph of horse with pemphigus foliaceous demonstrating a large subcorneal pustule with numerous acantholytic keratinocytes (arrow); magnification 100× (Rebecca Ruby, BVSc, MS, Cornell University).

7.3.2 Pemphigus vulgaris

7.3.2.1 Signalment and clinical signs

Pemphigus vulgaris (PV) is a very rare severe vesiculobullous and ulcerative autoimmune disease. It has been reported in humans, dogs, cats, a llama, a pig-tailed macaque and horses (Winfield, 2013). The most common presentation is ulceration, crusting and vesicle formation on the mucocutaneous junctions and oral mucosa. Corneal ulceration may also occur (Scott, 2011; Winfield, 2013). Ulcers coalesce and spread, leading to lesions that are larger than the original bullae, and may be painful and/or pruritic. Systemic signs of fever, anorexia, depression, dysphagia, and weight loss are common, the latter particularly with extensive oral involvement (Miller, 2013).

7.3.2.2 Immunologic mechanisms and etiologic associations

Pemphigus vulgaris may be caused by a *primary* autoimmune response against self-antigens, or *secondary* to an immune-response against nonself-antigens. In humans and dogs, PV may occur secondary to drug administration, and cessation of treatment is curative. Self-antigen desmoglein 3, a transmembrane desmosomal cadherin of keratinocytes, is the targeted antigen when PV is confined to oral mucous membranes in dogs and humans. In cases where PV involves haired skin, other antigens, such as Dsg-1, may be targeted. In a reported case of a Welsh pony stallion with PV, anti-Dsg-3 antibodies were measured in the serum (Winfield, 2013).

7.3.2.3 Diagnostics

Diagnosis of PV is made by history, physical examination and skin biopsy. The characteristic histopathologic finding in PV is a suprabasilar cleft with acantholysis, leading to vesicle or bulla formation. The bullae may separate from the basal cells, leaving a layer of rounded cells, often referred to as a *row of tombstones* (Winfield, 2013). Bullae are minimally inflamed when intact but secondary ulceration leads to increased inflammatory cells and exudation of fibrin and serum. Direct immunofluorescence or immunohistochemistry may be positive, and the presence of autoantibodies against Dsg-3 detected.

7.3.2.4 Treatment and prognosis

Pemphigus vulgaris holds a grave prognosis, with no successful treatment reported in horses (Scott, 2011).

7.3.3 Paraneoplastic pemphigus

Paraneoplastic pemphigus (PNP) occurs in humans and dogs. In people, most cases are associated with lymphoproliferative neoplasms (Zhu, 2007). In humans, PNP is characterized by five diagnostic criteria:

1 the presence of painful, progressive stomatitis and a polymorphous skin eruption;

2 histological evidence of suprabasalar acantholysis, multilevel apoptotic keratinocytes, with satellitosis and interface dermatitis;

3 presence of autoantibody detection in direct and/or indirect immunofluorescence studies;

4 detection of anti-plakin autoantibodies and/or anti-desmoglein antibodies by immunoblotting or immunoprecipitation; and

5 the presence of an associated neoplasm (Freedberg, 2003; Choi, 2012).

Three cases have been reported in dogs, which presented thymic lymphoma, thymoma and undifferentiated sarcoma, respectively (Olivry, 2006b). In two of the three dogs reported, circulating anti-plakin and anti-Dsg-3 autoantibodies were demonstrated (Olivry, 2006a).

7.3.3.1 Signalment and clinical signs

A single case of putative PNP has been reported in a six year old Tennessee Walking Horse gelding (Williams, 1995). Blisters and bullae were found within the oral cavity and lip, and a large sarcoma was found on the neck. The histologic findings from the oral lesions showed subepithelial clefts and vesicles, with destruction of the basement membrane, changes that were consistent with bullous pemphigoid. Results of autoantibody testing were equivocal. Indirect immunofluorescence indicated positive staining of the cell surface of keratinocytes and transitional epithelium of the urinary bladder, which is a pattern characteristic for pemphigus-like antibodies. Following surgical removal of the mass, the horse's attitude and oral lesions improved, and the horse was found to be clinically normal 14 months later. The authors concluded that this case should be classified as either paraneoplastic pemphigus or paraneoplastic pemphigoid, with the immunoprecipitation findings supporting paraneoplastic pemphigus, while the histologic findings were consistent with paraneoplastic pemphigoid. This case fulfilled four of the five criteria in human medicine, with inconsistent histopathologic findings.

7.3.3.2 Immunologic mechanisms and etiologic associations

The pathogenesis of PNP in humans is undetermined. Suggested mechanisms include epitope spreading, tumor antigen cross-reaction with epidermal antigens, and induction of autoreactive T lymphocytes with tumor-producing plakin proteins (Zhu, 2007).

7.3.3.3 Treatment and prognosis

Treatment includes removal or treatment of the neoplasm, and immunosuppressive therapy with high doses of corticosteroids (Williams, 1995; Scott, 2011). In general, the prognosis depends on the nature of the underlying neoplasm. PNP associated with malignant neoplasms has a poor prognosis and high mortality rate (up to 90%). Mortality frequently results from sepsis or multi-organ failure, particularly respiratory failure. The prognosis in dogs is poor, and all three reported cases resulted in death.

7.3.4 Bullous pemphigoid

Bullous pemphigoid (BP) is a rare vesiculobullous, supepithelial autoimmune skin and mucosal disease in horses. It is the most common autoimmune subepidermal bullous dermatosis in humans (Williams, 1995). Autoantibodies are directed at the epidermal-dermal junction against antigens at the basal cell hemidesmosomes. In humans, dogs, cats, pigs and horses, BP is characterized by the presence of skin fixed and circulating IgG autoantibodies that target two bullous pemphigoid antigens: BPAG1 or BP230, a 230 kDa intracytoplasmic protein of the plakin family; and BPAG2 of BP180, a 180 kDa transmembrane type XVII collagen.

7.3.4.1 Signalment and clinical signs

In the horse, BP is severe and rapidly progressive. Affected horses vary in age from 5–14 years, with no breed or sex predilection (Scott, 2011). Primary skin lesions include intact vesicles and bullae. However, these lesions are transient and are not commonly seen. Intact bulla may be observed in the pinna, which is protected. Painful epidermal collarettes, crusts and ulcerations at the sites of ruptured bulla may be prominent. In addition, lesions can occur in the oral cavity, mucocutaneous junctions of the lips, vulva, anus and eyelids, and in the gastrointestinal tract (White, 2009; Scott, 2011). Horses are systemically ill with signs of depression, anorexia, weight loss and/or pyrexia.

7.3.4.2 Immunologic mechanisms and etiologic associations

Antibodies have been detected in horses to BPAG2, a type XVII collagen that is present within the lamina lucida of the basement membrane zone (BMZ). It is also a constitutive transmembrane glycoprotein present in basal keratinocytes involved in junctional adhesion (Olivry, 2000). Antibody binding activates complement, causing mast cell degranulation, chemotaxis of eosinophils and neutrophils, release of tissue destructive enzymes, and injury to the BMZ. Drug administration (e.g., penicillins, sulfonamides and furosemide), ultraviolet light, and genetics are thought to be associated with the pathogenesis of this disease in humans (Freedberg, 2003; Scott, 2011). The cause of antibody production in BP is unknown in all species.

7.3.4.3 Diagnostics

Definitive diagnosis is based on history, physical examination, skin or mucosal biopsy, immunofluorescence or immunohistochemical testing. Histopathologically, the earliest observed change is subepidermal vacuolar alteration, followed by an intact epidermis above a clean space separating it from the dermis. There is subepidermal or subepithelial cleft and vesicle formation, which may extend to the follicular infundibula. Neutrophils and eosinophils are present along the base of the vesicle or bullae, and the dermis is generally minimally inflamed. Ulcerated lesions show marked increases in inflammation and fibrin. The dermal infiltrate consists of variable numbers of neutrophils, eosinophils and mononuclear cells, and it may be mild and perivascular (cell-poor) to moderate and interstitial (cell-rich).

Immunohistochemistry or direct immunofluorescence shows a linear deposition of immunoglobulin and, often, complement at the BMZ of the skin or mucosa (Olivry, 2000; Scott, 2011). Indirect immunofluorescence testing shows circulating basement membrane-specific IgG autoantibodies that target the NC16A domain of the BPAG2 type XVII collagen.

7.3.4.4 Treatment and prognosis

Early diagnosis and aggressive therapy with corticosteroids and azathioprine is probably required for the successful management of this disease in horses, along with avoidance of direct sunlight and discontinuation of any drugs that may be implicated in the pathogenesis (White, 2009; Scott, 2011). The prognosis for BP is poor, and all reported cases in horses have died prior to, or in spite of, treatment.

7.4 Cutaneous adverse drug reactions

Cutaneous adverse drug reactions are uncommon in horses (Cannon, 2003; Scott, 2011), independent of the route of administration (Cannon, 2003; Freedberg, 2003; Scott, 2011). Two major groups associated with adverse drug reactions are:
(a) those that are predictable, dose-dependent and related to the pharmacologic actions of the drug;
(b) those that are unpredictable, non-dose dependent, and related to the individual's immunologic response.

Predictable cutaneous reactions occur with anticancer and immunosuppressive drugs, and include alopecia, purpura, poor wound healing, and increased susceptibility to infections (Scott, 2011). Immunologic reaction may include any of the four hypersensitivity reactions (Scott, 2011; Ahmed, 2013).

7.4.1 Signalment and clinical signs

There are no age or gender predilections reported in horses (Cannon, 2003; White, 2009). Cutaneous adverse drug reactions can mimic any dermatosis (Freedberg, 2003; Ahmed, 2013). The most common cutaneous reactions associated with drug administration are contact dermatitis, exfoliative dermatitis, erythema multiforme and urticaria (Scott, 2011). Other reactions include: vesicular and ulcerative eruptions; severe pruritus; erythroderma; maculopapular rash; panniculitis; pemphigus foliaceous; sterile pyogranuloma; trichorrhexis; hypotrichosis; and tail head dermatitis (Scott, 2011). Fixed drug reactions have been reported to occur, and are most common on genital skin (Freedberg, 2033; Scott, 2011; Ahmed, 2013).

In horses, adverse cutaneous reactions are most commonly associated with a history of administration of sulfonamines, penicillins, phenylbutazone, ivermectin, diuretics, antipyretics, phenothiazines, and topical agents (Cannon, 2003; White, 2009; Scott, 2011). Typically, a reaction occurs 1–3 weeks after starting therapy. Some reactions may occur months after the drug was administered. Occasional drug eruptions, particularly those associated with vaccines or other injectable medications, may persist for weeks to months.

7.4.2 Immunologic mechanisms and etiologic associations

The pathogenesis of most drug eruptions is not understood, although the clinical features are often consistent with immune-mediated disease. The immune system may target the native drug, its metabolite, altered self-molecules or a combination of these factors (Freedberg, 2003). Drug reactions associated with sulfonamides and anticonvulsants are thought to be associated with oxidation by cytochrome P-450 into chemically reactive metabolites. This process may occur in the liver, with secondary transfer to the skin or in keratinocytes by epidermal cytochrome P-450. There is decreased detoxification of these reactive metabolites, which then bind to proteins and induce an immunologic response (Scott, 2011).

7.4.3 Diagnostics

There are no specific skin lesions, histopathologic changes or laboratory findings that indicate cutaneous adverse drug eruption. Definitive diagnosis is difficult, and a diagnosis of drug reaction is based on a good clinical history, ruling out other dermatoses, and general supporting histologic findings (Table 7.2).

7.4.4 Treatment and prognosis

The offending drug should be withdrawn, and chemically related compounds avoided. Clinical signs may need to be treated with topical or systemic therapy, as indicated, and response to glucocorticoid therapy may be poor. The prognosis is good when the initiating stimulus is identified and removed and there is not multi-organ involvement or extensive epidermal necrosis. Resolution of signs may occur from 48 hours to six months following cessation of the initiating factor.

7.5 Erythema multiforme

Erythema multiforme (EM) is an uncommon, acute, immune-mediated response that presents with cutaneous and/or mucosal lesions. It can be triggered by a variety of etiologies, and is often self-limiting. In humans, the condition is commonly divided as *erythema multiforme minor* and *major*, according to severity and mucosal involvement. EM minor is most commonly associated with viral infections (e.g., herpes simplex virus in human patients) (Samim, 2013), and EM major associated with drug eruptions (Scott, 2011).

7.5.1 Signalment and clinical signs

There are no known age, breed or gender predilections (Scott, 2011). In humans, the condition is more common in young adult females (Samim, 2013).

The classic characteristic lesion of EM in human patients is a *target* pattern lesion. In the early phases, the lesions are round edematous papules, surrounded by a blanching that resembles an insect bite or urticarial papule (Sokumbi, 2012). These papules then enlarge and develop concentric alterations of a targetoid lesion. Subsequently, there is central necrosis, followed by a dark red inflammatory zone, followed by a pale edematous ring and erythematous zone on the periphery.

In horses, lesions may vary from urticarial papules and plaques to vesicles and bullae, and to ulcerative mucosal lesions (Scott, 2011). Urticarial lesions do not pit with pressure, as in true urticaria. These lesions take on a target-like appearance, with peripheral expansion and central resolution, forming annular to arciform lesions (Figure 7.3a). The overlying skin and hair coat are usually normal. Horses with urticarial-like lesions are often asymptomatic. Those with more severe widespread lesions may have cutaneous pain, ulcerative lesions, and systemic signs of fever, depression and anorexia (Scott, 2011).

7.5.2 Immunologic mechanisms and etiologic associations

The pathogenesis of EM is not fully understood. It is thought to be the result of a host-specific cell-mediated hypersensitivity

Table 7.2 The diagnostic criteria and variable histologic patterns associated with cutaneous adverse drug reactions in horses.

Criteria for diagnosis	Histopathologic patterns associated with cutaneous adverse drug eruptions
• A drug history with the eruption occurring within the first 1–3 weeks of drug administration. • Prior exposure to the drug may have led to sensitization. • The suspected drug is known to cause similar cutaneous reactions. • The cutaneous reaction cannot be explained by the known pharmacologic actions of the drug. • Lack of alternative explanation's for the cutaneous eruption. • Resolution begins to occur within 1–2 weeks after discontinuation of the drug. • The reaction is reproduced with re-administration of the drug.	• Perivascular dermatitis • Interface dermatitis • Vasculitis • Intraepidermal vesiculopustular dermatitis • Subepidermal vesicular dermatitis • Follicular necrosis • Granulomatous mural folliculitis • Dermal eosinophilia • Erythema multiforme • Epitheliotropic lymphoma like reaction

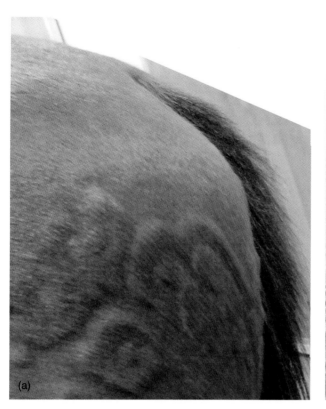
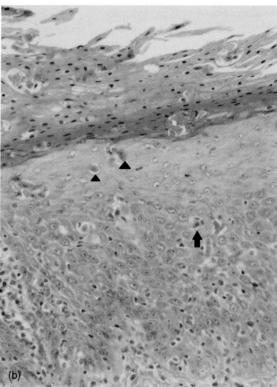

Figure 7.3 Erythema multiforme.
(a) Annular and arciform lesions over the rump (courtesy of Charlotte Herdan, BSc, BVSc, MANZCVS, MRCVS);
(b) Photomicrograph showing multi-level apoptotic keratinocytes (arrow heads) and satellitosis (arrow); satellitosis refers to lymphocytes surrounding apoptotic keratinocytes; magnification 200 × (Rebecca Ruby, BVSc, MS, Cornell University).

reaction. When keratinocytes are antigenically altered by insulting events (e.g., infections, drugs, food, neoplasia, or connective tissue disease), they become targets of cytotoxic T lymphocytes, leading to apoptosis and satellitosis (Scott, 2011; Sokumbi, 2012).

Most cases of EM in horses have been associated with drug administration, including potentiated sulfonamides, penicillins and ivermectin (Scott, 2011). Herpes virus infection, lymphoma, vaccinations, food and topical chemicals have also been reported to cause EM in horses (White, 2009; Scott, 2011). Often, an etiology is not identified, and many cases are qualified as idiopathic (Marshall, 1991). In one case report, an endocrine imbalance was suggested as a cause of EM in a post-partum mare (Oryan, 2010). Another case report attributed EM lesions to equid herpes virus 5 infection, with a lymphoplasmacytic histiocytic interface dermatitis, multi-level apoptotic keratinocytes and hydropic degeneration, and viral inclusion bodies observed histologically. The virus was identified by polymerase chain reaction (PCR) (Herder, 2012). The described horse had no respiratory disease, and the authors considered this a unique manifestation of EHV-5 infection.

In human patients, EM is similarly triggered by a wide range of events, including viral and bacterial infections, drug administration, autoimmune disease, radiation, immunization, malignancy, and menstruation (Freedburg, 2003). The most common cause is herpes simplex virus (HSV) infection. Following viremia, the viral DNA is transferred to keratinocytes in the epidermis and activates CD4+ T helper cells and the release of interferon gamma (IFN-gamma) (Sokumbi, 2012; Samim, 2013). In cases of drug-associated EM, inflammatory cytokine TNF-alpha, perforin and granzyme B are involved, suggesting a different immunologic mechanism. In human patients, there may be increased susceptibility to disease associated with certain MHC molecules (Samim, 2013).

7.5.3 Diagnostics

Definitive diagnosis is based on history, physical examination, and skin biopsy. EM has a cutaneous and mucosal reaction pattern, and a complete history is necessary for diagnosis. Histopathologic changes include multilevel single cell keratinocyte apoptosis of the epidermis and, sometimes, the follicular outer root sheath, with satellitosis of lymphocytes and macrophages, lymphoplasmacytic hydropic interface dermatitis, pigment dispersal to superficial dermal melanophages (pigmentary incontinence), and variable dermal edema and purpura (Figure 7.3b). There may be extensive keratinocyte apoptosis, leading to epidermal necrosis that can mimic toxic epidermal necrolysis (Stannard, 2000). In some cases, there may be severe subepidermal vesicles.

7.5.4 Treatment and prognosis

When identified, the underlying cause should be addressed or treated. Minor EM cases may spontaneously resolve within weeks to months and, anecdotally, pentoxifylline may help (Scott, 2011). The use of systemic corticosteroids and other immunomodulatory drugs is controversial, but may be needed in major EM, particularly when the underlying cause cannot be found. These cases have a poor prognosis.

7.6 Lupus erythematosus

Lupus erythematosus (LE) encompasses a group of diseases with different clinical syndromes that share a similar underlying autoimmune process (Scott, 2011). In human medicine, LE includes three major subtypes:

1 chronic cutaneous LE;
2 subacute cutaneous LE;
3 systemic or acute cutaneous LE.
  In horses, LE is divided into two forms:
1 discoid lupus erythematosus (DLE), which is confined to the skin;
2 systemic lupus erythematosus (SLE), which has dermal and systemic manifestations.
  Progression from DLE to SLE rarely, if ever, occurs (Scott, 2011). Five main characteristics of cutaneous LE are:
(a) photoaggravation;
(b) keratinocytes damage;
(c) lymphohistiocytic infiltrate;
(d) autoantibody production;
(e) antigen-antibody complex deposition (Freedburg, 2003; Winfield, 2013).

7.6.1 Systemic lupus erythematosus

Systemic lupus erythematosus (SLE) is a very rare multi-organ autoimmune disease of horses, with a wide variation in clinical presentation. Only two case reports have been published, although there are additional anecdotal cases known (Geor, 1990; Clark, 1998). The disease is characterized by a loss of self-tolerance, with production and activation of autoreactive T and B cells (Freedburg, 2003; Scott, 2011; Choi, 2012; Miller, 2013). Autoantibodies are directed at nucleic acids and their binding proteins.

7.6.1.1 Signalment and clinical signs

There are no known age, sex or breed predispositions (Scott, 2011). Cutaneous lesions include: lymphedema of the distal limbs; panniculitis; mucocutaneous ulceration; alopecia; scaling; leukoderma (face, neck, trunk); and exfoliative dermatitis. In addition, systemic signs include: polysynovitis; anemia; thrombocytopenia; purpura; glomerulonephritis; uveitis; peripheral lymphadenopathy; fever, anorexia; and weight loss.

7.6.1.2 Immunologic mechanisms and etiologic associations

The etiology is multifactorial and not well understood. Contributing factors include: genetic background; immunologic status (e.g., T cell deficiency, complement deficiency, B cell hyperactivity); concurrent viral infections; hormonal profiles; and ultraviolet light exposure (Fournel, 1992; Freedburg, 2003; Tizzard, 2009; Choi, 2012). Drugs and modified-live vaccines are known to either precipitate or antagonize SLE in human patients and dogs (Kass, 1985; Geor, 1990; Miller, 2013). Drugs have been suspected to precipitate SLE-like reactions in horses (Cannon, 2003).

Ultraviolet light penetrates the epidermis, causing cellular damage and enhanced expression of intercellular adhesion molecules (e.g., ICAM-1), and exposing intracellular self-antigens (e.g., Ro). Specific autoantibodies develop to these antigens, which attach to keratinocytes and induce antibody-dependent cell cytotoxicity through natural killer (NK) cells. Injured keratinocytes release IL-2 and other lymphocyte chemo-attractants, resulting in lymphocytic infiltrates (Miller, 2013).

Recent literature shows that there is a requirement for dendritic cells to stimulate autoreactive T and B cells (Choi, 2012), and for the release of IFN. This cytokine activates neutrophils and promotes their death through a process referred to as NETosis, which involves the production of a neutrophil extracellular trap (NET), a web-like structure formed by neutrophil DNA. In health, the NET is an effective method for entrapment and killing of bacteria; in SLE, it exposes abundant extracellular DNA for autoantibody production, creating a positive feedback loop.

In dogs, there is a systemic immune shift to absolute lymphopenia, and a greater decrease in CD4$^+$ T cells, with a resulting decrease in CD4$^+$/CD8$^+$ ratio (Miller, 2013). B cell hyperactivity leads to the production of autoantibodies, particularly against nuclear antigens (antinuclear antibodies, ANA), which may be measured. While there is direct damage from the presence of these antibodies, the most severe destruction occurs from a hypersensitivity reaction type III, with the deposition of antigen-antibody complexes in the BMZ and within the walls of dermal blood vessels.

7.6.1.3 Diagnostics

Definitive diagnosis is difficult, and depends on clinical signs, histopathological and clinicopathologic changes. A positive serum ANA titer supports diagnosis of SLE but must be interpreted along with other findings. In human and canine medicine, the criteria for diagnosis of SLE are a positive ANA test and the involvement of two or more body systems. The most common body systems affected in the horse are joints, skin, kidney, oral mucosa and the hematopoietic system (Scott, 2011). The following are proposed criteria for the diagnosis of equine SLE:

1 a positive ANA cell test;
2 minimum of two findings among: characteristic skin lesions; polyarthritis; immune-mediated hemolytic anemia; immune-mediated thrombocytopenia; or glomerulonephritis (proteinuria) (Scott, 2011).

Dermatohistopathologic findings are lichenoid or hydropic interface dermatitis of the epidermis and follicular outer root sheath, with subepidermal vacuolar alteration, dermal mucinosis, and thickening of the basement membrane with lymphohistiocytic to plasmacytic cellular infiltrates. In addition, apoptotic keratinocytes, predominantly within the stratum basale, and pigmentary incontinence may be observed. A *lupus band*, characterized by the deposition of immunoglobulin and/or complement in the BMZ, may be observed with direct immunoflouresence or immunohistochemistry.

7.6.1.4 Treatment and prognosis

Treatment involves immunosuppressive doses of systemic corticosteroids as described above (Scott, 2011). The addition of azathioprine and omega-3/6 fatty acids may help (Scott, 2011). These patients are at high risk for infections, which should be treated aggressively and promptly (Freedberg, 2003). In general, the earlier the diagnosis and treatment, the better the prognosis. However, prognosis varies depending on the number and type of body systems involved, and degree of damage.

7.6.2 Discoid lupus erythematosus

Discoid lupus erythematosus (DLE), or cutaneous lupus erythematosus, is a rare autoimmune dermatitis with no systemic involvement. There is current debate regarding the most appropriate nomenclature, and a suggestion for naming this condition as *photosensitive nasal dermatitis* has been made (Hargis, 2012).

7.6.2.1 Signalment and clinical signs

There are no breed or gender predilections, and most common affected age ranges from 1–14 years (Scott, 2011). Clinical signs may have gradual to rapid onset of typically symmetric skin lesions, beginning on the face, around lips, nostrils and periocular regions (White, 2009; Scott, 2011). These lesions consist of non-painful and non-puritic well-circumscribed areas of erythema, scaling and alopecia. Occasionally, crusts, erosions and leukotrichia may be observed. Over time, extension to other areas of the body may happen, including the neck, shoulders, perianal and perineal regions.

7.6.2.2 Diagnostics

Definitive diagnosis is based on clinical history, physical examination, histopathologic findings, and immunofluorescence or immunohistochemical testing. Dermatohistopathology reveals a hydropic and or lichenoid interface dermatitis, with apoptosis of the basal epidermal and follicular outer root sheath keratinocytes, pigmentary incontinence, focal thickening of the BMZ, subepidermal vacuolar alteration, variable degrees of mucinosis, and infiltration of lymphocytes, plasma cells and histiocytes around dermal vessels (Figure 7.4). Rarely, multinucleate giant cells are present (Scott, 2011). Immunoglobulin and/or complement deposition may be detected in the basement membrane, using immunohistochemical or direct immunoflouresence.

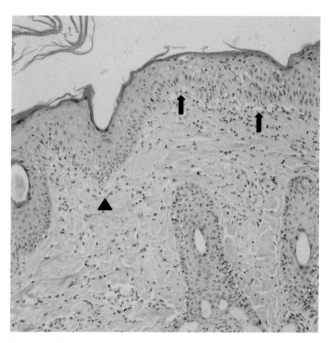

Figure 7.4 Cutaneous lupus erythematosus: photomicrograph showing subepidermal vacuolar alteration (arrow) and pigmentary incontinence (arrow head); magnification 100× (Rebecca Ruby, BVSc, MS, Cornell University).

7.6.2.3 Immunologic mechanisms and etiologic associations

The etiology is multifactorial and not well understood, and it follows the same principles for SLE described above. Clinical signs are exacerbated by exposure to ultraviolet light, which further suggests its implication.

7.6.2.4 Treatment and prognosis

Mild cases of DLE can often be controlled by avoidance of intense sunlight and use of topical sunscreens and glucocorticoids (Scott, 2011). Initial therapy may begin with more potent topical corticosteroids applied every 12 hours and, once the condition is in remission, milder formulations applied as needed. In some cases, systemic corticosteroids may be needed until remission is achieved, with topical agents used for maintenance. Omega-3/6 fatty acids may help. The prognosis is good with lifelong therapy and protection from ultraviolet light.

References

Ahmed, A., Pritchard, S. and Reichberg, J. (2013). A review of cutaneous drug eruptions. *Clinical Geriatric Medicine* **29**, 527–545.

Brenner, S., Bialy-Golan, A. and Ruocco, V. (1998). Drug-induced pemphigus. *Clinics in Dermatology* **16**, 393–397.

Cannon, A.G. and V.K. Affolter. (2003). Cutaneous adverse drug reactions. In: Robinson, N.E. (ed). *Current Therapy in Equine Medicine V*, 177. St. Louis.

Choi, J., Kim, S.T. and Craft, J. (2012). The pathogenesis of systemic lupus erythematosus—an update. *Current Opinion in Immunology* **24**(6), 651–657.

Choi, Y., Nam, K-H., Lee, J-B., Lee, J.Y., Ihm, C-W., Lee, S.E., Oh, S.H., Hashimoto, T. and Kim, S-C. (2012). Retrospective analysis of 12 Korean patients with paraneoplastic pemphigus. *The Journal of Dermatology* **39**(12), 973–981.

Clark, E.G. (1998). Equine systemic *lupus erythematosus*. *Canadian Veterinary Journal* **29**(7), pp. 595.

Di Zenzo, G., Thoma-Uszynski, S., Calabresi, V., Fontao, L., Hofmann, S.C., Lacour, J.P., Sera, F., Bruckner-Tuderman, L., Zambruno, G., Borradori, L. and Hertl, M. (2011). Demonstration of epitope-spreading phenomena in bullous pemphigoid: results of a prospective multicenter study. *Journal of Investigative Dermatology* **131**(11), 2271–2280.

Fournel, C., Chabanne, L., Caux, C., Faure, J-R., Rigal, D., Magnol, J-P. and Monier, J-C. (1992). Canine systemic lupus erythematosus. I: A study of 75 cases. *Lupus* **1**(3), 133–139.

Freedberg, I.M. (2003). *Fitzpatricks Dermatology in General Medicine*, sixth edition. New York, McGraw-Hill.

Geor, R.J., Clark, E.G., Haines, D.M. and Napier, P.G. (1990). Systemic lupus erythematosus in a filly. *Journal of American Veterinary Association* **197**(11), 1489–1492.

Grando, S.A. (2012). Pemphigus autoimmunity: hypotheses and realities. *Autoimmunity* **45**(1), 7–35.

Hargis, A.M., Clark, E.G., Duclos, D.D., Leclerc, S. and West, K. (2001). Spongiotic vesicular dermatitis as a cutaneous reaction pattern in seven horses. *Veterinary Dermatology* **12**(5), 291–296.

Hargis, A.M. and Ginn, P.E. (2012). The integument. In: Zachary, J.F. and McGavin, M.D. (eds). *Pathologic basis of veterinary disease*, fifth edition, pp. 972–1084. St. Louis, Elsevier.

Herder, V., Barsnick, R., Walliser, U., Teifke, J-P., König, P., Czerwinski, G., Hansmann, F., Baumgärtner, W. and Hewicker-Trautwein, M. (2012). Equid herpesvirus-5 dermatitis in a horse – Resembling herpes-associated *erythema multiforme*. *Veterinary Microbiology* **155**(2–4), 420–424.

Kass, P.H., Farver, T.B., Strombeck, D.R. and Ardans, A.A. (1985). Application of the log linear and logistic regression models in the prediction of systemic lupus erythematosus in the dog. *American Journal of Veterinary Research* **469**(11), 2340–2345.

Liska, D.A., Akucewich, L.H., Marsella, R., Maxwell, L.K., Barbara, J.E. and Cole, C.A. (2006). Pharmacokinetics of pentoxifylline and its 5-hydroxyhexyl metabolite after oral and intravenous administration of pentoxifylline to healthy adult horses. *American Journal of Veterinary Research* **67**(9), 1621–1627.

Marshall, C. (1991). Erythema multiforme in two horses. *Journal of the South African Veterinary Association* **62**(3), 133.

Miller, W.H. Jr. Griffin, C.E. and Campbell, K.L. (2013). Autoimmune and Immune-mediated dermatoses. In: *Muller and Kirk's Small Animal Dermatology*. Elsevier Health Sciences.

Miragliotta, V., Donadio, E., Felicioli, A., Podestà, A., Ricciardi, M.P., Ceccardi, S. and Abramo, F. (2006). Immunolocalisation of desmoglein-1 in equine muzzle skin. *Equine Veterinary Journal* **38**(5), 485–487.

Olivry, T. (2006b). A review of autoimmune skin diseases in domestic animals: I–superficial pemphigus. *Veterinary Dermatology* **17**(5), 291–305.

Olivry, T. and Linder, K.E. (2009). Dermatoses affecting desmosomes in animals: a mechanistic review of acantholytic blistering skin diseases. *Veterinary Dermatology* **20**(5–6), 313–326.

Olivry, T., Borrillo, A.K.G., Xu, L., Dunston, S.M., Slovis, N.M., Affolter, V.K., DeManuelle, T.C. and Chan, L.S. (2000). Equine bullous pemphigoid IgG autoantibodies target linear epitopes in the NC16A ectodomain of collagen XVII (BP180, BPAG2). *Veterinary Immunology and Immunopathology* **73**(1), 45–52.

Olivry, T., LaVoy, A., Dunston, S.M., Brown, R.S., Lennon, E.M., Warren, S.J., Prisayanh, P., Müller, E.J., Suter, M.M. and Dean, G.A. (2006a). Desmoglein-1 is a minor autoantigen in dogs with pemphigus foliaceus. *Veterinary Immunology and Immunopathology* **110**(3), 245–255.

Oryan, A., Ghane, M. and Ahmadi, N. (2010). Erythema multiforme and its clinicopathological disorders in a horse. *Comparative Clinical Pathology* **19**(2), 179–184.

Papich, M.G. (2007). *Saunders Handbook of Veterinary Drugs*, second edition. St. Louis, Saunders Elsevier.

Samim, F., Auluck, A., Zed, C. and Williams, M. (2013). Erythema multiforme: a review of epidemiology, pathogenesis, clinical features, and treatment. *Dental Clinics of North America* **57**, 583–596.

Scott, D.W. (1994). Marked acantholysis associated with dermatophytosis due to Trichophyton equinum in two horses. *Veterinary Dermatology* **5**(3), 105–110.

Scott, D.W. and Miller, W.H. Jr. (1998). Erythema multiforme in the horse: literature review and report of 9 cases (1988–1996). *Equine Practice* **20**, 6.

Scott, D.W. and Miller, W.H. (2011). Skin Immune System and Allergic Skin Diseases. In: *Equine Dermatology*, second edition. St. Louis, Saunders.

Sokumbi, O. and Wetter, D.A. (2012). Clinical features, diagnosis, and treatment of erythema multiforme: a review for the practicing dermatologist. *International Journal of Dermatology* **51**(8), 889–902.

Stannard, A.A. (2000). Immunologic Diseases. *Veterinary Dermatology* **11**(3), 163–178.

Tizzard, I.R. (2009). Autoimmunity: General Principles. In: *Veterinary Immunology: An Introduction VIII*. St. Louis, Saunders Elsevier.

Vandenabeele, S.I.J., White, S.D., Affolter, V.K., Kass, P.H. and Ihrke, P.J. (2004). Pemphigus foliaceus in the horse: a retrospective study of 20 cases. *Veterinary Dermatology* **15**(6), 381–388.

White, S.D. (2009). Diseases of the skin. In: Smith, B.P. (ed). *Large Animal Internal Medicine IV* pp. 1306–1338. St. Louis, Elsevier.

White, S.D., Maxwell, L.K., Szabo, N.J., Hawkins, J.L. and Kollias-Baker, C. (2005). Pharmacokinetics of azathioprine following single-dose intravenous and oral administration and effects of azathioprine following chronic oral administration in horses. *American Journal of Veterinary Research* **66**(9), 1578–1583.

Williams, M.A., Dowling, P.M., Angarano, D.W., Yu, A.A., DiFranco, B.J., Lenz, S.D. and Anhalt, G.J. (1995). Paraneoplastic bullous stomatitis in a horse. *Journal of the American Veterinary Medical Association* **207**(3), 331–334.

Winfield, L.D., White, S.D., Affolter, V.K., Renier, A.C., Dawson, D., Olivry, T., Outerbridge, C.A., Wang, Y.H., Iyori, K. and Nishifuji, K. (2013). *Pemphigus vulgaris* in a Welsh pony stallion: case report and demonstration of antidesmoglein autoantibodies. *Veterinary Dermatology* **24**(2), 269–e60.

Zabel, S., Mueller, R.S., Fieseler, K.V., Bettenay, S.V., Littlewood, J.D. and Wagner, R. (2005). Review of 15 cases of *pemphigus foliaceus* in horses and a survey of the literature. *Veterinary Record* **157**, 505–509.

Zhu, X. and Zhang, B. (2007). Paraneoplastic pemphigus. *The Journal of Dermatology* **34**(8), 503–511.

8 Serum Sickness

Lais R.R. Costa

8.1 Definition

Serum sickness is a systemic disease caused by the formation of immune complexes, where the antigen is soluble and exogenous in origin. The immune complexes are formed in the circulation and deposited typically in vessel walls of many tissues/organs, including glomeruli, synovial membrane, lymph nodes, and skin. Immune complex formation leads to inflammation at the site of deposition of immune complexes. Immune complex-mediated diseases are also referred to as hypersensitivity type III reactions.

Serum sickness was elucidated by the pediatrician Clemens von Pirquet in 1906, following his observations of the reactions associated with the administration of diphtheria antitoxin to children (Jackson, 2000; Silverstein, 2000). His statement: "*The conception that antibodies, which should protect against disease, are also responsible for disease, sounds at first absurd*" gave rise to the concept of allergy. Subsequently, numerous physicians described the syndrome in various clinical settings (Boots, 1923; Lawley, 1985).

8.2 Signalment and clinical signs

In immune complex-mediated diseases, immunoglobulin binds to exogenously administered soluble foreign antigens (proteins) to form circulating immune complexes that can deposit in a variety of capillaries. Blood is filtered at high pressure in the vascular beds of certain organs, including the kidneys, joints, skin and lymph nodes, and these vessels are particularly susceptible to deposition of immune-complexes. Tissues in their vicinity become damaged by the ensuing immune reaction.

The clinical signs include: fever; skin eruptions of purpura (purple-colored patches and eruptions on the skin and mucous membranes); lymphadenopathy; arthralgia and polysynovitis; albuminuria/proteinuria (glomerulonephritis); and acute renal failure. Signs may appear as early as seven days but, most commonly, 10–14 days after receiving the exogenous soluble foreign antigens (Kumar, 2010; Frank, 2014). Upon a second administration of the soluble foreign antigens, an accelerated systemic reaction occurs.

It appears that there is no known breed and sex predisposition to the development of antigen-antibody immune complex-mediated disease in horses (Swiderski, 1997, 2000). Neonates are thought to be less likely to develop the condition.

8.3 Immunologic mechanisms and etiologic associations

Serum sickness is a hypersensitivity reaction mediated by the formation of antigen-antibody immune-complexes within the circulation, and their deposition in vascular beds. Immunoglobulins of the IgM or IgG isotypes are the mostly involved in the binding to soluble exogenous immunogenic substances (Kumar, 2010; Frank, 2014). There are many factors that determine the formation and the deposition of these immune-complexes, including the quality of the antigens and immune-complexes and the condition of the circulation and vascular beds:

- High molecular weight foreign proteins are more immunogenic;
- multivalent antigens that bind multiple antibodies with different specificities form immune complex lattices;
- medium size complexes; and
- vascular beds, where the blood is filtered at high pressure, favor the deposition of immune-complexes.

However, one of the most important determinants is the relative concentration of antigens and antibodies (Kumar, 2010; Frank, 2014).

Initially, following administration of large amounts of immunogenic, soluble, exogenous antigens, the production of antibodies is small. Therefore, when antibodies first appear in the circulation, there is an excess of antigen, there is no cross-linking of antibodies, and the small number of immune-complexes neither deposit nor activate complement (Figure 8.1). Indeed, antigen-antibody immune-complexes are cleared from the circulation by the liver sinusoidal endothelial cells expressing Fc-gamma receptor II, which binds the antibody heavy chain constant region (Ganesan, 2012).

Increased production of antibodies leads to equivalence in the amount of antibodies and antigens in the circulation, and the formation of large antigen-antibody immune-complexes (lattice), which are efficiently removed by the cells of the

Equine Clinical Immunology, First Edition. Edited by M. Julia B. Felippe.
© 2016 John Wiley & Sons, Inc. Published 2016 by John Wiley & Sons, Inc.

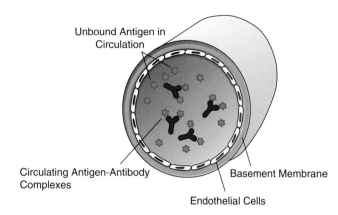

Figure 8.1 Initial phase of antigen-antibody complex formation following administration of immunogenic, soluble, exogenous antigenic substance. At first, there is an excess of antigen, relative to the amount of antibodies, and the small number of immune complexes neither deposit nor activate complement. They are cleared from the circulation by liver sinusoidal endothelial cells expressing Fc-gamma receptor (FcγR) II.

mononuclear phagocyte system (MPS), particularly macrophages in the red pulp of the spleen. As large immune-complexes activate complement, their removal is primarily mediated by the C3 receptor. The C3b component associated with large immune complexes bind to the C3b receptor on the surface of red blood cells, also leading to their removal by the MPS. Antibody excess is established as the amount of antigen is removed from the circulation by means of removal of large immune-complexes. This leads to saturation of the antigen valences and formation of medium-size immune-complexes, which remain in the circulation for longer, depositing along the endothelial surface of certain vascular beds, especially arterioles of glomeruli, synovial membrane and skin.

Medium-size immune complexes activate complement via C1q, initiating the cascade of sequential proteolytic cleavage that results in the formation of factors C3b, iC3b and C4b, and the release of factors C3a and C5a. Complement activation induces an inflammatory cascade that result in endothelial cell swelling and fibrin deposition, increased vascular permeability and chemoattraction of neutrophils (Figure 8.2). Deposition of immune-complexes and C3b in the endothelial basement

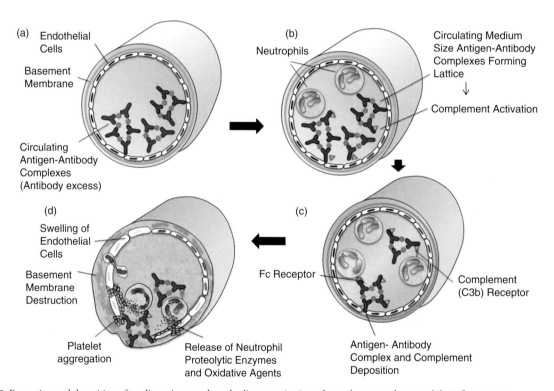

Figure 8.2 Formation and deposition of medium size complexes leading to activation of complement and neutrophilic inflammation.
(a) Once antibody excess is established, there is saturation of the antigen valences and formation of medium size immune complexes, which remain in the circulation longer and deposit along the endothelial surface of certain vascular beds (particularly arterioles of glomeruli, synovial membrane and skin).
(b) Medium-sized immune complexes efficiently activate complement via C1q, leading to the cascade of sequential proteolytic cleavage.
(c) Complement activation results in formation of factors C3b, iC3b and C4b and the release of factors C3a and C5a, leading to an inflammatory cascade with endothelial cell swelling and fibrin deposition, increased vascular permeability and chemoattraction of neutrophils.
(d) Deposition of immune complexes and C3b in the basement membrane is followed by platelet aggregation at the site of deposition. Recruited neutrophils become activated and pass across the basement membrane. Activated neutrophils release proteolytic enzymes and oxidative agents, with destruction of the basement membrane and surrounding tissues and, ultimately, necrotizing vasculitis.

membrane is followed by platelet aggregation at the site of deposition. Recruited neutrophils become activated and pass across the basement membrane. Activated neutrophils release proteolytic enzymes (including acid phosphatases, acid hydrolytic enzymes, cathepsins, elastase and collagenase) and oxidative agents. Enzymatic and oxidative damage mediated by neutrophils lead to destruction of the basement membrane and surrounding tissues, ultimately resulting in necrotizing vasculitis.

Etiologic associations of serum sickness reactions in humans have changed overtime. The condition was common in humans because of the wide use of xenogeneic serum to prevent or treat toxin-mediated and infectious diseases (Frank, 2014). Purified whole immunoglobulins obtained from horses vaccinated with rabies virus, tetanus, botulism, or diphtheria toxins, and snake and scorpion venoms, have been administered to humans for temporary protection. Moreover, equine anti-thymocyte globulin (ATG) and anti-lymphocyte globulin (ALG) have been used for the prevention of allograft rejection, and for treatment of aplastic anemia and myelodysplasia. Both ATG and ALG have been associated with serum sickness (Jackson, 2000).

Nowadays, antivenoms, anti-toxins and prevention of allograft rejection are still administered as polyclonal sera. However, they only contain the Fab fragments of the immunoglobulins, so they are minimally immunogenic. Presently, most cases of serum sickness in humans are reactions to drugs such as penicillin, cephalosporin and sulfonamides (Frank, 2014).

Similarly, horses receiving soluble exogenous immunogenic proteins (e.g. equine polyclonal antibody products, including snake antivenins; tetanus, botulinum, or *Clostrium difficile* antitoxins; hyperimmune plasma products against specific organisms [*Rhodococcus equi*, West Nile virus, gram negative bacteria]; and plasma and serum transfusions) have the potential to develop immune complex-mediated diseases. Despite the wide use of these products in equine medicine, adverse reactions have not been reported (Perkins, 2002; Tennent-Brown, 2009; Fielding *et al.*, 2011). Occasional reports of adverse reactions following intravenous plasma administration to adult horses and foals are immediate-hypersensitivity reactions (Hardefeldt, 2010; Reynolds, 2012; Rowlands, 2013). Determination of the incidence of systemic antigen-antibody immune-complex disease in horses following administration of exogenous immunogenic products would require a multi-institutional surveillance/vigilance system.

8.4 Diagnostics

Confirmation of immune complex-mediated disease can be challenging, and it is not typically performed in clinical practice. Tentative diagnosis of immune complex-mediated disease is based on history, clinical signs and laboratory findings of organ damage (e.g. glomerulonephritis albuminuria/proteinuria and azotemia indicating glomerulonephritis). In human patients,

a number of assays can be used for confirmation of immune complex-mediated disease, including (Frank, 2014):

(a) the detection of circulating immune-complexes using radio-immunoassay for IgG and IgM;

(b) detection of circulating immune-complexes bound to complement component C1q using radiolabeled 125I-C1q or enzyme-linked immunosorbent assay;

(c) the presence of C3-bound to immune-complexes (solid phase anti-C3 assay);

(d) measurement of C3 and C4 concentrations in serum, and low values of C3 and C4 are interpreted as an indirect indication of consumption of complement components.

None of these assays are specific for the antigen.

In horses, determination of complement components (C3 and C4) has been reported, but it is not routinely offered in diagnostic laboratories (Lavoie, 1989; Reis, 1989; Gardner, 2007). Measurement of C1q-binding has not been reported in horses. Instead, confirmation of the diagnosis of immune complex-mediated disease in horses is done by histolopathologic evaluation of tissue lesions.

Early histopathologic findings include the presence of electron-dense deposits in the endothelial basement membrane, which reveal immune-complexes, complement and fibrin deposition in the vessel wall. As the disease progresses, histopathologic findings include necrotizing vasculitis of small vessels with endothelial swelling and necrosis, fibrin deposition, platelet aggregation, neutrophilic infiltrate, and leukocytoclastic vasculitis.

8.5 Treatment and prevention

The management of serum sickness is focused on removal of the offending/triggering antigen, decreasing inflammation to halt tissue injury, and decreasing production of antibodies. In addition, appropriate supportive therapy is used to control clinical signs, particularly renal damage. When the offending antigen is known, serum sickness is self-limiting, as the administration of the foreign antigen is discontinued. Anti-inflammatory therapy might be accomplished by the use of glucocorticoids or nonsteroidal anti-inflammatory drugs.

If immunosuppressive therapy is contemplated, it is best achieved by administration of dexamethasone at 0.05–0.2 mg/kg IV or PO every 12 or 24 hours (Felippe, 2014). When signs of inflammation are resolved, the dose should be decreased by 10–20% every 24 to 48 hours. Therapy can be switched from dexamethasone to prednisolone initially, at 1 mg/kg PO every 12 or 24 hours, and gradually decreased to 0.2–0.5 mg/kg PO every 12, 24 or 48 hours. Long-term immunosuppressive therapy is rarely necessary. Patients receiving glucocorticoids should be monitored for side-effects of corticosteroid therapy, including evidence of polyuria and polydipsia, laminitis and secondary infection.

Prevention of serum sickness is accomplished by documentation of the offending antigen, and future avoidance of administration.

References

Boots, R.H., and Swift, H.F. (1923). The arthritis of serum sickness. *Journal of American Medical Association* **80**, 12–15.

Felippe, M.J.B. (2014). Immunotherapy. In: Sellon, D. and Long, M. (eds). *Equine Infectious Disease*, second edition, pp. 584–597. St. Louis, Saunders Elsevier.

Fielding, C.L., Pusterla, N., Magdesian, K.G., Higgins, J.C. and Meier, C.A. (2011). Rattlesnake envenomation in horses: 58 cases (1992–2009). *Journal of American Veterinary Medical Association* **238**, 631–635.

Frank, M.M., and Hester, C.G. (2014). Immune complex-mediated disease. In: Adkinson. N.F., Bochner, B.S., Burks, A.W., Busse, W.W., Holgate, S.T., Lemanske, R.F. and O'Hehir, R.E. (eds). *Middleton's Allergy Principles and Practice*, eighth edition, pp. 602–616. Philadelphia, Elsevier Saunders.

Ganesan, L.P., Kim, J., Wu, Y., Mohanty, S., Phillips, G.S., Birmingham, D.J., Robinson, J.M. and Anderson, C.L. (2012). FcγRIIb on liver sinusoidal endothelium clears small immune complexes. *Journal of Immunology* **189** (10), 4981–4988.

Gardner, R.B., Nydam, D.V., Luna, J.A. Bicalho, M.L., Matychak, M.B. and Flaminio, M.J. (2007). Serum opsonization capacity, phagocytosis, and oxidative burst activity in neonatal foals in the intensive care unit. *Journal of Veterinary Internal Medicine* **21** (4), 797–805.

Hardefeldt, L.Y., Keuler, N. and Peek, S.F. (2010). Incidence of transfusion reactions to commercial equine plasma. *Journal of Veterinary Emergency and Critical Care* **20** (4), 421–425.

Jackson, R. (2000). Serum sickness. *Journal of Cutaneous Medicine and Surgery* **4** (4), 223–225.

Kumar, V., Abbas, A.K., Fausto, N. and Aster, J.C. (2010). *Robbins and Cotran Pathologic Basis of Disease*, eighth edition, pp. 204–205. Philadelphia, Saunders Elsevier.

Lavoie, J.P., Spensley, M.S., Smith, B.P., Bowling, A.T. and Morse, S. (1989). Complement activity and selected hematologic variables in newborn foals fed bovine colostrum. *American Journal of Veterinary Research* **50** (9), 1532–1536.

Lawley, T.J., Bielory, L., Gascon, P., Yancey, K.B., Young, N.S. and Frank, M.M. (1985). A study of human serum sickness. *Journal of Investigative Dermatology* **85** (1 Suppl), 129s–132s.

Perkins, G.A., Yeager, A., Erb, H.N., Nydam, D.V., Divers, T.J. and Bowman, J.L. (2002). Survival of foals with experimentally induced *Rhodococcus equi* infection given either hyperimmune plasma containing *R. equi* antibody or normal equine plasma. *Veterinary Therapy* **3** (3), 334–346.

Reis, K.J. (1989). A hemolytic assay for the measurement of equine complement. *Veterinary Immunology and Immunopathology* **23** (1–2), 129–137.

Reynolds, N. (2012). Plasma transfusion reactions. http://www .veterinaryimmunogenics.com/News/TransfusionReactions

Rowlands, A, Lake Immunogenics, Inc., Ontario, NY and Wyatt, J. University of Rochester, Rochester, NY (personal communication).

Silverstein, A.M. (2000). Historical insight: Clemens Freiherr von Pirquet: explaining immune complex disease in 1906. *Nature Immunology* **1** (6), 453–455.

Swiderski, C. (1997). Hypersensitivity reactions. In: Reed, S. and Baily, W. (eds). *Equine Internal Medicine*, first edition, pp. 19–47. Philadelphia, WB Saunders.

Swiderski, C. (2000). Hypersensitivity disorders in horses. *Veterinary Clinics of North America: Equine Practice* **16**, 131–151.

Tennent-Brown, B. (2011). Plasma therapy in foals and adult horses. *Compendium: Continuing Education for Veterinarians* **33**, E1–4.

9 Vasculitis

James S. W. Prutton and Nicola Pusterla

9.1 Definition

Vasculitis results from different types of inflammatory mechanisms secondary to an infectious, toxic, neoplastic or systemic immunologic disorder (Morris, 1987). When an infectious etiology is involved, endothelial cell destruction can result from direct pathogen invasion, activation of neutrophils, and the release of proteolytic enzymes and free radicals that cause cell damage. Local vasculitis can also develop following injection of drugs (e.g., local anesthetics and vaccines) (Crowson, 2003). Alternatively, a secondary immune mechanism may cause endothelial cell damage, including *antibody-mediated* (auto-antibody binding or antibody-antigen immune-complex deposition) or *cellular-mediated* inflammation.

The immune-mediated response manifests at various blood vessels (veins, capillaries or arteries), with the most commonly affected vessels being the post-capillary venules (Mehregan, 1992; Knottenbelt, 2002). *Small vessel vasculitides* are the most common type of vasculitis, caused by deposition of auto-antibody or antibody-antigen immune-complex on the endothelium. Another mechanism described in human patients involves anti-neutrophil cytoplasm antibody (ANCA). Also, in human patients, *medium vessel vasculitis* causes artery aneurysms, and *large vessel vasculitis* can be caused by giant cell arteritis (Wilfong, 2013).

The clinical manifestations will depend on the vessels affected and the severity of the vascular damage. The apparent indiscriminate nature of vasculitis can lead either to a *localized* disease (one organ, most frequently cutaneous disease) or to a *multisystemic* disease, with the risk of renal failure (Morris, 1987).

9.2 Signalment and clinical signs

On initial presentation, a full history could help in determining possible triggering factors of immune-mediated vasculitis, including concurrent or historical disease, drug usage, vaccination, diet changes, and exposure to infectious organisms. A retrospective case series of vasculitis reported that affected horses commonly presented for photosensitization (White, 2009).

In systemic vasculitis, horses present with clinical signs including depression, anorexia, pyrexia, and mucosal petechiae and ecchymosis (Figure 9.1). Pyrexia has been seen as a negative indicator for prognosis (Morris, 1987). The edema can be localized to limbs, ventrum (Figure 9.2) or be generalized.

Cutaneous manifestations of vasculitis usually include erythema, crusts, scales, pruritus, oozing of serum, edema of the distal limbs, and necrosis (Figure 9.3). Often, the edema will be warm and painful on palpation; the patient may be refractory to exercise, requiring more intense treatment. Secondary cellulitis, thrombophlebitis, laminitis or pneumonia has been described (Smith, 2009).

9.3 Immunologic mechanisms and etiologic associations

The pathophysiology of immune-mediated vasculitis is often not clear, although it involves inflammation, vessel wall damage, and edema. Inflammation of the endothelial cells stimulates the release of vasoactive amines from platelets and expression of beta-2 integrin on the endothelium, which promotes the deposition of circulating *antibody-antigen immune-complexes* on the vascular walls (hypersensitivity type II). Consequently, this inflammatory process activates neutrophils and the complement pathway, and perpetuates endothelial damage (Jones, 2001; Danila, 2008). Similar events occur when there is direct binding of *auto-antibodies* to endothelial cells (hypersensitivity type II).

The binding of auto-antibodies or the deposition of immune-complexes on vessel walls is favored in areas of blood flow turbulence, vessel bifurcation and/or increased hydrostatic forces (Smith, 2009). In addition, it promotes: continuing activation of mesangial cells, macrophages and platelets; the upregulation of adhesion molecules, including leukocyte function antigen-1 (LFA-1), intracellular adhesion molecule-1 (ICAM-1), E-selectin and P-selectin that promote neutrophils diapedesis; and the production of inflammatory cytokines tumor necrosis alpha (TNF-alpha) and interleukin (IL)-1, chemokine IL-8, perforin, Fas ligand, proteolytic enzymes (lysosomal, elastase, collagenase), reactive oxygen species, thromboxane, nitrous oxide (NO), histamine, and platelet activating factor (PAF) (Sindrilaru, 2007). There is concurrent release of plasminogen activator inhibitor-1 (PAI-1) for increased thrombogenesis, and further slowing of the blood flow.

Equine Clinical Immunology, First Edition. Edited by M. Julia B. Felippe.
© 2016 John Wiley & Sons, Inc. Published 2016 by John Wiley & Sons, Inc.

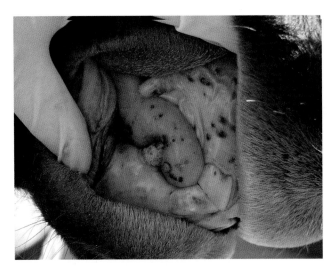

Figure 9.1 Vasculitis: mucosal petechiation and ecchymosis secondary to vasculitis in a horse (Nicola Pusterla, University of California-Davis).

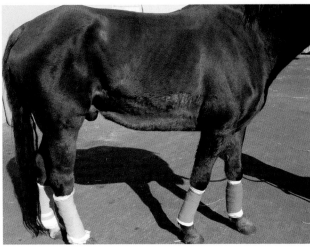

Figure 9.2 Vasculitis: ventral edema in a horse with vasculitis (Nicola Pusterla, University of California-Davis).

These mediators are responsible for the classical signs of vasculitis, including increased membrane permeability, edema and protein loss. The damage caused to the endothelial layer leads to exposure of subendothelial collagen and/or release of tissue factors, resulting in thromboembolic and ischemic events, with a net increase in vasoconstriction and platelet aggregation, and further tissue ischemia.

Cellular-mediated inflammation may occur upon T and B lymphocyte activation through molecular mimicry or super-antigens, which are pathogen antigens that cause polyclonal lymphocyte activation and massive cytokine release (Lidar, 2009). Th1 and Th2 type responses have both been implicated in vasculitides, with localized disease showing a predominantly Th1-based response, and systemic disease showing a Th2 response. In human patients with immune-mediated vasculitis, the expression of IL-18 (a Th1 and Th2 pro-inflammatory cytokine) is increased, which further exacerbates the immune response (Danila, 2008).

Histopathological evaluation of the affected tissue(s) is required to confirm vasculitis, and differentiation from a vasculopathy secondary to an ischemic event. The histological diagnosis describes endothelial necrosis, with varying degrees of involvement of neutrophils, eosinophils and lymphocytes (Pascoe, 1999; McGavin, 2007; White, 2009). A leukocytoclastic vasculitis is classified by the presence of neutrophil perivascular infiltration, with pyknosis and karyorrhexis inside and around the involved vessels, leading to endothelial cell swelling and necrosis, extravasation of erythrocytes and fibrinoid deposits (Mehregan, 1992; McGavin, 2007; Smith, 2009; Innerå, 2013; Figure 9.4). Immunohistochemistry can reveal antibodies within the vessel walls (Marti, 2003).

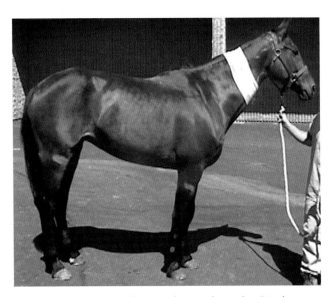

Figure 9.3 Vasculitis: limb edema in a horse with vasculitis (Nicola Pusterla, University of California-Davis).

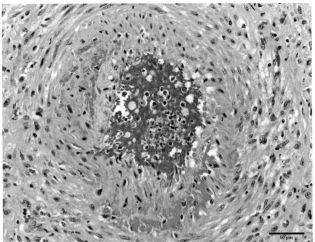

Figure 9.4 Vasculitis: histopathological image of vasculitis within the sciatic nerve showing leukocytoclasis and fibrinoid necrosis (hematoxylin and eosin stain) (Nicola Pusterla, University of California-Davis).

9.4 Diagnostics

Following a full history and preliminary clinical work-up, a biopsy of the affected area is essential in order to confirm vasculitis. Biopsies should be taken and stored in both formaldehyde (for histology) and Michel's transport medium (for immunohistochemistry). It is essential to take multiple samples from different sites, and to include recent lesions.

Blood work reflects inflammation associated with the inciting cause of the vasculitis, generally with neutrophilia and a high number of bands, hyperfibrinogenemia, hyperglobulinemia, anemia and thrombocytopenia. The anemia may be due to chronic disease or a hemolytic event, while thrombocytopenia is often due to consumption. Renal and liver function should be investigated with blood biochemistry, particularly in systemic vasculitis.

The list of differential diagnosis includes drug or vaccine response, pastern and cannon leukocytoclastic vasculitis, photo-activated vasculitis, purpura hemorrhagica, equine viral arteritis, equine infectious anemia, equine herpes virus-1, equine granulocytic anaplasmosis, endotoxemia, complement deficiency, serum sickness, African horse sickness, radiation injury, chemical and physical injury, poisoning, and localized thrombophlebitis (Jesty, 2006). Paraneoplastic vasculitis occurs in human patients and has also been reported in the horse (Finley, 1998).

9.5 Treatment

The treatment of vasculitis depends on the underlying disorder, degree and localization of histopathological changes, but it commonly involves immunosuppressive therapy. The aim of treatment is to remove the antigenic stimulus, thus stopping the ongoing inflammatory and immune responses.

The first step is to stop all drugs that are under administration, and assess what is required and what could be causing the vasculitis (Divers, 2003). Supportive care consists of hydrotherapy, pressure wraps, intravenous fluids and a tracheostomy, if indicated.

Anti-inflammatories are pivotal in the treatment of vasculitis, not only for pain relief but also to reduce local inflammation. Flunixin meglumine at 1.1 mg/kg IV or PO BID inhibits thromboxane production and, thus, reduces the risk of thrombus formation. It also reduces the expression of adhesion molecules on the surface of lymphocytes, minimizing the interaction with endothelial cells. When an immune-mediated process is identified, immunosuppression can be achieved with corticosteroids, initially dexamethasone at 0.05–0.2 mg/kg SID IV or PO. If the oral route is chosen, the dose should be increased, to account for the decreased oral bioavailability. Prednisolone at 0.5–2.0 mg/kg PO BID to SID may follow dexamethasone when inflammation is under control. Immunosuppressive drugs and the duration of treatment should be tailored to the severity of disease, and it may be required for many weeks, taking into account the approximately 30-day half-life of antibodies.

Treatment with corticosteroids includes the risk of increased susceptibility to infections, and laminitis, particularly in the case of vasculitis. Therefore, other types of immunomodulators may be necessary in combination with low-dose corticosteroids, or in their replacement. Azathioprine at 3 mg/kg PO SID inhibits the enzyme amidophosphoribosyltransferase required for purine nucleotide synthesis, and can be used as a maintenance therapy (Broussalis, 2013). Aurothioglucose, a gold salt, has also been used at 1 mg/kg IV SID, but it can take 16 weeks before a beneficial response is seen, and it is not widely available (Vandenabeele, 2004). Lidocaine at 1.3 mg/kg IV bolus, followed by 0.05 mg/kg/min IV constant rate infusion, can be used as an inhibitor of endotoxin, granulocyte infiltration, and myeloperoxidase activity.

In order to reduce the risk of thrombosis and ischemia, pentoxifylline at 8.4 mg/kg PO TID or BID has hemorheologic effects of red cell deformability and decreased blood viscosity. In addition, it inhibits inflammatory cell adhesion and the release of cytokines. The use of heparin or acetylsalicylic acid is questionable for the treatment of vasculitis, particularly in the case of thrombocytopenia, and low doses are reserved for cases with evidence of thrombophlebitis. Severe cases of vasculitis may require judicious fluid therapy to maintain tissue perfusion and renal function, with monitoring of edema due to increased endothelial permeability.

Antibiotic therapy should be started if clinically warranted and based on culture and sensitivity results if available. Antiviral therapy could be key to the treatment of early infection, e.g., EHV-1 (Wong, 2010).The most commonly used drugs in the treatment of vasculitis are listed in Table 9.1.

9.6 Thrombophlebitis

Risk factors associated with localized thrombophlebitis include catheter placement, type of material, size and duration, and types of medication for intravenous use. Concurrent diseases, including sepsis, endotoxemia, disseminated intravascular coagulation, coagulopathies, neoplasia and protein-losing (loss of protein C and antithrombin III) enteropathy/nephropathy represent risk factors associated with the development of thrombophlebitis (Dolente, 2005; Moreau, 2009). Septic thrombophlebitis can cause embolisms, generally in pulmonary or synovial tissues (Ryu, 2004).

Clinical signs include firm, warm and localized swelling over the vein, diffuse swelling and pain. These signs can worsen to depression, fever and complications associated with secondary emboli (Russell, 2010). Ultrasonography can demonstrate increased thickness of the vein wall, the presence of thrombi within the vein, and perivascular edema. A sterilely retrieved aspirate of the thrombus used for microbiological culture can

Table 9.1 Commonly used drugs with dosages for the treatment of vasculitis.

Drug	Dosage(s)	Route and duration of treatment
Anti-inflammatories		
Flunixin meglumine	1.1 mg/kg	PO or IV, BID
	0.3 mg/kg	PO or IV, TID
Dexamethasone	0.05-0.2 mg/kg	IM or IV, SID
Prednisolone acetate	0.5-2 mg/kg	PO, BID or SID
Immunomodulators		
Aurothioglucose (gold salts)	1 mg/kg	IV, SID
Azathioprine	3 mg/kg	PO, SID
Antithrombotics		
Pentoxyfilline	8.4 mg/kg	PO, TID or BID
Low molecular weight heparin	50 U/kg	SQ, SID
Unfractionated heparin	40-100 IU/kg	IV or SQ, TID or BID
Acetylsalicylic acid	15-20 mg/kg	PO, SID or EOD
Antiherpetic drugs		
Acyclovir	10-20 mg/kg	PO, TID
Valacyclovir	20-40 mg/kg	PO, TID or BID
Other		
Lidocaine	1.3 mg/kg	IV bolus prior to CRI, once
	0.05 mg/kg/min	IV, CRI

IV – intravenous; PO – per os or orally; SQ – subcutaneous; CRI – continuous rate infusion; SID – *semel in die* or once a day; BID – *bis in die* or twice a day; TID – *ter in die* or three times a day.

determine the presence of a septic process and can help with antibiotic treatment decisions (Klohnen, 2009).

9.7 Pastern and cannon leukocytoclastic vasculitis

Pastern and cannon leukocytoclastic vasculitis (PCLV) is a sporadic disease that affects non-pigmented skin. Antibody binding to the endothelium activates complement, causing cellular damage and necrosis. Clinical signs are acute onset of localized or diffuse erythema, oozing, crusting, edema and lameness (Pascoe, 1999). It can appear similar to idiopathic *grease heel* or *scratches* (Figure 9.5A and B).

Although located solely on non-pigmented skin, there does not appear to be a link with photosensitizing agents (Risberg, 2005). Instead, PCLV can often be associated with long-standing dermatophytosis, bacterial infection or chorioptic mange. A recent study postulated how the administration of progestin (Altrenogest) could have an immunosuppressive effect leading to an increased bacterial load within the pastern (Risberg, 2005).

Biopsy is critical to the diagnosis of this disease, with: histopathological evidence deep dermal and hypodermal foci of hemorrhage; moderate edema of the dermis; and neutrophil infiltration surrounding the vessels. Mostly, the tunica media of the arteries and arterioles is affected.

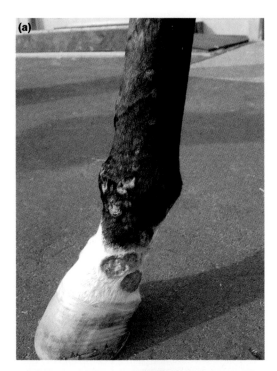

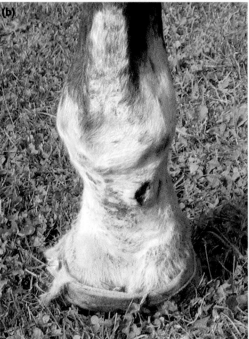

Figure 9.5 Leukocytoclastic vasculitis.
A) Horse with lesions typical for pastern and cannon leukocytoclastic vasculitis (Nicola Pusterla, University of California-Davis).
B) A case of pastern vasculitis under immunosuppressive treatment (courtesy of Amy Johnson, University of Pennsylvania).

9.8 Drug-induced vasculitis

The diagnosis of a drug-induced vasculitis is based on the temporal relationship between the clinical manifestation of vasculitis and the use of the offending drug. Several drugs have been linked to idiosyncratic drug reactions that include vasculitis in horses, including penicillin, potentiated sulfonamides, ceftiofur, rifampin, acepromazine, detomidine, and tiludronate (White, 2009). In addition, the use of the mycobacterial-derived cell wall extract for the treatment of sarcoids has been associated with vasculitis (White, 2009).

The mechanisms of drug-induced vasculitis in horses have not yet been elucidated. In the human medical field, certain drugs induce the production of IgG autoantibodies against antigens within the cytoplasm of neutrophils, a condition known as anti-neutrophil cytoplasm antibody (ANCA) (Harrison, 1989; Cuellar, 2002; Gao, 2009; Fukuhara, 2013). Multiple factors are likely to be involved in the production of ANCA and vasculitis. Some drugs may be metabolized by myeloperoxidase released from active neutrophils into cytotoxic compounds, or may act as haptens for myeloperoxidase (Jiang, 1994). Another proposed mechanism suggests that the offending drugs accumulate within neutrophils and bind to myeloperoxidase, altering its configuration. Drugs that have been associated with ANCA-vasculitis in human medicine include minocycline and sulfasalazine (Cuellar, 2002; Gao, 2009; Lenert, 2013).

Most common clinical sings include arthralgia, myalgia and skin rash (Radić, 2011). ANCA against myeloperoxidase can be detected using ELISA or immunofluorescence (Cambridge, 1994). Early lesions in skin biopsies show vascular endothelial swelling and necrosis. Lysed neutrophils will often be seen within the affected vessels (Harper, 2000).

9.9 Photo-activated vasculitis (photodynamic drugs)

Photo-activated vasculitis is seen when phylloerythrin accumulates within the skin, leading to photosensitization. Phylloerythrin exposure to light energy causes activation of electrons and free radical formation, with resulting damage to skin proteins, nucleic acids and receptor molecules.

Photosensitization can occur in two main ways (Pilsworth, 2007; White, 2009; Campbell, 2010):

1 Through the ingestion of plants or drugs containing photodynamic agents (e.g., St. John's Wort, mycotoxins from fungi, thiazides, tetracyclines, sulfonamides, furosemide).
2 Due to failure of the liver to detoxify phylloerythrin, a by-product of the digestion of chlorophyll that is normally conjugated within the liver and excreted in the bile.

Clinical sings include photophobia, discomfort, scratching, erythema, edema, serous exudation, scab formation, and skin necrosis. Initially, the lesions occur on the unpigmented or lightly pigmented skin, then spread to the rest of the body. Often, the lesions have secondary bacterial infections (Stegelmeier, 2002).

9.10 *Strongylus vulgaris*

Following ingestion, infective L3 phase larvae penetrate the mucosa of the small intestine, molt into L4 and begin to migrate via the submucosal arteries. The L4 then mature in the mesenteric artery roots for 3–4 months. The affected vessels will appear largely inflamed, with cellular infiltration, the development of adherent thrombi and infarction of the intestine (McGavin, 2007).

Although rarely seen in horses since the introduction of ivermectin, patients show anemia, hypoproteinemia and leucocytosis, and signs of sporadic or severe colic with a high prevalence of death. Fecal flotation may not correlate with the presence of larval forms in the mesenteric vessels, and definitive diagnosis is generally made at post-mortem.

9.11 Equine granulocytic anaplasmosis

Anaplasma phagocytophilum, a Gram-negative bacterium, is the causative agent of equine granulocytic anaplasmosis, a disease transmitted by *Ixodes* spp. ticks. *A. phagocytophilum* has been shown to infect endothelial cells and progenitor cells of the bone marrow, with a tropism towards cells of the hematopoietic and phagocytic system. The pathogen inhibits the release of TNF-alpha, IL-6, and IL-13, and reduces the IgE-dependant activation of mast cells (Ojogun, 2011). The reduction in the innate pro-inflammatory response is probably the reason why *A. phagocytophilum* can often show mild clinical signs.

Microscopic lesions occur within the kidneys, heart, muscular fascia and lung, although the majority are seen within the small arteries and veins of the legs (Franzén, 2007). The endothelial cells are swollen and the capillary walls are thickened. Necrotizing inflammation is seen in arterioles and capillaries often associated with perivascular and interstitial mononuclear cell infiltration and hemorrhage. The correlation between the vascular damage and the bacteria is not obvious, and it is thought that the bacteria could cause local inflammation, with oxidative and enzymatic damage (Lepidi, 2000).

Affected horses show fever, depression, anorexia, limb edema, petechiae, icterus, ataxia and reluctance to move. Rhabdomyolysis, myalgia and orchitis can also occur in the course of the disease (Nolen-Walston, 2004; Hilton, 2008). Hematological changes include anemia, thrombocytopenia, and leucopenia. Stained direct blood smears show small, round, dark purple dots within the cytoplasm of neutrophils and eosinophils. Polymerase chain reaction (PCR) of blood has been shown to be positive 2–3 days prior to the development of clinical signs, and to persist 4–9 days beyond abatement of clinical signs (Franzén, 2005). Serology can be performed to indicate a rising titer (Dzięgiel, 2013). Biopsies of the distal limbs show petechial hemorrhage and edema, along with proliferative and necrotizing vasculitis of small arteries and veins. Treatment is accomplished with oxytetracycline at 6.6–10 mg/kg SID for 5–10 days.

9.12 Equine viral arteritis

In equine viral arteritis (EVA), the virus replicates within lung macrophages and endothelial cells, including small blood vessels, mesothelium and smooth muscle of the tunica media in smaller arteries. Infection induces natural killer (NK) cell response, with lysis of the infected cells by perforins. In addition, infected macrophages secrete pro-inflammatory cytokines (e.g., TNF-alpha, IL-1beta, IL-6) and chemokine (e.g., IL-8), and up-regulate adhesion molecules, leading to further leukocyte infiltration, cytokine release, necrosis, increased endothelial permeability, hemorrhage, and edema.

The clinical signs vary from subclinical infection to influenza-like illness, with panvasculitis, edema, hemorrhage, interstitial pneumonia in the neonatal foal, and abortion in pregnant mares due to lethal fetal infection (Piero, 1997; Del Piero, 2000; McGavin, 2007). Pyrexia, depression, anorexia, dependant edema, gait stiffness, conjunctivitis, respiratory distress and urticaria have also been reported.

Biopsies can be used to confirm the presence of vasculitis, characterized by fibrinoid necrosis of the tunica media, abundant vascular and perivascular lymphocytic and granulocytic infiltration with karyorrhexis, loss of endothelium and formation of large fibrinocellular stratified thrombi (Smith, 2009). Diagnosis of EVA is supported by seroconversion (virus neutralization assay or ELISA), and/or virus isolation, using RT-PCR performed on nasopharyngeal or conjunctival swabs, citrate or EDTA blood samples, semen, or aborted fetuses.

9.13 Equine herpesvirus-1

Equine herpevirus-1 (EHV-1) is an endotheliotropic and lymphotropic virus, with an active lytic or a latent phase (Allen, 2008; Pusterla, 2010). Infection requires viral attachment to the cell membrane with fusion and penetration, followed by translocation of viral DNA to the nucleus, replication of viral DNA leading to synthesis of viral proteins, and capsid assembly, which results in egress from and lysis of the host cell, including endothelial cells (Goehring, 2010).

The damage within the microvasculature leads to inflammation, microthrombi, extravasation of mononuclear cells, perivascular cuffing, and local hemorrhage (Lunn, 2009). The inflammatory cuffing extends into the adventitia, media and intima of the vessel wall (Allen, 2006). It is thought that immune-complexes and cytokines (IL-2 and IFN-gamma) from cytotoxic T cells influence the severity and propagation of the disease (Borchers, 2006; Luce, 2007; Ma, 2013). Glycoprotein production (gI and gE) is also involved in antibody-antigen immune-complex deposition within vessel walls, activation of complement and release of lysosomal enzymes, with subsequent vasculitis and hemorrhage.

The central nervous system infection involves a primary vasculitis and secondary thrombo-ischemic event following endothelial cell infection. Uterine infection involves lysis of the endothelial cells, particularly the small arteriolar branches of the glandular layer of the endometrium at the base of the microcotyledons (Reed, 2004). Myelomalacia, abortion in the last third of gestation or stillbirth is secondary to ischemic events with hypoxic degeneration (Allen, 2006; Henninger, 2007; Gilkerson, 2008).

Polymerase chain reaction has become a rapid and sensitive method for the detection of EHV-1 in both nasal secretions and blood in early infection (Burgess, 2012). Immunofluorescence and histopathology can be used to detect EHV-1 in aborted fetal and post-mortem samples. Treatment with acyclovir at 10–20 mg/kg PO TID, or valacyclovir at 20–40 mg/kg PO TID or BID, has been attempted.

9.14 African horse sickness

African horse sickness is caused by an orbivirus from the family *Reoviridae*. This is one of the most important equine diseases seen in Africa, but with potential to spread to other parts of the world through insect vectors (Maclachlan, 2010). Viral replication occurs in the endothelial cells, pulmonary intravascular macrophages, interstitial macrophages and fibroblasts, leading to endothelial damage, neutrophil sequestration and changes in pulmonary microvasculature. Initial replication occurs in the regional lymph nodes, and a primary viremia spreads the virus to lungs, spleen and other lymphoid tissues. In peripheral blood, the virus is associated with red cells and monocytes. It is possible that the association of the African horse sickness virus to red cell wall reduces antibody production (Ellor, 2004; Aklilu, 2012).

There are four forms of the disease (Ellor, 2004; Weyer, 2013; Finno, 2009):

1 *Horse sickness form*, with mild fever, edema of supraorbital fossae, and low fatality rate.
2 *Cardiac subacute form*, with fever that lasts several weeks, profound subcutaneous edema of the head, neck and chest (never in the lower limbs), petechiation and hemorrhage of the sclera; colic is often, and fatality rate is over 50%.
3 *Mixed form*, with fever, respiratory distress with large amounts of hemorrhagic froth coming from the mouth and nose, generalized edema, and fatality rate is higher than 90%.
4 *Pulmonary form*, with severe respiratory signs of tachypnea, dyspnea, coughing, nasal discharge, fever, and fatality rate 95%.

Quantitative PCR is the main diagnostic technique, and a sandwich ELISA can be used for rapid identification of African horse sickness virus antigen in solid tissue samples. Clinical signs are pathognomonic for the disease, and the severity and rapid progression to death often negates the need for an ante-mortem diagnosis. Vaccination is essential because of the overall high fatality of this disease (Crafford, 2013).

References

Aklilu, N., Batten, C., Gelaye, E., Jenberie, S., Ayelet, G., Wilson, A., Belay, A., Asfaw, Y., Oura, C., Maan, S., Bachanek-Bankowska, K. and Mertens, P.P.C. (2012). African horse sickness outbreaks caused by multiple virus types in Ethiopia. *Transboundary and Emerging Diseases* **61**, 1–8.

Allen, G.P. and Breathnach, C.C. (2006). Quantification by real-time PCR of the magnitude and duration of leucocyte-associated viraemia in horses infected with neuropathogenic vs. non-neuropathogenic strains of EHV-1. *Equine Veterinary Journal* **38**(3), 252–257.

Allen, G.P., Bolin, D.C., Bryant, U., Carter, C.N., Giles, R.C., Harrison, L.R., Hong, C.B., Jackson, C.B., Poonacha, K., Wharton, R. and Williams, N.M. (2008). Prevalence of latent, neuropathogenic equine herpesvirus-1 in the Thoroughbred broodmare population of central Kentucky. *Equine Veterinary Journal* **40**(2), 105–110.

Borchers, K., Thein, P. and Sterner-Kock, A. (2006). Pathogenesis of equine herpesvirus-associated neurological disease: a revised explanation. *Equine Veterinary Journal* **38**(3), 283–287.

Broaddus, C., Balasuriya, U.B.R., White, J.L.R., Timoney, P.F., Funk, R.A. and Holyoak, G.R. (2011). Evaluation of the safety of vaccinating mares against equine viral arteritis during mid or late gestation or during the immediate postpartum period. *Journal of American Veterinary Medical Association* **238**(6), 741–750.

Broussalis, E., Trinka, E., Kraus, J., McCoy, M., and Killer, M. (2013). Treatment strategies for vasculitis that affects the nervous system. *Drug Discovery Today* **18**, 1–17.

Burgess, B.A., Tokateloff, N., Manning, S., Lohmann, K., Lunn, D.P., Hussey, S.B. and Morley, P.S. (2012). Nasal shedding of equine herpesvirus-1 from horses in an outbreak of equine herpes myeloencephalopathy in Western Canada. *Journal of Veterinary Internal Medicine* **26**(2), 384–392.

Cambridge, G., Wallace, H., Bernstein, R.M. and Leaker, B. (1994). Autoantibodies to myeloperoxidase in idiopathic and drug-induced systemic lupus erythematosus and vasculitis. *Rheumatology* **33**(2), 109–114.

Campbell, W.M., Dombroski, G.S., Sharma, I., Partridge, A.C. and Collett, M.G. (2010). Photodynamic chlorophyll a metabolites, including phytoporphyrin (phylloerythrin), in the blood of photosensitive livestock: overview and measurement. *New Zealand Veterinary Journal* **58**(3), 146–154.

Crafford, J.E., Lourens, C.W., Gardner, I.A., Maclachlan, N.J. and Guthrie, A.J. (2013). Passive transfer and rate of decay of maternal antibody against African horse sickness virus in South African thoroughbred foals. *Equine Veterinary Journal* **45**(5), 604–607.

Crowson, A.N., Mihm, M.C. Jr. and Magro. C.M. (2003). Cutaneous vasculitis: a review. *Journal of Cutaneous Pathology* **30**(3), 161–173.

Cuellar, M.L. (2002). Drug-induced vasculitis. *Current Rheumatology Reports* **4**(1), 55–59.

Danila, M.I., and Bridges. S.L. (2008). Update on pathogenic mechanisms of systemic necrotizing vasculitis. *Current Rheumatology Reports* **10**(6), 430–435.

Del Piero, F. (2000). Equine viral arteritis. *Veterinary Pathology* **37**, 287–396.

Divers, T.J. (2003). Prevention and treatment of thrombosis, phlebitis, and laminitis in horses with gastrointestinal diseases. *Veterinary Clinics of North America: Equine Practice* **19**(3), 779–790.

Dolente, B.A., Beech. J., Lindborg. S. and Smith, G. (2005). Evaluation of risk factors for development of catheter-associated jugular thrombophlebitis in horses: 50 cases (1993–1998). *Journal of American Veterinary Medical Association* **227**(7), 1134–1141.

Dzięgiel, B., Adaszek, L., Kalinowski, M. and Winiarczyk, S. (2013). Equine granulocytic anaplasmosis. *Research in Veterinary Science* **95** (2), 316–320.

Ellor, P.S.M. and Amblin, C.H. (2004). Review article African horse sickness. *Veterinary Research* **35**(4), 445–466.

Finley, M.R., Rebhun, W.C., Dee, A. and Lanstemo, I. (1998). Paraneoplastic pruritus and alopecia in a horse with diffuse lymphoma. *Journal of American Veterinary Medical Association* **213**(1), 102–4.

Finno, C.J., Spier, S.J. and Valberg, S.J. (2009). Equine diseases caused by known genetic mutations. *Veterinary Journal* **179**(3), 336–347.

Franzén, P., Aspan, A., Egenvall, A., Gunnarsson, A., Åberg, L. and Pringle, J. (2005). Acute clinical, hematologic, serologic, and polymerase chain reaction findings in horses experimentally infected with a European strain of *Anaplasma phagocytophilum*. *Journal of Veterinary Internal Medicine* **19**(2), 232–239.

Franzén, P., Berg, A., Aspan, A., Gunnarsson, A. and Pringle, J. (2007). Death of a horse infected experimentally with *Anaplasma phagocytophilum*. *Veterinary Record* **160**(4), 122–125.

Fukuhara, A., Tanino, Y., Sato, S., Ishii, T., Nikaido, T., Kanazawa, K., Saito, J., Ishida, T., Kanno, M., Watanabe, T. and Munakata, M. (2013). Systemic vasculitis associated with anti-neutrophil cytoplasmic antibodies against bactericidal/permeability increasing protein. *Internal Medicine* **52**(10), 1095–1099.

Gaffo, A.L. (2013). Thrombosis in vasculitis. *Best Practices and Research: Clinical Rheumatology* **27**(1), 57–67.

Gao, Y. and Zhao, M.H. (2009). Review article: Drug-induced anti-neutrophil cytoplasmic antibody-associated vasculitis. *Nephrology* **14** (1), 33–41.

Garcia-Seco, E., Costa, L.R.R., McClure-Blackmer, J.M. and Foil, C.S. (2002). Necrotising vasculitis without subcutaneous oedema in a miniature horse. *Equine Veterinary Education* **14**(5), 243–246.

Gilkerson, J.R. (2008). Equine herpesvirus neurological disease. *Equine Veterinary Journal* **40**(2), 102–103.

Goehring, L.S., Landolt, G.A. and Morley, P.S. (2010). Detection and management of an outbreak of equine herpesvirus type 1 infection and associated neurological disease in a veterinary teaching hospital. *Journal of Veterinary Internal Medicine* **24**(5), 1176–1183.

Guillevin, L. (2013). Infections in vasculitis. *Best Practices in Research Clinical Rheumatology* **27**(1), 19–31.

Hall, J.E. (2011). *Guyton and Hall Textbook of Medical Physiology*, 12th edition. Philadelphia, Elsevier Saunders.

Harper, L. and Savage, C.O.S. (2000). Pathogenesis of ANCA-associated systemic vasculitis. *Journal of Pathology* **190**(3), 349–359.

Harrison, D.J. and Kharbanda, R. (1989). Autoantibodies to neutrophil cytoplasmic antigens in systemic vasculitis have the same target specificity. *Journal of Pathology* **158**(3), 233–238.

Henninger, R.W., Reed, S.M., Saville, W.J., Allen, G.P., Hass, G.F., Kohn, C.W. and Sofaly, C. (2007). Outbreak of neurologic disease caused by equine herpesvirus-1 at a university equestrian center. *Journal of Veterinary Internal Medicine* **21**(1), 157–165.

Hilton, H., Madigan, J.E. and Aleman, M. (2008). Rhabdomyolysis associated with *Anaplasma phagocytophilum* infection in a horse. *Journal of Veterinary Internal Medicine* **22**(4), 1061–1064.

Innerå, M. (2013). Cutaneous vasculitis in small animals. *Veterinary Clinics of North America: Small Animal Practice* **43**(1), 113–134.

Jesty, S.A. and Reef, V.B. (2006). Septicemia and cardiovascular infections in horses. *Veterinary Clinics of North America: Equine Practice* **22**(2), 481–495.

Jiang, X., Khursigara, G. and Rubin, R.L. (1994). Transformation of lupus-inducing drugs to cytotoxic products by activated neutrophils. *Science* **266**(5186), 810–813.

Jones, S.L., Sharief, Y. and Chilcoat, C.D. (2001). Signaling mechanism for equine neutrophil activation by immune complexes. *Veterinary Immunology and Immunopathology* **82**(1), 87–100.

Klohnen, A. (2009). New perspectives in postoperative complications after abdominal surgery. *Veterinary Clinics of North America: Equine Practice* **25**(2), 341–350.

Knottenbelt, D.C. (2002). Vasculitis: just what does it mean? *Equine Veterinary Education* **14**(5), 247–251.

Lenert, P., Icardi, M. and Dahmoush, L. (2013). ANA (+) ANCA (+) systemic vasculitis associated with the use of minocycline: case-based review. *Clinical Rheumatology* **32**(7), 1–8.

Lepidi, H., Bunnell, J.E., Martin, M.E., Madigan, J.E., Stuen, S. and Dumler, J.S. (2000). Comparative pathology, and immunohistology associated with clinical illness after *Ehrlichia phagocytophila*-group infections. *American Journal of Tropical Medicine and Hygiene* **62**(1), 29–37.

Lidar, M., Lipschitz, N., Langevitz, P. and Shoenfeld, Y. (2009). The infectious etiology of vasculitis. *Autoimmunity* **42**(5), 432–438.

Luce, R., Shepherd, M., Paillot, R., Blacklaws, B., Wood, J.L.N. and Kydd, J.H. (2007). Equine herpesvirus-1-specific interferon gamma (IFNγ) synthesis by peripheral blood mononuclear cells in thoroughbred horses. *Equine Veterinary Journal* **39**(3), 202–209.

Lunn, D.P., Davis-Poynter, N., Flaminio, M.J.B.F., Horohov, D.W., Osterrieder, K., Pusterla, N. and Townsend, H.G. (2009). Equine herpesvirus-1 consensus statement. *Journal of Veterinary Internal Medicine* **23**(3), 450–461.

Ma, G., Azab, W. and Osterrieder, N. (2013). Equine herpesviruses type 1 (EHV-1) and 4 (EHV-4)-masters of co-evolution and a constant threat to equids and beyond. *Veterinary Microbiology* **167** (1–2), 123–134.

Maclachlan, N.J. and Guthrie, A.J. (2010). Re-emergence of bluetongue, African horse sickness, and other orbivirus diseases. *Veterinary Research* **41**(6), 35.

Marti, E., Horohov, D.W., Antzak, D.F., Lazary, S. and Paul Lunn, D. (2003). Advances in equine immunology: Havemeyer workshop reports from Santa Fe, New Mexico, and Hortobagy, *Hungary. Veterinary Immunology and Immunopathology* **91**(3), 233–243.

McGavin, M.D. and Zachary, J.F. (2007). *Pathologic Basis of Veterinary Disease*, fourth edition. St Louis, Elsevier Mosby.

Mehregan, D.R., Hall, M.J. and Gibson, L.E. (1992). Urticarial vasculitis: a histopathologic and clinical review of 72 cases. *Journal of American Academy of Dermatology* **26**(3), 441–448.

Moreau, P. and Lavoie, J.P. (2009). Evaluation of athletic performance in horses with jugular vein thrombophlebitis: 91 cases (1988–2005).

Journal of American Veterinary Medical Association **235**(9), 1073–1078.

Morris, D.D. (1987). Cutaneous vasculitis in horses: 19 cases (1978–1985). *Journal of American Veterinary Medical Association* **191**(4), 460.

Nolen-Walston, R.D., D'Oench, S.M., Hanelt, L.M., Sharkey, L.C. and Paradis, M.R. (2004). Acute recumbency associated with *Anaplasma phagocytophilum* infection in a horse. *Journal of American Veterinary Medical Association* **224**(12), 1964–1966.

Ojogun, N., Barnstein, B., Huang, B., Oskeritzian, C.A., Homeister, J.W., Miller, D., Ryan, J.J. and Carlyon, J.A. (2011). Anaplasma phagocytophilum infects mast cells via alpha1,3-fucosylated but not sialylated glycans and inhibits IgE-mediated cytokine production and histamine release. *Infection and Immunity* **79**(7), 2717–2726.

Pascoe, R.R.R. and Knottenbelt, D.C. (1999). *Manual of Equine Dermatology*. Hong Kong, WB Saunders.

Piero, F.D. (2000). Equine viral arteritis. *Veterinary Pathology* **37**(4), 287–296.

Piero, F.D., Wilkins, P.A., Lopez, J.W., Glaser, A.L., Dubovi, E.J., Schlafer, D.H. and Lein, D.H. (1997). Equine viral arteritis in newborn foals: clinical, pathological, serological, microbiological and immunohistochemical observations. *Equine Veterinary Journal* **29** (3), 178–185.

Pilsworth, R. and Knottenbelt, D. (2007). Photosensitisation and sunburn. *Equine Veterinary Education* **19**(1), 32–33.

Pusterla, N. Hussey, S.B., Mapes, S., Johnson, C., Collier, J.R., Hill, J., Lunn, D.P. and Wilson, W.D. (2010). Molecular investigation of the viral kinetics of equine herpesvirus-1 in blood and nasal secretions of horses after corticosteroid-induced recrudescence of latent infection. *Journal of Veterinary Internal Medicine* **24**(5), 1153–1157.

Pusterla, N., Watson, J.L., Affolter, V.K., Magdesian, K.G., Wilson, W.D. and Carlson, G.P. (2003). *Purpura haemorrhagica* in 53 horses. *Veterinary Record* **153**(4), 118–121.

Radić, M. (2011). Drug-Induced Vasculitis. In: Amezcua-Guerra, L.M. (ed). *Advances in the Etiology Pathogenesis and Pathology of Vasculitis*. East Providence, InTech.

Reed, S.M. and Toribio, R.E. (2004). Equine herpesvirus 1 and 4. *Veterinary Clinics of North America: Equine Practice* **20**(3), 631–642.

Risberg, Å.I., Webb, C., Cooley, A., Peek, S. and Darien, B. (2005). Leucocytoclastic vasculitis associated with *Staphylococcus intermedius* in the pastern of a horse. *Veterinary Record* **156** (23), 740–743.

Russell, T.M., Kearney, C. and Pollock, P.J. (2010). Surgical treatment of septic jugular thrombophlebitis in nine horses. *Veterinary Surgery* **39** (5), 627–630.

Ryu, S., Kim, J., Bak, U., Lee, C. and Lee, Y.L. (2004). A hematogenic pleuropneumonia caused by postoperative septic thrombophlebitis in a Thoroughbred gelding. *Journal of Veterinary Science* **5**(1), 75–77.

Sellon, D.C. and Long, M.T. (2007). *Equine Infectious Diseases*. St Louis, Elsevier Saunders.

Sindrilaru, A., Seeliger, S., Ehrchen, J.M., Peters, T., Roth, J., Scharffetter-Kochanek, K. and Sunderkötter, C.H. (2007). Site of blood vessel damage and relevance of CD18 in a murine model of immune complex-mediated vasculitis. *Journal of Investigation in Dermatology*, **127**(2), 447–454.

Smith, B.P. (2009). *Large Animal Internal Medicine*, fourth edition. St Louis, Elsevier Mosby.

Stegelmeier, B.L. (2002). Equine photosensitization. *Clinical Techniques in Equine Practice* **1**(2), 81–88.

Sweeney, C.R., Timoney, J.F., Newton, J.R. and Hines, M.T. (2005). *Streptococcus equi* infections in horses: guidelines for treatment, control, and prevention of strangles. *Journal of Veterinary Internal Medicine* **19**(1), 123–134.

Vandenabeele, S.I.J., White, S.D., Affolter, V.K., Kass, P.H. and Ihrke, P.J. (2004). *Pemphigus foliaceus* in the horse: a retrospective study of 20 cases. *Veterinary Dermatology* **15**(16), 381–388.

Weyer, C.T., Quan, M., Joone, C., Lourens, C.W., MacLachlan, N.J. and Guthrie, A.J. (2013). African horse sickness in naturally infected, immunised horses. *Equine Veterinary Journal* **45**(1), 117–119.

White, S.D., Affolter, V.K., Dewey, J., Kass, P.H., Outerbridge, C. and Ihrke, P.J. (2009). Cutaneous vasculitis in equines: a retrospective study of 72 cases. *Veterinary Dermatology* **20** (5–6), 600–606.

Wilfong, E.M. and Seo, P. (2013). Vasculitis in the intensive care unit. *Best Practice and Research: Clinical Rheumatology* **27**(1), 95–106.

Wong, D.M., Maxwell, L.K. and Wilkins, P.A. (2010). Use of antiviral medications against equine herpes virus associated disorders. *Equine Veterinary Education* **22**(5), 244–252.

10 Purpura Hemorrhagica

Laszlo M. Hunyadi and Nicola Pusterla

10.1 Definition

Equine purpura hemorrhagica (PH) is an acute, non-contagious, aseptic necrotizing vasculitis, characterized by edema and petechial or ecchymotic hemorrhage of the mucosa and subcutaneous tissue (Pusterla, 2003). The exact pathogenesis of PH is not fully understood at this time, but the vasculitis appears to be caused by the deposition of antigen-antibody immune complexes on blood vessel walls. Although the prevalence is unknown, PH is often associated with infection or vaccination against *Streptococcus equi* subsp. *equi* (*S. equi*). Purpura hemorrhagica can also occur with other infections, including equine influenza, equine viral arteritis, equine herpes virus type 1, *Streptococcus equi* subsp. *zooepidemicus*, *Rhodococcus equi* and *Corynebacterium pseudotuberculosis*. However, in some cases, the disease occurs in the absence of any known or documented infection (Pusterla, 2003).

10.2 Signalment and clinical signs

There are no breed or gender predilections reported for PH, and most affected horses tend to be older than two years (Pusterla, 2003). Clinical signs usually develop acutely within 2–4 weeks after a respiratory infection, and can vary from a mild transient reaction to a severe fatal disease.

Typical clinical signs include urticaria followed by pitting edema of the distal limbs (Figures 10.1 and 10.2), head and ventrum, and petechial/ecchymoses of the mucosal membranes (Figure 10.3). Severe head edema can cause difficulty in breathing and eating, leading to anorexia, lethargy, and weight loss (Radostits, 2007). General edema can result in exudation, ulceration, crusting, and eventually sloughing of the skin. Affected horses are often depressed, febrile, tachycardic, tachypnic, stiff and reluctant to move (Reed, 2010). The vasculitis can also affect other organ systems, including the gastrointestinal tract, lungs, and muscles. Some horses develop colic or diarrhea due to hemorrhage, infarction, edema or necrosis of the intestinal wall. Fatality usually results from severe pneumonia, cardiac arrhythmias, renal failure, gastrointestinal complications, or severe muscle infarctions (Kaese, 2005).

10.3 Immunologic mechanisms and etiologic associations

The risk of developing PH after exposure to *S. equi* or vaccination with *S. equi* M-protein (SeM) is not well understood. A pre-existing high IgA serum antibody titer against the SeM or culture supernatant proteins may predispose horses to the development of PH (Heath, 1991). High IgA titers have been reported in horses with PH, compared with titers in horses recently infected with *S. equi* or horses with an unknown history of infection. Increased IgG titers in horses with PH typically coincide with improved clinical signs and recovery. Since IgA and M-like proteins have been found in the sera of horses diagnosed with PH, it is believed that IgA are involved in the pathophysiology of disease.

It is not understood why horses have high concentrations of IgA and low concentrations of IgG during the acute stages of PH. Current hypothesis include:

(a) uncontrolled expansion of B cell populations that produce IgA in response to *S. equi* antigen;
(b) failure of the liver's ability to remove IgA;
(c) delayed production of IgG in response to novel antigen;
(d) defective or suppressed production of IgG; and
(e) neutralization or excess utilization of IgG.

Purpura hemorrhagica has been compared to Henoch-Schönlein purpura (HSP), an antigen-antibody immune-complex-mediated disease in human patients. In the case of HSP, it is suspected that microbes introduced through the respiratory tract may activate a subgroup of T cells that secrete TGF-beta, which facilitates isotype switching to IgA. A similar mechanism may lead to the increase in IgA seen in horses with PH (Yang, 2008). These IgA antibody-antigen immune-complexes may then bind to the endothelial cells, and lead to endothelial cell lysis via the activation of complement and endothelial cell production of IL-8. Chemokine IL-8 is known to attract and activate neutrophils to release reactive oxygen metabolites and granule proteases, which further damage endothelial cells. Further investigations are needed to explore the mechanisms involved in both HSP and equine PH, including variations of disease-associated genes, identification of the microbes that induce and trigger PH in horses, and

Equine Clinical Immunology, First Edition. Edited by M. Julia B. Felippe.
© 2016 John Wiley & Sons, Inc. Published 2016 by John Wiley & Sons, Inc.

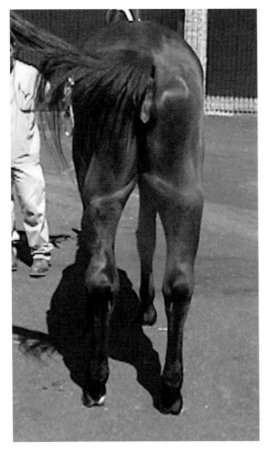

Figure 10.1 Purpura hemorrhagica: limb edema in a horse affected with purpura hemorrhagica (Nicola Pusterla, University of California-Davis).

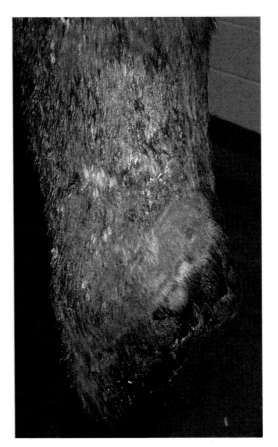

Figure 10.2 Purpura hemorrhagica: limb edema in a horse affected with purpura hemorrhagica. Note the exudation and crusts (Julia Felippe, Cornell University).

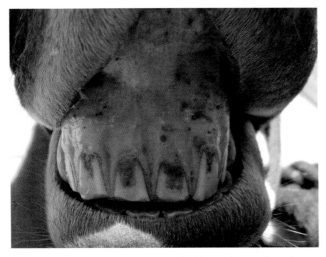

Figure 10.3 Purpura hemorrhagica: petechial hemorrhage in the oral mucosa in a horse affected with purpura hemorrhagica (Nicola Pusterla, University of California-Davis).

determination of IgA reactive PH-specific epitopes (Yang, 2008; Saulsbury, 2010).

10.4 Diagnostics

The diagnosis of PH is based on history of a recent respiratory tract infection, clinical signs (including edema and mucosal hemorrhage), and exclusion of other causes of vasculitis (Pusterla, 2003). Confirmation of the diagnosis requires a skin biopsy taken early in the disease process and before the administration of corticosteroids (Radostits, 2007). Histology shows leukocytoclastic vasculitis with the presence of an inflammatory infiltrate of neutrophils, nuclear fragmentation, extravasation of erythrocytes, and necrosis of vessel walls (Figure 10.4).

Leukocytoclastic vasculitis, also known as hypersensitivity vasculitis, is a small-vessel inflammatory disease mediated by deposition of antibody-antigen immune-complexes, characteristic of hypersensitivity type III. In the pathogenesis of leukocytoclastic vasculitis, activated neutrophils that express adhesion molecules adhere to activated endothelial cells and infiltrate into the vessel walls, with consequent release of their lytic enzymes.

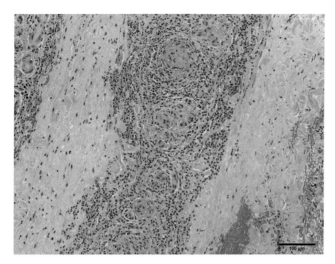

Figure 10.4 Purpura hemorrhagica: photomicrograph of a cutaneous biopsy showing histological evidence of a leukocytoclastic vasculitis with necrosis of blood vessel walls and neutrophil infiltration from a horse affected with purpura hemorrhagica (hematoxylin and eosin stain) (Nicola Pusterla, University of California-Davis).

Table 10.1 Commonly used drugs with dosages for the treatment of equine purpura hemorrhagica.

Drug	Dosage	Route and duration of treatment
Anti–inflammatories		
Flunixin meglumine	1.1 mg/kg	BID, PO or IV
Phenylbutazone	2.2 mg/kg	BID, PO or IV
Immunomodulators		
Dexamethasone	0.05–0.25 mg/kg	BID or SID, IM or IV
Prednisolone acetate	0.5–2 mg/kg	BID or SID, PO
Antithrombotics		
Pentoxyfilline	8.4 mg/kg	TID or BID, PO
Low molecular weight heparin	50 U/kg	SID, SQ
Unfractionated heparin	40–100 IU/kg	TID or BOD, IV or SC
Acetylsalicylic acid	15–20 mg/kg	SID or every other day, PO
Antimicrobial drugs		
Potassium penicillin	22,000 IU/kg	QID, IV
Procaine penicillin	22,000 IU/kg	BID, IM
Trimethoprim sulfamethoxazole	30 mg/kg	BID, PO
Ceftiofur sodium	2.2 mg/kg	BID or SID, IV, IM, or SC

IV – intravenous; IM – intramuscular; SC – subcutaneous; PO – *per os* or orally; SID – *semel in die* or once a day; BID – *bis in die* or twice a day; TID – *ter in die* or three times a day; QID – *quarter in die* or four times a day.

Antibody-antigen immune-complexes that are present in the sera of horses with PH are composed predominantly of antibodies of the IgA or IgM isotype, complexed with SeM antigen (Reed, 2010). An ELISA detecting antibodies directed against the SeM protein of *S. equi* can also be used to assess a horse's response to vaccination and the risk for developing PH (Sweeny, 2005). IgA titers to the SeM and other nonspecific proteins in the *S. equi* are significantly greater than titers in horses with uncomplicated strangles. Elevated IgA titers to *S. equi*, and IgG-SeM titers greater than 6400, are generally suggestive of PH (Reed, 2010).

Complete blood counts typically reveal a chronic inflammatory process, with mild to moderate anemia, leukocytosis, neutrophilia, hyperproteinemia, hyperglobulinemia and hyper-fibrinogenemia (Pusterla, 2003). Clotting profiles and platelet counts are usually normal, but thrombocytopenia has been reported in a few cases. Biochemical panels often reveal high levels of muscle enzymes, including aspartate aminotransferase and creatine kinase, indicating a myopathy secondary to a vascular inflammatory reaction. Similar lesions may occur in other organs, such as liver and kidneys, leading to increased liver enzymes and azotemia, respectively (Pusterla, 2003; Radostits, 2007; Reed, 2010; Sellon, 2007; Smith, 2009).

10.5 Treatment and prevention

The mainstay treatment protocol for treating PH is aimed at reducing the inflammation associated with the blood vessel walls, removing the inciting cause, and providing supportive care (Table 10.1).

Reducing the inflammation of blood vessel walls involves reducing the immune response and removing the antigenic stimulus. Dexamethasone is initially administered at 0.05–0.2 mg/kg SID IV or PO until inflammation is reduced. Prednisolone at 0.5–2.0 mg/kg PO BID to SID can be used as a maintenance dose after the initial dexamethasone treatment. Immunosuppressive dose and duration of treatment should be tailored to the severity of the disease, and it may be required for many weeks, taking into account the approximately 30-day half-life of antibodies. In addition to corticosteroids, non-steroidal anti-inflammatory drugs, such as phenylbutazone or flunixin meglumine, aid in reducing inflammation and providing analgesia (Pusterla, 2003; Radostits, 2007; Reed, 2010; Sellon, 2007; Smith, 2009).

One of the most difficult goals of treatment for PH is removing the source of the antigenic stimulus, especially when the inciting infectious organism is unknown. Since PH is frequently related to *S. equi* infection, horses are commonly treated with penicillin. Treatment with penicillin is recommended until clinical signs resolve, usually within 1–3 weeks (Pusterla, 2003; Radostits, 2007; Reed, 2010; Sellon, 2007; Smith, 2009). Other antimicrobial options to treat *S. equi* are potentiated sulfas (e.g., trimethoprim-sulfamethoxazole), and cephalosporins (e.g., ceftiofur).

Typical supportive care consists of bandaging swollen legs, caring for wounds, cold hydrotherapy and intravenous fluid administration. For horses with or in respiratory distress, tracheotomy may be required. Dysphagic horses with severe head swelling or pharyngeal inflammation may need enteral feeding via nasogastric intubation (Pusterla, 2003; Radostits, 2007; Reed, 2010; Sellon, 2007; Smith, 2009). Anti-thrombotic agents for the prevention of thromboembolic complications have also been used in a clinical setting, including pentoxifylline at 8.4 mg/kg PO TID or BID, acetylsalicylic acid, and unfractionated or low molecular weight heparin.

The prognosis and clinical outcome improves with early and aggressive treatment. However, the immunological response of each individual horse, the severity of the vasculitis, and the triggering antigenic stimulus, determine most accurately the outcome of the disease. The clinical outcome also depends on the extent of the internal organs affected, and the time and nature of the treatment. The case fatality rate with appropriate treatment has been estimated to be 10%. Immunosuppression by prolonged treatment, ranging from 2–4 weeks with corticosteroids, has been shown to decrease the rate of relapse. Antimicrobials are typically administered until clinical signs subside, with an average duration of treatment being three weeks (Pusterla, 2003; Radostits, 2007; Reed, 2010; Sellon, 2007; Smith, 2009).

Since there are no exact causes of PH known, there are no specific preventative measures. Reducing the incidence of upper respiratory tract infections such as *S. equi* can be helpful. Special care and consideration should be given to the use of vaccines containing SeM or avirulent *S. equi* in horses with low risk for strangles, or in horses with recent strangles infection. Although a causative relationship between vaccine administration and development of PH has not been shown, there is circumstantial evidence supporting an association between the two. In endemic areas, it is advised to measure serum antibodies to SeM before vaccine administration, and to avoid vaccinating horses with antibody titers greater than 3200 (Sweeny, 2005; Waller, 2011; Boyle, 2009).

Take home message

Equine purpura hemorrhagica is an acute, non-contagious, aseptic necrotizing vasculitis, characterized by fever, depression, edema, and petechial or ecchymotic hemorrhage of the mucosa and subcutaneous tissues. General edema can result in exudation, ulceration, crusting and, eventually, sloughing of the skin.

Purpura hemorrhagica is caused by a hypersensitivity type III reaction involving antigen-antibody immune-complex deposition in vessels. Antibodies are often produced against pathogens (commonly, in the horse, *Streptococcus equi* subsp. *equi*).

IgA may be involved in the pathophysiology of disease. High IgA titers have been reported in horses with purpura hemorrhagica, compared with titers in horses recently infected with *S. equi* or horses with an unknown history of infection. Elevated *S. equi*-specific IgA titers, and IgG-SeM titers greater than 6400 are suggestive of purpura hemorrhagica.

Histology reveals small vessel leukocytoclastic vasculitis secondary to a hypersensitivity type III reaction, mediated by deposition of antibody-antigen immune-complexes in small vessel basement membrane. Antibodies attract neutrophils and activate complement, resulting in necrosis and extravasation of erythrocytes.

Treatment aims at removing the inciting cause (treating infection), preventing the activation of immune cells, decreasing inflammation (immunosuppression), and providing supportive care.

References

Boyle, A.G., Sweeny, C.R., Kristula, M., Boston, R. and Smith, G. (2009). Factors associated with likelihood of horses having a high serum *Streptococcus equi* SeM-specific antibody titer. *Journal of American Veterinary Association* **235**(8), 973–977.

Heath, S.E., Geor, R.J., Tabel, H. and McIntosh, K. (1991). Unusual Patterns of serum antibodies to *Streptococcus equi* in two horses with purpura hemorrhagica. *Journal of Veterinary Internal Medicine* **5**(5), 263–267.

Kaese, H.J., Valberg, S.J., Hayden, D.W., Wilson, J.H., Charlton, P., Ames, T.R. and Al-Ghamdi, G.M. (2005). Infarctive purpura hemorrhagica in five horses. *Journal of American Veterinary Association* **226**(11), 1893–1898.

Pusterla, N., Watson, J.L., Affolter, V.K., Magdesian, K.G., Wilson, W.D. and Carlson, G.P. (2003). Purpura hemorrhagica in 53 horses. *Veterinary Record* **153**(4), 118–121.

Radostits, O.M., Gay, C.C., Hinchcliff, K.W. and Constable, P.D. (eds, 2007). *Purpura Hemorrhagica.* In: *Veterinary Medicine. A Textbook of the Diseases of Cattle Sheep Pigs Goats and Horses*, tenth edition, pp. 1925–1929. St. Louis, Elsevier Saunders.

Reed, S.M., Bayly, W.M. and Sellon, D.C. (eds, 2010). *Purpura Hemorrhagica.* In: *Equine Internal Medicine* third edition, pp. 309–310. St. Louis, Elsevier Saunders.

Saulsbury, F.T. (2010). Henoch-Schönlein Purpura. *Current Opinions in Rheumatology* **22**(5), 598–602.

Sellon, D.C. and Long, M.T. (eds, 2007). Immune-Mediated Complications of *S. equi*: *Purpura Hemorrhagica.* In: *Equine Infectious Diseases*, pp. 249–250. St. Louis, Elsevier Saunders.

Smith, B.P. and Sweeny, C.R. (eds, 2009). *Streptococcus equi* infection (Strangles): Purpura hemorrhagica. In: *Large Animal Internal Medicine*, fourth edition, pp. 553–536. St. Louis, Mosby Elsevier.

Sweeny, C.R., Timoney, J.F., Newton, J.R. and Hines, M.T. (2005). *Streptococcus equi* infections in horses: guidelines for treatment, control, and prevention of strangles. *Journal of Veterinary Internal Medicine* **19**(1), 123–134.

Waller, A.S., Pailot, R. and Timoney, J.F. (2011). *Streptococcus equi*: a pathogen restricted to one host. *Journal of Medical Microbiology* **60**(9), 1231–1240.

Yang, Y.H., Chuang, Y.H., Wang, L.C., Huang, H.Y., Gershwin, M.E. and Chiang, B.L. (2008). The immunobiology of Henoch-Schönlein purpura. *Autoimmunity Reviews* **7**(3), 179–184.

11 Glomerulonephritis

M. Julia B. Felippe

11.1 Definition

Immune-mediated glomerulonephritis is progressive inflammation and injury of the glomeruli, caused by humoral and cellular immunity, with consequent increased permeability to proteins through the podocyte gaps that line the glomerulus.

The deposition of antibody to the glomerular basement membrane is the pathologic basis of glomerulonephritis. Chronic infections (including *Leptospira pomona*, equine infectious anemia virus, and *Streptococcus* spp.) favor the production of antigen-antibody immune-complexes. In addition, antibody can be produced directly to the endothelial epitopes (e.g., exposed collagen), and idiopathic etiologies are possible (Banks, 1972a; Roberts, 1982; Divers, 1992). The deposition of antibodies to the glomerular subendothelial space, mesangium or basement membrane attracts neutrophils and complement, and their activation and cytokine release recruit macrophages and lymphocytes, which further propagate the inflammation. Tissue damage results from activated-complement cell destruction, activity of metalloproteases and reactive oxygen species (Klahr, 1988). The inflammatory mediators also stimulate proliferation of mesangial cells (Banks, 1972b).

Other local and systemic effects are caused by the increased production of platelet activating factor (PAF), thromboxane A2, rennin and angiotensin II, during renal injury (Klahr, 2000). Persistent activation of platelets and complement promotes intravascular coagulation and glomerular injury. Mesangial fibrosis and sclerosis contribute to glomerular hypertension, with additional protein loss (Floege, 1993).

In human medicine, glomerulonephritis is classified as:
(a) Asymptomatic proteinuria that accompanies other systemic diseases.
(b) Nephrotic syndrome, characterized by proteinuria, hypoproteinemia, peripheral edema, and hyperlipidemia.
(c) Acute nephritic syndrome, characterized by sudden onset of proteinuria, hematuria, and azotemia (acute renal failure).
(d) chronic renal failure due to loss of glomerular mass.

Glomerulonephritis can also be secondary to other types (non-antibody-mediated) of vascular disorders, including ischemia, toxins, and infections that affect large areas of the kidneys and cause generalized failure (both tubulointerstitial and glomerular).

11.2 Signalment and clinical signs

In horses, glomerulonephritis can be clinical or subclinical, secondary to other disease processes, and an incidental finding in necropsy and histopathology. Glomerulonephritis rarely progresses to chronic renal failure. Proteinuria and hematuria are the hallmark clinical signs, with consequent rapid weight loss, hypoproteinemia (particularly albumin), and tissue edema. The inflammation can be focal, or may affect both kidneys. Hyperlipidemia and hypercholesteremia may develop secondary to hepatic lipoprotein production, to compensate low plasma oncotic pressure and urinary losses of regulatory proteins that control lipid homeostasis. Reports have included young and adult female and male horses of different breeds.

11.3 Immunologic mechanisms and etiologic associations

Glomerulonephritis may be mesangioproliferative or non-proliferative (membranous, with thickening of the glomerular basement membrane and capillary walls). Combination membranoproliferative lesions are also possible (Banks, 1972b; Walduogeal, 1983). Histological evaluation shows increased cellularity of the glomerular tufts, with expansion of the mesangial matrix, synechiae to the Bowman's capsule, sclerosis and atrophy. In addition, capillary basement membranes are thickened.

Immunofluorescence can be used to identify the presence of antibody on the glomerular basement membrane. A linear pattern of staining suggests direct *in situ* antibody deposition, while an irregular or granular pattern suggests deposition of antigen-antibody immune-complexes (Banks, 1972b). Antibodies can be of IgG, IgM and/IgA isotypes, and complement is also present (Wilkinson, 1985; McSloy, 2007). Deposition of group-C streptococcal antigen-IgG immune-complexes has been reported in horses; in this case, a history of respiratory disease caused by *S. equi subspecies zooepidemicus* was associated with the renal disease (Divers, 1992).

In a report of mesangioproliferative glomerulonephritis in horses using electron microscopy, intracapillary electron-dense

Equine Clinical Immunology, First Edition. Edited by M. Julia B. Felippe.
© 2016 John Wiley & Sons, Inc. Published 2016 by John Wiley & Sons, Inc.

fibrillary deposits were seen in the glomeruli of some horses, and intracellular rhomboid crystalline deposits (cryoglobulins) in the glomeruli of one horse (McCausland, 1976; Osborne, 1977; Sabnis, 1984). Cryoglobulins, serum antibodies that precipitate under cold conditions, are involved in small-to-medium vessel vasculitis in human patients with infections (*Mycoplasma* spp., *Streptococcus* spp., hepatitis C virus), multiple myeloma and leukemias, and autoimmune diseases (e.g., systemic lupus erythematosus, rheumatoid arthritis). The cryoglobulins are IgG against the Fc portion of antibodies (either against IgG, or against IgM and IgA), and they form immune-complexes.

Take home message

Immune-mediated glomerulonephritis is a progressive inflammation and injury of the glomeruli caused by humoral and cellular immunity, with consequent increased permeability to proteins.

The deposition of antibodies to the glomerular subendothelial space, mesangium or basement membrane attracts neutrophils and complement, and their activation and cytokine release recruit macrophages and lymphocytes, which further propagate the inflammation.

Glomerulonephritis can be classified as:

a. asymptomatic proteinuria that accompanies other systemic diseases;
b. nephrotic syndrome characterized by proteinuria, hypoproteinemia, peripheral edema, and hyperlipidemia;
c. acute nephritic syndrome characterized by sudden onset of proteinuria, hematuria, and azotemia (acute renal failure); and
d. chronic renal failure due to loss of glomerular mass.

Glomerulonephritis is also classified as mesangioproliferative or non-proliferative, or a combination of both.

Immunosuppressive therapy may be effective in controlling kidney damage and in promoting improvement of clinical signs (e.g., edema, hypertension and proteinuria).

11.4 Diagnostics

Basic blood work may reveal inflammatory response to an insulting infection and/or tissue damage, with neutrophilia, hyperglobulinemia, and hyperfibrinogenemia. Blood biochemistry may indicate hypoproteinemia due to hypoalbuminemia, hyperlipidemia and hypercholesteremia. Low levels of antithrombin III in the blood alert for a hypercoagulable state. Azotemia is rare in glomerulonephritis, but may be present when glomerular filtration rate is below 25% of normal. Urinalysis indicates proteinuria and lipiduria, and a urine protein: creatinine ratio higher than 2.0 supports glomerular protein loss (van Biervliet, 2002).

Systemic hypertension may indicate glomerular hypertension due to mesangial proliferation and capillary thrombosis. Kidney ultrasonography can evaluate signs of advanced disease (smaller size, decreased corticomedullary image contrast), and renal biopsy and histology (including electron microscopy, and immunofluorescence for antibody and complement) informs about type and severity of disease. Serologic testing for streptococcal M-protein is indicated.

11.5 Treatment and prognosis

Immunosuppressive therapy may be effective in controlling kidney damage and promoting improvement of clinical signs (e.g., edema, hypertension and proteinuria). However, when discontinued, the disease may progress and clinical signs return. In post-infectious glomerulonephritis, immunosuppressive therapy should be in place along with antimicrobials, at least until elimination of the insulting infection, and perhaps for some time beyond that, in order to allow a significant decrease in antigen-specific antibody titers (e.g., half-life of IgG is 28–32 days). In other forms of glomerulonephritis (e.g., *in situ* direct antibody binding, idiopathic), prolonged treatment may be needed indefinitely, with drug doses tailored to the patient, and a possibility of relapses.

Dexamethasone, initially at 0.1 mg/kg IV SID for 5–7 days, then a decreased dose at 0.05 mg/dL, has been reported effective in the treatment of glomerulonephritis. The dose should be further reduced, or replaced by prednisolone at 0.5 to 1.0 mg/kg PO BID or SID, according to clinical signs and blood work/urinalysis parameters. The use of glucocorticoids has some risks, as they can stimulate glomerular hypertrophy and increase thrombosis and azotemia. In human medicine, some patients require the combination of glucocorticoids and alkylating agents (e.g., cyclophosphamide) and, occasionally, plasmapheresis (Pani, 2013).

Protein intake in the diet should be reduced to 1.3 g of crude protein/kg/day, using about 6 kg of late-growth grass hay and 2 kg of 12% protein senior feed. Low-dose aspirin therapy at 4 mg/kg PO SID or every other day is an option when there are concerns of hypercoagulability, and angiotensin-converting enzyme (ACE) inhibitors (e.g., enalapril) in the case of hypertension. Prognosis is poor.

References

Banks, K.L. and Henson, J.B. (1972b). Immunologically mediated glomerulitis of horses. II. Antiglomerular basement membrane antibody and other mechanisms of spontaneous disease. *Laboratory Investigation* **26**(6), 708–715.

Banks, K.L., Henson, J.B. and McGuire, T.C. (1972a). Immunologically mediated glomerulitis of horses. I. Pathogenesis in persistent infection by equine infectious anemia virus. *Laboratory Investigation* **26**(6), 701–707.

Divers, T.J., Timoney, J.F., Lewis, R.M. and Smith, C.A. (1992). Equine glomerulonephritis and renal failure associated with complexes of group-C streptococcal antigen and IgG antibody. *Veterinary Immunology and Immunopathology* **32**(1–2), 93–102.

Floege, J., Eng, E., Young, B.A. and Johnson, R.J. (1993). Factors involved in the regulation of mesangial cell proliferation *in vitro* and *in vivo*. *Kidney International Supplement* **39**, S47–S54.

Klahr, S., Schreiner, G. and Ichikawa, I. (1988). The progression of renal disease. *New England Journal of Medicine* **318**(25), 1657–1666.

Klahr, S. and Morrissey, J. (2000). The role of vasoactive compounds, growth factors and cytokines in the progression of renal disease. *Kidney International Supplement* **75**, S7–S14.

McCausland I.P. and Milestone, B.A. (1976). Diffuse mesangioproliferative glomerulonephritis in a horse. *New Zealand Veterinary Journal* **24**(10), 239–241.

McSloy, A., Poulsen, K., Fisher, P.J., Armien, A., Chilton, J.A. and Peek, S. (2007). Diagnosis and treatment of a selective immunoglobulin M glomerulonephropathy in a quarter horse gelding. *Journal of Veterinary Internal Medicine* **21**(4), 874–877.

Osborne, C.A., Hammer, R.F., Stevens, J.B., Resnick, J.S. and Michael, A.F. (1977). The glomerulus in health and disease: a comparative review of domestic animals and man. *Advanced Veterinary Science Compendium Medicine* **21**, 207–285.

Pani, A. (2013). Standard immunosuppressive therapy of immune-mediated glomerular diseases. *Autoimmunity Review* **12**(8), 848–853.

Roberts, M.C. and Kelly, W.R. (1982). Renal dysfunction in a case of *purpura haemorrhagica* in a horse. *Veterinary Record* **110**(7), 144–146.

Sabnis, S.G., Gunsond, E. and Antonovycth, T. (1984). Some unusual features of mesangioproliferative glomerulonephritis in horses. *Veterinary Pathology* **21**(6), 574–558.

van Biervliet, J., Divers, T.J., Porter, B. and Huxtable, C. (2002). Glomerulonephritis in horses. *Compendium on Continued Education for Practicing Veterinarian* **24**(1–2), 892–902.

Walduogeal, A., Wild, P. and Wegmannc, H. (1983). Membranoproliferative glomerulonephritis in a horse. *Veterinary Pathology* **20**(4), 500–503.

Wilkinson, J.E., Smith, C.A., Castleman, W.L. and Lewis, R.M. (1985). Fibrillary deposits in glomerulonephritis in a horse. *Veterinary Pathology* **22**(6), 647–649.

12

Inflammatory and Immune-Mediated Muscle Disorders

Sian Durward-Akhurst and Stephanie J. Valberg

12.1 Definition

A suspicion of inflammatory myopathy in horses arises from clinical history, physical exam findings, hematologic findings, serum biochemistry profile, and bacterial cultures/PCR or serum titers. Further support for a diagnosis of an inflammatory myopathy is provided by muscle biopsies. The key muscle biopsy finding that indicates an inflammatory myopathy is the presence of lymphocytes and macrophages within myofibers. A vasculitis is also a common accompanying finding.

In human and canine medicine, subdivision of inflammatory myopathies into infectious, paraneoplastic, or primary immune-mediated disorders is possible, based on the clinical work-up, supporting serology and specificity of muscle biopsy findings (Evans, 2004; Stenzel, 2012). In horses, inflammatory myopathies are not as well characterized, and it is difficult to clearly discern whether myositis arises as a secondary consequence of an infection, or represents a primary immune-mediated disorder. Nevertheless, for the purposes of stimulating more thought with regard to immune-mediated disorders in horses, this chapter will include inflammatory myopathies linked to the immune response to concurrent infections (e.g., infarctive purpura hemorrhagica, *Streptococcus equi* rhabdomyolysis) and those likely triggered by autoimmunity or an aberrant immune response (e.g., immune-mediated myositis in Quarter Horse-related breeds, systemic calcinosis, inflammatory/immune mediated myositis, and sarcoystis myositis).

12.2 Infarctive purpura hemorrhagica

Infarctive purpura hemorrhagica (IPH) represents a severe form of vasculitis associated with purpura hemorrhagica that produces ischemia and complete infarction of portions of the skeletal muscle, in addition to other organs.

12.2.1 Signalment and clinical signs

Horses with IPH most often have a history of a preceding infection, often involving *S. equi*. However, other viral and bacterial agents have been implicated, as well as vaccination against *S. equi* (Pusterla, 2003). There is no known breed, gender or age predilection. The primary presenting complaint is often painful lameness, accompanied by limb swelling and muscle stiffness, and some cases present with signs of abdominal pain (Kaese, 2005).

Physical examination reveals classic signs of purpura hemorrhagica such as petechiae, depression, and moderate well-demarcated limb edema; in addition, horses with IPH will have focal firm swellings within the pectoral, hind limb adductor and gaskin muscles (Kaese, 2005; Figure 12.1 a, b). Other clinical signs include oral infarctions resembling ulcers, signs of severe colic, and hemorrhagic gastric reflux.

12.2.2 Diagnostics

Hematologic and biochemical abnormalities are generally similar to other cases of purpura hemorrhagica, and include a leukocytosis characterized by neutrophilia with a left shift and toxic changes, hyperglobulinemia and hypoalbuminemia (Kaese, 2005; Pusterla, 2003). While many cases of purpura hemorrhagica have mild elevations in serum creatine kinase (CK < 3000 U/L), cases of IPH have marked elevations in serum CK activity (> 47,000 U/L), and aspartate aminotransferase (AST) is usually over 960 U/L (Kaese, 2005; Pusterla, 2003). ELISA titers for *S. equi* serum M protein (SeM) are usually markedly elevated.

Peritoneal fluid obtained by abdominocentesis may be normal or may be serosanguinous, with increased total protein, total nucleated cell and red blood cell counts if gastrointestinal infarction is present. Ultrasonographic examination of swollen muscles reveals focal hypoechoic lesions within the muscle tissue. Since infarctions are focal, it can be difficult to ensure that a biopsy sample is obtained from abnormal muscle tissue. Samples from palpably normal muscle tissues show no pathologic abnormalities, whereas definitive histopathologic findings include a leukocytoclastic vasculitis and acute coagulative necrosis of whole muscle fascicles (Figure 12.2 a, b).

Equine Clinical Immunology, First Edition. Edited by M. Julia B. Felippe.
© 2016 John Wiley & Sons, Inc. Published 2016 by John Wiley & Sons, Inc.

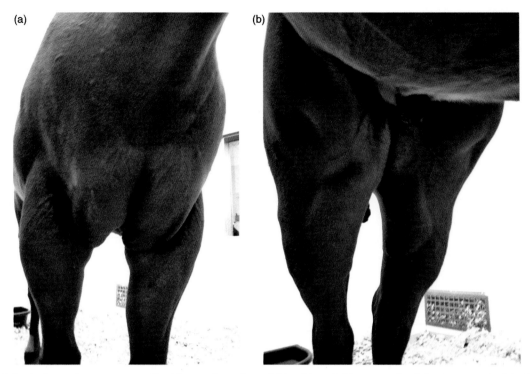

Figure 12.1 Infarctive hemorrhagic purpura: swollen **(a)** pectoral muscles, and **(b)** gaskin and adductor muscles. Infarctions occur in skeletal muscles that are commonly compressed when horses are recumbent (Stephanie Valberg, University of Minnesota).

12.2.3 Immunologic mechanisms and etiologic associations

IPH resembles Henoch-Schönlein purpura in humans, which is characterized by infarctive vasculitis of the skin, kidneys and gastrointestinal tract, due to IgA immune complex deposition (Kauffmann, 1980). IgM- or IgA-streptococcal M protein immune complexes are present in high levels in the sera of horses with purpura hemorrhagica. These immune complexes deposit along the vessels and activate complement, leading to a leuko-cytoclastic vasculitis, vascular necrosis, occlusion and, when severe, infarction (Galan, 1985). Infarctions are most extensive in skeletal muscles that are compressed during recumbency, such as the pectorals, gaskins and adductor muscles (Kaese, 2005). Infarction of other tissues, such as the skin, gastrointestinal tract, pancreas and lungs are often found at post-mortem, and S. equi abscessation of one or more lymph nodes is usually present.

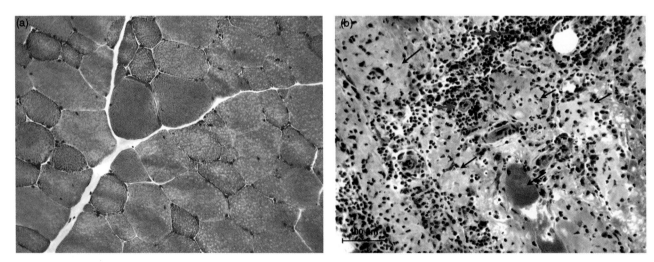

Figure 12.2 Infarctive hemorrhagic purpura: hematoxylin and eosin stains of (a) a cross-section of normal equine skeletal muscle, and (b) infracted area of skeletal muscle, with complete coagulative necrosis of muscle fibers (black arrows), and leukocytoclastic vasculitis comprised of neutrophils and lymphocytes (grey horizontal arrows) (Stephanie Valberg, University of Minnesota).

12.2.4 Treatment and prognosis

Early recognition of signs and aggressive antibiotic and corticosteroid treatment are essential to fight the high fatality rate with IHP. Treatment of Henoch-Schönlein purpura in humans, including cases with intestinal infarctions, involves plasmapheresis or high-dose intravenous pulse therapy, with methylprednisolone, followed by oral corticosteroids plus immunosuppressive agents such as cyclophosphamide and azathioprine (Kauffmann, 1981). One horse with IPH was successfully treated with intravenous potassium penicillin, nonsteroidal antiinflammatories, and three weeks of dexamethasone tapering treatment (from 0.1 to 0.07 mg/kg IV SID), followed by an overlapping tenweek tapering course of oral prednisolone (starting at 2 mg/kg SID PO) (Kaese, 2005).

12.3 Rhabdomyolysis associated with *Streptococcus equi*

Young Quarter Horses are susceptible to severe acute generalized rhabdomyolysis during a concurrent *S. equi* infection (Sponseller, 2005). These horses have an inflammatory leukogram and marked elevations in serum CK and AST activities. Mortality is high, due to the severity of rhabdomyolysis and unrelenting pain.

12.3.1 Signalment and clinical signs

To date, reported cases of *S. equi* rhabdomyolysis have been Quarter Horses of both genders that are less than seven years old (Sponseller, 2005). Clinical signs of upper respiratory tract infection, such as pyrexia, purulent nasal discharge, mandibular lymphadenopathy and/or guttural pouch empyema are present. Within seven days, affected horses develop a stiff gait, which rapidly progresses to markedly firm, swollen, and painful epaxial and gluteal muscles. The majority of affected horses progress to recumbency and are unable to stand. The severe and unrelenting pain usually requires euthanasia within 48 hours of becoming recumbent.

12.3.2 Immunologic mechanisms and etiologic associations

The precise inflammatory or immunologic mechanism for rhabdomyolysis is not known. At this time there, are two proposed etiologies. The first proposes a *toxic shock-like reaction*, due to the stimulation of the immune system by streptococcal superantigens (Sponseller, 2005). Superantigens cause non-specific activation of T cells, leading to polyclonal T cell activation and a massive inflammatory cytokine release. Subsequent further activation of the immune system produces an uncontrolled generalized inflammatory response, which can lead to multiple organ dysfunction and extensive tissue necrosis (Gardam, 1998; Schlievert, 1993).

Toxic shock syndrome occurs in humans secondary to streptococcal group A infection (Breiman, 1993). *S. equi* has four

known superantigens: SePE-H, SePE-I, *speLSe*, and *speMSe* (Artiushin, 2002; Proft and Fraser, 2003, 2007Proft, 2003, 2007). There have been two reports of toxic shock syndrome in horses: one secondary to pericardial effusion and *Streptococcus imitis* bacteremia; and the other secondary to *Staphylococcus aureus* pneumonia (Dolente, 2000; Holbrook, 2003). No studies have measured the extent of the cytokine response in horses affected by *S. equi* rhabdomyolysis.

The second proposed cause of rhabdomyolysis with *S. equi* infection is a *bacteremia*, with secondary multiplication of *S. equi* in skeletal muscle and myodegeneration from *S. equi* proteases (e.g., streptokinase, streptolysin S or an unidentified cytotoxic protein) (Sponseller, 2005; Timoney, 2004). *S. equi* has not been cultured from, or identified by, PCR amplification in skeletal muscle from affected horses; however, *S. equi* bacteria have been identified in affected muscle, using immunofluorescent stains for both Lancefield group C carbohydrate and *S. equi* M protein (SeM) (Sponseller, 2005).

There is currently no evidence that the *S. equi* involved in rhabdomyolysis is an atypical and more virulent genetic strain of *S. equi*. Muscles from horses with *S. equi* rhabdomyolysis have no evidence of neutrophilic infiltrates, which may reflect low numbers of bacteria or inhibition of neutrophil chemotaxis. Humans with necrotizing myositis secondary to group A *Streptococcus* have numerous bacteria in skeletal muscle, but a general absence of neutrophilic inflammation, explained by a streptococcal protease that degrades the chemotaxin interleukin 8 (IL-8) (Hidalgo-Grass, 2004). It is of note, however that, in the small number of equine cases that have been tested, no proteolytic activity was present in affected muscles (Sponseller, 2005).

12.3.3 Diagnostics

Hematologic abnormalities include mature neutrophilia and hyperfibrinogenemia. Serum CK activity is usually >100,000 U/L, with or without an accompanying elevation in serum AST activity. Titers to the M protein of *S. equi* are usually low, unless horses have been recently vaccinated (Quist, 2011; Sponseller, 2005). Endoscopy of the upper respiratory tract shows retropharyngeal lymphadenopathy and/or guttural pouch empyema, with a positive bacterial culture and PCR for *S. equi*. Urinalysis is usually consistent with rhabdomyolysis and dehydration, with significant myoglobinuria and hypersthenuria.

Muscle biopsies, when taken within a few days of rhabdomyolysis development, confirm acute extensive myodegeneration, with very few cellular infiltrates of macrophages. The sublumbar muscles are usually most severely affected and have more macrophage infiltration at post-mortem. Lymphocytic infiltrates are not a feature of muscle histopathology with this condition (Quist, 2011; Sponseller, 2005).

12.3.4 Treatment and prognosis

Early recognition of the signs of muscle stiffness, and quick assessment of the extent of rhabdomyolysis via serum CK activity, are critical for a successful outcome. To date, the mortality rate has been very high for reported cases. Current recommendations include flushing infected guttural pouches, draining abscessed lymph nodes, and treating *S. equi* infection using antimicrobials. Treatment with penicillin has not impacted the outcome of most equine cases of *S. equi* rhabdomyolysis (Quist, 2011; Sponseller, 2005).

In human medicine and in mouse models of *Streptococcus pyogenes* myositis, treatment with penicillin is associated with mortality rates of up to 85% (Adams, 1985). The high failure rate of penicillin treatment, despite sensitivity, is attributed to low levels of bacterial turnover, minimizing the inhibitory effect of penicillin on bacterial cell wall biosynthesis (Eagle, 1952). Experimental models *S. pyogenes* myositis in mice found that clindamycin, which impairs protein synthesis, dramatically improved survival rates (Stevens, 1988). Clindamycin, however, is contraindicated in horses, due to the risk of fatal colitis. The use of other macrolides, such as azithromycin combined with rifampin, may be an alternative antibiotic approach for *S. equi* rhabdomyolysis in foals, as safety in adult horses needs to be further studied (LeClere, 2012).

Nonsteroidal antiinflammatories (NSAID) and, possibly, high doses of short-acting corticosteroids, may assist in controlling the inflammatory response with *S. equi* infection. Analgesia is extremely important, as unrelenting pain is a major challenge. Constant rate infusions of lidocaine, detomidine, morphine, or ketamine may provide better relief from anxiety and pain than periodic injections of tranquilizers or NSAIDs.

Horses should be placed in a deeply bedded stall and moved from side to side every four hours if they are unable to rise. Some horses may benefit from a sling, if they will bear weight on their hindlimbs when assisted to stand. Treating horses prior to recumbency improves outcome. One case that was successfully treated developed moderate atrophy of the gluteal muscles, which resolved by three months post-discharge (Sponseller, 2005).

12.4 Immune-mediated myositis in Quarter Horse-related breeds

Immune-mediated Myositis (IMM) in Quarter Horse-related breeds results in: malaise; rapid, pronounced atrophy, particularly affecting epaxial and gluteal muscles; and high serum CK and AST activities (Lewis, 2007). Treatment with antiinflammatory doses of corticosteroids halts muscle atrophy, and the musculature regenerates over time. Other breeds of horses occasionally develop focal or multifocal muscle atrophy, with an inflammatory or immune mediated basis, and these cases are described in the section on uncharacterized immune-mediated and inflammatory myopathies.

12.4.1 Signalment and clinical signs

Generalized IMM usually affects horses of Quarter Horse-related breeds that are either younger than eight years old or older than 16 years, without gender predilection (Lewis, 2007). A history of exposure to a triggering factor exists in only approximately one-third of cases. The known triggering factor is usually exposure to *S. equi*, another respiratory pathogen, or possibly vaccination (Lewis, 2007). The most prominent clinical sign is dramatic muscle atrophy, particularly of the epaxial and gluteal muscles, accompanied by stiffness and general malaise (Figure 12.3 a, b). Muscle atrophy is usually rapid, and may progress to involve 40% of the horse's muscle mass within a week. Horses can develop generalized weakness, leading to frequent periods of recumbency. Muscle atrophy often persists for months before a gradual increase in muscle mass occurs.

12.4.2 Immunologic mechanisms and etiologic associations

Equine IMM bears some similarities to human and canine forms of immune-mediated myositis, but there are also many differences (Pumarola, 2004; Shelton, 2007). In Quarter Horse-related

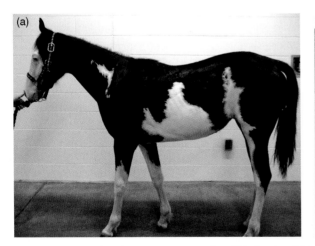
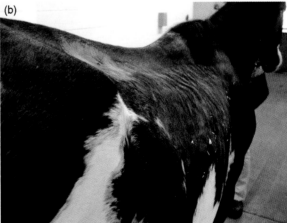

Figure 12.3 Immune-mediated myositis: severe atrophy of (**a**) gluteal and (**b**) epaxial muscles in an American Paint horse with immune-mediated myositis. Muscle mass recovered after treatment with prednisolone (Anna Firshman, University of Minnesota).

breeds, there is a distinct predilection for the epaxial and gluteal muscles, whereas the semimembranosus muscle is usually spared. The reason for this predilection is unknown. Acutely, lymphocytic infiltrates within myofibers and around vessels have a high T lymphocyte CD4$^+$/CD8$^+$ ratio (Lewis, 2007). This finding is similar to dermatomyositis (DM) in humans, and canine masticatory muscle myositis. However, unlike patients with DM, large numbers of B cells are not observed in affected muscles of horses (Dalakas, 2005; Evans, 2004). Furthermore, unlike canine masticatory muscle myositis, specific binding of IgG to myofibers is not present in epaxial or gluteal muscles of horses with IMM (Evans, 2004; Pumarola, 2004; Shelton, 1987).

One of the possible mechanisms for the development of IMM is the loss of self-tolerance to antigens expressed by muscle cells (Engel, 2004). Myoblasts and myotubes do not normally express detectable major histocompatibility (MHC) class II molecules and, therefore, do not present immunogenic peptides to lympho-cytes (Engel, 2004). Cytokines such as IFN-gamma, however, can induce myoblasts to express MHC class II molecules, potentially resulting in presentation of not only bacterial or viral antigens, but also autoantigens to CD4$^+$ cells (Bao, 1990; Hohlfeld, 1990).

MHC class II expression has been identified in myofibers of dogs with IMM but has not yet been studied in horses with IMM (Pumarola, 2004). It is possible that horses with IMM have altered autoantigen expression, by target or antigen-presenting cells, that changes the normal state of T cell tolerance. Alterna-tively, loss of self-tolerance could occur as a result of activation of otherwise inactivated autoreactive T cells by:

1 shared epitopes with an infectious agent causing antigenic mimicry;

2 microbial superantigens produced by infectious agents; or

3 high concentrations of cytokines, such as IL-2 (Engel, 2004).

The ability of locally produced cytokines to induce proteolysis and muscle catabolism may also contribute to the rapid onset of muscle atrophy (Creus, 2009).

There is strong evidence of a genetic susceptibility to partic-ular forms of immune-mediated myositis in humans and dogs, and this condition could potentially exist within the Quarter Horse breed (Massey, 2013; Rothwell, 2013). Variations in the MHC locus, particularly of the MHC class II molecule, have been found to be highly associated with human autoimmune diseases (Gregersen, 2009).

12.4.3 Diagnostics

Hematologic abnormalities are uncommon with IMM unless there is a concurrent infectious process. During the *acute* phase of muscle atrophy, serum CK and AST activities are moderately to markedly elevated; however, during the later phase of *chronic* atrophy, serum CK and AST activities can be normal.

The most useful diagnostic test during the acute phase of the disease is a muscle biopsy of the epaxial and/or gluteal muscles (Lewis, 2007). Several formalin-fixed Trucut samples from the epaxial or gluteal muscles are often sufficient to establish a clinical diagnosis. Histologic abnormalities include infiltration of the myofibers by lymphocytes, a lymphocytic vasculitis, anguloid atrophy of the myofibers, fiber necrosis and, in some cases, multinucleated giant cells (Figure 12.4 a, b). Impor-tantly, biopsies taken several weeks after the onset of atrophy may just have nonspecific findings of myogenic atrophy, without evidence of the hallmark feature of lymphocytic infiltrates. Biopsies of the semitendinosus or membranosus muscles are usually not helpful in establishing a diagnosis; they are often normal, or have evidence of atrophy and mild inflammatory cell infiltration.

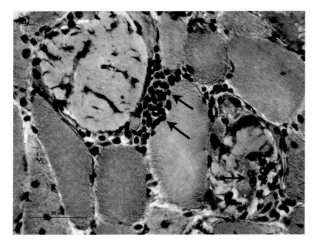
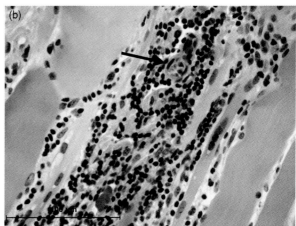

Figure 12.4 Immune-mediated myositis.
(a) Cross-section of epaxial muscle, stained with hematoxylin and eosin, showing invasion of a healthy muscle fiber by lymphocytes (arrow) and presence of macrophages in a degenerating muscle fiber (red horizontal arrow).
(b) Lymphocytic vasculitis within skeletal muscle (arrows) (Stephanie Valberg, University of Minnesota).

12.4.4 Treatment and prognosis

Appropriate antimicrobials should be selected if there is evidence of concurrent infection. Corticosteroids are the mainstay of treatment and, unlike immune-mediated disorders in humans and dogs, anti-inflammatory, rather than immunosuppressive, doses are effective (Evans, 2004). Recommended dosages are dexamethasone at 0.05 mg/kg IV for three days, followed by prednisolone at 1 mg/kg PO for 7–10 days, with tapering by 100 mg/week over one month (Lewis, 2007).

Prevention is challenging, because only a small proportion of affected horses have a history of a triggering factor. Preventing exposure to respiratory infections where possible is recommended, and spacing out vaccines to prevent a surge of inflammatory cytokines, avoiding immune stimulants, and monitoring closely in order to institute treatment early if recurring signs of atrophy develop, are also recommended.

Malaise often resolves rapidly following treatment with corticosteroids, and muscle atrophy quickly ceases. Serum CK activity often returns to normal levels after 7–10 days of corticosteroid treatment. Recovery of the muscle mass is more gradual, and usually takes 2–3 months; some focal residual muscle atrophy can remain (Lewis, 2007). Horses that are not treated with corticosteroids may develop extensive muscle atrophy but, in many cases, muscle mass will gradually recover. Recurrence of atrophy in susceptible horses occurs in about 40% of cases, and these horses may require repeated bouts of corticosteroid treatment.

12.5 Systemic calcinosis

A novel fatal syndrome of systemic dystrophic calcification, called systemic calcinosis or calciphylaxis, has been described in horses that share a similar initial presentation to generalized IMM (Fales-Williams, 2008; Tan, 2010). In addition to signs of malaise, mild fever, stiffness, and muscle atrophy, horses have characteristic hyperfibrinogenemia and hyperphosphatemia, leading to dystrophic calcification of many tissues and diverse organ failure.

12.5.1 Signalment and clinical signs

All horses reported with systemic calcinosis have been of Quarter Horse related breeds and under nine years old (Fales-Williams, 2008; Tan, 2010). Initial clinical signs usually include a mild fever, malaise, stiffness, and loss of muscle mass, particularly over the lumbar and gluteal area (Figure 12.5). Many horses have evidence of a cough, tachypnea and mild ventral edema. As the disease progresses, a variety of signs can develop, such as progressive weakness, inability to remain standing, respiratory distress, laminitis, or gastrointestinal inflammation. Whether these signs are a direct result of systemic dystrophic calcification, or an underlying precipitating inflammatory disease, is unclear.

There can be a wide range of hematologic abnormalities, depending on the underlying disease process that precedes

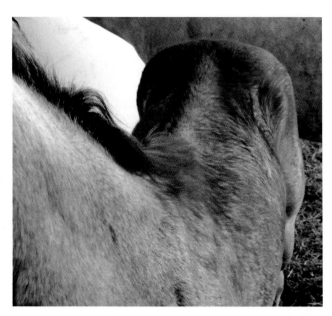

Figure 12.5 Systemic calcinosis: severe atrophy of epaxial muscles in a foal that developed systemic calcinosis (Rebecca Funk, Virginia Maryland College of Veterinary Medicine).

dystrophic calcification. The most consistent alterations in the hemogram are hyperfibrinogenemia and mild leukocytosis. In the biochemistry profile, the product of calcium (Ca) multiplied by phosphorus (P) is more than 65, and serum CK activities are at least three times higher than the normal range (Tan, 2010).

12.5.2 Immunologic mechanisms and etiologic associations

Systemic calcinosis occurs in humans, particularly those on dialysis due to renal failure (Khafif, 1990). In human medicine, a $Ca \times P$ equaling more than 65 is used as an indicator of a potential risk of dystrophic calcification (Carter, 2013). $Ca \times P$ higher than 66 was present in the case reports of horses that developed systemic dystrophic calcification. The reason for the elevated $Ca \times P$ in horses with systemic calcinosis is not known, but there is a strong suspicion that an inflammatory process could be the trigger.

Synergistic effects of cytokines such as TNF-alpha and IL-6 on activation of the receptor activator of nuclear factor kappa B ligand (RANK-L) have been reported, which lead to enhanced bone resorption (Lam, 2000). RANKL/RANK signaling regulates the formation of multinucleated osteoclasts from their precursors, as well as their activation and survival in normal bone remodeling. The combined impact of activation of RANK-L is to increase resorption of bone, which may lead to hyperphosphatemia.

Hyperphosphatemia, in turn, can induce dystrophic calcification through four different processes (Llach, 1999; Tan, 2010; Watson, 1997):

1 Passive calcium phosphate deposition from phosphate supersaturation in the blood.

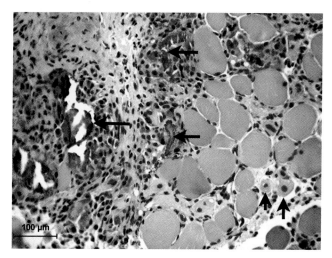

Figure 12.6 Systemic calcinosis: presence of calcified myofibers (horizontal arrows), fibrosis and regenerating fibers (vertical arrows) in skeletal muscle of a horse with systemic calcinosis (Stephanie Valberg, University of Minnesota).

2 An active process promoting the conversion of smooth muscle cells to osteogenic cell types.

3 Directly increasing parathyroid hormone secretion and transcription.

4 interference with renal production of 1,25-dihydroxyvitamin D levels, which has been associated with increased coronary artery calcification in humans.

12.5.3 Diagnostics

Systemic calcinosis should be suspected if a horse presents with muscle atrophy, malaise, respiratory distress or renal insufficiency, and with evidence of hyperfibrinogenemia and an elevated product of Ca times P in the blood work.

The histopathologic findings in muscle biopsies resemble those of IMM. However, multinucleated giant cells are consistently present, along with dystrophic calcification of muscle fibers (Tan, 2010; Figure 12.6). At post-mortem, dystrophic calcification is also evident in one or all of the following tissues, in addition to skeletal muscle: the alveoli in pulmonary tissue; cardiac myofibers; renal tubules; and tunica intima of blood vessels. In one case, dramatic lesions of arterial medial calcification of the aorta, coronary, and pulmonary arteries were reported (Fales-Williams, 2008).

12.5.4 Treatment and prognosis

This condition is often associated with a fatal outcome. Horses are usually submitted to euthanasia, due to progressive weakness, an inability to remain standing, respiratory distress, laminitis, or other underlying disease. Treatment is largely directed toward controlling the initial inflammatory condition, although the use of corticocosteroids is somewhat controversial. In human medicine, corticosteroid treatment has been implicated as a triggering mechanism for systemic calcinosis. In horses, however, the clinical signs that precede systemic calcinosis so

closely resemble IMM, a corticosteroid responsive disease, that corticosteroid treatment is often instituted when signs of rapid muscle atrophy develop.

12.6 Uncharacterized immune-mediated and inflammatory myopathies

There are individual cases of myositis in horses that could have an inflammatory or immune-mediated basis. One case report of focal myositis in a 16 year old pony describes a progressive symmetrical bilateral reduction of muscles over a three-month period in the mid-neck region (Barrott, 2004). The pony had normal serum CK and AST activities. The diagnosis was made on the basis of the presence of multifocal interstitial aggregates of lymphocytes and plasma cells, with few admixed histiocytes and focally numerous eosinophils, predominantly in perivascular locations. Parasitic causes were considered unlikely, due to regular deworming history and lack of *Sarcocystis* within the muscle biopsy. Muscle mass returned to normal following treatment with dexamethasone. Another brief mention of a horse with multifocal atrophy that had changes consistent with immune-mediated myositis on the muscle biopsy is mentioned in a review article (Beech, 2000).

Within the Neuromuscular Diagnostic Laboratory database at the University of Minnesota, a small number of horses of breeds other than Quarter Horses with a suspected inflammatory or immune-mediated etiology have been identified. These included an Anglo-Arabian, a mixed-breed pony, a Percheron, a Warmblood, and two Thoroughbred horses. The common clinical presentation was muscle atrophy, and the suspicion of an inflammatory/immune process was based on the presence of lymphocytic infiltrates in muscle biopsy specimens. Two of the horses had acute and severe atrophy, while the other horses had a more gradual onset of atrophy. The atrophied muscles were predominantly the gluteal and epaxial muscles, and two horses had additional muscle groups involved. A variable degree of lymphocytic infiltration of muscle fibers and lymphocytic vasculitis was present in muscle biopsies. Two of these horses had a history of hematologic abnormalities consistent with a recent infection. None of these cases were reported to have elevated serum CK or AST activities. The pathophysiology of the disease in this subset of horses is unknown.

12.7 Sarcocystis myositis

A small number of sarcocysts are a common finding in equine muscles biopsies and, under normal circumstances, these cysts are not associated with an inflammatory reaction, but are incidental findings. They are usually *Sarcocystis bertrami*, *S. equicanis*, or *S. fayeri*, and dogs serve as the definitive host (Tinling, 1980). There is, however, a report of an inflammatory myositis associated with sarcocysts within skeletal muscle in a

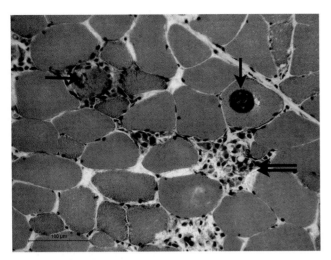

Figure 12.7 *Sarcocystis* myositis: acute skeletal muscle fiber degeneration (horizontal arrow) and macrophage infiltration of a degenerate muscle fiber (double arrow) in a skeletal muscle sample, with *Sarcocysts* present in myofibers (vertical arrow) (Stephanie Valberg, University of Minnesota).

horse, and two further cases have been noted by the Neuromuscular Diagnostic Laboratory at the University of Minnesota (Traub-Dargatz, 1994).

Malaise, anorexia, weakness, asymmetric atrophy of some muscles, and symmetric atrophy of gluteal, epaxial and quadriceps muscles, have been reported. Few abnormalities were evident in the hematologic or biochemical profiles. Diagnosis of sarcocystosis is based on history, clinical signs, and serologic titers, as well as the demonstration of an inflammatory reaction (lymphocytes and macrophages, with or without eosinophils) associated with immature cysts in muscle biopsies (Figure 12.7). It is unclear why a small number of horses develop a profound inflammatory response to sarcocysts within skeletal muscle. Exposure to large numbers of the sporozoan parasite in canine feces, or immunosuppression, may be factors that contributed to myositis (Cawthorn, 1990).

Treatment with antiprotozoal drugs such as pyremethamine/trimethoprim-sulfa was successful in one case, and the more recently available diclazuril product may be another potential treatment (Traub-Dargatz, 1994).

References

Adams, E.M., Gudmundsson, S., Yocum, D.E., Haselby, R.C., Craig, W.A. and Sundstrom, W.R. (1985). Streptococcal myositis. *Archives of Internal Medicine* **145**, 1020–1023.

Artiushin, S.C., Timoney, J.F., Sheoran, A.S. and Muthupalani, S.K. (2002). Characterization and immunogenicity of pyrogenic mitogens SePE-H and SePE-I of *Streptococcus equi*. *Microbial Pathogenesis* **32**, 71–85.

Bao, S.S., King, N.J. and dos Remedios, C.G. (1990). Elevated MHC class I and II antigens in cultured human embryonic myoblasts following stimulation with gamma-interferon. *Immunology & Cell Biology* **68** (Pt 4), 235–241.

Barrott, M.J., Brooks, H.W. and McGowan, C.M. (2004). Suspected immune-mediated myositis in a pony. *Equine Veterinary Education* **16**(2), 80–83.

Beech, J. (2000). Equine muscle disorders 2. *Equine Veterinary Education* **12**, 208–213.

Breiman, R.F., Davis, J.P., Facklam, R.R., Gray, B.M., Hoge, C.W., Kaplan, E.L., Mortimer, E.A., Schlievert, P.M., Schwartz, B., Stevens, D.L. and Todd, J.K. (1993). Defining the group A streptococcal toxic shock syndrome. Rationale and consensus definition. *Journal of American Medical Association* **269**, 390–391.

Carter, T. and Ratnam, S. (2013). Calciphylaxis: a devastating complication of derangements of calcium-phosphorus metabolism – a case report and review of the literature. *Nephrology Nursing Journal* **40**, 431–435.

Cawthorn, R.J., Clark, M., Hudson, R. and Friesen, D. (1990). Histological and ultrastructural appearance of severe Sarcocystis fayeri infection in a malnourished horse. *Journal of Veterinary Diagnostic Investigation* **2**, 342–345.

Creus, K.K., De, P.B., Werbrouck, B.F., Vervaet, V., Weis, J. and De Bleecker, J.L. (2009). Distribution of the NF-kappaB complex in the inflammatory exudates characterizing the idiopathic inflammatory myopathies. *Annals of the New York Academy of Sciences* **1173**, 370–377.

Dalakas, M.C. (2005). Autoimmune muscular pathologies. *Neurological Sciences* **26** Suppl 1, S7–S8.

Dolente, B.A., Seco, O.M. and Lewis, M.L. (2000). Streptococcal toxic shock in a horse. *Journal of the American Veterinary Medical Association* **217**, 64–7, 30.

Eagle, H. (1952). Experimental approach to the problem of treatment failure with penicillin. I. Group A streptococcal infection in mice. *American Journal of Medicine* **13**, 389–399.

Engel, A.G. and Hohlfeld, R. (2004). The Polymyositis and Dermatomyositis Syndromes. In: Engel, A.G. and Franzini-Armstrong, C. (eds). *Myology: Basic and Clinical*, 1321–1366. McGraw-Hill, New York.

Evans, J., Levesque, D. and Shelton, G.D. (2004). Canine inflammatory myopathies: a clinicopathologic review of 200 cases. *Journal of Veterinary Internal Medicine* **18**, 679–691.

Fales-Williams, A., Sponseller, B. and Flaherty, H. (2008). Idiopathic arterial medial calcification of the thoracic arteries in an adult horse. *Journal of Veterinary Diagnostic Investigation* **20**, 692–697.

Galan, J.E. and Timoney, J.F. (1985). Immune complexes in purpura hemorrhagica of the horse contain IgA and M antigen of *Streptococcus equi*. *Journal of Immunology* **135**, 3134–3137.

Gardam, M.A., Low, D.E., Saginur, R. and Miller, M.A. (1998). Group B streptococcal necrotizing fasciitis and streptococcal toxic shock-like syndrome in adults. *Archives of Internal Medicine* **158**, 1704–1708.

Gregersen, P.K. and Olsson, L.M. (2009). Recent advances in the genetics of autoimmune disease. *Annual Review of Immunology* **27**, 363–391.

Hidalgo-Grass, C., Dan-Goor, M., Maly, A., Eran, Y., Kwinn, L.A., Nizet, V., Ravins, M., Jaffe, J., Peyser, A., Moses, A.E. and Hanski, E. (2004). Effect of a bacterial pheromone peptide on host chemokine degradation in group A streptococcal necrotising soft-tissue infections. *Lancet* **363**, 696–703.

Hohlfeld, R. and Engel, A.G. (1990). Induction of HLA-DR expression on human myoblasts with interferon-gamma. *American Journal of Pathology* **136**, 503–508.

Holbrook, T.C., Munday, J.S., Brown, C.A., Glover, B., Schlievert, P.M. and Sanchez, S. (2003). Toxic shock syndrome in a horse with *Staphylococcus aureus* pneumonia. *Journal of the American Veterinary Medical Association* **222**, 620–622.

Kaese, H.J., Valberg, S.J., Hayden, D.W., Wilson, J.H., Charlton, P., Ames, T.R. and Al-Ghamdi, G.M. (2005). Infarctive *purpura hemorrhagica* in five horses. *Journal of the American Veterinary Medical Association* **226**, 1893–8, 1845.

Kauffmann, R.H. and Houwert, D.A. (1981). Plasmapheresis in rapidly progressive Henoch-Schoenlein glomerulonephritis and the effect on circulating IgA immune complexes. *Clinical Nephrology* **16**, 155–160.

Kauffmann, R.H., Herrmann, W.A., Meyer, C.J., Daha, M.R. and Van Es, L.A. (1980). Circulating IgA-immune complexes in Henoch-Schonlein purpura. A longitudinal study of their relationship to disease activity and vascular deposition of IgA. *American Journal of Medicine* **69**, 859–866.

Khafif, R.A., DeLima, C., Silverberg, A. and Frankel, R. (1990). Calciphylaxis and systemic calcinosis. Collective review. *Archives of Internal Medicine* **150**, 956–959.

Lam, J., Takeshita, S., Barker, J.E., Kanagawa, O., Ross, F.P. and Teitelbaum, S.L. (2000). TNF-alpha induces osteoclastogenesis by direct stimulation of macrophages exposed to permissive levels of RANK ligand. *Journal of Clinical Investigation* **106**, 1481–1488.

Leclere, M., Magdesian, K.G., Cole, C.A., Szabo, N.J., Ruby, R.E., Rhodes, D.M., Edman, J., Vale, A., Wilson, W.D. and Tell, L.A. (2012). Pharmacokinetics and preliminary safety evaluation of azithromycin in adult horses. *Journal of Veterinary Pharmacology and Therapeutics* **35**(6), 541–9.

Lewis, S.S., Valberg, S.J. and Nielsen, I.L. (2007). Suspected immune-mediated myositis in horses. *Journal of Veterinary Internal Medicine* **21**, 495–503.

Llach, F. (1999). Hyperphosphatemia in end-stage renal disease patients: pathophysiological consequences. *Kidney International Supplements* **73**, S31–S37.

Massey, J., Rothwell, S., Rusbridge, C., Tauro, A., Addicott, D., Chinoy, H., Cooper, R.G., Ollier, W.E. and Kennedy, L.J. (2013). Association of an MHC class II haplotype with increased risk of polymyositis in Hungarian Vizsla dogs. *PLoS One* **8**, e56490.

Proft, T. and Fraser, J.D. (2003). Bacterial superantigens. *Clinical and Experimental Immunology* **133**, 299–306.

Proft, T. and Fraser, J.D. (2007). Streptococcal superantigens. *Chemical Immunology and Allergy* **93**, 1–23.

Pumarola, M., Moore, P.F. and Shelton, G.D. (2004). Canine inflammatory myopathy: analysis of cellular infiltrates. *Muscle & Nerve* **29**, 782–789.

Pusterla, N., Watson, J.L., Affolter, V.K., Magdesian, K.G., Wilson, W.D. and Carlson, G.P. (2003). *Purpura haemorrhagica* in 53 horses. *Veterinary Record* **153**, 118–121.

Quist, E.M., Dougherty, J.J., Chaffin, M.K. and Porter, B.F. (2011). Equine rhabdomyolysis. *Veterinary Pathology* **48**, E52–E58.

Rothwell, S., Cooper, R.G., Lamb, J.A. and Chinoy, H. (2013). Entering a new phase of immunogenetics in the idiopathic inflammatory myopathies. *Current Opinion in Rheumatology* **25**, 735–741.

Schlievert, P.M. (1993). Role of superantigens in human disease. *Journal of Infectious Diseases* **167**, 997–1002.

Shelton, G.D. (2007). From dog to man: the broad spectrum of inflammatory myopathies. *Neuromuscular Disorders* **17**, 663–670.

Shelton, G.D. and Cardinet, G.H., III (1987). Pathophysiologic basis of canine muscle disorders. *Journal of Veterinary Internal Medicine* **1**, 36–44.

Sponseller, B.T., Valberg, S.J., Tennent-Brown, B.S., Foreman, J.H., Kumar, P. and Timoney, J.F. (2005). Severe acute rhabdomyolysis associated with *Streptococcus equi* infection in four horses. *Journal of the American Veterinary Medical Association* **227**, 1800–1804.

Stenzel, W., Goebel, H.H. and Aronica, E. (2012). Review: immune-mediated necrotizing myopathies – a heterogeneous group of diseases with specific myopathological features. *Neuropathology and Applied Neurobiology* **38**, 632–646.

Stevens, D.L., Gibbons, A.E., Bergstrom, R. and Winn, V. (1988). The Eagle effect revisited: efficacy of clindamycin, erythromycin, and penicillin in the treatment of streptococcal myositis. *Journal of Infectious Diseases* **158**, 23–28.

Tan, J.Y., Valberg, S.J., Sebastian, M.M., Davis, G.D., Kelly, J.R., Goehring, L.S., Harland, M.M., Kuebelbeck, K.L., Waldridge, B.M., Newton, J.C. and Reimer, J.M. (2010). Suspected systemic calcinosis and calciphylaxis in 5 horses. *Canadian Veterinary Journal* **51**, 993–999.

Timoney, J.F. (2004). The pathogenic equine streptococci. *Veterinary Research* **35**, 397–409.

Tinling, S.P., Cardinet, G.H., III Blythe, L.L., Cohen, M. and Vonderfecht, S.L. (1980). A light and electron microscopic study of sarcocysts in a horse. *Journal of Parasitology* **66**, 458–465.

Traub-Dargatz, J.L., Schlipf, J.W., Jr. Granstrom, D.E., Ingram, J.T., Shelton, G.D., Getzy, D.M., Lappin, M.R. and Baker, D.C. (1994). Multifocal myositis associated with *Sarcocystis* spp. in a horse. *Journal of the American Veterinary Medical Association* **205**, 1574–1576.

Watson, K.E., Abrolat, M.L., Malone, L.L., Hoeg, J.M., Doherty, T., Detrano, R. and Demer, L.L. (1997). Active serum vitamin D levels are inversely correlated with coronary calcification. *Circulation* **96**, 1755–1760.

13 Granulomatous Diseases

Lais R.R. Costa

13.1 Definition

Hypersensitivity reactions, also known as immunopathologic reactions, are undesirable, inappropriate or exaggerated immunologic responses that directly injure bodily tissues. When the damage is mediated by immune cells, as opposed to soluble factors, the condition is referred to as cell-mediated hypersensitivity, or delayed-type hypersensitivity reaction. These reactions, also known as hypersensitivity type IV reactions, consist of sensitization of T cells, which lead to the establishment of chronic inflammatory response. Typically, the inflammatory response is characterized by prominent macrophage activation, although other inflammatory cells might also be involved. Hypersensitivity type IV reactions might be further classified according to the cytokine profiles and cells involved in the immunopathology, including macrophage-derived, neutrophil-derived or eosinophil-derived tissue damage, or cytotoxic CD8[+] T lymphocyte-derived apoptosis of the target cells caused by perforin and granzyme B (Sell, 1978; Sell, 1996; Uzzaman, 2012).

Cell-mediated immunopathologic reactions often develop within 24–48 hours (hence the delayed-type hypersensitivity designation) following re-exposure to the triggering/offending antigen (Ag), which is generally environmental or self in origin. Microbial and parasitic Ags can also trigger cell-mediated immunopathologic reactions, resulting in chronic inflammatory disease, the classical examples of which are *Mycobacterium tuberculosis* and *Mycobacterium leprae*. In some cases, the exaggerated cell-mediated response against microbial Ags might lead to elimination of the microorganism while, in others, the responses may simply limit dissemination of the infection while allowing the microbe to persist locally. Exaggerated cell-mediated immune reactions can occur without protective immunity, yet can lead to tissue damage.

13.2 Signalment and clinical signs

The clinical manifestations of cell-mediated immunopathologic reactions are dependent upon the nature and site(s) of tissue injury. The immune response is characterized by chronic inflammation, with infiltration of mononuclear cells (large numbers of macrophages and some lymphocytes), tissue necrosis, fibrosis, and angiogenesis. Other types of inflammatory cells may be recruited, including neutrophils, eosinophils, basophils, mast cells and plasma cells. The cell-mediated immunopathologic reactions may also be characterized by granuloma formation. Granulomas are circumscribed collections of macrophages, epithelioid cells, and multinucleated giant cells, characterizing a focal, chronic inflammatory response.

13.3 Immunologic mechanisms and etiologic associations

The etiology of cell-mediated immunopathologic reactions are generally divided into environmental, self or microbial, although the etiologic/triggering agents are often not known (Table 13.1).

Cell-mediated immunopathologic reactions are typically triggered by the presence of an Ag that is taken up by an antigen presenting cell (APC, principally a macrophage or dendritic cell), processed and presented via the major histocompatibility complex (MHC) class II molecule to CD4[+] T cells that can recognize the foreign peptides (Figure 13.1). Thus antigen peptides originated from exogenous proteins, either environmental or derived from extracellular pathogens, are loaded into MHC Class II molecules and lead to sensitization of CD4[+] T cells.

In contrast, antigen peptides originated from endogenous proteins, either self or derived from intracellular pathogens, are loaded into MHC Class I molecules and presented to CD8[+] T cells. Some APCs are capable of cross-presentation, where antigen peptides originated from exogenous foreign proteins are presented on MHC class II molecules to CD4[+] T cells (Joffre, 2012).

The CD4[+] T cells then differentiate into either T helper (Th) subsets, Th1 or Th17 or Th2, depending on the type of Ag and the additional cytokines produced by the APC. In the presence of IL-12 secreted by APCs, Ag-specific CD4[+] T cells become activated as Th1 cells, secrete interferon-gamma (IFN-gamma), and undergo clonal expansion (Cohn, 2014; Lambrecht, 2014). CD4[+] T cells may instead differentiate into Ag-specific Th2 or Th17, depending on the type of antigen and APC activation (Figure 13.2).

Equine Clinical Immunology, First Edition. Edited by M. Julia B. Felippe.
© 2016 John Wiley & Sons, Inc. Published 2016 by John Wiley & Sons, Inc.

Table 13.1 Proposed etiologic associations of conditions involving cell-mediated immunopathologic reactions in horses: T cell response leads to chronic inflammation, tissue injury and, in most conditions, granuloma formation.

Organ/tissue	Condition	Proposed triggering agents/Ags
Systemic	Equine sarcoidosis	Unknown; except one report of association with consumption of vetch, *Vicia* sp., and one report of association with *Mycobacterium* spp.
	Other multisystemic granulomatous disease	Microbial: *Coccidioides*, *Mycobacterium avium* subsp. *avium* (aka MAA causing disseminated granulomatous disease, also referred to as atypical tuberculosis); *Blastomyces* spp.; repeated immunostimulation with Bacillus Calmette-Guerin
Skin	Hypersensitivity to insect bite	Environmental: salivary Ags of biting insects especially from *Culicoides spp.*, and possibly *Simulium spp., Stomoxys calcitrans* and *Haematobia irritans*.
	Allergic contact dermatitis	Environmental: non-irritant agents, such as electrophilic metals (e.g., cobalt, nickel, chromium and zinc), dyes, preservatives or accelerator present in various items. Items reported to be associated with allergic contact dermatitis in horses include pasture plants (e.g., buttercups or *Rannunculus* spp.), bedding, products for topical use (soaps, shampoos, sprays, rinses, insect repellents), grooming aids, blankets, tack, cotton, jute.
	Erythema multiforme	Multiple etiologic associations that lead to alterations of keratinocytes, including drugs (e g., potentiated sulfonamides, penicillin, ivermectin), infection (e.g., herpes virus), vaccination, neoplasia (e.g., lymphoma), topical products. In many cases, the cause remains unknown (idiopathic)
	Equine collagenolytic granulomas	Undetermined etiology: possibly associated with insect bites, and injection administration
	Granulomatous ulcerative dermatitis	Microbial: *including Basidiobolus* (zygomycosis), *Pythium insidiosum* (pythiosis), *Absidia corymbifera* (mucormycosis), *Nocardia* (nocardiosis or eumycotic mycetoma), *Actinomyces* (actinomycotic mycetoma), *Staphylococcus* (bacterial pseudomacetoma or botryomycosis), *Candida* spp. (nodular candidiasis), *Sporothrix skenchii* (sporotricosis), *Trichophyton equinum* (dermatophytic pseudomycetoma), Parasitic: *Habronema* larvae (habronemiasis) Unknown (sterile granulomas)
Respiratory	Ulcerative granulomas of nasal and nasopharyngeal mucosa	Microbial: including *Conidiobolus, Cryptococcus* spp.
	Hypersensitivity pneumonitis	Environmental: including inhalation of organic Ags such as protein Ags from chicken/bird, weevils/insects in grains, and fungal spores
	Recurrent airway obstruction	Environmental: inhalation of organic Ags in hay or pasture, especially molds, and possibly plants grains
	Pyogranulomatous bronchopneumonia	Microbial: *Rhodococcus equi*
	Granulomatous pneumonia	Microbial: including *Coccidioiodes, Aspergillus, Pneumocystis (carinii) jiroveci; Histoplasma, Cryptococcus*, and repeated injections of Bacillus Calmette-Guerin Environmental: crystalline silicates (Silicosis) Unknown causes (idiopathic)
Digestive	Chronic idiopathic inflammatory bowel diseases	Unknown: possible association with aluminum
Nervous	Polyneuritis equi	Self (axonal proteins, myelin)
Muscle	Immune-mediated myositis	Unknown
Eye	Equine recurrent uveitis	Self (retinal proteins) or microbial (leptospiral Ags)
	Immune-mediated keratopathy	Unknown

Ags – antigens. Data from Swiderski, 1997, 2000; Lunn, 2010; Tizard, 2013. Scott 2010; Woods 1992; Oliveira-Filho 2012; Reeder 2014; Mathison 1995.

After the initial exposure (also referred to as the sensitization phase), Ag-specific long-lived memory CD4$^+$ or CD8$^+$ T cells are generated, and these become activated when re-exposed to the respective triggering antigen. APCs can also determine whether an immune reaction is long-lived. For example, some APCs protect effector T cells from suppression, as in the case of the long-lived response following exposure to mycobacterial adjuvants (Kumar, 2010b). T cell-mediated immune responses might be a double-edged sword; on the one hand, they provide protection from disease but, on the other hand, they lead to the development of delayed immunopathologic reaction.

Upon re-exposure, exogenous Ags are captured and processed by the APCs, and are presented to T-cells in the context of MHC Class II. This interaction results in IL-1 production by APC, and production of IL-2 by the T cell, leading to clonal expansion of the antigen-specific T-cell already committed to a particular Th subset.

Clonal expansion of Th1, Th17 or Th2 cells culminates with the production of large amounts of subset-specific cytokine profiles and results in an inflammatory reaction (Figure 13.3). The cascade of cytokines recruits non-specific circulating leukocytes, including monocytes, segmented neutrophils, eosinophils, basophils, mast cells and lymphocytes, to infiltrate the

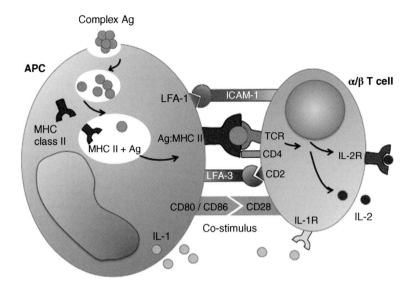

Figure 13.1 Interaction of antigen presenting cells and T lymphocytes.

Cell-mediated immunopathologic reactions are mediated by alpha/beta (α/β) T cell receptors (TCR) that recognize antigen (Ag) fragments in the context of the major histocompatibility complex (MHC) molecules. Antigen recognition by α/β T cells requires two signals. One signal is the Ag-specific binding of the α/β heterodimer TCR to the Ag fragment coupled with the MHC molecule. This binding is stabilized by the binding of the CD4 receptor to the MHC class II molecule, and by the binding of the accessory molecules CD2 and ICAM-1, on the surface of T cells, to the LFA-3 and LFA-1 on the cell surface of antigen-presenting cells (APC), respectively. The co-stimulatory signal is through the binding of CD28 and CD40L on T cells to CD80/CD86 and CD40 on the surface of APC. Interleukin (IL)-1, produced and released by APC, results in stimulation of IL-1 receptors (IL-1R) on the surface of T cells. T cell activation leads to expression IL-2 receptor (IL-2 R) and production of IL-2, resulting in autocrine and paracrine effect leading to clonal expansion of the Ag-specific T cell.

site. Following infiltration, these chemoattracted cells also produce inflammatory mediators and cytokines, which amplify the inflammatory reaction (Figure 13.3). The CD4$^+$ Th1 and Th17 subsets contribute to organ-specific disease, in which chronic inflammation is the prominent aspect of the pathology. The inflammatory reaction associated with Th1 cells is dominated by activated macrophages, leading to granulomatous inflammation. However, the reaction triggered by Th17 cells has a prominent neutrophil component

accompanying the mononuclear phagocyte infiltrate, leading to pyogranulomatous inflammation (Kumar, 2010a).

Chronic inflammatory response, the hallmark of delayed immunopathologic reactions, is characterized by: prominent infiltration of mononuclear cells (mononuclear phagocytes, lymphocytes and sometimes plasma cells); tissue destruction induced by the inflammatory cells and their mediators; and concurrent replacement of damaged tissue with proliferation of connective tissue (fibrosis) and proliferation of small blood

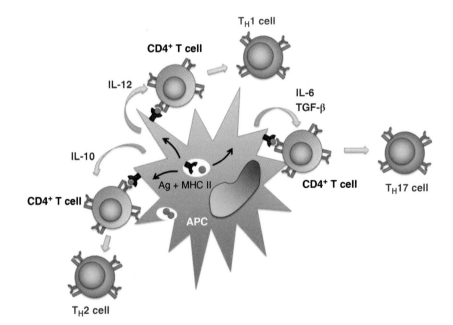

Figure 13.2 Sensitization phase of cell-mediated immunopathologic reactions.

Antigen (Ag) is processed and presented in the context of major histocompatibility complex (MHC) molecule on the surface of antigen-presenting cells (APCs), leading to activation of antigen-specific T cells. The cytokine milieu, largely dictated by the particular APC, leads to differentiation of the Ag-specific T cell into specific subsets of T helper (Th) cells. Differentiation into Th1 cells occurs in the presence of IL-12; differentiation of Th17 occurs in the presence of IL-6 and TGF-beta; and differentiation of Th2 occurs in the presence of IL-10. Sensitization phase is followed by the development of memory T cells.

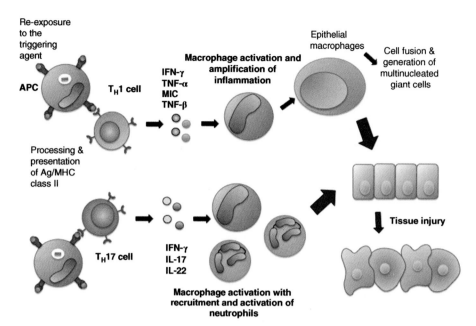

Figure 13.3 Effector phase of cell-mediated immunopathologic reactions.
Upon re-exposure to the triggering/offending agent, antigen (Ag) is processed and presented in the context of major histocompatibility complex (MHC) molecule on the surface of antigen presenting cells (APC), leading to activation and clonal expansion of Ag-specific memory T cells already committed to a T helper (Th) cell subset. Th cell activation culminates with the production of large amounts of subset-specific cytokine profiles, resulting in recruitment of non-specific circulating leukocytes, including monocytes, segmented neutrophils and eosinophils, to infiltrate the site. These chemoattracted cells also produce inflammatory mediators, chemokines and cytokines, which amplify the inflammatory reaction and contribute to organ-specific disease. For example, the inflammatory reaction associated with T cells of the Th1 subset is dominated by activated macrophages, leading to granulomatous inflammation, while the reaction triggered by Th17 cells has a prominent neutrophil component accompanying the mononuclear phagocyte infiltrate, leading to pyogranulomatous inflammation. The CD4$^+$ Th2 subset leads to delayed phase of antibody-mediated reactions, which accompany IgE-mediated reactions.

vessels (angiogenesis) (Kumar, 2010a). The chronic mononuclear phagocyte stimulation leads to the appearance of numerous epithelioid cells (also referred to as epithelioid histiocytes). These are activated macrophages acquiring elongated shape; with fine granular eosinophilic cytoplasma and central oval to elongated nucleus, thus resembling epithelial cells. As these self-perpetuating reactions progress, the epithelioid cells fuse to form multinucleated histiocytic giant cells (Cohen, 2009; Kumar, 2010a).

13.4 Diagnostics

The diagnosis of cell-mediated immunopathologic reactions is based on history, clinical presentation and histopathologic evaluation of biopsy specimen of lesion(s). Histolopathological evaluation defines the inflammatory infiltrate:

(a) If it is composed of lymphocytes and macrophages, it is described as granulomatous inflammatory infiltrate.
(b) When there is concomitant pronounced neutrophilic inflammation, the inflammatory reaction is described as pyogranulomatous.

(c) When there is concomitant prominent infiltration of eosinophilis, the lesion is described as eosinophilic granulomatous reaction.

In order to investigate for microbial or parasitic etiology, special histologic staining techniques are indicated. For example, the Grocott (or Gomori) methenamine silver (also referred to as GMS) staining facilitates the detection and evaluation of hyphae. It is, therefore, commonly used in cases when *Pythium, Basidiobolus, Conidiobolus, Aspergillus, Cryptococcus,* and branched filament fungi are suspected. Acid-fast staining should be considered in cases of multisystemic granulomatous diseases, in order to determine whether mycobacteria are involved. Immunohistochemistry to highlight specific markers on biopsied specimens can provide further characterization of the etiologic agent and cellular infiltrate. Suspected fungal and bacterial etiologies should be further evaluated with fungal and bacterial cultures of specimens, including tissue biopsy, pleural or peritoneal fluids, granules, or exudate from granulomas.

Determination of the cause of granulomatous pneumonia relies on cytologic evaluation, bacterial and fungal cultures of tracheobronchial aspirate, obtained from horses with pulmonary imaging suggestive of granuloma formation. Transcutaneous sampling of pulmonary lesions, including lung biopsies for histologic evaluation, and biopsy or fine needle aspirate for bacterial and fungal cultures, are rarely necessary for definitive diagnosis, but may be recommended in some cases.

13.5 Treatment and prevention

Management of delayed hypersensitivity reactions is focused on elimination of the underlying cause (i.e., eliminating exposure to the offending/triggering Ag), controlling clinical signs and minimizing complications. Ideally, therapy will moderate the cellular immune response in order to halt tissue injury.

Conditions associated with an environmental etiology are aimed at avoidance of the triggering agent. Conditions involving self-antigens and auto-immunity are managed with immuno-suppressive therapy. An exaggerated cell-mediated response against a microbial antigen aimed at eliminating the microbe, despite being harmful to the host may, in fact, be preventing the development of a disseminated infection. Therefore, before considering immunosuppressive treatment in these cases, it is important to establish the appropriate treatment aimed at eliminating the infectious or parasitic agent, thus decreasing the risk of dissemination of the infection upon immuno-suppression (Costa, 2012a, 2012b; Giguere, 2013; Davis, 2014; Sellon, 2014; Stewart, 2014).

The most commonly used immunosuppressant drugs in horses are the glucocorticoids (Lunn, 2010; Felippe, 2014). Initial immunosuppression is achieved by administration of dexamethasone at 0.05–0.2 mg/kg IV or PO every 12 or 24 hours. When signs of inflammation are resolved, the dose should be decreased by 10–20% every 24–48 hours. Therapy can be switched from dexamethasone to prednisolone, initially at 1 mg/kg PO every 12 or 24 hours, and gradually decreased to 0.2–0.5 mg/kg PO every 12, 24 or 48 hours over a period of two weeks, if clinical signs do not recur. Four to six weeks of immunosuppressive therapy may be required for treatment of delayed hypersensitivity, and a maintenance dose of predniso-lone may be required. Patients should be monitored for side-effects of corticosteroid therapy, including evidence of polyuria and polydipsia, laminitis and secondary infection.

Another immunosuppressive drug that might be used in horses for the treatment of immune-mediated diseases is aza-thioprine, instead of, or in conjunction with, corticosteroid therapy. Azathioprine causes immunosuppression, most notably by inhibiting purine synthesis, thus impeding cell proliferation, and by interfering with T-lymphocyte signaling pathways (Divers, 2010). Adequate immunosuppression by azathioprine is achieved at 3 mg/kg PO every 12 hours. It has been used for the management of various types of immune-mediate conditions, including inflammatory bowel diseases and polyneuritis equi. Long-term administration of azathioprine rarely causes side-effects of secondary infection due to immunosuppression,

anemia, leukopenia, alopecia and hepatotoxicity (White, 2005; Divers, 2010).

13.6 Types of cell-mediated hypersensitivity reactions

13.6.1 Multisystemic granulomatous diseases

Multisystemic granulomatous diseases may be associated with microbial, non-microbial or unknown Ag. The most common conditions in horses include equine sarcoidosis, coccidioido-mycosis, and disseminated mycobacterial disease. Repeated immunostimulation with Bacillus Calmette-Guerin has been reported to be a cause of widespread granulomatous disease in a horse (van de Boom, 2008). Other causes of multisystemic granulomatous diseases, including disseminated histoplasmosis, are not presented in this chapter.

13.6.1.1 Equine sarcoidosis

∗ Equine sarcoidosis, also referred to as idiopathic systemic granulomatous disease, affects adult horses generally older than four years of age, but shows no breed or sex predisposition. Clinical signs include multifocal skin lesions, ranging from scaling and crusting to nodular masses, accompanied by granulomatous lesions involving internal organs, most often lungs, lymph nodes and liver, and occasionally the gastrointestinal tract. Common signs include weight loss, anorexia, icterus, low-grade fever and peripheral lymphadenopathy. Respiratory distress, diarrhea, exercise intolerance and lameness are not uncommon (Spiegel, 2006; Reijerkerk, 2009; Sloet van Oldruitenborgh-Oosterbaan, 2013). Signs of central nervous system dysfunction, including cervical stiffness, head pressing and convulsion, have been reported (Peters, 2003). The etiology of sarcoidosis is unknown; although etiologic association have been reported. These include one report of association with consumption of vetch, *Vicia sp.* (Woods, 1992), and one report of association with *Mycobacterium spp.* infection (Oliveira-Filho, 2012).

Lesions in affected organs/tissues (most often skin, lymph nodes, and lungs and, less often, spleen, liver, and endocardium) are characterized by multifocal infiltrates of macrophages, lymphocytes and plasma cells, admixed with varying numbers of multinucleated giant cells, epithelioid macrophages, and fibrosis (Spiegel, 2006; Reijerkerk, 2009; Sloet van Oldruitenborgh-Oosterbaan, 2013).

Diagnosis of equine sarcoidosis is made by the clinical appearance and history of exfoliative dermatitis and weight loss, in conjunction with histopathology of lesions and ruling out other causes of granulomatous disease. Histopathologic evaluation of affected tissues (generally skin, lymph nodes and lungs) show lymphohistiocytic infiltrates, epithelioid macrophages, multinucleated giant cells and fibrosis (Reijerkerk, 2009).

Clinical management of equine sarcoidosis is challenging, regardless of whether it presents as generalized or a localized condition. Treatment of equine sarcoidosis often consists of administration of corticosteroids (e.g., dexamethasone, prednisolone) for a prolonged period of time, ranging from months to years (Spiegel, 2006; Reijerkerk, 2009; Sloet van Oldruitenborgh-Oosterbaan, 2013). Response to treatment is variable, and spontaneous remission or lack of progression may be observed in some affected horses.

13.6.1.2 Coccidioidomycosis

Coccidioidomycosis generally occurs in horses under eight years of age, with no known breed predisposition, although Arabians are overrepresented (Long, 2014; Ziemer, 1992). Females are also overrepresented. A seasonal trend of fall to winter has been reported. The most consistent signs are weight loss, intermittent febrile episodes and respiratory disease, with chronic cough, tachypnea, and discomfort associated with pleural effusion. Lymphohematogenous dissemination leads to: lameness, due to osteomyelitis; abortion, due to placentitis; and colic and peritoneal effusion, due to abdominal involvement. The percutaneous route of infection shows subcutaneous draining tracts (Long, 2014).

Coccidioidomycosis is characterized by granulomatous to pyogranulomatous inflammation in various anatomical sites, including the lungs, pleural cavity, mediastinum and thoracic lymph nodes, bone, skin and abdominal organs, peritoneum and mammary glands (Long, 2014). The immunological response, and the mechanism mediating immunopathology and immunity in equine coccidioidomycosis, are not completely understood, and most of what is known stems from studies in humans and laboratory animals. Cell-mediated immunity is critical in controlling the disease, and humoral response appears to be immunosuppressive (Long, 2014). Although humoral immune response against *Coccidioides* develops, it is not protective, and serum levels of polyclonal IgG are, in fact, indicative of active, progressive disease (Long, 2014). The lack of a protective response may be associated with a diminished expression of IL-12 receptor in APCs, and down-regulation of Th1 response by perigranulomatous B cells and CD4[+] T cells that secrete the anti-inflammatory cytokine IL-10 (Li, 2005).

The organism (arthroconidia) triggers a strong neutrophilic response, with activation of neutrophils leading to enhanced phagocytosis and oxidative burst. Nevertheless, 80% of the arthroconidia survive, allowing maturation of the organism into spherules, which are impervious to the fungicidal activity of neutrophils (Long, 2014). Likewise, the organism triggers strong activation of monocytes/macrophages, with enhanced phagocytosis. However, 99% of the organisms survive, by inhibiting phagosome-lysosome fusion, an ability similar to that of mycobacteria (Long, 2014). Thus, *Coccidioides* induces strong pyogranulomatous reaction, which is inefficient in eliminating the organism.

Diagnosis of coccidioidomycosis can be challenging, requiring multiple tests, including cytology and culture of tracheobronchial washes, culture and histologic evaluation of tissues, and serology. The organism can be seen with hematoxylin-eosin staining, although GMS staining, periodic acid-Schiff (PAS) staining and calcofluor white fluorescent staining may improve diagnosis (Long, 2014). Gram staining does not stain *Coccidioides* spp. The culture is carried out on conventional culture media, although media containing antibiotics can enhance the chance of growing *Coccidioides*. Serum titers of IgG antibodies correlate with the severity of disease: high or rising titers are indicative of worsening, and falling titers are indicative of resolution of disease. High serum antibody titers, greater than 1:16, are associated with disseminated coccidioidomycosis, whereas lower titers are associated with localized infection (Long, 2014).

13.6.1.3 Disseminated mycobacterial infection

Disseminated mycobacterial infections in horses are generally caused by *Mycobacterium avium*, and are characterized by a robust granulomatous inflammatory response (Pavlik, 2004). Disseminated mycobacterial infection tends to occur in horses between 1–6 years old. No sex or breed predisposition is reported (Oaks, 2007). The nonspecific signs have an insidious onset and include depression, intermittent febrile episodes and weight loss. Signs are slowly progressive over months and, by the time of diagnosis, the patient is generally emaciated. Lymphoadenopathy involving both thoracic and abdominal cavities is common. Chronic diarrhea is associated with the involvement of the small intestine, cecum or colon. Respiratory signs are rarely seen, despite pulmonary involvement being common.

The mechanisms mediating immunopathology of mycobacterial infection are associated with the strong activation of mononuclear phagocytes and survival of the organism within the mononuclear phagocyte by inhibition of phagosome-lysosome fusion (Oaks, 2007; Valledor, 2010). The granulomatous inflammation, consisting of macrophages, multinucleated giant cells and epithelioid macrophages, forms multifocal to miliary nodules, some of which contain caseous necrosis or are ulcerated (Pavlik, 2004; Oaks, 2007).

13.6.2 Skin granulomatous diseases
13.6.2.1 Allergic contact dermatitis

Allergic contact dermatitis, also referred to as contact hypersensitivity, is a cutaneous delayed type hypersensitivity reaction produced by exposure of the external skin surface to non-irritant compounds, such as dyes and electrophilic metals (Nixon, 2014; Reeder, 2014).

No age, sex or breed predisposition has been reported. It is characterized by skin lesions, either maculopapular (small, discolored, palpable bumps of the skin) or lichenified (thickening and hardening of the skin, giving a wrinkled, leathery appearance), accompanied by varying degrees of pruritis (Scott, 2010).

Compounds that are not antigenic act as a hapten, thus associating with a carrier protein. Electrophilic metals readily ionize and react with proteins, forming complexes that are phagocytosed and processed by Langerhans cells (LC) (Yoshihisa, 2012). Activated LCs migrate via afferent lymphatic vessels to draining lymph nodes, for presentation to, and activation of, T cells (sensitization phase) (Nixon, 2014; Reeder, 2014). Re-exposure to the contact allergen elicits antigen presentation by LCs and activation of specific T cells, leading to a cascade of cytokine and chemokine release, culminating with amplification of the inflammatory response. Allergic contact dermatitis is characterized by perivascular lymphocytic inflammation, with neutrophilic infiltration, spongiosis (epidermal intercellular edema) and lymphocytic exocytosis (intraepithelial lymphocytes).

Diagnosis of allergic contact dermatitis can be challenging. Patch testing (sometimes referred to as epicutaneous test) reproduces the exposure mode in allergic contact dermatitis and it is, therefore, the best confirmatory test (Nixon, 2014; Reeder, 2014). Patch testing consists of challenging the animal with the suspected allergen/hapten by applying it to a small, circumscribed area of intact healthy skin. Upon re-exposure to the substance, a reaction at the site of application will usually develop within 48–72 hours (Reeder, 2014).

Management of allergic contact dermatitis includes avoidance of the offending compound, which may suffice to resolve the problem (Reeder, 2014). Topical corticosteroids can be applied if affected areas are small, whereas systemic corticosteroids, often given orally, are recommended for larger or multifocal lesions.

13.6.2.2 Equine collagenolytic granuloma

Equine collagenolytic granuloma, also referred to as eosinophilic granuloma or nodular necrobiosis, is a non-ulcerative cutaneous nodular dermatosis, characterized by the predominance of eosinophils and the presence of collagen necrosis (Mathison, 1995; Scott, 2010). No breed, sex or age predisposition has been reported. Eosinophilic granuloma is suspected on the basis of a history and clinical finding of non-pruritic, non-painful, non-ulcerated, slow-progressing skin nodules, ranging in size from 0.5–10 cm, located most commonly on the neck, withers, and dorsal trunk. Initially, the nodules are soft and, over weeks to months, they progress to firm, haired, circumscribed, non-painful and non-pruritic masses (Scott, 2010). The etiology of equine collagenolytic granuloma is not known but, in several cases, etiological associations with injection administration or insect bites have been presented. (Mathison, 1995; Slovis, 1999).

The diagnosis is confirmed by histopathology of a representative biopsy of the lesions or exfoliative cytology (Mathison, 1995; Scott, 2010). Histopathologic evaluation reveals eosinophilic granulomatous reaction surrounding areas of degenerated collagen. Exfoliative cytology reveals eosinophils, lymphocytes and macrophages.

Treatment of eosinophilic granuloma depends on the location, number and type of lesions. Because the condition does not cause pain or pruritus, the lesions might be left untreated. If treatment is contemplated. The therapeutic options include: surgical excision of a single lesion; intralesional injection of corticosteroids (e.g., triamcinolone or methylprednisolone); and/or systemic corticosteroids, if multiple lesions are present (Mathison, 1995, Scott, 2010).

13.6.2.3 Ulcerative granuloma

Ulcerative granulomas of the skin are cell-mediated immunopathologic reactions to microbial and parasitic agents, and include nocardiosis, basidiobolomycosis, pythiosis, habronemiasis, mucormycosis, eumycotic and actinomycotic mycetomas. No breed, sex or age predisposition has been reported. It manifests with an insidious onset of single or multiple nodular skin lesions that erode to ulcerative areas, with moderate to severe pruritis and oozing of serosanguinous discharge (Miller, 1984; Gaastra, 2010; Costa, 2012a, 2012b). Mycetomas, basidiobolomycosis and pythiosis are characterized by the presence of draining tracts, with the discharge containing granules (Miller, 1984; Costa, 2012a, 2012b; Scott, 2010).

In most cases, the granulomas of the skin and mucosa are ulcerative, and the inflammatory infiltrate is composed mostly of numerous macrophages, neutrophils, eosinophils, mast cells, whereas lymphocytes and plasma cells are scattered throughout the lesion (Miller, 1984; Gaastra, 2010; Rommel Max, 2010; Grooters, 2014; Stewart, 2014). These lesions are often described as eosinophilic granulomatous inflammation with necrosis and fibrosis (Groters, 2014). The etiologic agent may be seen in the necrotic areas. The amount of edema, fibrosis, and the number of macrophages and multinucleated giant cells surrounding the necrotic centers varies according to the etiologic agent.

Determination of the etiology of ulcerative granulomas of the skin and mucosa requires collection of representative biopsies for histologic evaluation and aerobic bacterial and fungal cultures. Not all granulomatous lesions are the result of immunopathologic reactions to microbial and parasitic agents. Histologic evaluation of sections should be stained with hematoxylin-eosin and other special stainings (e.g., GMS and PAS). Differential diagnoses of ulcerative granuloma include: exuberant granulation tissue; cutaneous habronemiasis; foreign body granuloma; zygomycosis; pythiosis; ulcerated neoplasia such as sarcoid and squamous cell carcinoma; cutaneous nocardiosis (generally distal limb); bacterial pseudomycetoma or botryomycosis (limb, lips, head, mammary area, scrotum); cutaneous actinomycosis (generally head and neck); phaeohyphomycoses and eumycotic mycetomas (Costa, 2012a, 2012b).

In the case of fungal granuloma, the hyphae are often embedded in an amorphous cement-like substance known as Splendore-Hoeppli material. Immunohistochemistry of biopsy specimens is often recommended for confirmation of pythiosis, but it is not available for basidiobolomycosis and conidiobolomycosis (Grooters, 2014; Stewart, 2014). Confirmation of the causative fungal organism is best obtained by culture and identification of the reproductive structures (conidia and zygospores). Serology maybe used for confirmation of pythiosis.

The treatment of ulcerative granulomas of the skin, nasal and nasopharyngeal mucosa depends on the etiology (Costa, 2012a, 2012b; Grooters, 2014, Stewart, 2014). Treatment of fungal granulomas and pythiosis requires a combination of surgical resection and medical management with anti-fungal drugs and, possibly, immunotherapy with autologous vaccine (Gaastra, 2010; Grooters, 2014). Treatment should be instituted as soon as possible, due to rapid progression of the infection; the longer the duration of infection, the poorer the prognosis. The location of the lesion(s) greatly influence prognosis. Immunosuppressive therapies in the treatment of ulcerative granulomas of skin, nasal and nasopharyngeal mucosa are rarely used.

13.6.3 Respiratory granulomatous diseases

13.6.3.1 Ulcerative granulomas of nasal and nasopharyngeal mucosa

Ulcerative granulomas of nasal passage and nasopharyngeal mucosa include conidiobolomycosis and cryptococcosis. No breed, sex or age predisposition has been reported. Clinical signs manifest as insidious onset of serosanguinous nasal discharge, and dyspnea associated with upper respiratory tract obstruction (Miller, 1984; Costa, 2012a, 2012b; Rommel Max, 2010; Grooters, 2014; Stewart, 2014). The immunopathology, diagnosis and treatment of ulcerative granulomas of the mucosa of the nasal passages and nasopharynx are discussed in detail under the previous section, because they are similar to the ulcerative granulomas of the skin.

13.6.3.2 Granulomatous pneumonia

Granulomatous pneumonia has been reported with various etiologic associations, including silicosis, coccidioidomycosis, aspergillosis, pneumocystosis, histoplasmosis, cryptococcosis, adverse reaction to immunostimulants and idiopathic (Mansmann, 1992; Byars, 2009). Clinical signs often include intermittent fever, weight loss, anorexia and cachexia (Mansmann, 1992). No breed, sex or age predisposition has been reported.

13.6.3.3 Pneumoconiosis or pulmonary silicosis

Pneumoconiosis in horses is caused by inhalation of small inorganic (silicate) particles that deposit in the lower respiratory tract and are engulfed by alveolar macrophages – hence, the designation of "pulmonary silicosis". No breed, sex or age predisposition has been reported. Patients tend to be mostly middle-aged horses. Clinical signs of pulmonary silicosis include exercise intolerance, tachypnea, increased respiratory effort, and flared nostrils and weight loss, and they may be manifested months to years after the exposure to silica (Marsh, 2014). Intermittent lameness, characterized by stiffness and reluctance to move, associated with bone fragility, due to osteoporosis of the scapula, pelvis, ribs and vertebrae, and known as silicate

associated osteoporosis, has been reported concurrently with pulmonary silicosis (Durham, 2009; Arens, 2011).

Pneumoconiosis is characterized by widespread granulomatous fibrosing bronchiolitis. The peribronchiolar granulomatous inflammation consists of macrophages that contain heterogeneous pigmented or clear crystals, a small number of lymphocytes, and coalescence of contiguous fibrotic parenchyma (Durham, 2009; Arens, 2011; Marsh, 2014).

Diagnosis is based on history, clinical presentation, and thoracic imaging consistent with interstitial/granulomatous pulmonary disease. Cytologic evaluation of samples obtained from tracheobronchial aspirate or bronchoalveolar lavage fluid obtained from horses reveals granulomatous inflammation and the presence of birefringent crystals within macrophages (Durham, 2009; Arens, 2011; Marsh, 2014).

Typically, the onset of disease is insidious and, by the time of diagnosis, the process is so advanced that treatment is often unrewarding and prognosis is poor. If treatment is attempted, it consists of immunosuppressive therapy with corticosteroids (Durham, 2009; Arens, 2011; Marsh, 2014).

13.6.3.4 Aspergillosis

Pulmonary aspergillosis is characterized by multifocal pyogranulomatous inflammation of the pulmonary parenchyma, often occurring as a result of hematogenous spread, associated with loss of integrity of the gastrointestinal barrier, as well as through inhalation (Hattel, 1991; Sweeney, 1999; Sellon, 2014).

Pulmonary aspergillosis may be accompanied by nasal discharge, nasal plaques, tachypnea and dyspnea. No breed, sex or age predisposition has been reported.

13.6.3.5 Hypersensitivity pneumonitis

Hypersensitivity pneumonitis, also referred to as allergic alveolitis or Farmer's lung, is associated with inhalation of organic dust. The condition affects adult horses, without obvious breed or sex predisposition. Clinical signs include exercise intolerance, dyspnea, labored breathing, weight loss and fever (Moore, 2004; Mansmann, 1992).

Environmental Ags trigger a lymphocytic/plasmacytic bronchiolitis and a lymphocytic interstitial pneumonia, accompanied by granuloma formation and fibrosis (Moore, 2004; Mansmann, 1992).

13.6.3.6 Pyogranulomatous bronchopneumonia

Pyogranulomatous bronchopneumonia in foals is typically caused by virulent strains of *Rhodococcus equi*. Closely related to *Mycobacterium*, *Corynebacterium* and *Nocardia*, *R. equi* has a complex mycolic acid-containing cell wall that functions as a barrier for survival within macrophages (Hines, 2014). Infection by *R. equi* typically manifests as pulmonary disease characterized by chronic multiple miliary pyogranulomatous lesions (often most severe in the cranioventral portions of the lung), accompanied by lymphoadenitis, although abdominal involvement (especially mesenteric lymph nodes) is not uncommon.

Occasionally, widespread infection associated with hematogenous dissemination of the organism occurs.

Rhodococcus equi infections affect foals between 1–6 months old, and no breed or sex predisposition has been documented. Clinical signs include insidious, chronic pneumonia, manifested initially by fever, lethargy and coughing, progressing to anorexia, tachypnea, labored breathing (flared nostrils and pronounced abdominal excursion during respiration) and tachycardia. Nasal discharge, failure to grow and weight loss may be present (Giguere, 2011a; Hines, 2014).

Virulent strains of *R. equi* cause chronic, progressive granulomatous to pyogranulomatous reaction in foals, whereas immunocompetent adult horses are resistant to infection (Hines, 2014). The virulence of *R. equi* involves various virulence plasmids, and pathogenesis involves all branches of the immune system. Activated macrophages and neutrophils are important in controlling establishment of *R. equi* infection, and failure in neutrophil induction and activated macrophage killing is thought to allow replication of *R. equi* within non-activated resident macrophages (Kanaly, 1995; Hines, 2014). Antibodies, especially isotypes capable of opsonization and complement fixation, are thought to play an important role in prevention of establishment of *R. equi* infection, and failure to produce or transfer these antibodies though colostrum most likely predisposes to infection. However, cell-mediated immunity involving both CD4$^+$ (in particular, the Th1 subset) and CD8$^+$ T lymphocytes is thought to be crucial for the clearance of intracellular *R. equi*, and their failure leads to the development of infection (Kanaly, 1995; Hines, 2014).

Diagnostic confirmation of *R. equi* as the cause of pyogranulomatous pneumonia in foals includes history, clinical signs and age of the foal, and is best confirmed by bacterial culture or amplification of the virulence-associated protein A (*vap A*) gene by polymerase chain reaction (PCR) of tracheobronchial aspirate (Giguere, 2011b). Serologic tests for *R. equi* have low sensitivity and/or specificity and are, therefore, not good indicators of disease.

Treatment of pyogranulomatous pneumonia associated with *R. equi* infection requires antimicrobials and supportive care. Oxygen therapy may also be necessary. Current recommendations on the antimicrobial choice for the treatment of *R. equi* infection can be found elsewhere. (Giguere, 2011b, 2013; Hines, 2014) No immunomodulation is recommended, except judicious use of non-steroid anti-inflammatory drugs (Giguere, 2011b; Hines, 2014). Prevention of *R. equi* should include decreasing the environmental contamination, although early detection of diseased individuals appears to be the most feasible and crucial. The clinical effectiveness of passive humoral protection against *R. equi* infection is controversial (Giguere, 2011b). However, hyperimmune plasma transfusion may be beneficial before exposure to *R. equi* (i.e., in the first days of life), as opsonization of *R. equi* is essential for neutrophil function preventing the establishment of infection.

13.6.4 Gastrointestinal granulomatous diseases

13.6.4.1 Chronic idiopathic inflammatory bowel diseases

Chronic idiopathic inflammatory bowel diseases, also referred to as inflammatory bowel diseases, consist of a group of conditions characterized by infiltration of the bowel wall with immune cell types. Specific conditions include granulomatous enteritis (GE), multisystemic eosinophilic epitheliotropic disease (MEED), lymphocytic-plasmacytic enterocolitis, and idiopathic eosinophilic enterocolitis. No sex predisposition has been reported to any of these conditions, and cases of GE and MEED are most often reported in young horses.

Standardbred horses are predisposed to GE and MEED, and Thoroughbreds are predisposed to MEED. Signs may include recurrent episodes of colic, depression, weight loss, hypoproteinemia due to hypoalbuminemia, and impaired glucose or xylose absorption (Schumacher, 2000; Kalck, 2009; Scott, 1999; Sanchez, 2010). The etiology of chronic inflammatory bowel diseases is largely unknown. A cluster of equine cases of inflammatory bowel diseases has suggested a possible association of with aluminum ingestion (Fogarty, 1998). In laboratory animals, aluminum was shown to cause enhanced intestinal mucosa inflammation and decreased healing in a murine model of colitis, and was thus implicated as a risk factor for inflammatory bowel diseases (Pineton de Chambrun, 2014).

Granulomatous enteritis is characterized by diffuse granulomatous inflammation and the presence of epithelioid macrophages and giant cells in the intestinal wall (Schumacher, 2000; Kalck, 2009; Scott, 1999; Sanchez, 2010). Multisystemic eosinophilic epitheliotropic disease is characterized by segmental or multifocal granulomas, with lymphocytic and pronounced eosinophilic infiltration of the intestinal mucosa and submucosa (Schumacher, 2000; Kalck, 2009; Scott, 1999; Sanchez, 2010). Idiopathic eosinophilic enterocolitis is characterized by pronounced eosinophilic infiltration of all layers of the intestinal wall, in addition to lymphocytic infiltration (Schumacher, 2000). Lymphocytic-plasmacytic enteropathy is characterized by infiltration of lamina propria with lymphocytes and plasma cells (Schumacher, 2000; Kalck, 2009; Scott, 1999; Sanchez, 2010).

Management of chronic idiopathic inflammatory bowel diseases can be challenging, because these conditions are not particularly responsive to any form of treatment. However, a combination of immunomodulation and, if possible, surgical resection of the affected portion of the intestine, may be attempted.

13.6.5 Neurologic granulomatous diseases

13.6.5.1 Polyneuritis equi

Polyneuritis equi, previously called neuritis of the cauda equina, affects adult horses without breed or sex predisposition. It is an insidious, progressive dysfunction of the nerves of the cauda equina and cranial nerves. Clinical signs include: dysuria; urinary incontinence; initial hyperesthesia of the tail, followed by hypoesthesia of the tail; absence or diminished tail, anal, and perineal tone; hypotonicity and possibly atrophy of gluteal, semimembranosus/semitendinosus muscles; paresis and ataxia of the pelvic limbs; and paralysis of one or more cranial nerves (Rousseaux, 1984; van Galen, 2008; Aleman, 2009). Cranial nerve involvement is generally asymmetrical, often of the trigeminal (CN V), facial (CN VII), vestibulocochlear (CN VIII) nerves, and manifests as facial paralysis, abnormal mastication, and masseter atrophy.

Polyneuritis equi is a mixed immunopathologic condition characterized by perineural inflammatory infiltrate of mostly T and B lymphocytes, macrophages and giant cells, but may also include plasma cells, eosinophils and neutrophils (Rousseaux, 1984; van Galen, 2008; Aleman, 2009). The granulomatous inflammation of the nerve roots is associated with hemorrhage, demyelination, axonal degeneration and fibrosis. Antibodies to P2 myelin are produced, indicating a mixed, complex immunopathology that culminates with the progressive, insidious radiculoneuritis (van Galen, 2008, Aleman, 2009).

Diagnosis of polyneuritis equi is largely based on clinical presentation and careful neurologic evaluation, and by ruling-out other conditions, including sacral trauma at the level of S2 vertebra, equine herpes virus myeloencephalopathy, equine protozoa myeloencephalitis, West Nile virus encephalitis, and rabies (Vatistas, 1991, 1995; Hahn, 2008; van Galen, 2008). Ante-mortem confirmation of polyneuritis equi is possible by histologic evaluation of a biopsy of the sacrocaudalis dorsalis lateralis muscle, which contains nerve branches arising from the cauda equina (Aleman, 2009). The diagnosis of polyneuritis equi is confirmed by demonstration of excessive epineural and perineural fibrosis, neurogenic pattern of myofiber atrophy and prominent macrophage infiltration, accompanied by mononuclear cells composed of $CD8^+$ cytotoxic T lymphocytes, $CD4^+$ helper T lymphocytes and plasma cells.

Management of polyneuritis equi is largely supportive, because immunomodulation is generally not effective in halting the progression of the disease. Immunosuppression might be attempted with systemic corticosteroids, with or without azathioprine. Prognosis of polyneuritis equi is poor.

References

Aleman, M., Katzman, S.A., Vaughan, B., Hodges, J., Crabbs, T.A., Christopher, M.M., Shelton, G.D. and Higgins, R.J. (2009). Ante-mortem diagnosis of *polyneuritis equi*. *Journal of Veterinary Internal Medicine* 23, 665–668.

Arens, A.M., Barr, B., Puchalski, S.M., Poppenga, R., Kulin, R.M., Anderson, J. and Stover, S.M. (2011). Osteoporosis associated with pulmonary silicosis in an equine bone fragility syndrome. *Veterinary Pathology* 48, 593–615

Byars, T.D. (2009). Granulomatous lung disease. In: Robinson, N.E. and Sprayberry, K. (eds). *Current Therapy in Equine Medicine* volume 6, pp. 297–298. St. Louis, Saunders, Elsevier.

Chinen, J., Fleisher, T.A., and Shearer, W.T. (2014). Adaptive Immunity. In: Adkinson, N.F., Bochner, B.S., Burks, A.W., Busse, W.W., Holgate, S.T., Lemanske, R.F. and O'Hehir, R.E. (eds). *Middleton's Allergy Principles and Practice*, eighth edition, pp. 20–29. Philadelphia, Elsevier Saunders.

Cohen, R.D., Scott, D.W. and Erb, H.N. (2009). Prevalence, number and morphological types of multinucleated histiocytic giant cells in equine inflammatory dermatoses: A retrospective light microscopic study of skin biopsy specimens from 362 horses. *Equine Veterinary Journal* 41, 406–409.

Cohn, L. and Ray, A. (2014). Biology of lymphocytes. In: Adkinson, N.F., Bochner, B.S., Burks, A.W., Busse, W.W., Holgate, S.T., Lemanske, R.F. and O'Hehir, R.E. (eds). *Middleton's Allergy Principles and Practice*, eighth edition, pp. 271–282. Philadelphia, Elsevier Saunders.

Costa, L.R.R. (2012a). Zygomycosis. In: Wilson, D.A. (ed). *Clinical Veterinary Advisor; The Horse*, pp. 657–659. St. Louis, Elsevier Saunders.

Costa, L.R.R. (2012b). Pythiosis. In: Wilson, D.A. (ed). *Clinical Veterinary Advisor; The Horse*, pp. 485–487. St. Louis, Elsevier Saunders.

Davis, J.L. and Papich, M.G. (2014). Antimicrobial Therapy. In: Sellon, D. and Long, M. (eds). *Equine Infectious Disease*, second edition, pp. 571–584. St. Louis, Saunders Elsevier.

Divers, T.J. (2010). Azathioprine – a useful treatment for immune-mediated disorders in the horse? *Equine Veterinary Education* 22, 501–502.

Durham, M. (2009). The silicosis and osteoporosis syndrome. In: Robinson, N.E. and Sprayberry, K. (eds). *Current Therapy in Equine Medicine* volume 6, pp. 303–306. St Louis, Saunders, Elsevier.

Felippe, M.J.B. (2014). Immunotherapy. In: Sellon, D. and Long, M. (eds). *Equine Infectious Disease*, second edition, pp. 584–597. St. Louis, Saunders Elsevier.

Fogarty, U., Perl, D., Good, P., Ensley, S., Seawright, A. and Noonan, A. (1998). A cluster of equine granulomatous enteritis cases: the link with aluminium. *Veterinary and Human Toxicology* 40, 297–305.

Gaastra, W., Lipmanb, L.J.A., De Cockc, A.W.A.M., Exelb, T.K., Peggeb, R.B.G., Scheurwaterb, J., Vilelad, R. and Mendoza, L. (2010). *Pythium insidiosum*: An overview. *Veterinary Microbiology* 146, 1–16.

Giguere, S., Cohen, N.D., Chaffin, M.K., Hines, S.A., Hondalus, M.K., Prescott, J.F. and Slovis, N.M. (2011a). *Rhodococcus equi*: Clinical manifestations, virulence, and immunity. *Journal of Veterinary Internal Medicine* 25, 1221–1230.

Giguere, S., Cohen, N.D., Chaffin, M.K., Slovis, N.M., Hondalus, M.K., Hines, S.A. and Prescott, J.F. (2011b). Diagnosis, treatment, control, and prevention of infections caused by Rhodococcus equi in foals. *Journal of Veterinary Internal Medicine* 25, 1209–1220.

Giguère, S. and Afonso, T. (2013). Antimicrobial Drug Use in Horses. In: Giguère, S., Prescott, J. F. and Dowling, P.M. (eds). *Antimicrobial Therapy in Veterinary Medicine*, fifth edition. Hoboken, John Wiley & Sons.

Grooters, A. (2014). Pythiosis and Zygomycosis. In: Sellon, D. and Long, M. (eds). *Equine Infectious Disease*, second edition, pp. 415–420. St. Louis, Saunders Elsevier.

Hahn, C.N. (2008). *Polyneuritis equi*: the role of T-lymphocytes and importance of differential clinical signs. *Equine Veterinary Journal* 40, 100. (DOI: 10.2746/042516408X276924).

Hattel, A.L., Drake, T.R., Anderholm, B.J. and McAllister, E.S. (1991). Pulmonary aspergillosis associated with acute enteritis in a horse. *JAVMA* 199, 589–590.

Hines, M. (2014). Rhodococcus equi. In: Sellon, D. and Long, M. (eds). *Equine Infectious Disease*, second edition, pp. 287–301. St. Louis, Saunders Elsevier.

Joffre, O.P., Segura, E., Savina, A. and Amigoretta, S. (2012). Cross-presentation by dendritic cells. *Nature Reviews Immunology* **12**, 557–569. (DOI: 10.1038/nri3254)

Kalck, K.A. (2009). Inflammatory bowel disease in horses. *Veterinary Clinics of North America: Equine Practice* **25**, 303–315.

Kanaly, S.T., Hines, S.A. and Palmer, G.H. (1995). Cytokine modulation alters pulmonary clearance of *Rhodococcus equi* and development of granulomatous pneumonia. *Infection and Immunity* **63**, 3037–3041.

Kumar, V., Abbas, A.K., Fausto, N. and Aster, J.C. (2010a). *Robbins and Cotran Pathologic Basis of Disease*, eighth edition, pp 43–78. Philadelphia, Saunders Elsevier.

Kumar, V., Abbas, A.K., Fausto, N. and Aster, J.C. (2010b). *Robbins and Cotran Pathologic Basis of Disease*, eighth edition, pp 183–258. Philadelphia, Saunders Elsevier.

Lambrecht, B.N. and Hammad, H. (2014). Antigen-Presenting Dendritic Cells. In: Adkinson, N.F., Bochner, B.S., Burks, A.W., Busse, W.W., Holgate, S.T., Lemanske, R.F. and O'Hehir, R.E. (eds). *Middleton's Allergy Principles and Practice*, eighth edition, pp. 215–227. Philadelphia, Elsevier Saunders.

Li, L. (2005). *Immunopathology of Coccidioidal Granulomata and the Regulation of Interleukin-12 Signal Transduction in Human Coccidioidomycosis*. 126 pp. Tuscon, The University of Arizona.

Long, M.T., Pappagianis, D. and Higgins, J. (2014). Coccidioidomycosis. In: Sellon, D. and Long, M. (eds). *Equine Infectious Disease*, second edition, pp. 399–406. St. Louis, Saunders Elsevier.

Lunn, P. and Horohov, D. (2010). The Equine Immune System. In: Reed, S.M., Bayly, W.M. and Sellon, D.C. (es). *Equine Internal Medicine*, third edition, pp. 2–56. Philadelphia, Saunders.

Mansmann, R.A. (1992). Granulomatous Pneumonia. In: Colahan, P. T., Mayhew, I. G., Merritt, A. M. and Moore, J. N. (eds). *Equine Medicine and Surgery*, fourth edition, pp. 449–451. Goleta, American Veterinary Publications.

Marsh, P.S. (2014). Pneumoconiosis (Silicosis). In: Smith, B.P. (ed). *Large Animal Internal Medicine*, fifth edition, pp. 540–541. St. Louis, Elsevier Mosby.

Mathison, P.T. (1995). Equine nodular dermatoses. *Veterinary Clinics of North America: Equine Practice* **11**, 75–89.

Miller, R.I. and Campbell, R.S.F. (1984). The comparative pathology of equine cutaneous phycomycosis. *Veterinary Pathology* **21**, 325–332.

Moore, J.E., Matsuda, M., Yamamoto, S., Buckley, T. and Millar, B.C. (2004). Hypersensitivity pneumonitis in the horse: an under-diagnosed condition? *Journal of Equine Veterinary Science* **24**, 510–511.

Nixon, R.L. and Diepgen, T. (2014). Contact Dermatitis. In: Adkinson, N.F., Bochner, B.S., Burks, A.W., Busse, W.W., Holgate, S.T., Lemanske, R.F. and O'Hehir, R.E. (eds). *Middleton's Allergy Principles and Practice*, eighth edition, pp. 565–574. Philadelphia, Elsevier Saunders.

Oaks, J.L. (2007). Mycobacterial Infections. In: Sellon, D. and Long, M. (eds). *Equine Infectious Disease*, second edition, pp. 296–300. St. Louis, Elsevier.

Oliveira-Filho, J.P., Monteiro, L.N., Delfiol, D.J.Z., Sequeira, J.L., Amorim, R.M., Fabris, V.E., Del Piero, F. and Borges, A.S. (2012). Mycobacterium DNA detection in liver and skin of a horse with generalized sarcoidosis. *Journal of Veterinary Diagnostic Investigation* **24**, 596.

Pavlik, I., Jahn, P., Dvorska, L., Bartos, M., Novotny, L. and Halouzka, R. (2004). Mycobacterial infections in horses: a review of the literature. *Veterinary Medicine – Czech* **49**, 427–440.

Peters, M., Graf, G. and Pohlenz, J. (2003). Idiopathic systemic granulomatous disease with encephalitis in a horse. *Journal of Veterinary Medicine Series A* **50**, 108–112.

Pineton de Chambrun, G., Body-Malapel, M., Frey-Wagner, I., Djouina, M., Deknuydt, F., Atrott, K., Esquerre, N., Altare, F., Neut, C., Arrieta, M.C., Kanneganti, T.D., Rogler, G., Colombel, J.F., Cortot, A., Desreumaux, P. and Vignal, C. (2014). Aluminum enhances inflammation and decreases mucosal healing in experimental colitis in mice. *Mucosal Immunology* **7**, 589–601.

Reeder, C. and Griffin, J. (2014). Equine allergic dermatitis. In: Noli, C., Foster, A.P. and Rosenkrantz, W. (eds). *Veterinary Allergy*, pp 387. St. Louis, Wiley.

Reijerkerk, E.P.R., Veldhuis Kroeze, E.J.B. and Sloet van Oldruitenborgh-Oosterbaan, M.M. (2009). Equine sarcoidosis. *Sarcoidosis Vasculitis and Diffuse Lung Diseases* **26**, 20–23.

Rommel Max, T.S.L., DeFrancisco, A.L. and Singh, K. (2010). Vet med today: pathology in practice. *JAVMA* **236**, 831–833.

Rousseaux, C.G., Futcher, K.G., Clark, E.G. and Naylor, J.M. (1984). *Cauda equina* neuritis: A chronic idiopathic polyneuritis in two horses. *Canadian Veterinary Journal* **25**, 214–218.

Sanchez, L.C. (2010). Diseases Associated with Malabsorption and Maldigestion. In: Reed, S.M., Bayly, W.M. and Sellon, D.C. (eds). *Equine Internal Medicine*, third edition, pp. 850–856. Philadelphia, Saunders.

Schumacher, J., Edwards, J.F. and Cohen, N.D. (2000). Chronic idiopathic inflammatory bowel diseases of the horse. *Journal of Veterinary Internal Medicine* **14**, 258–65.

Scott, E.A., Heidel, J.R., Snyder, S.P., Ramirez, S. and Whitler, W.A. (1999). Inflammatory bowel disease in horses: 11 cases (1988–1998). *JAVMA* **214**, 1527–1530.

Scott D.W. and Miller, W.H. Jr. (2010). *Equine Dermatology*, second edition. St. Louis, Elsevier Saunders.

Sell, S. (1978). Immunopathology. *American Journal of Pathology* **90**, 215–280.

Sell, S. and Max, E.E. (1996). Delayed-type hypersensitivity. In: Sell, S. (ed). *Immunology Immunopathology and Immunity*, sixth edition, pp. 431–451. Washington, ASM Press.

Sellon, D.C. and Kohn, C. (2014). Aspergillosis. In: Sellon, D. and Long, M. (eds). *Equine Infectious Disease*, second edition, pp. 421–434. St. Louis, Saunders Elsevier.

Sloet van Oldruitenborgh-Oosterbaan, M.M. and Grinwis, G.C.M. (2013). Equine sarcoidosis: Clinical signs, diagnosis, treatment and outcome of 22 cases. *Veterinary Dermatology* **24**, 218–224. (DOI: 10.1111/j.1365-3164.2012.01108.x)

Slovis, N.M., Watson, J.L., Affolter, V.K. and Stannard, A.A. (1999). Injection site eosinophilic granulomas and collagenolysis in 3 horses. *Journal of Veterinary Internal Medicine* **13**, 606–612.

Spiegel, I.B., White, S.D., Foley, J.E., Drazenovich, N.L., Ihrke, P.J. and Affolter, V.K. (2006). A retrospective study of cutaneous equine sarcoidosis and its potential infectious aetiological agents. *Veterinary Dermatology* **17**, 51–62.

Stewart, A.J. (2014). Fungal Infections of the Equine Respiratory Tract. In: Smith, B.P. (ed). *Large Animal Internal Medicine*, fifth edition, pp. 494–504. St. Louis, Elsevier Mosby.

Sweeney, C.R. and Habecker, P.L. (1999). Pulmonary aspergillosis in horses: 29 cases (1974–1997). *JAVMA* **214**, 808–811.

Swiderski, C. (1997). Hypersensitivity reactions. In: Reed, S.M., Bayly, W.M. and Sellon, D.C. (eds). *Equine Internal Medicine*, third edition, pp. 19–47. Philadelphia, WB Saunders.

Swiderski, C. (2000). Hypersensitivity disorders in horses. *Veterinary Clinics of North America: Equine Practice* **16**, 131–151.

Tizard, I.R. (2013). *Veterinary Immunology*, ninth edition, St. Louis, Elsevier.

Uzzaman, A. and Cho, S.H. (2012). Classification of hypersensitivity reactions. *Allergy and Asthma Proceedings* **33**, S96–S99.

Valledor, A.F., Lloberas, J. and Celada, A. (2010). Macrophage Foam Cells. eLS (DOI: 10.1002/9780470015902.a0020730)

Van den Boom, R., Veldhuis Kroeze, E.J.B., Klein, W.R., Houwers, D.J., van der Zanden, A.G.M. and Sloet van Oldruitenborgh-Oosterbaan, M.M. (2008). Granulomatous pneumonia, lymphadenopathy, and hepatopathy in an adult horse with repeated injection of BCG. *Journal of Veterinary Internal Medicine* **22**, 1056–1060.

Van Galen, G., Cassart, D., Sandersen, C., Delguste, C., Nollet, H., Amory, H. and Ducatelle, R. (2008). The composition of the inflammatory infiltrate in three cases of *polyneuritis equi*. *Equine Veterinary Journal* **40**, 185–188.

Vazquez-Boland, J.A., Giguere, S., Hapeshi, A., MacArthur, I., Anastasi, E. and Valero-Rello, A. (2013). *Rhodococcus equi*: the many facets of a pathogenic actinomycete. *Veterinary Microbiology* **167**, 9–33. (DOI: 10.1016/j.vetmic.2013.06.016)

Vatistas, N., Mayhew, I.G., Whitwell, K.E. and Bell, B.T.L. (1991). *Polyneuritis equi*: a clinical review incorporating a case report of a horse displaying unconventional signs. *Progress in Veterinary Neurology* **2**, 67–72.

Vatistas, N. and Mayhew, I.G. (1995). Differential diagnosis of polyneuritis equi. *In Practice* **17**, 26–29. (DOI: 10.1136/inpract.17.1.26)

White, S.D., Maxwell, L.K., Szabo. N.J., Hawkins, J.L. and Kollias-Baker. C. (2005). Pharmacokinetics of azathioprine following single-dose intravenous and oral administration and effects of azathioprine following chronic oral administration in horses. *American Journal of Veterinary Research* **66**, 1578–1583.

Woods, L.W., Johnson, B., Hietala, S.K., Galey, F.D. and Gillen, D. (1992). Systemic granulomatous disease in a horse grazing pasture containing vetch (*Vicia* sp.). *Journal of Veterinary Diagnostic Investigation* **4**, 356–360.

Yoshihisa, Y. and Shimizu, T. (2012). Metal allergy and systemic contact dermatitis: an overview. *Dermatology Research and Practice* Article ID 749561. (DOI: 10.1155/2012/749561).

Ziemer E.L., Pappagianis, D., Madigan, J.E., Mansmann, R.A. and Hoffman, K.D. (1992). Coccidioidomycosis in horses: 15 cases (1975–1984). *JAVMA* **201**, 910–916.

14 Chronic Inflammatory Bowel Disease

Gillian A. Perkins

14.1 Definition

Equine Chronic Inflammatory Bowel Disease (CIBD) is a malabsorptive and maldigestive disorder. CIBD is characterized by dysfunction of the gastrointestinal (GI) tract, due to infiltration of the mucosa and submucosa with populations of eosinophils, lymphocytes, plasma cells, basophils or macrophages. Therefore, CIBD has been grouped into eosinophilic enteritis, lymphocytic enteritis, plasmacytic enteritis, and granulomatous enteritis. These conditions may involve both the small and large intestines of the horse. In addition, there may be systemic inflammation and other organ systems involved, as in the case of multisystemic epitheliotropic eosinophilic disease (MEED) or a more localized inflammation, as in focal eosinophilic enteritis (Edwards, 2000; Southwood, 2000; Archer, 2006; Bosseler, 2013).

CIBD is a complex disease, and the phenotypic characterization probably has many underlying causes. A limited number of studies address CIBD in the horse, including single and multiple case reports, with a description of the clinical signs, diagnostic testing and outcomes, and a focus on ruling out various infectious disease etiologies. Further work is necessary to investigate the GI immune system and microbiota in horses with CIBD, in comparison with healthy normal horses.

14.2 Signalment and clinical signs

CIBD is often reported in younger horses, but can affect any age and breed (Scott, 1999; Kemper, 2000; Schumacher, 2000; Kalck, 2009). Both eosinophilic and granulomatous enteritis have been reported in Standardbred horses, including pairs of siblings (Lindberg, 1985).

Horses with CIBD can range from having mild and unapparent disease, to severe weight loss and intermittent colic. The dysfunction of the GI tract can result in malabsorption and maldigestion, or may be associated with dysbiosis and alterations in gas production. Thus, the clinical signs are mostly associated with malabsorption, leading to hypoproteinemia, dependent edema and weight loss. In addition, mild recurrent colic, with or without endotoxemia has been reported. Horses with focal eosinophilic enteritis may have acute and severe obstructive intestinal disease, due to severe segmental thickening of the GI tract (Edwards, 2000; Southwood, 2000; Swain, 2003). When the colon is involved, the horse may have soft feces or diarrhea.

14.3 Immunologic mechanisms and etiologic associations

14.3.1 Gut immune system

CIBD involves a complex interplay among host genetics, the immune system, intestinal microbiota, dietary constituents, and environmental triggers of intestinal inflammation. There is limited knowledge of these factors in equine CIBD, and much of the information discussed below comes from studies evaluating canine and human IBD.

The gastrointestinal mucosal immune system is highly complex and must be tolerant of food antigens and commensal organisms, but also must be able to respond rapidly and adequately to pathogenic microbes. There are innate physical factors that protect the GI mucosa: the mucosal epithelium and enterocytes, which are held together by tight junctions; mucus secreted by goblet cells, which coats the epithelium; and antimicrobial peptides, secreted by paneth cells. In addition, there are the various parts of the local immune system, consisting of the gut-associated lymphoid tissue and the laminia propria, Peyer's patches, lymphoid follicles, and mesenteric lymph nodes.

Antigen-presenting cells, most commonly dendritic cells, are continuously sampling antigens from the intestinal lumen through pattern recognition receptors (Allenspach, 2011). The antigen pattern determines the type of activation of the antigen presenting cell and, consequently, the direction of the adaptive immune response towards eradication or tolerance. For instance, if rotavirus is recognized, the T-helper 1 (Th1) pathway is favored, producing IFN-gamma, which leads to reduced rotavirus replication, the destruction of infected cells, and development of protective immunity (Holloway, 2013). The Th2 pathway is initiated when parasite antigens, such as

Equine Clinical Immunology, First Edition. Edited by M. Julia B. Felippe.

Parascaris equorum and small strongles, are recognized, and cytokines secreted (e.g., IL-4, IL-5), recruiting eosinophils, basophils and mast cells. Bacteria such as *Salmonella* spp. may induce a proinflammatory response, characterized by Th17 and cytokines IL-17 and IL-23. In the case of commensal bacteria, the pattern recognition receptors are thought to stimulate the naïve T cells to differentiate into T regulatory cells, which counteract any pro-inflammatory cytokines produced by Th17 cells.

A delicate balance exists between inflammation and tolerance in the GI mucosal immune system. Any defect along the entire pathway from the intestinal barrier to the mesenteric lymph node can result in inappropriate and overacting responses (Allenspach, 2011). These responses result in intestinal inflammation, characterized by epithelial damage and ulceration, recruitment of inflammatory cells, and villous atrophy.

Mucosal secretory immunoglobulin A (IgA) is a major player of the GI immune system, but has not been extensively studied in the horse. IgA is the most abundantly produced immuno-globulin and accounts for about 80% of the total body immunoglobulin, with primary distribution in the mucosal surfaces. Gastrointestinal IgA is produced in a dimeric form (two IgA molecules joined by a J chain) by the Peyer's patches, lamina propria, and intestinal lymphoid follicles, and is transported transepithelially into the gastrointestinal lumen. The IgA intra-luminally binds to pathogens and prevents them from crossing the mucosal epithelial barrier. Equine IgA has been evaluated in serum, mammary secretions, nasal secretions, and gastro-intestinal tissue sections (Browning, 1991; Sheoran, 2000; Breathnach, 2001; Nunn, 2007). To date, little is known about the role of GI mucosal IgA and CIBD in horses.

14.3.2 Microbiota

With the advent of culture-independent technologies that sequence the 16S ribosomal RNA (rRNA) found in all bacteria, otherwise known as next generation sequencing, the complex and diverse equine GI microbiome is being revealed. Most studies have utilized fecal samples, due to ease of sampling and clinical application, although few horses have been studied to date. Diet, stabling and management have effects on the microbiota (Daly, 2012; O'Donnell, 2013; Dougal, 2014). Despite the diversity of bacteria found by next generation sequencing in the equine feces, the core microbiome defined as the microbiota consistently identified in healthy horses appears to be relatively small, and about 10–15% of the bacteria identified have been shared among all horses irrespective of feed or geographical location. (O'Donnell, 2013). As expected, horses with colitis have a shift in their microbiome towards less diversity, and antibiotics disrupt the normal GI microbiota (Costa, 2012; Daly, 2012).

How does the gut microbiota relate to CIBD and do bacteria play a role in CIBD in horses or other mammals? No single pathogen has been implicated as the cause of CIBD in horses to date. *Mycobacterium paratuberculosis*, which causes Johne's disease in ruminants, characterized by granulomatous inflammation

of the ileum, has not been identified in the horse. *Mycobacterium avium* subspecies *avium* is a rare cause of granulomatous disease in the horse, and has only been reported in Europe (Ryhner, 2009). It has been determined that Boxer dogs with granulomatous colitis have an adherent and invasive *E. coli* that lacks genes associated with virulence present in diarrheagenic *E.coli*. This condition, formerly treated unsuccessfully with steroids, is now treated with chronic antimicrobials, with positive outcomes (Craven, 2011). Further investigation is warranted into the equine intestinal microbiome and its relationship to CIBD, which will hopefully improve our understanding of the disease and treatment plans for these horses.

14.3.3 Parasites

The horse is constantly exposed to parasites and is intermittently treated with antihelmintics. There may be a subset of horses that have an overzealous response to parasites due to deworming protocols or other factors. The role that parasites play in CIBD is not fully understood.

14.3.4 Diet

The diet most certainly plays a role in GI disease and CIBD, but limited information is available about this association in the horse. A group of warm blood horses with CIBD responded favorably to a gluten-restricted diet (fed haylage, alfalfa and black crushed oats). Most of these horses did not have anti-gluten antibody concentrations (recombinant human tissue-transglutaminase (rhTGA) IgA antibody) that were higher than control animals fed a gluten-rich diet. The exception was one Friesian stallion, which had originally a very high rhTGA concentration and, after a half a year of gluten-poor diet, showed an improvement in rhTGA antibody concentrations, duodenal histopathology and total protein. This syndrome in the horse seems to be a gluten-sensitive enteropathy, which could involve immune and non-immune mechanisms (van der Kolk, 2012).

14.3.5 Genetics

Many different genetic loci representing defects in innate immunity have been linked with IBD in people. Many dog breeds are predisposed to IBD, including the Boxer, with granulomatous colitis, and the German Shepherd, with anti-biotic responsive enteropathy. In addition, Standardbred and Thoroughbred horses have been reported with IBD (Lindberg, 1985), but the small number of cases reported for CIBD in horses limits our ability to determine a genetic predisposition.

14.3.6 Etiological associations based on type of inflammatory cells
14.3.6.1 Eosinophilic enteritis and multisystemic eosinophilic epitheliotropic disease (MEEDS)

Eosinophilic enteritis can happen in isolation or be part of a multisystemic eosinophilic epitheliotropic disease (MEEDS), which generally involves the skin, gastrointestinal tract, liver, and pancreas. Horses with MEEDS do not usually have a peripheral eosinophilia.

MEEDS is a rare equine disease affecting young to middle aged horses in a variety of horse breeds (Nimmo Wilkie, 1985; Breider, 1985; Gibson, 1987; Sanford, 1989; Schumacher, 1991; Hillyer, 1992; Henson, 2002; Swain, 2003; Carmalt, 2004; Singh, 2006; Bosseler, 2013). The etiology is unknown, although parasitic, allergic, toxic, and viral causes have been suggested. In addition, a horse with MEEDS was diagnosed with T cell lymphosarcoma consisting of two discrete jejunal masses that were found on necropsy examination. It was suggested that the T lymphocytes secreted IL-5, which triggered the differentiation and activation of eosinophils at other sites of the GI tract, pancreas, and lungs (La Perle, 1998). Another horse with MEEDS had multiple colonic nematode parasites, encysted within submucosal eosinophilic abscesses, identified as *Strongylus edentatus*, suggesting that the multisystemic signs could be a result of a hypersensitivity reaction to parasite antigens (Cohen, 1992).

Segmental eosinophilic enteritis (also known as idiopathic focal eosinophilic enteritis, IFEE) and colitis have also been reported to cause obstructive colic, resulting in exploratory laparotomy and resection of the affected segment (Edwards, 2000; Southwood, 2000; Stanar, 2002; Archer, 2006; Makinen, 2008). Two out of 22 horses with eosinophilic colitis had microscopic evidence of helminth involvement (Edwards, 2000), while no evidence of endoparasites was noted in 23 horses with IFEE (Makinen, 2008). The inability to find parasites in these horses could be due to the chronicity of the disease process, anthelmintic use and the absorption of parasites.

14.3.6.2 Lymphocytic and plasmacytic enteritis

Lymphocytic and plasmacytic enteritis is characterized by a moderate to severe infiltration of lymphocytes or plasma cells, accompanied by varying degrees of villus blunting, fusion or atrophy, and the presence of mucosal and/or submucosal edema (MacAllister, 1990; Kemper, 2000). The causes remain unknown, and are similar to the other types of IBDs. Chronic diarrhea and small intestinal infiltration with lymphocytes and plasma cells could be a premalignant phase of intestinal lymphoma, although this association has not been documented in the horse (Kemper, 2000).

14.3.6.3 Granulomatous enteritis and idiopathic systemic granulomatous disease

Granulomatous enteritis is characterized by sheets of macrophages or epithelioid cells and circumscribed granulomas in the mucosa or submucosa of the intestine. These histologic findings are similar to Crohn's disease in human patients, and to Johne's disease in cattle. While *Mycobacterium paratuberculosis* has not been identified in horses, *M. avium* has been reported in Europe (Ryhner, 2009). Granulomatous enteritis has also been associated with high levels of aluminum, hairy vetch ingestion, or infections with *Listeria monocytogenes*,

Salmonella typimurium and cyathostomes (Anderson, 1983; Fogarty, 1998; Nemeth, 2013). The compromised GI mucosal barrier may also allow for bacterial translocation and bacteremia (Johnson, 1993).

Equine idiopathic systemic granulomatous disease, also known as sarcoidosis, is characterized by exofoliative dermatitis, severe wasting, and granulomatous inflammation of multiple organ systems, sometimes including the GI tract (Sargent, 2007). This disease is rare in horses. The initiator of inflammation in the gut is probably the same as that which triggers the inflammation in the other areas of the body. It is hypothesized to be associated with EHV-1, EHV-2, and *Borrelia* spp. or secondary to immune stimulants such as *Bacillus* Calmette-Guérin (BCG), although reactions to BCG have not involved the GI tract (Sargent, 2007).

Take home message

CIBD is characterized by dysfunction of the gastrointestinal tract due to infiltration of the mucosa and submucosa with populations of eosinophils, lymphocytes, plasma cells, basophils or macrophages.

More commonly, CIBD affects the small intestine, but it can also involve the large intestine.

Clinical signs relate to malabsorption and maldigestion, leading to hypoproteinemia, dependent edema, weight loss, mild recurrent colic, and soft feces or diarrhea (when the colon is involved).

Thickened loops of intestine can be palpable on rectal palpation, or observed with transabdominal ultrasonographic examination. Lymphadenopathy may also be detected.

A glucose absorption test can confirm malabsorption.

The confirmatory diagnosis is provided by the intestinal biopsy histology. Duodenal mucosal biopsy may be obtained via gastroduodenoscopy, left flank laparotomy/laparoscopy or exploratory laparotomy. Rectal mucosal biopsy may be diagnostic in 50% of cases.

To date, no single pathogen has been implicated as the cause of CIBD in horses.

Tentative treatment of CIBD is aimed at decreasing the horse's exposure to dietary, parasitic or environmental allergens, coupled with immunosuppression.

14.4 Diagnostics

The physical examination of a horse with CIBD often reveals limb and ventral edema, and moderate to poor body condition. Thickened loops of intestine can be palpable on rectal examination. Abdominal ultrasonographic examination may reveal diffuse or segmental thickening of the small intestinal wall (> 3 mm) and/or colon and cecum. In addition, lymphadenopathy can be appreciated on ultrasonographic examination.

Horses with clinical signs consistent with CIBD often have a hypoproteinemia characterized by decreased concentrations of both albumin and globulin. Proteinuria should be ruled out to confirm that a protein-losing nephropathy is not responsible for the hypoproteinemia. A glucose absorption test can confirm the inability of the intestines to absorb the nutrient tested. In healthy horses, administration of 1 g/kg of glucose as a 20% solution by nasogastric tube results in maximum plasma glucose levels (> 85% baseline) at 120 minutes (Roberts, 1979). In general, abdominocentesis does not reveal any significant findings, except in horses with eosinophilic enteritis. Many of these tests can be used for supporting diagnosis, as well as for monitoring the response to treatment.

Confirmatory diagnosis is provided by the intestinal biopsy histology. The least invasive means of obtaining an intestinal mucosal biopsy from a horse includes duodenal biopsy via gastroduodenoscopy, or rectal mucosal biopsy, both done in a standing sedated horse (Lindberg, 1996; Divers, 2006). Unfortunately, rectal mucosal biopsies are only diagnostic in about 50% of CIBD horses, because the disease is often limited to the small intestine (Lindberg, 1985; Schumacher, 2000). If a diagnosis is not made based on the duodenal and rectal biopsies, then an intestinal biopsy can be attempted through a left flank laparotomy/laparoscopy, although sometimes with difficulty to access the affected GI segment. Exploratory laparotomy and full-thickness intestinal biopsies can also be performed.

The diagnosis of CIBD is confirmed by histopathology, and is generally characterized by the inflammatory cell infiltrate seen within the mucosal epithelium and lamina propria of the small intestine. Normal intestinal histopathology will reveal a range of inflammatory cells, making the diagnosis difficult. Severe inflammatory reactions with more than four cell-layers thick, are considered abnormal. However, less inflammation could also be considered abnormal.

Two studies evaluated the normal inflammatory cell counts in the small intestine (jejunum, duodenum) in the villous and intercryptal lamina propria in a total of 17 horses (Packer, 2005; Divers, 2006). The majority of cells were T and B cells; in general, very few eosinophils were seen in the villous lamina propria and twice as many were seen in the intercryptal region. In another study, particular attention was paid to the presence of eosinophils throughout the normal equine gastrointestinal tract, and in horses exposed to *Strongylus vulgaris* (Rotting, 2008). In normal horses, the highest numbers of eosinophils were found in the cecum, ascending and transverse colon, and the lowest in the stomach and the small colon. This distribution closely resembles the typical distribution of encysted cyathostomes. Nevertheless, helminth naïve horses showed similar numbers of eosinophils throughout the gastrointestinal tract, suggesting that the presence and distribution of eosinophils within the intestinal mucosa in horses is independent of parasite challenge.

The histological variation of the rectum has not been studied extensively. Some key points regarding equine rectal mucosal histopathology include:

1 Neutrophils within the surface epithelium or crypts are not present in control specimens.
2 Scattered neutrophils are seen in the lamina propria.
3 Cellularity (lymphocytes and plasma cells) of the lamina propria in healthy controls is considered slight to moderate.
4 Various degrees of eosinophil infiltration of the lamina propria are a common finding in healthy control specimens (sometimes higher than affected cases).
5 Changes in goblet cell populations, with either loss of mucus or hyperplasia, is associated with inflammation in some cases.
6 Simple proctatitis (lymphocytes and plasma cells) is a non-specific finding, and could suggest IBD further upstream of any cell type.

The World Small Animal Veterinary Association (WSAVA) Gastrointestinal Standardization Group developed a set of histopathological standards for the diagnosis of gastrointestinal inflammation in endoscopic biopsy samples from dogs and cats. This document divides the gastrointestinal tract into three distinct regions: stomach, small intestine and colon. It also provides examples of normal and mild to marked changes in various categories of injury and inflammation in the gut (Day, 2008). The duodenal histopathology is evaluated for surface epithelial injury, inflammation, villous stunting, crypt distension, lacteal dilation, and mucosal fibrosis. The colonic histopathology is evaluated for surface epithelial injury, crypt hyperplasia, crypt dilation/distortion, and fibrosis/atrophy. Further evaluation of the differences between normal and abnormal intestinal and colonic inflammation is warranted in the horse.

In general, a diagnosis of CIBD is confirmed, based on the histopathological findings of the intestine, followed by exclusion of various infectious diseases, in particular *Lawsonia intracellularis*, *Salmonella* spp., and gastrointestinal parasites, including ascarids and cyathostomes.

14.5 Treatment and prognosis

Treatment of CIBD is aimed at decreasing the horse's exposure to dietary, parasitic or environmental/nutritional allergens, coupled with immunosuppression. In addition, the balance of bacterial communities within the gut may also contribute to this inflammatory condition, and antimicrobials may be indicated. The lack of overall understanding of the exact etiopathogenesis of this disease makes treatment more of a trial, followed by response assessment.

The role of gastrointestinal parasites in equine CIBD is unknown and, initially, horses should be treated for encysted small strongyles, using fenbedazole (10 mg/kg PO SID for five days) or moxidectin (400 mcg/kg PO once) prior to any other treatments. Administration of a daily-dewormer, such as pyrantel tartrate, could also be tried in order to limit continued exposure to parasites (Kalck, 2009).

Dietary modification or exclusion can be attempted. In general, any dietary modification should be tried for 4–6 weeks prior to making any conclusions or re-introducing a new feedstuff. If a gluten allergy or sensitivity is suspected, then avoiding wheat and mixed feeds, and feeding grasses, alfalfa and oats, can be attempted (van der Kolk, 2012).

As most of these horses are in poor body condition, the diet should be enhanced in order to achieve weight gain. A highly digestible and well-balanced feed, with smaller amounts fed more frequently, along with a high quality fiber, are recommended. Corn oil for fat may be added to the diet, and simplification of any nutritional supplements should be made (Kalck, 2009). Nutritional deficiencies should be addressed; for example, the author has seen cases of lower motor neuron disease (vitamin E deficiency) secondary to IBD. The role of pre- and probiotics in the treatment of CIBD is unknown.

Corticosteroids have been the mainstay of therapy for CIBD in horses. When horses have documented malabsorption, the recommendation is to begin the therapy with parenteral corticosteroids at immunosuppressive dosages (dexamethasone at 0.05–0.1 mg/kg IV SID), with tapering over time and in response to treatment (Duryea, 1997; Barr, 2006; Kalck, 2009). The benefits of therapy need to be weighed against the possible side-effects, such as insulin resistance and laminitis, as well as a predisposition to secondary infections. Azathioprine may be administered in combination or alone, in order to cause immunosuppression. However, it has not been evaluated in cases of CIBD (White, 2005).

Olsalazine sodium has been used therapeutically against inflammatory bowel disease in humans, despite poor bioavailability. Bacteria in the colon split this prodrug into two molecules of 5-aminosalicyclic acid that act locally to reduce inflammation. A single dose of 30 mg/kg, administered by nasogastric tubes in the fasted horse, has been shown to be safe, although its use in cases of equine CIBD has not been evaluated (Knoll, 2002).

The antimicrobial metronidazole has been recommended for equine CIBD because of its effects on anaerobic bacteria in the gut (e.g., potentially *Clostridium* spp.), as well as anti-inflammatory effects (Barr, 2006; Mair, 2006). Other potential treatments for CIBD include anabolic steroids, antibiotics, and iodochlorhyroxyquin. However, there is no evidence to suggest that these treatments would be effective (Mair, 2006).

Surgical resection of focal eosinophilic enteritis can be curative either alone, or in combination with corticosteroid therapy, with good prognosis (Edwards, 2000; Southwood, 2000; Archer, 2006).

If the horse is diagnosed with lymphoma, then chemotherapy can be attempted, to prolong the horse's life.

The prognosis for CIBD in horses is generally poor, with most published reports ending with a description of a necropsy examination. However, treatment successes occur, with estimates of half of the horses showing improvement or resolution of clinical signs. Occasionally, horses with CIBD may require lifelong, low-dose treatment with corticosteroids in order to remain symptom-free (Mair, 2006; Kalck, 2009).

References

Allenspach, K. (2011). Clinical immunology and immunopathology of the canine and feline intestine. *The Veterinary Clinics of North America. Small Animal Practice* **41**, 345–360.

Archer, D.C., Barrie Edwards, G., Kelly, D.F., French, N.P. and Proudman, C.J. (2006). Obstruction of equine small intestine associated with focal idiopathic eosinophilic enteritis: an emerging disease? *Veterinary Journal* **171**, 504–512.

Anderson, C.A. and Divers, T.J. (1983). Systemic granulomatous inflammation in a horse grazing hairy vetch. *Journal of American Veterinary Medical Association* **183**, 569–570.

Barr, B.S. (2006). Infiltrative intestinal disease. *The Veterinary Clinics of North America. Equine Practice* **22**, e1–7.

Bosseler, L., Verryken, K., Bauwens, C., de Vries, C., Deprez, P., Ducatelle, R. and Vandenabeele, S. (2013). Equine multisystemic eosinophilic epitheliotropic disease: a case report and review of literature. *New Zealand Veterinary Journal* **61**, 177–182.

Breathnach, C.C., Yeargan, M.R., Sheoran, A.S. and Allen, G.P. (2001). The mucosal humoral immune response of the horse to infective challenge and vaccination with equine herpesvirus-1 antigens. *Equine Veterinary Journal* **33**, 651–657.

Breider, M.A., Kiely, R.G. and Edwards, J.F. (1985). Chronic eosinophilic pancreatitis and ulcerative colitis in a horse. *Journal of the American Veterinary Medical Association* **186**, 809–811.

Browning, G.F., Chalmers, R.M., Sale, C.S., Fitzgerald, T.A. and Snodgrass, D.R. (1991). Homotypic and heterotypic serum and milk antibody to rotavirus in normal, infected and vaccinated horses. *Veterinary Microbiology* **27**, 231–244.

Carmalt, J. (2004). Multisystemic eosinophilic disease in a Quarter Horse. *Equine Veterinary Journal* **16**, 231–234.

Cohen, N.D., Loy, J.K., Lay, J.C., Craig, T.M. and McMullan, W.C. (1992). Eosinophilic gastroenteritis with encapsulated nematodes in a horse. *Journal of the American Veterinary Medical Association* **200**, 1518–1520.

Costa, M.C., Arroyo, L.G., Allen-Vercoe, E., Stampfli, H.R., Kim, P.T., Sturgeon, A. and Weese, J.S. (2012). Comparison of the fecal microbiota of healthy horses and horses with colitis by high throughput sequencing of the V3-V5 region of the 16S rRNA gene. *PLoS One* **7**, e41484.

Craven, M., Mansfield, C.S. and Simpson, K.W. (2011). Granulomatous colitis of boxer dogs. *The Veterinary Clinics of North America. Small Animal Practice* **41**, 433–445.

Daly, K., Proudman, C.J., Duncan, S.H., Flint, H.J., Dyer, J. and Shirazi-Beechey, S.P. (2012). Alterations in microbiota and fermentation products in equine large intestine in response to dietary variation and intestinal disease. *The British Journal of Nutrition* **107**, 989–995.

Day, M.J., Bilzer, T., Mansell, J., Wilcock, B., Hall, E.J., Jergens, A., Minami, T., Willard, M. and Washabau, R. World Small Animal Veterinary Association Gastrointestinal Standardization Group. (2008). Histopathological standards for the diagnosis of gastrointestinal inflammation in endoscopic biopsy samples from the dog and cat: a report from the World Small Animal Veterinary Association Gastrointestinal Standardization Group. *Journal of Comparative Pathology* **138** (Suppl 1), S1–43.

Divers, T.J., Pelligrini-Masini, A. and McDonough, S. (2006). Diagnosis of inflammatory bowel disease in a Hackney pony by gastroduodenal endoscopy and biopsy and successful treatment with corticosteroids. *Equine Veterinary Education* **18**, 284–287.

Dougal, K., de la Fuente, G., Harris, P.A., Girdwood, S.E., Pinloche, E., Geor, R.J., Nielsen, B.D., Schott, H.C., 2nd, Elzinga, S. and Newbold, C.J. (2014). Characterisation of the faecal bacterial community in adult and elderly horses fed a high fibre, high oil or high starch diet using 454 pyrosequencing. *PLoS One* **9**, e87424.

Duryea, J.H., Ainsworth, D.M., Mauldin, E.A., Cooper, B.J. and Edwards, R.B., 3rd. (1997). Clinical remission of granulomatous enteritis in a standardbred gelding following long-term dexamethasone administration. *Equine Veterinary Journal* **29**, 164–167.

Edwards, G.B., Kelly, D.F. and Proudman, C.J. (2000). Segmental eosinophilic colitis: a review of 22 cases. *Equine Veterinary Journal Suppl* (32), 86–93.

Fogarty, U., Perl, D., Good, P., Ensley, S., Seawright, A. and Noonan, J. (1998). A cluster of equine granulomatous enteritis cases: the link with aluminium. *Veterinary and Human Toxicology* **40**, 297–305.

Gibson, K.T. and Alders, R.G. (1987). Eosinophilic enterocolitis and dermatitis in two horses. *Equine Veterinary Journal* **19**, 247–252.

Henson, F.M.D., Milner, P.I. and Sheldon, O. (2002). Multisystemic eosinophilic epitheliotrophic disease in a Welsh pony. *Equine Veterinary Education* **14**, 176–178.

Hillyer, M.H. and Mair, T.S. (1992). Multisystemic eosinophilic epitheliotropic disease in a horse: attempted treatment with hydroxyurea and dexamethasone. *The Veterinary Record* **130**, 392–395.

Holloway, G. and Coulson, B.S. (2013). Innate cellular responses to rotavirus infection. *The Journal of General Virology* **94**, 1151–1160.

Johnson, P.J. and Goetz, T.E. (1993). Granulomatous enteritis and Campylobacter bacteremia in a horse. *Journal of the American Veterinary Medical Association* **203**, 1039–1042.

Kalck, K.A. (2009). Inflammatory bowel disease in horses. *The Veterinary Clinics of North America. Equine Practice* **25**, 303–315.

Kemper, D.L., Perkins, G.A., Schumacher, J., Edwards, J.F., Valentine, B.A., Divers, T.J. and Cohen, N.D. (2000). Equine lymphocytic-plasmacytic enterocolitis: a retrospective study of 14 cases. *Equine Veterinary Journal Suppl* (32), 108–112.

Knoll, U., Strauhs, P., Schusser, G. and Ungemach, F.R. (2002). Study of the plasma pharmacokinetics and faecal excretion of the prodrug olsalazine and its metabolites after oral administration to horses. *Journal of Veterinary Pharmacology and Therapeutics* **25**, 135–143.

La Perle, K.M., Piercy, R.J., Long, J.F. and Blomme, E.A. (1998). Multisystemic, eosinophilic, epitheliotropic disease with intestinal lymphosarcoma in a horse. *Veterinary Pathology* **35**, 144–146.

Lindberg, R., Nygren, A. and Persson, S.G. (1996). Rectal biopsy diagnosis in horses with clinical signs of intestinal disorders: a retrospective study of 116 cases. *Equine Veterinary Journal* **28**, 275–284.

Lindberg, R., Persson, S.G., Jones, B., Thoren-Tolling, K. and Ederoth, M. (1985). Clinical and pathophysiological features of granulomatous enteritis and eosinophilic granulomatosis in the horse. *Zentralblatt für Veterinärmedizin. Reihe A* **32**, 526–539.

MacAllister, C.G., Mosier, D., Qualls, C.W., Jr. and Cowell, R.L. (1990). Lymphocytic-plasmacytic enteritis in two horses. *Journal of the American Veterinary Medical Association* **196**, 1995–1998.

Mair, T.S., Pearson, G.R. and Divers, T.J. (2006). Malabsorption syndromes in the horse. *Equine Veterinary Education* **18**, 299–308.

Makinen, P.E., Archer, D.C., Baptiste, K.E., Malbon, A., Proudman, C.J. and Kipar, A. (2008). Characterisation of the inflammatory reaction in equine idiopathic focal eosinophilic enteritis and diffuse eosinophilic enteritis. *Equine Veterinary Journal* **40**, 386–392.

Nemeth, N.M., Blas-Machado, U., Hopkins, B.A., Phillips, A., Butler, A.M. and Sanchez, S. (2013). Granulomatous typhlocolitis, lymphangitis, and lymphadenitis in a horse infected with Listeria monocytogenes, Salmonella Typhimurium, and cyathostomes. *Veterinary Pathology* **50**, 252–255.

Nimmo Wilkie, J.S., Yager, J.A., Nation, P.N., Clark, E.G., Townsend, H.G. and Baird, J.D. (1985). Chronic eosinophilic dermatitis: a manifestation of a multisystemic, eosinophilic, epitheliotropic disease in five horses. *Veterinary Pathology* **22**, 297–305.

Nunn, F.G., Pirie, R.S., McGorum, B., Wernery, U. and Poxton, I.R. (2007). Preliminary study of mucosal IgA in the equine small intestine: specific IgA in cases of acute grass sickness and controls. *Equine Veterinary Journal* **39**, 457–460.

O'Donnell, M.M., Harris, H.M., Jeffery, I.B., Claesson, M.J., Younge, B., O'Toole, P.W. and Ross, R.P. (2013). The core faecal bacterial microbiome of Irish Thoroughbred racehorses. *Letters in Applied Microbiology* **57**, 492–501.

Packer, M., Patterson-Kane, J.C., Smith, K.C. and Durham, A.E. (2005). Quantification of immune cell populations in the lamina propria of equine jejunal biopsy specimens. *Journal of Comparative Pathology* **132**, 90–95.

Roberts, M.C. and Norman, P. (1979). A re-evaluation of the D (+) xylose absorption test in the horse. *Equine Veterinary Journal* **11**, 239–243.

Rotting, A.K., Freeman, D.E., Constable, P.D., Eurell, J.A. and Wallig, M.A. (2008). Mucosal distribution of eosinophilic granulocytes within the gastrointestinal tract of horses. *American Journal of Veterinary Research* **69**, 874–879.

Rotting, A.K., Freeman, D.E., Constable, P.D., Moore, R.M., Eurell, J.C., Wallig, M.A. and Hubert, J.D. (2008). The effects of Strongylus vulgaris parasitism on eosinophil distribution and accumulation in equine large intestinal mucosa. *Equine Veterinary Journal* **40**, 379–384.

Ryhner, T., Wittenbrink, M., Nitzl, D., Zeller, S., Gygax, D. and Wehrli Eser, M. (2009). Infection with Mycobacterium avium subspecies avium in a 10 year old Freiberger mare. *Schweizer Archiv für Tierheilkunde* **151**, 443–447.

Sanford, S.E. (1989). Multisystemic eosinophilic epitheliotropic disease in a horse. *Canadian Veterinary Journal* **30**, 253–254.

Sargent, S.J., Buchanan, B.R., Frank, L.A., Sommardahl, C.S., Kania, S.A. and Rotstein, D.S. (2007). Idiopathic systemic granulomatous disease. *Compendium Equine Continuing Education* **2**, 23–30.

Schumacher, J., Spano, J.S., Oliver, J.L. and Smith, R.A. (1991). Hypereosinophilic syndrome in an American Paint Horse. *Journal of Equine Veterinary Science* **11**, 346–348.

Schumacher, J., Edwards, J.F. and Cohen, N.D. (2000). Chronic idiopathic inflammatory bowel diseases of the horse. *Journal of Veterinary Internal Medicine* **14**, 258–265.

Scott, E.A., Heidel, J.R., Snyder, S.P., Ramirez, S. and Whitler, W.A. (1999). Inflammatory bowel disease in horses: 11 cases (1988–1998). *Journal of the American Veterinary Medical Association* **214**, 1527–1530.

Sheoran, A.S., Timoney, J.F., Holmes, M.A., Karzenski, S.S. and Crisman, M.V. (2000). Immunoglobulin isotypes in sera and nasal mucosal secretions and their neonatal transfer and distribution in horses. *American Journal of Veterinary Research* **61**, 1099–1105.

Singh, K., Holbrook, T.C., Gilliam, L.L., Cruz, R.J., Duffy, J. and Confer, A.W. (2006). Severe pulmonary disease due to multisystemic eosinophilic epitheliotropic disease in a horse. *Veterinary Pathology* **43**, 189–193.

Southwood, L.L., Kawcak, C.E., Trotter, G.W., Stashak, T.S. and Frisbie, D.D. (2000). Idiopathic focal eosinophilic enteritis associated with small intestinal obstruction in 6 horses. *Veterinary Surgery* **29**, 415–419.

Stanar, L.S., Little, D., Redding, W.R. and Jones, S.L. (2002). Idiopathic eosinophilic enteritis in a 10-week-old colt. *Compendium* **24**, 342–347.

Swain, J.M., Licka, T., Rhind, S.M. and Hudson, N.P. (2003). Multifocal eosinophilic enteritis associated with a small intestinal obstruction in a standardbred horse. *Veterinary Record* **152**, 648–651.

van der Kolk, J.H., van Putten, L.A., Mulder, C.J., Grinwis, G.C., Reijm, M., Butler, C.M. and von Blomberg, B.M. (2012). Gluten-dependent antibodies in horses with inflammatory small bowel disease (ISBD). *Veterinary Quarterly* **32**, 3–11.

White, S.D., Maxwell, L.K., Szabo, N.J., Hawkins, J.L. and Kollias-Baker, C. (2005). Pharmacokinetics of azathioprine following single-dose intravenous and oral administration and effects of azathioprine following chronic oral administration in horses. *American Journal of Veterinary Research* **66**, 1578–1583.

15 Recurrent Uveitis

Brian C. Gilger

15.1 Definition

Equine recurrent uveitis (ERU, also known as moon blindness, iridocyclitis and periodic ophthalmia) is a very common cause of vision loss in horses throughout the world (Deeg, 2008, 2008b; Gilger, 2010a; Lowe, 2010). Equine recurrent uveitis is characterized by multiple recurrent bouts of inflammation of the iris, ciliary body, and choroid (uveitis), followed by variable length periods of inflammatory remission. The uveitis bouts are spontaneous in occurrence and are not associated with recurrent trauma or other primary ocular disease, such as corneal ulceration, neoplasia, or infectious endophthalmitis.

When making the diagnosis of ERU, one should carefully differentiate from other causes of uveitis and recurrent ocular inflammation. ERU is now considered a classic immune-mediated disease, with several important initiators of the immune response (Dick, 1998; Kalsow, 1998; Gilger, 1999, 2008; Deeg, 2001, 2002a, 2002b, 2006a, 2006b; Zipplies, 2012). In most horses with ERU, treatment is not directed at these initial underlying causes, since they are usually resolved, but at managing the ongoing immune-mediated disease.

15.2 Signalment and clinical signs

Horses can develop ERU at any age, but the peak time of the initial uveitis episode is 4–6 years old. Development of ERU appears not to be gender specific; however, the Appaloosa, Warmblood, and American Quarter Horse are predisposed breeds (Dwyer, 1995; Deeg, 2004; Gilger, 2010a, 2011; Lowe, 2010).

Three clinical syndromes that are most commonly observed in ERU include *classic*, *insidious*, and *posterior* ERU (Gilger, 2011). *Classic ERU* is most common and is characterized by active inflammatory episodes in the eye, followed by periods of minimal, chronic ocular inflammation. The acute, *active phase* of *ERU* predominantly involves inflammation of the iris, ciliary body, and choroid, with concurrent involvement of the cornea, anterior chamber, lens, retina, and vitreous (Figure 15.1). Typical clinical signs of active ERU include photophobia, blepharospasm, corneal edema, aqueous flare, hypopyon, miosis, vitreous haze, and chorioretinitis.

Substantial corneal cloudiness or cellular infiltrate is not typical of ERU and, if these signs are present, primary (usually infectious) keratitis may be the underlying cause of the uveitis (i.e., it would be considered *secondary* uveitis). In ERU, signs of active, acute uveitis will recede after a period of 10–21 days (this period can be shortened with appropriate anti-inflammatory therapy), and the disease enters a *quiescent or chronic* phase. The clinical signs of chronic ERU include corneal edema, iris fibrosis and hyperpigmentation, posterior synechia, corpora nigra degeneration (smooth edges), miosis, cataract formation, vitreous degeneration and discoloration, and peripapillary retinal degeneration (Figure 15.2). The quiescent phase is generally followed by further, increasingly severe, episodes of active uveitis, and it is the recurrent, progressive nature of the disease that is responsible for the development of cataract, intraocular adhesions, phthisis bulbi, and blindness.

In the second syndrome, the *insidious* type of ERU, the inflammation remains at a constant, low-grade level that leads over time to chronic clinical signs of ERU. In nearly all horses with this syndrome, overt discomfort is not observed by the owners, and the first notable abnormality is the development of a cataract or blindness. This syndrome of ERU is most commonly seen in Appaloosa and draft breed horses.

The *posterior* type of ERU has clinical signs existing entirely in the vitreous and retina, with little or no anterior signs of uveitis (Gilger, 2011). In this syndrome, there are vitreal opacities, retinal inflammation (with or without detachment), and degeneration. Posterior ERU is most common in Warmblood horses.

15.3 Immunologic mechanisms and etiologic associations

15.3.1 Primary uveitis

Equine recurrent uveitis is a non-specific immune-mediated disease that results in recurrent or persistent inflammatory episodes in the eye. To diagnose the syndrome of ERU, the clinician must differentiate it from non-ERU primary uveitis. There is a long list of infectious and non-infectious agents responsible for causing primary uveitis in the horse. Although

Equine Clinical Immunology, First Edition. Edited by M. Julia B. Felippe.
© 2016 John Wiley & Sons, Inc. Published 2016 by John Wiley & Sons, Inc.

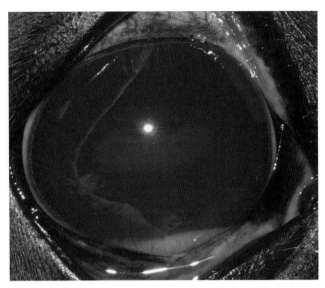

Figure 15.1 Equine eye demonstrating clinical signs of the acute, active phase of ERU. There is miosis, aqueous flare, hypopyon, anterior chamber fibrin, and diffuse mild corneal edema (B. Gilger, North Carolina State University).

any of these causes of uveitis may allow horses to develop ERU, not all of these acute uveitis cases will develop into ERU.

Several organisms have been associated with the initiation of equine uveitis. In some instances – but not all – the uveitis associated with these systemic infections may develop into immune-mediated uveitis or ERU. One of the most common systemic diseases associated with equine recurrent uveitis is leptospirosis (Halliwell, 1985; Davidson, 1987; Sillerud, 1987; Dwyer, 1995; Faber, 2000). Roberts demonstrated that ERU could develop after primary systemic infection and primary

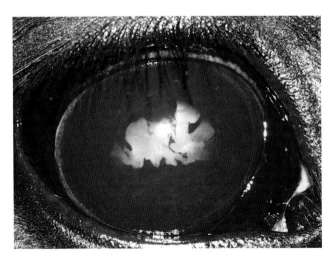

Figure 15.2 Equine eye with clinical signs typical of chronic recurrent uveitis. There is corpora nigra atrophy, iris fibrosis and hyperpigmentation, posterior synechia, miosis, and cataract formation (B. Gilger, North Carolina State University).

acute uveitis of leptospirosis. However, ERU typically did not develop until one year after the systemic infection had resolved (Roberts, 1971).

Recent studies have shown that antibodies against leptospiral lipoproteins (i.e., LruA, LruB, LruC) are detected in the eyes of uveitic horses, and that these antibodies demonstrate an *in vitro* cross-reactivity with components of equine lens, ciliary body, and retina (Verma, 2008, 2010, 2012a). The authors of these studies concluded that LruA and LruB share immune epitopes with equine ocular proteins, suggesting that cross-reactive antibody interactions may contribute to immunopathogenesis of *Leptospira*-associated ERU (Verma, 2010). It has also been shown that sera from humans who have leptospiral uveitis, and some with Fuchs uveitis or Behcet's syndrome, may also contain antibodies against LruA and LruB (Verma, 2008). It is possible that the initial leptospiral infection and subsequent primary uveitis produces antibodies against LruA and LruB, and these antibodies cross react with proteins in the equine eye to initiate the immunopathogenesis of ERU (Verma, 2010, 2012a). A recent study has suggested that the actual persistence or sequestration of leptospiral bacteria does not play a direct role in the pathogenesis of ERU (Gilger, 2008).

Another systemic disease associated with equine uveitis includes onchocerciasis, which is much less common now, with the widespread use of ivermectin. In this case, the inciting cause for the uveitis is the inflammatory reaction associated with dead and dying onchocerca larvae in the cornea after treatment with the antihelmintic therapy. Other systemic causes of uveitis include *Streptococcus equi* infection, brucellosis, toxoplasmosis, equine herpes virus (EHV-1, EHV-2), equine viral arteritis, parainfluenza type 3, generalized septicemia, endotoxemia, neoplasia, and tooth root abscess.

Take home message

Primary equine uveitis, which can be caused by several systemic diseases, is different than the immunologic syndrome of ERU.

15.3.2 Recurrent episodes of uveitis

The uveal tract of the eye contains most of the blood supply, and is in direct contact with peripheral vasculature. Therefore, diseases of the systemic circulation (e.g., bacteremia and septicemia) will also affect the uveal blood circulation. There is a barrier between this blood circulation and the internal aspects of the eye, called the *blood-ocular barrier*. This consists of the blood-aqueous barrier (i.e., tight junctions between the non-pigmented epithelial cells of the ciliary body and non-fenestrated iridal blood vessels) and the blood-retinal barrier (i.e., tight junctions between the cells of the retinal pigmented epithelium (RPE) and non-fenestrated retinal vessels). These semipermeable barriers normally prevent large molecules and cells from entering the eye, and help the intraocular fluids to remain clear. The blood-ocular barrier also limits the immune

Table 15.1 Suspected antigens associated with the immunopathogenesis of equine recurrent uveitis.

Suspected antigen	Method	Induce ERU-like disease experimentally?	Reference
Retinal S-Antigen	*In vitro* stimulation of vitreal lymphocytes	weak, epitope spreading	Deeg 2001 Deeg 2004
Interphotoreceptor retinoid-binding protein (IRBP)	*In vitro* stimulation of vitreal lymphocytes	yes	Deeg, 2001 Deeg, 2002b
Cellular retinaldehyde-binding protein (CRALBP)	Retinal proteome	yes	Deeg, 2009
Malate dehydrogenase (MDH)	Retinal proteome	no	Deeg, 2009
Neurofilament medium (NF-M)	Mass spectrometry and ELISA; IHC	–	Swadzba, 2012
LruA, LruB, LruC (leptospiral antigens that cross-react with equine ocular tissue)	Screening LruA, LruB, LruC antibodies with protein extracts and eye fluids from ERU horses	–	Verma 2010 Verma, 2012b

ELISA – enzyme-linked immunosorbent assay; IHC – Immunohistochemistry; ERU – equine recurrent uveitis

response to the internal aspects of the eye, causing the eye to be considered an immune-privileged site.

In cases of trauma or inflammation, these barriers can be disrupted, allowing blood products and cells to enter the eye. Aqueous flare, cell accumulations, and haze in the aqueous or vitreous, are clinically observable signs of the disruption of the blood-ocular barrier that occurs in uveitis. Disruption of the barrier enables the activation of various host immune responses, including production of antibodies to self-antigens not normally recognized by the horses' own immune system, as well as the production of antibodies to foreign antigens inside the eye (Gilger, 2011).

In ERU eyes, infiltrating inflammatory cells were found to be predominantly CD4$^+$ T cells (i.e., 48% CD4$^+$ and 18% CD8$^+$ in the ciliary body stroma) using immunohistochemistry. However, very few inflammatory cells were observed in the normal eyes (Gilger, 1999). These CD4$^+$ T cells secrete proinflammatory cytokines such as interleukin 2 (IL-2) and interferon-gamma (IFN-gamma), a phenotype called TH1 helper cell. Recently, it was demonstrated using immunohistochemistry that eyes with ERU were positive for IL-17 and IL-23 within the cytoplasm of non-pigmented ciliary epithelial cells and mononuclear inflammatory cells infiltrating the iris and ciliary body. These findings strongly suggest that Th17 cells also play a role in the pathogenesis of ERU (Regan, 2012).

The origin and recurrence of immune-mediated uveitis can be explained by the concepts of molecular mimicry, bystander activation, and epitope spreading (Deeg, 2001, 2006a, 2006b, 2008; Gilger, 2011). *Epitope spreading* is defined as the diversification of epitope specificity from the initial focused, dominant, epitope-specific immune response, directed against a self- or foreign protein to cryptic epitopes on that protein (intramolecular spreading) or other proteins (intermolecular spreading) (Deeg, 2006a, 2008). Epitope spreading has been confirmed in a high percentage of cases of ERU (Deeg, 2006a).

In most autoimmune diseases, several autoantigens (Table 15.1) participate in the pathogenesis, and epitope spreading is accountable for disease induction, progression, and inflammatory relapses (Deeg, 2006a, 2008). Shifts in immunoreactivity could account for the remitting/relapsing character of ERU. Genetic background and antigens encountered influence the direction and extent of epitope reactivity, and they probably play an important role in the heterogeneous clinical manifestations of ERU (Gilger, 2011). An immune response to cellular retinaldehyde-binding protein (CRALBP) (Deeg, 2006b) was detectable in a large percentage of ERU cases, and is thus considered a novel uveitis autoantigen. CRALBP and interphotoreceptor retinoid-binding protein (IRBP) demonstrated 100% uveitogenicity in the horse, and both autoantigens were capable of causing clinical recurrent uveitis in the horse (Deeg, 2006b) that closely resembled the clinical course of spontaneous ERU. Other autoantigens have been determined to play a role in the immunopathogensis of some horses with ERU (Table 15.1).

15.4 Diagnostics

15.4.1 Primary uveitis

Primary, acute uveitis (inflammation of the uveal tract) must be distinguished from the chronic, recurrent form (ERU). The clinician should not assume that every case of uveitis is ERU. As the name suggests, ERU is characterized by multiple, recurrent episodes of uveitis, whereas acute uveitis is limited to a single event. There is no age, breed, or sex predisposition for acute anterior uveitis. Typical clinical signs associated with acute anterior uveitis are all due to damage of the anterior uvea and subsequent compromise of the blood-aqueous barrier. They include photophobia, blepharospasm, corneal edema, aqueous flare, hypopyon, miosis, vitreous haze, and chorioretinitis.

Diagnostic testing for primary equine uveitis may help determine the underlying cause of a specific episode of acute anterior uveitis. The testing would include complete blood count, serum chemistry profiles, serologic tests for specific infectious organisms (such as *Leptospira*), and conjunctival biopsies for detection of *Onchocerca* microfilaria. For *Leptospira*, concurrent aqueous humor and serum serology is recommended, to determine if there is intraocular production of anti-leptospiral antibodies (Gilger, 2008). Detection of intraocular (aqueous or vitreous humor) organism DNA using PCR should also be done, when available. A positive C value (intraocular titer greater than serum titer), and detection of organism DNA, is strongly suggestive that the organism is playing a causative role in the uveitis (Gilger, 2008).

15.4.2 Recurrent episodes of uveitis

The clinical diagnosis of the syndrome of ERU is based on the presence of characteristic clinical signs (corneal edema, aqueous flare, posterior synechia, corpora nigra atrophy, cataract formation, vitreous degeneration, retinal edema or degeneration, with or without signs of associated ocular discomfort, including epiphora, periocular swelling, and blepharospasm) *and* history of documented recurrent or persistent episodes of uveitis. Both features are required to make this clinical diagnosis, especially to differentiate from non-ERU uveitis and other causes of recurrent or persistent ocular inflammation, such as herpes virus keratitis or immune-mediated keratitis.

> **Take home message**
>
> The clinical diagnosis of the syndrome of ERU is made by observing the characteristic clinical signs of acute and/or chronic uveitis *with* a documented history of recurrent or persistent episodes of uveitis.

15.5 Treatment and prevention

Treatment of primary uveitis is a combination of specific treatment of the underlying cause of the inflammation, and also anti-inflammatory treatment of the uveitis.

The main goals of therapy for ERU are to preserve vision and reduce and control ocular inflammation, in an attempt to limit permanent damage to the eye. In horses where a definite inciting cause has been identified, treatment is directed at eliminating the primary problem, and initial tests to isolate an inciting agent are performed. Due to the likely immune-mediated underlying pathogenesis, however, an inciting cause cannot be identified in most cases. Therefore, therapy is directed at the allaying of symptoms and reducing ocular inflammation.

Vision loss is a common long-term manifestation of ERU and, therefore, initial therapy must be aggressive. In acute cases, treatment, in the form of systemic and local therapy, consisting of antibiotics, corticosteroids and anti-inflammatory drugs, is used many times simultaneously. In severe cases, local subconjunctival or intravitreal injections of corticosteroids may be indicated as an adjunct to therapy. Many horses respond well to intermittent topical and/or systemic therapy of their active episodes of ERU. Other horses, however, do not respond to traditional therapy, and may experience frequent recurrences of uveitis. The reader is directed to recent comprehensive descriptions of equine therapies for additional details (Gilger, 2011). Traditional treatments used for ERU (i.e., corticosteroids and non-steroidal anti-inflammatory medications) are aimed at reducing inflammation and minimizing permanent ocular damage at each active episode. They are less effective in preventing recurrence of disease.

Cyclosporine (CsA) has been used to help prevent recurrent episodes of uveitis in ERU. CsA blocks the transcription of interleuken-2, a major initiator of uveitis, through the inhibition of calcineurin. Therefore, CsA may be the ideal drug to prevent the activation of T lymphocytes and recurrence of uveitis. CsA-releasing devices, placed in or near the suprachoroidal space or intravitreally, have been used in horses with chronic ERU for nearly ten years (Gilger, 2000a, 2000b, 2001, 2006).

Recently, data from 186 eyes of 156 horses that had CsA devices implanted for ERU were reviewed (Gilger, 2010b). Mean follow-up was 29 months (1–7 years). Horses with implants had significantly fewer flares after surgery (mean 0.05 flares/month) than prior to implantation. Overall, 79.9% were visual at the last follow-up time (Gilger, 2010b). These results suggest that the suprachoroidal placement of the CsA device result in excellent long-term control of ERU (Gilger, 2010b).

> **Take home message**
>
> Because ERU is an immune-mediated disease, an inciting cause cannot be identified in most cases. Therefore, therapy is directed at the allaying of symptoms and reducing ocular inflammation.

15.6 Prognosis and clinical outcomes

There is very little information in the literature that defines the prognosis and outcome of horses with ERU. Most valid information has been reported by Dr. Ann Dwyer (Gilger, 2011). In Dr. Dwyer's study, she reviewed the prevalence of unilateral and bilateral disease and the overall visual prognosis of horses with ERU.

In this study of 160 horses, 50% of the leptospiral-associated cases had unilateral disease and 50% had bilateral disease, but over 80% of the Appaloosas had bilateral disease. Horses that were seronegative to leptospirosis and were not Appaloosas had predominately unilateral disease (i.e., 62% unilateral disease). Dr. Dwyer also noted that if ERU was unilateral, and no bouts of inflammation were observed in the opposite eye for two years after the initial process, it was uncommon for uveitis to show up later in the contralateral eye (Gilger, 2011).

The prognosis for vision is guarded in horses with ERU that have had multiple or frequent episodes of uveitis. Dr. Dwyer estimates, in her practice, that vision-threatening ERU affects at least 1–2% of the horses (Gilger, 2011). In Dr. Dwyer's study, the analysis of the visual outcome of 160 horses with ERU, followed over 11 years, revealed that 56% horses lost vision in one or both eyes, and 20% of the cases became completely blind (Dwyer, 1995; Gilger, 2011).

References

Davidson, M.G., Nasisse, M.P. and Roberts, S.M. (1987). Immuno-diagnosis of leptospiral uveitis in two horses. *Equine Veterinary Journal* **19**(2), 155–157.

Deeg, C.A. (2008a). Ocular immunology in equine recurrent uveitis. *Veterinary Ophthalmology* **11**(Suppl 1), 61–65.

Deeg, C.A. (2009). A proteomic approach for studying the pathogenesis of spontaneous equine recurrent uveitis (ERU). *Veterinary Immunology and Immunopathology* **128**(1–3), 132–136.

Deeg, C.A., Kaspers, B., Gerhards, H., Thurau, S.R., Wollanke, B. and Wildner, G. (2001). Immune responses to retinal autoantigens and peptides in equine recurrent uveitis. *Investigative Ophthalmology & Visual Science* **42**(2), 393–398.

Deeg, C.A., Ehrenhofer, M., Thurau, S.R., Reese, S., Wildner, G. and Kaspers, B. (2002a). Immunopathology of recurrent uveitis in spontaneously diseased horses. *Experimental Eye Research* **75**(2), 127–133.

Deeg, C.A., Thurau, S.R., Gerhards, H., Ehrenhofer, M., Wildner, G. and Kaspers, B. (2002b). Uveitis in horses induced by interphotoreceptor retinoid-binding protein is similar to the spontaneous disease. *European Journal of Immunology* **32**(9), 2598–2606.

Deeg, C.A., Marti, E., Gaillard, C. and Kaspers, B. (2004). Equine recurrent uveitis is strongly associated with the MHC class I haplotype ELA-A9. *Equine Veterinary Journal* **36**(1), 73–75.

Deeg, C.A., Amann, B., Raith, A.J. and Kaspers, B. (2006a). Inter- and intramolecular epitope spreading in equine recurrent uveitis. *Investigative Ophthalmology & Visual Science* **47**(2), 652–656.

Deeg, C.A., Pompetzki, D., Raith, A.J., Hauck, S.M., Amann, B., Suppmann, S., Goebel, T.W., Olazabal, U., Gerhards, H., Reese, S., Stangassinger, M., Kaspers, B. and Ueffing, M. (2006b). Identification and functional validation of novel autoantigens in equine uveitis. *Molecular & Cellular Proteomics* **5**(8), 1462–1470.

Deeg, C.A., Hauck, S.M., Amann, B., Pompetzki, D., Altmann, F., Raith, A., Schmalzl, T., Stangassinger, M. and Ueffing, M. (2008b). Equine recurrent uveitis – a spontaneous horse model of uveitis. *Ophthalmic Research* **40**(3–4), 151–153.

Dick, A.D. (1998). Understanding uveitis through the eyes of a horse: relevance of models of ocular inflammation to human disease. *Ocular immunology and inflammation* **6**(4), 211–214.

Dwyer, A.E., Crockett, R.S. and Kalsow, C.M. (1995). Association of leptospiral seroreactivity and breed with uveitis and blindness in horses: 372 cases (1986–1993). *Journal of the American Veterinary Medical Association* **207**(10), 1327–1331.

Faber, N.A., Crawford, M., LeFebvre, R.B., Buyukmihci, N.C., Madigan, J.E. and Willits, N.H. (2000). Detection of Leptospira spp. in the aqueous humor of horses with naturally acquired recurrent uveitis. *Journal of Clinical Microbiology* **38**(7), 2731–2733.

Gilger, B.C. (2010a). Equine recurrent uveitis: the viewpoint from the USA. *Equine Veterinary Journal Suppl* (37), 57–61.

Gilger, B.C. and Deeg, C. (2011). Equine Recurrent Uveitis. In: Gilger, B. (ed.) *Equine Ophthalmology*, 317–349. Philadelphia, Elsevier.

Gilger, B.C., Malok, E., Cutter, K.V., Stewart, T., Horohov, D.W. and Allen, J.B. (1999). Characterization of T-lymphocytes in the anterior uvea of eyes with chronic equine recurrent uveitis. *Veterinary Immunology and Immunopathology* b (1), 17–28.

Gilger, B.C., Malok, E., Stewart, T., Ashton, P., Smith, T., Jaffe, G.J. and Allen, J.B. (2000a). Long-term effect on the equine eye of an intra-vitreal device used for sustained release of cyclosporine A. *Veterinary Ophthalmology* **3**(2–3), 105–110.

Gilger, B.C., Malok, E., Stewart, T., Horohov, D., Ashton, P., Smith, T., Jaffe, G.J. and Allen, J.B. (2000b). Effect of an intravitreal cyclosporine implant on experimental uveitis in horses. *Veterinary Immunology and Immunopathology* **76**(3–4), 239–255.

Gilger, B.C., Wilkie, D.A., Davidson, M.G. and Allen, J.B. (2001). Use of an intravitreal sustained-release cyclosporine delivery device for treatment of equine recurrent uveitis. *American Journal of Veterinary Research* **62**(12), 1892–1896.

Gilger, B.C., Salmon, J.H., Wilkie, D.A., Cruysberg, L.P., Kim, J., Hayat, M., Kim, H., Kim, S., Yuan, P., Lee, S.S., Harrington, S.M., Murray, P.R., Edelhauser, H.F., Csaky, K.G. and Robinson, M.R. (2006). A novel bioerodible deep scleral lamellar cyclosporine implant for uveitis. *Investigative Ophthalmology & Visual Science* **47**(6), 2596–2605.

Gilger, B., Salmon, J., Yi, N.Y., Barden, C.A., Chandler, H.L., Wendt, J.A. and Colitz, C.M. (2008). Role of Bacteria in Recurrent Uveitis in Eyes of Horses from Southeastern United States. *American Journal of Veterinary Research* **69**(10), 1329–1335.

Gilger, B.C., Wilkie, D.A., Clode, A.B., McMullen R.J., Jr. Utter, M.E., Komaromy, A.M., Brooks, D.E. and Salmon, J.H. (2010b). Long-term outcome after implantation of a suprachoroidal cyclosporine drug delivery device in horses with recurrent uveitis. *Veterinary Ophthalmology* **13**(5), 294–300.

Halliwell, R.E., Brim, T.A., Hines, M.T., Wolf, D. and White, F.H. (1985). Studies on equine recurrent uveitis. II: The role of infection with Leptospira interrogans serovar pomona. *Current Eye Research* **4**(10), 1033–1040.

Kalsow, C.M. and Dwyer, A.E. (1998). Retinal immunopathology in horses with uveitis. *Ocular immunology and inflammation* **6**(4), 239–251.

Lowe, R.C. (2010). Equine uveitis: a UK perspective. *Equine Veterinary Journal Suppl* (37), 46–49.

Regan, D.P., Aarnio, M.C., Davis, W.S., Carmichael, K.P., Vandenplas, M.L., Lauderdale, J.D. and Moore, P.A. (2012). Characterization of cytokines associated with Th17 cells in the eyes of horses with recurrent uveitis. *Veterinary Ophthalmology* **15**(3), 145–152.

Roberts, S.R. (1971). Chorioretinitis in a band of horses. *Journal of the American Veterinary Medical Association* **158**(12), 2043–2046.

Sillerud, C.L., Bey, R.F., Ball, M. and Bistner, S.I. (1987). Serologic correlation of suspected Leptospira interrogans serovar pomona-induced uveitis in a group of horses. *Journal of the American Veterinary Medical Association* **191**(12), 1576–1578.

Swadzba, M.E., Hirmer, S., Amann, B., Hauck, S.M. and Deeg, C.A. (2012). Vitreal IgM autoantibodies target neurofilament medium in a spontaneous model of autoimmune uveitis. *Investigative Ophthalmology & Visual Science* **53**(1), 294–300.

Verma, A. and Stevenson, B. (2012a). Leptospiral uveitis – there is more to it than meets the eye! *Zoonoses Public Health* **59**(Suppl 2), 132–141.

Verma, A., Rathinam, S.R., Priya, C.G., Muthukkaruppan, V.R., Stevenson, B. and Timoney, J.F. (2008). LruA and LruB antibodies in sera of humans with leptospiral uveitis. *Clinical and Vaccine Immunology* **15**(6), 1019–1023.

Verma, A., Kumar, P., Babb, K., Timoney, J.F. and Stevenson, B. (2010). Cross-reactivity of antibodies against leptospiral recurrent uveitis-associated proteins A and B (LruA and LruB) with eye proteins. *PLoS Neglected Tropical Diseases* **4**(8), e778.

Verma, A., Matsunaga, J., Artiushin, S., Pinne, M., Houwers, D.J., Haake, D.A., Stevenson, B. and Timoney, J.F. (2012b). Antibodies to a novel leptospiral protein, LruC, in the eye fluids and sera of horses with Leptospira-associated uveitis. *Clinical and Vaccine Immunology* **19**(3), 452–456.

Zipplies, J.K., Hauck, S.M., Eberhardt, C., Hirmer, S., Amann, B., Stangassinger, M., Ueffing, M. and Deeg, C.A. (2012). Miscellaneous vitreous-derived IgM antibodies target numerous retinal proteins in equine recurrent uveitis. *Veterinary Ophthalmology* **15**(Suppl 2), 57–64.

16

Recurrent Airway Obstruction and Summer Pasture-Associated Obstructive Pulmonary Disease

Michela Bullone and Jean-Pierre Lavoie

16.1 Definition

Heaves, also known as recurrent airway obstruction (RAO) and formerly as chronic obstructive pulmonary disease (COPD), and summer pasture-associated obstructive pulmonary disease (SPAOPD), are incurable allergy-like diseases affecting adult horses exposed to the barn dusts or airborne antigens present at pasture, respectively. Both host- and environment-derived factors are important determinants of these diseases, with a genetic predisposition present at least in some families.

Horses affected with these conditions present episodes of respiratory distress at rest, induced by ill-defined environmental triggers. Bronchospasm, airway tissue remodeling, neutrophilic inflammation and mucus secretions are characteristic findings. The clinical history suggests that antigen-specific immune responses underlie the diseases' pathogenesis and development. Indeed, antigen avoidance strategies are the only effective means at controlling airway inflammation in affected horses. These findings, combined, suggest that a late-phase allergic response contributes to the pathophysiology of these conditions. Corticosteroids and bronchodilators improve clinical signs, but do not adequately control the neutrophilic airway inflammation when horses are kept in the offending environment. Antiallergic medications and hyposensitization are not considered effective therapeutic modalities for these conditions.

16.2 Signalment and clinical signs

Heaves and SPAOPD are obstructive pulmonary diseases with distinct seasonality and geographic occurrences (Seahorn, 1993; Leguillette, 2003). Heaves is associated with exposure to hay and straw, and is more common in the winter months in regions with temperate climates, when horses are stabled for extended periods. SPAOPD was described firstly in Louisiana (Beadle, 1983), and has been since reported in Europe (Mair, 1996). SPAOPD exacerbations are more commonly observed during summer, when horses are kept on pasture.

The two diseases are not mutually exclusive, as they may occasionally be observed in the same animal (Thurlbeck, 1964; Lowell, 1964; Dixon, 1990). Heaves has been estimated to affect 10–20% of the adult equine population in areas of temperate climates, while no prevalence data is currently available for SPAOPD (Hotchkiss, 2007; Ramseyer, 2007). Reported onset of the disease is usually seven years of age or older. The hereditability of heaves has been demonstrated at least in some lineages/families, and the existence of genetic loci associated with heaves has been shown (Gerber, 1989; Marti, 1991). Both genders may be affected, with one study suggesting that females are at greater risk than males for developing the disease (Couetil, 2003). Conflicting data exist concerning breed predisposition, with Thoroughbred horses possibly more at risk than other breeds (Couetil, 2003).

When symptomatic, horses with heaves or SPAOPD present non-specific clinical signs indicative of lower airway diseases. Episodes of occasional or paroxysmal non-productive cough are common. Increased expiratory effort and respiratory frequency are observed during exacerbation. Mild serous, seromucous or mucopurulent nasal discharge, from one or both nostrils, may be seen. In severe cases, extended head and neck positioning are noticed, with flared nostrils and markedly increased abdominal expiratory effort. Anal cranio-caudal movements, synchronized with the respiration, indicate an increased respiratory abdominal effort. Flatulence may occur in these animals, concomitantly with coughing episodes.

The strong and continuous respiratory effort during expiration can lead to a *heaves line*, corresponding to hypertrophy of the external abdominal oblique muscle. Lung auscultation reveals wheezes and crackles in all lung fields, even in the absence of a rebreathing bag, or may sound silent. Thoracic percussion can identify increased lung field area due to air trapping.

Horses with mild heaves and SPAOPD generally do not show systemic signs of illness, and affected animals are alert, responsive to environmental stimuli, and have good appetite. Severely affected animals might be febrile and anorexic, developing rapid

Equine Clinical Immunology, First Edition. Edited by M. Julia B. Felippe.
© 2016 John Wiley & Sons, Inc. Published 2016 by John Wiley & Sons, Inc.

weight loss. Tachycardia and pulmonary hypertension may also develop during crisis, disappearing with remission of the disease. The frequency of acute episodes affecting these horses is variable, and reflects changes in the level of antigenic exposure; when heaves-susceptible horses are kept in the offending environment, airway obstruction is persistent (Jean, 1999). In some cases, it can take four weeks or more before clinical signs develop (Grunig, 1989; Leclere, 2012).

Reversibility of airway obstruction in absence of antigenic stimulation may delay disease recognition and prompt diagnosis. The disease may be undetected during pre-purchase examination, for instance, as horses in clinical remission may be indistinguishable from healthy horses on the basis of their respiratory pattern or respiratory frequency at rest (Leclere, 2011). Nevertheless, the identification of a *heaves line* may be suggestive of the disease. Also, during remission, coughing episodes when exercising or eating are common, as well as exercise-intolerance during demanding athletic activity. Thoracic auscultation is then often unremarkable. Tissue remodeling, especially when affecting airway smooth muscle bundles in the bronchial walls, is only partially reversed with one-year antigen withdrawal alone, and by a six-month corticosteroid treatment (Leclere, 2012), suggesting that residual structural alterations are maintained, even in horses in prolonged remission.

16.3 Immunologic mechanisms and etiologic associations

Both environmental and inherited factors, as well as allergy-associated mechanisms, have been implicated as contributing factors to heaves. Less information is available regarding SPAOPD, but increasing evidence suggests that these two diseases share common pathophysiological responses, albeit to different antigens. Clinical presentation and airway neutrophilic inflammatory profiles (Figure 16.1) are similar in the two diseases, and the finding that they may coexist in the same animal suggests that common mechanisms lead to their development (Lowell, 1964; Dixon, 1990). Antigen-specific and acquired immune responses evoking allergy likely play a role in disease progression, as well as innate immune mechanisms against highly phylogenetically conserved noxious antigens, such as endotoxins.

Genome-wide association studies have explored possible gene contributions in the two diseases, but the paucity of data and differences in methodologies prevent conclusive comparisons to date. Overall, genes associated with smooth muscle remodeling and leukotrienes metabolism were shown to be up-regulated in heaves, as well as the expression of IL-4 receptor and interacting proteins in a family of Swiss horses (Racine, 2011; Klukowska-Rotzler, 2012a; Lavoie, 2012). In SPAOPD, genes implicated in immune defense and in the modulation of inflammation were up-regulated (Venugopal, 2010). No direct gene up-regulation

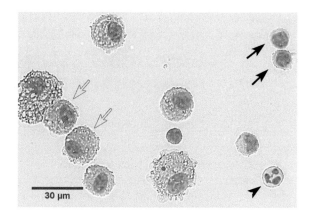

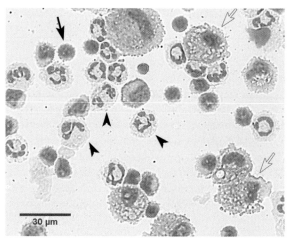

Figure 16.1 Bronchoalveolar fluid cytology from a healthy horse (upper panel) and a horse with heaves in exacerbation of the disease (lower panel). In healthy horses, the predominant cell types found in the BALF are macrophages (white arrows) and lymphocytes (black arrows). In heaves, neutrophils (arrow heads) are the predominant cell population.

overlap exists in the two diseases, but some of the genes up-regulated in SPAOPD code for proteins interacting with the IL-4 receptor (Racine, 2011).

Finally, heaves and SPAOPD are likely to be clinical syndromes resulting from various immunological mechanisms responding to diverse stimuli, probably interacting synergistically and leading to a similar clinical presentation.

16.3.1 Acquired immune mechanisms
16.3.1.1 Heaves and type I hypersensitivity
A type I hypersensitivity reaction (allergy) has been suggested as one immunologic mechanism responsible for heaves and SPAOPD, due to their strong association with moldy hay and pasturing, respectively. However, the typical immediate clinical response induced within minutes of exposure to allergens is not obvious in these conditions, and the involvement of allergy mediators as IgE, mast cells, and eosinophils in heaves requires better understanding. Nevertheless, an increased expression of IL-4, a Th2-type cytokine required for allergic diseases, and gene

polymorphisms of the IL-4 receptor, have been observed in some horses with heaves.

Allergy is defined as a type I hypersensitivity disorder of the immune system, characterized by an IgE-mediated overwhelming response to specific allergens. It is an acquired condition and, therefore, requires initial sensitization of the host's immune system (Uzzaman, 2012), starting with the presentation of the allergen by dendritic cells and macrophages to CD4[+] helper T lymphocytes. This induces an initial Th2-type immune response, with B cell production of specific IgE antibodies that circulate into the bloodstream and bind to high affinity receptor for IgE (Fc-epsilon-RI) on mast cells and basophils (Alphonse, 2008; Lavoie-Lamoureux, 2010). These metachromatic cells are normally present and quiescent in connective tissue and mucosae. They contain heterogeneous histamine and heparin-rich basophilic granules in the cytoplasm, together with lipid bodies in which arachidonic acid and its leukotriene metabolites are stored, for rapid secretion following cell activation (Amin, 2012). Cell activation is fast, because all it takes is the allergen binding to the already cell receptor-bound IgE for the release of the vasoactive metabolites.

When a sensitized host is exposed to the allergen again, an exacerbated biphasic response takes place. Within minutes following the binding of the allergen to receptors, activation and degranulation of mast cells and basophils results in the early phase or immediate allergic response, characterized in the lung by acute bronchoconstriction and inflammation. A later phase response develops typically 2–8 hours afterwards. Lymphocytes, particularly CD4[+] Th2 subsets, are recruited and release cytokines that contribute to the sustained inflammatory response. Neutrophils and eosinophils are then the predominant effector cells, likely aimed at neutralizing noxious antigens that started the initial immune reaction. In allergy, this response is often exaggerated or chronic, and it may result in tissue damage.

In heaves, inhalation of organic dust, derived primarily from hay, induces respiratory clinical signs. Several fungal spores, molds and mites are likely to be implicated (McGorum, 1993a; Pirie, 2002a, 2002b; Simonen-Jokinen, 2005; Laan, 2006a), but hay pollen less likely so (Lowell, 1964). In SPAOPD, one study identified an association between acute clinical signs and exposure to high environmental counts of fungal spores and grass pollen grains (Costa, 2006). The duration of antigen exposure required before heaves-affected horses develop acute clinical signs may vary from hours to days.

Although there have been indications of allergy-like mechanism involvement in heaves (Lowell, 1964), clinical signs associated with the expected early phase response are not common in these horses. In SPAOPD, complete unawareness of the causative factors triggering the respiratory response complicates the understanding of the kinetics of the disease. However, the delay of at least few hours between hay or pasture exposure and clinical signs argues against the presence of an immediate allergic response. Intriguingly, a subclinical and immediate (10–20 min post-antigen challenge) response, consisting of

increased pulmonary reactivity and histamine bronchoalveolar lavage fluid (BALF) concentration, has been observed in healthy horses, but not in heaves-affected horses (Deaton, 2007). The authors suggested that the lack of this *normal* response contributes to an increase in antigen deposition in the peripheral airways which, in turn, could induce an exaggerated late-phase response, as observed in affected horses.

The role of IgE in these conditions is indeed debated (Wagner, 2009). Higher concentrations of IgE specific to *Aspergillus fumigatus* and *Saccharopolyspora rectivirgula* (*Microspora faeni*) are present in BALF of heaves-affected horses, compared with controls (Halliwell, 1993; Dixon, 1996; Schmallenbach, 1998), while serum IgE concentrations are generally similar or show high variability in the two groups of horses (Halliwell, 1993; Schmallenbach, 1998; Eder, 2000; Kunzle, 2007). In SPAOPD, a study investigating the levels of IgE in tracheal wash aspirates found no differences between control and affected horses during the symptomatic and asymptomatic phases of the disease (Seahorn, 1997).

It has been speculated that there might be high and low IgE responders in the equine heaves population (Eder, 2000), as seen in human asthmatics, which could potentially bias IgE-related data interpretation. Serum IgE concentrations may not coincide with the manifestation of clinical allergic diseases but, rather, may indicate sensitization to given allergens (Pastorello, 1995). Also, serum IgE concentrations can be influenced by the degree of intestinal parasitism, as well as stable-specific environments (Eder, 2000). Therefore, current findings suggest that sensitization to hay molds and fungi is common in the horse population, and subjects developing heaves or SPAOPD tend to have higher IgE titers to these antigens. Whether IgE contributes to the initiation of the disease and to its clinical exacerbation, once established, remains to be ascertained.

While airway luminal mast cells are not increased in BAL fluids in heaves, they are present in increased number within the airway wall, particularly within the epithelium (Kaup, 1990; Winder, 1990; van der Haegen, 2005; Dacre, 2007; Deaton, 2007). Histamine, tryptase, leukotriene 4 and 5-hydroxytryptophan, four inflammatory mediators secreted by mast cells, are reported to increase in respiratory secretions, BALF, urine, or plasma of heaves-affected horses in response to natural antigen challenge (Olszewski, 1999; Dacre, 2007). Histamine concentration is increased in the airway epithelial lining fluid five hours after antigen challenge in heaves-affected horses, but not in controls, and it does not vary when measured in BALF (McGorum, 1993b; Deaton, 2007). Also, tissue mast cells have been found to be positively correlated with the degree of airway wall fibrosis and luminal neutrophilia, suggesting that they are at least partly involved (van der Haegen, 2005; Dacre, 2007; Kunzle, 2007).

Although mast cell activation by IgE has not been confirmed in heaves, a recent study (Moran, 2012) demonstrated that serum immunoglobulins (most likely IgE) from *A. fumigatus*-sensitized heaves-affected horses, but not from controls or from unsensitized horses with heaves, can activate mast cells and induce their degranulation in presence of *A. fumigatus* antigens. Also, *A. fumigatus* and *Alternaria tenius* extracts caused significantly higher histamine release from BAL cells from heaves-affected horses, both in remission and in exacerbation, compared to BALF cells from controls (Hare, 1999). Finally, blood basophils in heaves have increased sensitivity to *Mucor* spp. when compared to those of healthy horses (Dirscherl, 1993).

In summary, although IgE-mediated mast cell and basophil activation is unlikely to be the central triggering event in the cascade leading to clinical presentation of heaves, a certain degree of specificity is inherent in the pulmonary and systemic response to environmental antigens, possibly involving receptor-associated events (Figure 16.2).

16.3.1.2 The clinical response in heaves is reminiscent of a late-phase allergic response

Unlike the early allergic response that develops within minutes after antigen exposure and is short-lived, a late-phase response takes place a few hours after exposure to the allergens, and is sustained. It was initially believed that mediators released by mast cells and basophils during the early allergic response (cytokines, histamine, leukotriens, proteases) were responsible and required to trigger a late-response, via eosinophil recruitment and activation. Also, cytokines released by T cells – in particular, Th2 cells – might be sufficient to induce this response, even in absence of an IgE-mediated early phase response (Watanabe, 1995a, 1995b, 1997; Meyts, 2008; Nabe, 2011, 2013). Indeed, lymphocytes are recruited and activated into rodent models of asthmatic lung soon after the first antigenic challenge, and their presence *in situ* precedes neutrophil mobilization into the lungs (Watanabe, 1995a, 1995b; Meyts, 2008). However, no differences between groups have been observed in CD4$^+$ T cell numbers or in CD4$^+$:CD8$^+$ T cell ratio in BALF between horses with heaves and controls, even after antigen challenge in earlier studies (McGorum, 1993c; Watson, 1997).

The mechanisms by which lymphocytes induce a later asthmatic response are not clear, although it is generally accepted that it results from the release of immunoregulatory cytokines by CD4$^+$ Th2 cells (He, 2011). These findings support the hypothesis that allergic-mediated mechanisms in which the late-phase response predominates clinically might contribute to the pathogenesis of heaves. Indeed, a prominently neutrophilic inflammation is detected in BAL of affected horses, starting from 4–5 hours post challenge, and clinically evident pulmonary dysfunction arises hours to days after antigen exposure (Fairbairn, 1993; Brazil, 2005).

Based on gene expression studies, heaves and SPAOPD have been associated with predominant Th2-type immune response (Lavoie, 2001; Cordeau, 2004), or with a mixed Th1-Th2 response (Beadle, 2002; Kleiber, 2005). BAL lymphocytes of heaves-affected horses chronically exposed to hay, but not control horses, showed an increased expression of Th2-type cytokines, which coincided with disease exacerbation (Lavoie, 2001; Cordeau, 2004). Additional support for a role of the Th2-type response is the finding of increased expression of Th2-type receptors on neutrophils of horses with heaves, a polymorphism in the IL-4 receptors in some family of affected horses, and the increased expression of TSLP (thymic stromal lymphopoietin), previously identified as a central cytokine in driving Th2 cell differentiation (Dewachi, 2006; Jost, 2007; Racine, 2011; Klukowska-Rotzler et al., 2012a, 2012b). However, other studies failed to identify a predominant Th2 or even Th1 responses, suggesting a complex regulation process (Beadle, 2002; Ainsworth, 2003; Horohov, 2005).

The finding that the expression of the Th1- and Th2-type cytokines varies with disease stages suggests that the timing of the sampling may contribute to these differences (Cordeau, 2004; Horohov, 2005). In addition, IL-17, which promotes neutrophil chemotaxis and activation, has been shown at the mRNA level to be increased in BALF cells of horses during disease exacerbations (Debrue, 2005; Ainsworth, 2006). IL-17 has been associated with other respiratory neutrophilic diseases, including COPD and severe asthma in human patients (Nakagome, 2012; Halwani, 2013). In horses with heaves, airway mononuclear cells have enhanced expression of IL-17 mRNA when exposed to air dust *in vitro* (Ainsworth, 2007). Interestingly, Th17 and Th2 responses have been shown to act concurrently (Barboza, 2013; Ji, 2013), but whether T lymphocytes were the source of expression of this cytokine in heaves remains to be determined. To summarize, while several lines of evidence suggest a contribution of Th2-type cytokines in heaves and SPAOPD, up-regulation of Th1 and Th17 immune response may also be involved.

In conclusion, due to the lack of a clinical early phase response, heaves and SPAOPD cannot be defined as *true* type I hypersensitivities, although there are evidences of an allergic component to the pathogenesis of the diseases. IgE and mast cells, but not eosinophils, probably play a role in the development of the disease, but no clinical evidence exist that their functional blockage would inhibit the disease expression. Furthermore, clinical response to drugs commonly employed for the treatment of acute allergic response, such as antihistamine, is generally considered to be poor. Nevertheless, a Th2 and a Th17 driven immune response, alone or combined, could explain most of the clinical and pathological manifestations associated with these diseases.

> **Take home message**
>
> Heaves and SPAOPD are predominantly neutrophil-mediated diseases, whose pathogenetic features partly overlap those of type I hypersensitivity. However, they cannot be defined as *true* allergies, because of the lack of an early allergic response and of a clear involvement of IgE and mast cell-mediated mechanisms.

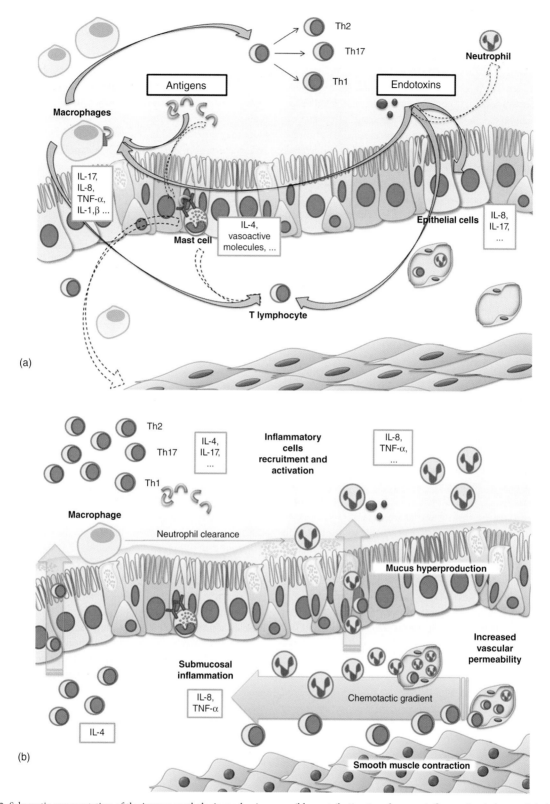

Figure 16.2 Schematic representation of the immunopathologic mechanisms possibly contributing to pulmonary inflammation in heaves. Inhaled antigens first come into contact with bronchial epithelium and immune cells normally present in the airway lumen.

(a) In heaves, it is likely that both of these cell types interact with antigens in an exaggerated way, inducing an aberrant inflammatory response. Endotoxins are antigens capable of inducing an inflammatory response even in healthy subjects and, for this reason they have been represented separately from other environmental antigens. In this simplified model, inflammation is induced and maintained mainly by activated lymphocytes via antigen presentation by macrophages, and is amplified by neutrophils and possibly mast cells, secreting chemotactic and vasoactive agents, fostering inflammatory cell recruitment, and further activation.

(b) The effects of such chronic stimulation produce structural and functional changes at the bronchial level, with epithelial hyperplasia of mucus producing cells, submucosal inflammation and edema, as well as smooth muscle contraction. All together, these phenomena lead to airway obstruction.

16.3.1.3 Heaves and type III hypersensitivity

Earlier reports suggested that a type III hypersensitivity reaction, involving antigen-antibody complexes, was the pathophysiological mechanism leading to heaves (Asmundsson, 1983; Robinson, 2001). Indeed, a delayed neutrophilic lung inflammation occurring following dust inhalation is a typical feature of human allergic pneumonitis. In human patients, this condition develops as a consequence of prolonged antigen exposure and high levels of antibody production in sensitized subjects (Lacasse, 2006). Moreover, the Gram-positive rod *Saccharopolyspora rectivirgula*, commonly present in moldy hay, has been recognized as one of the main triggering factors of one type of human allergic pneumonitis known as farmer's lung disease (Ranalli, 1999), and evidence exists that supports its involvement in the pathogenesis of heaves (Khan, 1985; Halliwell, 1993; McGorum, 1993a). However, unlike allergic pneumonitis, heaves and SPAOPD are not associated with alveolar inflammation, pulmonary granuloma formation and fever, which are the hallmark of this disease in human subjects. Also, precipitating antibodies generally employed for the detection of allergic pneumonitis were not found in the serum or lung tissue of heaves affected horses (Lawson, 1979; Bourré, 1992), discrediting type III hypersensitivity as the pathological mechanism leading to heaves development.

16.3.2 Innate immune mechanisms

16.3.2.1 Epithelial cells

Bronchial epithelial cells act as physical and chemical barriers of the airways, protecting from external irritants and pathogens. They are also immunologically active cells, able to interact with and respond to the surrounding environment by secreting several immunomodulatory molecules that act in both paracrine and autocrine manners (Blume, 2012). Bronchial epithelial cells obtained from horses with heaves before and after antigenic challenge showed increased expression of transcription factors involved in regulation of immune responses (NF-kappaB, AP-1 and CREB), compared with healthy controls (Bureau, 2000; Couetil, 2006a). However, no differences were observed when protein expression of IL-6, IL-10 and TNF-alpha, and gene expression of CXCL1 and TLR4, were measured in bronchial epithelium of heaves-affected and healthy control horses early after antigen challenge (Riihimaki, 2008). TSLP gene expression was increased to the same extent in bronchial epithelial cell cultures from both heaves-affected and control horses when different antigenic stimuli were applied for a few hours (Klukowska-Rotzler, 2012b). However, bronchial brush-derived epithelial cells were obtained later on in the development of the disease (i.e. after 14 days of antigen exposure) showed an increased expression of IL-8 and TLR-4, but not TLR2 compared to controls (Ainsworth, 2006; Berndt, 2007, 2009), suggesting that the epithelial cells do not initiate the inflammatory responses, but probably contribute in its maintenance.

16.3.2.2 Macrophages

Alveolar macrophages are, with lymphocytes, the most abundant cells in BALF of healthy horses, and are likely to be among the first immune cells coming into contact with inhaled antigens. In heaves, their responses appear to be dependent on the antigenic environment they are exposed to (Parbhakar, 2005; Laan, 2006a; Joubert, 2011; Aharonson-Raz, 2012). When exposed *ex vivo* to different antigenic stimuli, the response of BALF mononuclear cells (macrophages and lymphocytes) from horses with heaves differs from those of healthy horses only for their increased expression of IL-17 and CXCL2 at six hours, but not at 24 hours post-challenge, suggesting priming of these cells (Ainsworth, 2007). However, macrophages luminal recruitment is observed after airway neutrophil luminal peak, and there is evidence that macrophages instead play a role in neutrophil clearance and resolution of the inflammatory process (Brazil, 2005). Also, the inflammatory response of both equine and human alveolar macrophages and blood monocytes is modulated in the presence of IL-4 (Jackson, 2004; Varin, 2009). It is, therefore, tempting to speculate that macrophages act as a first-line defense early in disease development and subsequently shift their phenotype, inhibiting the initial inflammatory response. However, more studies are needed to clarify the role of macrophages in heaves.

16.3.2.3 Neutrophils

In heaves, neutrophil migration into the bronchial lumen is evident starting 4–5 hours after antigen exposure (Fairbairn, 1993; Brazil, 2005), often before clinical symptoms are detectable. This is reminiscent of the late-phase response of allergic diseases, during which neutrophils and eosinophils infiltrate the affected tissue. Neutrophils are the predominant (up to 80%) cells found in BALF of heaves- and SPAOPD-affected horses during disease exacerbations. Airway cells expressing IL-8, the most potent neutrophil chemotactic factor, are numerous, and include bronchial epithelial cells, macrophages, endothelial cells, and neutrophils themselves (Franchini, 1998; Ainsworth, 2006; Lavoie-Lamoureux, 2010). Also, stimulated smooth muscle cells have been shown to produce IL-8 in humans (Fong, 2000), but this would likely result in neutrophil accumulation in submucosal tissues, more than in airway lumen. Despite this evidence, the factors initiating and promoting airway neutrophilia in horses with heaves are still unclear.

Blood and airway neutrophils are activated in heaves, even during disease remission (Tremblay, 1993; Marr, 1997; Pellegrini, 1998; Lavoie-Lamoureux, 2012a). Neutrophil priming and activation occur mainly as a consequence of the innate immune response, following exposure to unspecific stimuli such as bacterial antigens or pro-inflammatory mediators. Activated neutrophils can synthesize pro-inflammatory cytokines, reactive oxygen species, nitric oxide, proteases, microbicidal products, lipid mediators and other histotoxins. Many of these are increased in heaves (Art, 2006; Venugopal, 2013), which supports an important role of neutrophils in bronchial tissue remodeling. Neutrophil products can degrade structural components of the airway wall (e.g., elastin, collagen), reducing airway tone and, possibly, exacerbating airway occlusion during bronchospasm (Winder, 2001; Klebanoff, 2005). The increased elastase concentration observed in BALF from horses with heaves compared with controls indicates enhanced neutrophil activation (Brazil, 2005; Deaton, 2005).

IL-4 is increased in BALF cells of heaves-affected horses (Lavoie, 2001), and it can activate equine neutrophils, promoting their chemotaxis and inducing the expression of mixed inflammatory proteins, including IL-8 and TNF-alpha, while markedly inhibiting IL-1beta (Lavoie-Lamoureux, 2010). In horses with heaves, peripheral blood neutrophils have shown up-regulation of selected Th2-type receptors (including IL-4 type I receptor (IL-4Ralpha) and CD23 (Fc-epsilon-RII)), compared with healthy control horses, and these differences were further accentuated during stabling (Dewachi, 2006). Nevertheless, when the expression of pro-inflammatory and chemotactic cytokines in peripheral neutrophils from heaves-affected and healthy horses was investigated after five hours of antigenic challenge, no differences were detected (Joubert, 2008).

Neutrophil apoptosis is recognized as an important mechanism for the resolution of inflammation. Several mediators implicated in heaves, such as IL-8, granulocyte-macrophage colony-stimulating factor (GM-CSF), and lipopolysaccharide (LPS), have been reported to increase neutrophil half-life, possibly by reducing the neutrophil apoptotic rate (Brazil, 2005). In horses with heaves undergoing acute antigen exposure, apoptosis of neutrophils peaks soon after these cells reach their maximal concentrations in BALF, and this phenomenon is accompanied by an increase in neutrophil phagocytosis by macrophages compared to normal conditions but unable to counterbalance the increased neutrophil influx (Figure 16.3; Brazil, 2005). The resulting decreased neutrophil clearance could then contribute to persistent airway inflammation and chronic disease. In horses with heaves, reduced apoptosis of BALF granulocytes has been reported during disease exacerbation, compared with controls, but peripheral granulocyte apoptotic rates were similar between the two groups, despite priming of peripheral neutrophils (Turlej, 2001; Lavoie-Lamoureux, 2012a). The treatment of equine BALF granulocytes with an antibody against GM-CSF reduced significantly their survival, restoring the normal apoptotic rate within 48 hours (Turlej, 2001).

Airway neutrophils are consistently present in affected horses, and may contribute to bronchospasm, increased mucus production, and other clinical signs present in heaves through the release of their various proinflammatory mediators (Macdowell, 2007). Nevertheless, numerous studies have shown that, while corticosteroids improved clinical signs, luminal neutrophilic inflammation persisted in heaves, even after the administration of inhaled corticosteroids for up to six months (Couetil, 2005, 2006b; Miskovic, 2007; Leclere, 2012). Persistence of neutrophils in the airways of horses with heaves does not necessarily imply their contribution to disease chronicity, as corticosteroids

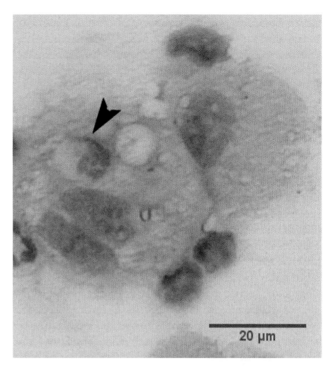

Figure 16.3 Macrophages are involved in neutrophil clearance from the airway lumen. A neutrophil (arrow head) is still identifiable within the cytoplasm of a macrophage

downregulate their inflammatory response while also decreasing their apoptosis (Hirsch, 2012).

Finally, also healthy horses, when exposed to antigen challenge, also develop a significant, while usually temporary and self-limiting, bronchial luminal neutrophilia in the absence of clinical signs. However, airway neutrophils from healthy horses are likely to be in a reduced state of activation compared with those of heaves-affected animals (Tremblay, 1993; Leclere, 2011). These findings suggest that the role of neutrophils and other inflammatory cells in heaves is significant but complex, and requires further elucidation.

16.3.3 Nonspecific immune response contribution

Endotoxins are present at variable concentrations in dusty stable environments (Pomorska, 2007; Aharonson-Raz, 2012). They bind to TLR-4 receptors on various epithelial and immune cell types, inducing an inflammatory response. Inhalation of LPS at low concentrations causes neutrophilic inflammation in horses, while respiratory dysfunction only at high concentrations (Pirie, 2001). LPS challenge increases matrix metalloproteinase 9 (MMP-9) in BALF of both heaves-affected and control horses in a dose-dependent manner, while hay exposure induces the same changes only in heaves-affected horses (Nevalainen, 2002; Simonen-Jokinen, 2005). Endotoxins have also been shown to act synergistically with other mold and fungal particles in heaves exacerbation, and they are an insufficient stimulus for disease development alone (Pirie, 2001, 2003).

Interestingly, *ex vivo* LPS stimulation of neutrophils from heaves-affected horses in remission induces an increased inflammatory response compared with control horses, indicating either an intrinsic defect in modulating immune responses or cellular priming caused by persistent systemic inflammation (Lavoie-Lamoureux, 2012a). Mast cells can also be activated by endotoxins via its binding to TLR-receptors (Saluja, 2012). TLR-4 has been shown to be present in equine lung tissue (Singh Suri, 2006), but no studies have specifically investigated its expression in equine mast cells at present. In conclusion, LPS represents a non-specific inflammatory airway stimulus in horses, but not sufficient alone to explain clinical exacerbations of heaves. Evidence exists suggesting that endotoxins act synergistically in heaves development, and that affected horses could be more sensitive than healthy subjects to this type of insult.

Because of their abundance in moldy hay, *Alternaria alternata* and *Aspergillus fumigatus* have been the fungi most commonly studied and linked to heaves pathogenesis. In SPAOPD, different subsets of fungal spores (mainly *Curvularia spp.*, *Drechslera* (*Helminthosporium*), *Nigrospora spp.* and *Basidiospore*) and grass pollens have been implicated as causative agents in disease exacerbations (Costa, 2006). Although a direct link has not been established between specific fungal species and equine recurrent airway obstructive diseases, it is generally accepted that environmental air dusts (mainly fungal spores) play a role in disease pathogenesis.

In general, Th1-type cell-mediated immunity is required for clearance of fungal infections, while Th2-type immunity usually results in susceptibility to infection, or development of an allergic type response (Blanco, 2008; Sorrell, 2009). In heaves and SPAOPD, the lack of clinical fungal infections, the BALF neutrophilia and the increased amount of IgE and Th2-type immune response lead to the conclusion that despite equine lungs are frequently contaminated by fungal microorganisms, innate immunity is involved and effective in their clearance, and possibly also in the development of an allergic response.

Anecdotal clinical field impression has lead to the suggestion that viral infections may trigger inflammatory events leading to heaves (Gerber, 1973). Although never thoroughly investigated, this hypothesis is supported by the higher titers to equine influenza A1 virus found in both tracheal mucus and serum of heaves-affected horses, compared with controls (Thorsen, 1983). Rhinovirus infections are considered important triggers for disease exacerbation in human asthma. As respiratory viruses are widely spread in the horse population, their possible role, along with that of other respiratory virus, in heaves and SPAOPD, warrants further investigations.

16.4 Diagnostics

Clinical diagnosis of heaves and SPAOPD is based on the recurrent presence of labored breathing at rest, often in association with cough, bilateral nasal discharge, and exercise intolerance when susceptible horses are exposed to the offending environmental antigens (stabling and hay feeding in heaves, pasturing during spring and summer months in SPAOPD). Mildly affected horses usually appear otherwise healthy, and do not exhibit signs of infection or systemic involvement. However, severely affected horses often present weight loss, and may be intermittently febrile.

Clinical score systems, based on the degree of respiratory effort at rest, allow response to therapy to be assessed, but fail to differentiate healthy horses from horses with heaves in clinical remission (Robinson, 2000; Pirie, 2001). Thoracic auscultation reveals wheezes and crackles during disease exacerbation. Lungs may be silent with severe airway obstruction due to increased air trapping. Lung function testing during disease exacerbation indicates increased lower airway resistance, elastance (decreased lung compliance), and airway hyperreactivity.

Normal BALF cytology reveals macrophages and lymphocytes as the predominant cells, with negligible proportions of other cell types. Heaves and SPAOPD are diffuse lung diseases, making the sample site relatively insignificant. The presence of neutrophilic inflammation (usually > 20%) in BALF cytology, during disease exacerbation, is a characteristic finding in heaves and SPAOPD, but is not specific for these conditions. Increased neutrophil percentage in BALF can also be observed in healthy horses, when stabled and fed hay (Tremblay, 1993). However, airway neutrophilia tend to be less severe in healthy animals, and it is believed to be self-limiting.

The neutrophil count of severely affected horses can occasionally be lower than expected (sometimes < 10%), probably because of proximal bronchial collapse despite low suction pressure during sample collection, and poor representation of the alveolar space. In addition, BALF cytology alone does not allow differentiating healthy horses from horses with heaves or SPAOPD during disease remission induced by antigen avoidance strategies (Jean, 1999). The low and variable yields of fluid recovered using BAL prevent an accurate assessment of the absolute numbers of cells but, in general, all cell types are increased in numbers.

Recent findings in our laboratory suggest that heterogeneity of lung neutrophilic, mastocytic, and eosinophilic inflammation may occasionally be present in heaves (Figure 16.4). These cell types may also be increased in IAD, suggesting that different inflammatory subsets may lead to similar clinical signs and vice versa, as recently reported in human asthma (Wenzel, 2012). For these reasons, the results of pulmonary cytology must be interpreted in conjunction with clinical signs. Importantly, the pulmonary neutrophilia observed in heaves and SPAOPD should not reflect lung bacterial infection.

The cytological findings in tracheal washes of both healthy and heaves-affected horses are unspecific, and vary widely among subjects, questioning their use as a reliable diagnostic tool in equine respiratory pathologies (Larson, 1985; Derksen, 1989). The presence of free or intracellular bacteria in these samples must be interpreted in light of the clinical signs. In the absence of fever, anorexia, and abnormal leukogram, the

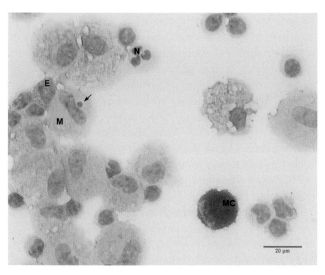

Figure 16.4 Neutrophils are normally the predominant inflammatory cell type found in bronchoalveolar fluid cytology in horses with heaves during disease exacerbations. However, in some heaves-affected horses, mast cells or eosinophils may be increased.
N – neutrophil; E – eosinophils; MC – mast cell; M – macrophage. The arrow indicates a cell phagocytized into a macrophage.

identification of bacteria is most likely to represent secondary colonization of the large airways, due to reduced mucociliary clearance. Similarly, the presence of fungal elements, even when phagocytized, reflects environmental fungal exposure, and is not indicative of fungal pneumonia in heaves.

Hematology and serum biochemistry results are within normal reference ranges, although serum protein and other markers of systemic inflammation have been shown to increase during disease exacerbations in heaves (Lavoie-Lamoureux, 2012b). Arterial blood gas analysis reveals significantly low PaO_2 in heaves-affected horses during exacerbation periods, in comparison with healthy horses and horses with heaves during remission (Art, 2006).

Endoscopy can assist in the diagnosis, although findings are non-specific. In one study, tracheal and bronchial mucus were increased in horses with heaves during exacerbation periods, compared with healthy horses, and also correlated with BALF neutrophil percentage (Koblinger, 2011). The respiratory mucosa may appear inflamed, with increased blood vessels visible through the respiratory epithelium. The main carina may be thickened, especially during exacerbations, possibly as a consequence of tissue edema induced by inflammation (Koch, 2007; Koblinger, 2011). Dynamic collapse of trachea and bronchi may be observed during coughing episodes, causing impact lesions with severe post-traumatic inflammation and mild local hemorrhages.

Bronchiectasis is a common sequela of severe heaves (Lavoie, 2004), and presents endoscopically as enlarged and deformed airways. Radiographic study of the thorax can reveal an increased bronchointerstitial pattern and/or bronchiectasic regions. Hyperinflation of the lung during exacerbations of the diseases can temporarily flatten the diaphragmatic silhouette, or make it concave. Emphysematous bullae are rare, even in severe cases, and can be detected radiographically as localized radiolucent areas within the pulmonary parenchyma. Ultrasonographic examination may reveal diffuse irregularities of the visceral pleura (comet tails). Ventilation-perfusion studies performed using scintigraphy allowed differentiation of heaves-affected horses from healthy horses, even when in remission (Votion, 1999a). However, limited availability of the equipment and associated costs prevent scintigraphy from becoming part of the routine diagnostic protocols for heaves or SPAOPD.

Intradermal allergen testing has been evaluated as a diagnostic tool in heaves, given its allergic-like pathogenesis. In one study (Lorch, 2001), affected horses tended to have more positive skin reactions, compared with matched controls 30 minutes and four hours after intradermic inoculation of the allergens. However, intradermal allergen testing failed to differentiate healthy horses from horses with heaves (Eder, 2001), and the response appeared to reflect the level of environmental allergens. Serum antibody titers against common antigens were reported inconsistently to be different in heaves-affected and healthy horses (Halliwell, 1993; Schmallenbach, 1998; Eder, 2000; Lorch, 2001; Kunzle, 2007; Tahon, 2009; Moran, 2010). Results of a recent study highlighted how equine serum antibodies directed against *Aspergillus fumigatus* promoted murine mast cell activation and degranulation (Moran, 2012). However, for the reasons listed above, intradermal allergen testing and serum antibody titers are not considered valuable diagnostic tools for the diagnosis of heaves and SPAOPD at the present time.

Recent studies of two large populations of horses have identified two chromosome regions encoding for several interleukins as significantly associated with heaves (Swinburne, 2009). Fine mapping of one of these regions identified a single-nucleotide polymorphism that was significantly related to heaves, probably representing a mutation with regulatory effect for the disease (Shakhsi-Niaei, 2012). Sequencing and analysis of IL-4 receptor gene seems to support a role for this molecule in heaves development (Jost, 2007; Klukowska-Rotzler et al., 2012a, 2012c). Genetic tests, however, are not yet available for general screening, and it is possible that their findings are not applicable to all heaves-affected horses, given the heterogeneity of the inflammatory response.

16.4.1 Differential diagnosis

Horses with heaves present with unspecific clinical signs that are shared by other diseases of the lower respiratory tract. Nevertheless, a history of labored breathing at rest (dyspnea) intermittently occurring over a 3 month period, or more, and absence of clinical signs of infection support the diagnosis of heaves.

The absence of respiratory stridor, predominant expiratory efforts, and abnormal lung sounds help ruling out upper airway obstruction and suggest lower respiratory tract disease. Bronchopneumonia and pleuropneumonia are the first diseases to rule out when examining a horse in respiratory distress. Fever, depression, anorexia and altered hemogram are typical signs of infectious bronchopneumonia. A careful auscultation of the thorax, thoracic radiographs and ultrasound examination can reveal pleural effusion, areas of consolidated lung and, possibly, pulmonary abscesses.

Equine multinodular pulmonary fibrosis is a recently described interstitial disease of horses, with possible association with equine herpesvirus-5 or asinine herpesvirus-5 infections (Williams, 2007; Wong, 2008; Back, 2012). The clinical presentation of affected animals may be similar to those found in heaves and SPAOPD, but the presence of radio-dense nodules on thoracic radiographs is characteristic of this condition. Likewise, thoracic neoplastic conditions, despite being rarely described in horses, may cause clinical signs resembling heaves. Radiographic and ultrasound examination may help in the diagnosis, as well as cytological evaluation of lower airway specimens, pleural effusion when present, and histologic findings from endobronchial or pulmonary biopsies (Mair, 1993; Davis, 2013; Bullone, 2014).

Chicken hypersensitivity pneumonitis is a rare and intriguing condition in horses, which develops when horses are stabled with, or close to, chickens. It causes a bronchointerstitial lung disease, clinically similar to heaves, and may affect horses of all ages. Removing causal allergens from the environment helps reducing clinical signs (Mansmann, 1975).

Similarly to heaves and SPAOPD, horses with *Dictyocaulus arnfieldi* infection may present with paroxysmal coughing, crackles and wheezes on thoracic auscultation, and increased respiratory effort at rest. Clinical diagnosis of lungworm disease is based on a history of contact with mules or donkeys and, occasionally, on the presence of eosinophils and immature *Dictyocaulus arnfieldi* in tracheal aspirates (MacKay, 1979; George, 1981). Clinical signs resolve with regular deworming (Britt, 1985).

Finally, IAD affects horses of all ages and does not cause labored breathing at rest. Common clinical signs are frequent coughing episodes, increased mucus production, and/or decreased athletic performances. Currently, there is no means to identify horses with IAD that will progress into heaves or SPAOPD over time.

Take home message

Heaves and SPAOPD can be diagnosed clinically in horses showing chronic (three months or more) respiratory distress, which is reversible by environmental changes and generally not accompanied by major alterations in blood parameters or physiological variables. BALF neutrophilia is a common finding.

16.5   Treatments and prevention

There are no known cures for heaves and SPAOPD. The cornerstone of management is currently based on antigen avoidance, and administration of corticosteroids and bronchodilators.

16.5.1   Environmental control

Reduction of environmental antigen (e.g., dust, molds, mites, pollens) exposure is paramount for the successful long-term management of horses with heaves or SPAOPD. In heaves, remission of clinical signs and airway inflammation is best achieved by placing affected horses on pasture all year long (Vandenput, 1998; Votion, 1999b). However, climatic or environmental conditions often do not allow this option in countries with a temperate climate. Supplementation of diet with hay while on pasture may lead to airway neutrophilia (Tremblay, 1993). Exposure to airborne stable dusts should be reduced to a minimum by changing food and bedding materials, decreasing hay movements and handling, and increasing ventilation. The replacement of hay by cube or pelleted hay, or possibly pasteurized hay, are effective therapies, although hay cubes or pellets could promote stereotypic behavior in some horses, by reducing the time they spend grazing (Elia, 2010). Hay silage has been associated with botulism in unvaccinated horses (Galey, 2001) and the efficacy of pasteurized hay at preventing the disease is not proven.

In SPAOPD, affected horses should be removed from pasture and placed in a low-dust environment during exacerbation periods (Beadle, 1983; Horohov, 2005). Even when antigen avoidance regimens are strictly implemented, the reversal of clinical signs of heaves and SPAOPD may take four weeks or more, and control of the airway inflammation may take even longer (Beadle, 1983; Dixon, 1995; Horohov, 2005; Leclere, 2012).

16.5.2   Anti-inflammatory drugs

Inflammation is believed to play a central role in the pathophysiology of heaves and SPAOPD, as suggested by the marked increase in neutrophil percentage in BALF during disease exacerbations. Only corticosteroids show effectiveness in controlling clinical signs. Leukotriene receptor antagonists and phosphodiesterase inhibitors were ineffective in preventing heaves exacerbations, despite promising results in *in vitro* studies (Rickards, 2001, 2003; Lavoie, 2002, 2006; Cesarini, 2006; Dunkel, 2009, 2010). Cromones are a group of compounds that prevent the release of inflammatory mediators from mast cells and other granulocytes. They have been shown to be effective as a preventive therapy in heaves, but are uncommonly used in clinical settings, due to limited effectiveness and availability (Thomson, 1981; Soma, 1987; Hare, 1994).

Whether administered systemically or by inhalation, corticosteroids are the most effective medication for the control of clinical signs in heaves and SPAOPD. Dexamethasone, prednisolone, isoflupredone, triamcinolone, beclomethasone and fluticasone are the most commonly used molecules. Partial and transient improvement may be observed within a few hours (Cornelisse, 2004), although the maximal control of airway obstruction usually requires a week or more. Histologic analysis of bronchial and pulmonary tissue after prolonged treatment with antigen avoidance, alone or combined with inhaled corticosteroids, showed a partial but significant reversibility of tissue remodeling.

When not combined with antigen avoidance strategies, only short residual effects are observed after drug administration is discontinued. Control of pulmonary neutrophilia with these drugs remains modest, if any (Ammann, 1998; Rush, 1998a; Couetil, 2006b; Lavoie, 2006), which is not due to an inherent resistance of equine neutrophils to corticosteroids (Lecoq, 2009; Hirsch, 2012).

While uncommon, systemic administration of corticosteroids to horses has been associated with several adverse effects, including adrenocortical suppression (Rush, 1998b; Picandet, 2003), laminitis (Eustace, 1990; Ryu, 2004), hepatopathy (Cohen, 1992; Ryu, 2004), muscle wasting (Cohen, 1992), altered bone metabolism (Lepage, 1993), and increased susceptibility to infection (Edington, 1985; Mair, 1996; Cutler, 2001; Fortier, 2013). They also affect the immune function, as they cause transient peripheral neutrophilia and lymphopenia (Targowski, 1975; Burguez, 1983), and may decrease the antibody response to vaccination (Slack, 2000).

On the other hand, inhaled corticosteroids have few systemic effects in horses with heaves, as shown by the absence of detectable clinical adverse effects, or alteration of lymphocyte subpopulations and function, circulating neutrophil gene expression, and primary and anamnestic immune responses to vaccination after up to one year of inhaled fluticasone administration (Dauvillier, 2011). Nevertheless, inhaled corticosteroids have been associated with a decrease in serum cortisol due to adrenocortical suppression (Rush, 1997; Laan, 2004; Munoz, 2015).

16.5.3 Bronchodilators

Bronchodilators with demonstrated efficacy for the treatment of horses with heaves include inhaled and systemic beta2-agonists and anticholinergic drugs. Inhaled β2-agonist administration results in a significant improvement of airway function (Derksen, 1999; Camargo, 2007; Bertin, 2011). Clenbuterol, a systemic beta2-agonist, improves clinical signs in approximately 75% of affected horses (Erichsen, 1994) and, in addition to its bronchodilator effect, clenbuterol also increases mucociliary clearance (Turgut, 1989). However, tachyphylaxis develops with prolonged administration (Read, 2012). Bronchodilators are rarely administered alone, given their lack of anti-inflammatory properties, although one study suggested that clenbuterol administration provides anti-inflammatory effects on bronchial inflammation (Laan, 2006b). Inhaled β-agonists alone have a rapid onset of action, but a short duration, which requires multiple daily administrations.

The systemically administered anticholinergic agents atropine and N-butylscopolammonium bromide are very effective at relieving airway obstruction in heaves and SPAOPD (Beadle, 1983; Thomson, 1983; Couetil, 2012). Atropine is likely to be the most potent bronchodilator in heaves, but its use is limited by its severe gastrointestinal side effects

(Ducharme, 1983). Inhaled anticholinergic drug ipratropium and revatropate may be valid alternatives, although they may occasionally reduce gastrointestinal sound score and oral mucous membranes hydration in treated horses (McGorum, 2013). Inhaled ipratropium has rapid onset of action, and dose-dependent effects lasting 4–6 hours (Robinson, 1993; Duvivier, 1999). N-butylscopolammonium bromide has bronchodilatory effects comparable to those of atropine, with reduced side effects (Couetil, 2012; De Lagarde, 2014). Nevertheless, its effects are short-lived, making this drug suitable only for assessing the reversibility of airway obstruction in research settings.

> ### Take home message
>
> The most efficacious long-term treatment for horses with heaves (and SPAOPD) is the implementation of antigen-avoidance strategies. Corticosteroids control the clinical signs, but their effect on inflammation is minimal if horses are not removed from the offending environment. Antihistamines, cysteinyl leukotriene inhibitors, and hyposensitization have no proven clinical efficacy.

The severe airway obstruction observed in heaves and SPAOPD is reversible and associated with low mortality rates. However, these are debilitating diseases, leading to early retirement from athletic life, or euthanasia due to lack of use. Clinical signs generally wane and wax, alternating periods of remission with periods of exacerbations, reflecting variable antigenic exposure. Death or euthanasia due to rapidly progressing cases, or unresponsiveness to antigen avoidance and corticosteroids, are very rare. Glucocorticoid resistance has been reported in one horse with heaves (Stamper, 2002). It has also been hypothesized that bronchiectasis and mucus plugs into the airways would decrease the response to treatments (Lavoie, 2004).

Affected horses are considered incurable, but exacerbation management is generally achieved successfully by environmental control, pharmacologic therapies, and client education. A survey indicated that 78% of horses diagnosed with heaves experienced period of disease exacerbation, even with environmental changes (Ainsworth, 1998). These results indicate the difficulty in applying effective and sustainable antigen avoidance strategies.

References

Asmundsson, T., Gunnarsson, E. and Johannesson, T. (1983). "Hay-sickness" in Icelandic horses: precipitin tests and other studies. *Equine Veterinary Journal* **15**, 229–232.

Aharonson-Raz, K., Lohmann, K. L., Townsend, H. G., Marques, F. and Singh, B. (2012). Pulmonary intravascular macrophages as proinflammatory cells in heaves, an asthma-like equine disease. *American Journal of Physiological Society Lung Cellular and Molecular Physiology* **303**(3), L189–198.

Ainsworth, D. M., Eicker, S. W. and Bennett, B. J. (1998). *Outcome of horses diagnosed with and treated for heaves.* World Equine Airway Symposium, Guelph, Canada.

Ainsworth, D. M., Grunig, G., Matychak, M. B., Young, J., Wagner, B., Erb, H. N. and Antczak, D. F. (2003). Recurrent airway obstruction (RAO) in horses is characterized by IFN-gamma and IL-8 production in bronchoalveolar lavage cells. *Veterinary Immunology and Immunopathology* **96**(1–2), 83–91.

Ainsworth, D. M., Wagner, B., Franchini, M., Grunig, G., Erb, H. N. and Tan, J. Y. (2006). Time-dependent alterations in gene expression of interleukin-8 in the bronchial epithelium of horses with recurrent airway obstruction. *American Journal of Veterinary Research* **67**(4), 669–677.

Ainsworth, D. M., Wagner, B., Erb, H. N., Young, J. C. and Retallick, D. E. (2007). Effects of *In vitro* exposure to hay dust on expression of interleukin-17, -23, -8, and -1beta and chemokine (C-X-C motif) ligand 2 by pulmonary mononuclear cells isolated from horses chronically affected with recurrent airway disease. *American Journal of Veterinary Research* **68**(12), 1361–1369.

Alphonse, M. P., Saffar, A. S., Shan, L., HayGlass, K. T., Simons, F. E. and Gounni, A. S. (2008). Regulation of the high affinity IgE receptor (Fc epsilonRI) in human neutrophils: role of seasonal allergen exposure and Th-2 cytokines. *PLoS One* **3**(4), e1921.

Amin, K. (2012). The role of mast cells in allergic inflammation. *Respiratory Medicine* **106**(1), 9–14.

Ammann, V. J., Vrins, A. A. and Lavoie, J. P. (1998). Effects of inhaled beclomethasone dipropionate on respiratory function in horses with chronic obstructive pulmonary disease (COPD). *Equine Veterinary Journal* **30**(2), 152–157.

Art, T., Franck, T., Lekeux, P., de Moffarts, B., Couetil, L., Becker, M., Kohnen, S., Deby-Dupont, G. and Serteyn, D. (2006). Myeloperoxidase concentration in bronchoalveolar lavage fluid from healthy horses and those with recurrent airway obstruction. *Canadian Journal of Veterinary Research* **70**(4), 291–296.

Back, H., Kendall, A., Grandon, R., Ullman, K., Treiberg-Berndtsson, L., Stahl, K. and Pringle, J. (2012). Equine multinodular pulmonary fibrosis in association with asinine herpesvirus type 5 and equine herpesvirus type 5: a case report. *Acta Veterinaria Scandinavica* **54**, 57.

Barboza, R., Camara, N. O., Gomes, E., Sa-Nunes, A., Florsheim, E., Mirotti, L., Labrada, A., Alcantara-Neves, N. M. and Russo, M. (2013). Endotoxin Exposure during Sensitization to Allergens Shifts TH2 Immunity Towards a TH17-Mediated Airway Neutrophilic Inflammation: Role of TLR4 and TLR2. *PLoS One* **8**(6), e67115.

Beadle, R. E. (1983). Summer pasture-associated obstructive pulmonary disease. In: Robinson, N. E. (ed). *Current Therapy in Equine Medicine.* Philadelphia, W.B. Saunders Co., 512–516.

Beadle, R. E., Horohov, D. W. and Gaunt, S. D. (2002). Interleukin-4 and interferon-gamma gene expression in summer pasture-associated obstructive pulmonary disease affected horses. *Equine Veterinary Journal* **34**(4), 389–394.

Berndt, A., Derksen, F. J., Venta, P. J., Ewart, S., Yuzbasiyan-Gurkan, V. and Robinson, N. E. (2007). Elevated amount of Toll-like receptor 4 mRNA in bronchial epithelial cells is associated with airway inflammation in horses with recurrent airway obstruction. *American Journal of Physiological Society Lung Cellular and Molecular Physiology* **292**(4), L936–943.

Berndt, A., Derksen, F. J., Venta, P. J., Karmaus, W., Ewart, S., Yuzbasiyan-Gurkan, V. and Robinson, N. E. (2009). Expression of toll-like receptor 2 mRNA in bronchial epithelial cells is not induced in RAO-affected horses. *Equine Veterinary Journal* **41**(1), 76–81.

Bertin, F. R., Ivester, K. M. and Couetil, L. L. (2011). Comparative efficacy of inhaled albuterol between two hand-held delivery devices in horses with recurrent airway obstruction. *Equine Veterinary Journal* **43**(4), 393–398.

Blanco, J. L. and Garcia, M. E. (2008). Immune response to fungal infections. *Veterinary Immunology and Immunopathology* **125**(1–2), 47–70.

Blume, C., Swindle, E. J., Dennison, P., Jayasekera, N. P., Dudley, S., Monk, P., Behrendt, H., Schmidt-Weber, C. B., Holgate, S. T., Howarth, P. H., Traidl-Hoffmann, C. and Davies, D. E. (2012). Barrier responses of human bronchial epithelial cells to grass pollen exposure. *European Respiratory Journal* **42**(1), 87–97.

Bourré, L., Vrins, A., Cormier, Y. and Lavoie, J. (1992). Comparaison des titres sériques d'anticorps anti-*Micropolyspora faeni* chez des chevaux atteints de M.P.V.R. et chez des chevaux contrôles. *Méd Vét Québec* **22**, 133.

Brazil, T. J., Dagleish, M. P., McGorum, B. C., Dixon, P. M., Haslett, C. and Chilvers, E. R. (2005). Kinetics of pulmonary neutrophil recruitment and clearance in a natural and spontaneously resolving model of airway inflammation. *Clinical & Experimental Allergy* **35**(7), 854–865.

Britt, D. P. and Preston, J. M. (1985). Efficacy of ivermectin against Dictyocaulus arnfieldi in ponies. *Veterinary Record* **116**(13), 343–345.

Bullone, M., M. Chevigny, M. Allano, J. G. Martin and J. P. Lavoie (2014). Technical and physiological determinants of airway smooth muscle mass in endobronchial biopsy samples of asthmatic horses. *Journal of Applied Physiology (1985)* **117** (7): 806–815.

Bureau, F., Bonizzi, G., Kirschvink, N., Delhalle, S., Desmecht, D., Merville, M. P., Bours, V. and Lekeux, P. (2000). Correlation between nuclear factor-kappaB activity in bronchial brushing samples and lung dysfunction in an animal model of asthma. *American Journal of Respiratory and Critical Care Medicine* **161**(4 Pt 1), 1314–1321.

Burguez, P. N., Ousey, J., Cash, R. S. and Rossdale, P. D. (1983). Changes in blood neutrophil and lymphocyte counts following administration of cortisol to horses and foals. *Equine Veterinary Journal* **15**(1), 58–60.

Camargo, F. C., Robinson, N. E., Berney, C., Eberhart, S., Baker, S., Detolve, P., Derksen, F. J., Lehner, A. F., Hughes, C. and Tobin, T. (2007). Trimetoquinol: bronchodilator effects in horses with heaves following aerosolised and oral administration. *Equine Veterinary Journal* **39**(3), 215–220.

Cesarini, C., Hamilton, E., Picandet, V. and Lavoie, J. P. (2006). Theophylline does not potentiate the effects of a low dose of dexamethasone in horses with recurrent airway obstruction. *Equine Veterinary Journal* **38**(6), 570–573.

Cohen, N. D. and Carter, G. K. (1992). Steroid hepatopathy in a horse with glucocorticoid-induced hyperadrenocorticism. *Journal of the American Veterinary Medical Association* **200**(11), 1682–1684.

Cordeau, M. E., Joubert, P., Dewachi, O., Hamid, Q. and Lavoie, J. P. (2004). IL-4, IL-5 and IFN-gamma mRNA expression in pulmonary lymphocytes in equine heaves. *Veterinary Immunology and Immunopathology* **97**(1–2), 87–96.

Cornelisse, C.J., Robinson, N.E., Berney, C.E., Kobe, C.A., Boruta, D.T. and Derksen, F.J. (2004). Efficacy of oral and intravenous dexamethasone in horses with recurrent airway obstruction. *Equine Veterinary Journal* **36**(5), 426–430.

Costa, L.R., Johnson, J.R., Baur, M.E. and Beadle, R.E. (2006). Temporal clinical exacerbation of summer pasture-associated recurrent airway obstruction and relationship with climate and aeroallergens in horses. *American Journal of Veterinary Research* **67**(9), 1635–1642.

Couetil, L.L. and Ward, M.P. (2003). Analysis of risk factors for recurrent airway obstruction in North American horses: 1,444 cases (1990–1999). *Journal of the American Veterinary Medical Association* **223**(11), 1645–1650.

Couetil, L.L., Chilcoat, C.D., DeNicola, D.B., Clark, S.P., Glickman, N.W. and Glickman, L.T. (2005). Randomized, controlled study of inhaled fluticasone propionate, oral administration of prednisone, and environmental management of horses with recurrent airway obstruction. *American Journal of Veterinary Research* **66**(10), 1665–1674.

Couetil, L.L., Art, T., de Moffarts, B., Becker, M., Melotte, D., Jaspar, F., Bureau, F. and Lekeux, P. (2006a). DNA binding activity of transcription factors in bronchial cells of horses with recurrent airway obstruction. *Veterinary Immunology and Immunopathology* **113** (1–2), 11–20.

Couetil, L.L., Art, T., de Moffarts, B., Becker, M., Melotte, D., Jaspar, F., Bureau, F. and Lekeux, P. (2006b). Effect of beclomethasone dipropionate and dexamethasone isonicotinate on lung function, bronchoalveolar lavage fluid cytology, and transcription factor expression in airways of horses with recurrent airway obstruction. *Journal of Veterinary Internal Medicine* **20**(2), 399–406.

Couetil, L., Hammer, J., Miskovic Feutz, M., Nogradi, N., Perez-Moreno, C. and Ivester, K. (2012). Effects of N-butylscopolammonium bromide on lung function in horses with recurrent airway obstruction. *Journal of Veterinary Internal Medicine* **26**(6), 1433–1438.

Cutler, T.J., MacKay, R.J., Ginn, P.E., Gillis, K., Tanhauser, S.M., LeRay, E.V., Dame, J.B. and Greiner, E.C. (2001). Immunoconversion against Sarcocystis neurona in normal and dexamethasone-treated horses challenged with S. neurona sporocysts. *Veterinary Parasitology* **95**(2–4), 197–210.

Dacre, K.J., McGorum, B.C., Marlin, D.J., Bartner, L.R., Brown, J.K., Shaw, D.J., Robinson, N.E., Deaton, C. and Pemberton, A.D. (2007). Organic dust exposure increases mast cell tryptase in bronchoalveolar lavage fluid and airway epithelium of heaves horses. *Clinical & Experimental Allergy* **37**(12), 1809–1818.

Dauvillier, J., Felippe, M.J., Lunn, D.P., Lavoie-Lamoureux, A., Leclere, M., Beauchamp, G. and Lavoie, J.P. (2011). Effect of long-term fluticasone treatment on immune function in horses with heaves. *Journal of Veterinary Internal Medicine* **25**(3), 549–557.

Davis, E. G. and Rush, B. R. (2013). Diagnostic challenges: Equine thoracic neoplasia. *Equine Veterinary Education* **25**(2), 96–107.

de Lagarde, M., N. Rodrigues, M. Chevigny, G. Beauchamp, B. Albrecht and J. P. Lavoie (2014). N-butylscopolammonium bromide causes fewer side effects than atropine when assessing bronchoconstriction reversibility in horses with heaves. *Equine Veterinary Journal* **46** (4): 474–478.

Deaton, C. M., Marlin, D. J., Smith, N. C., Roberts, C. A., Harris, P. A., Schroter, R. C. and Kelly, F. J. (2005). Antioxidant and inflammatory responses of healthy horses and horses affected by recurrent airway obstruction to inhaled ozone. *Equine Veterinary Journal* **37**(3), 243–249.

Deaton, C. M., Deaton, L., Jose-Cunilleras, E., Vincent, T. L., Baird, A. W., Dacre, K. and Marlin, D. J. (2007). Early onset airway obstruction in response to organic dust in the horse. *Journal of Applied Physiology* **102**(3), 1071–1077.

Debrue, M., Hamilton, E., Joubert, P., Lajoie-Kadoch, S. and Lavoie, J. P. (2005). Chronic exacerbation of equine heaves is associated with an increased expression of interleukin-17 mRNA in bronchoalveolar lavage cells. *Veterinary Immunology and Immunopathology* **105** (1–2), 25–31.

Derksen, F. J., Brown, C. M., Sonea, I., Darien, B. J. and Robinson, N. E. (1989). Comparison of transtracheal aspirate and bronchoalveolar lavage cytology in 50 horses with chronic lung disease. *Equine Veterinary Journal* **21**(1), 23–26.

Derksen, F. J., M. A. Olszewski, N. E. Robinson, C. Berney, J. E. Hakala, C. J. Matson and D. T. Ruth (1999). Aerosolized albuterol sulfate used as a bronchodilator in horses with recurrent airway obstruction. *American Journal of Veterinary Research* **60** (6): 689–693.

Dewachi, O., Joubert, P., Hamid, Q. and Lavoie, J. P. (2006). Expression of interleukin (IL)-5 and IL-9 receptors on neutrophils of horses with heaves. *Veterinary Immunology and Immunopathology* **109**(1–2), 31–36.

Dirscherl, P., Grabner, A. and Buschmann, H. (1993). Responsiveness of basophil granulocytes of horses suffering from chronic obstructive pulmonary disease to various allergens. *Veterinary Immunology and Immunopathology* **38**(3–4), 217–227.

Dixon, P. M. and McGorum, B. (1990). Pasture-associated seasonal respiratory disease in two horses. *Veterinary Record* **126**(1), 9–12.

Dixon, P. M., Railton, D. I., McGorum, B. C. and Tothill, S. (1995). Equine pulmonary disease: a case control study of 300 referred cases. Part 4: Treatments and re-examination findings. *Equine Veterinary Journal* **27**(6), 436–439.

Dixon, P.M., McGorum, B.C., Marley, C., Halliwell, R.E., Matthews, A.G. and Morris, J.R. (1996). Effects of equine influenza and tetanus vaccination on pulmonary function in normal and chronic obstructive pulmonary disease affected horses. *Equine Veterinary Journal* **28**, 157–160.

Ducharme, N. G. and Fubini, S. L. (1983). Gastrointestinal complications associated with the use of atropine in horses. *JAVMA* **182**(3), 229–231.

Dunkel, B., Rickards, K. J., Werling, D., Page, C. P. and Cunningham, F. M. (2009). Neutrophil and platelet activation in equine recurrent airway obstruction is associated with increased neutrophil CD13 expression, but not platelet CD41/61 and CD62P or neutrophil-platelet aggregate formation. *Veterinary Immunology and Immunopathology* **131**(1–2), 25–32.

Dunkel, B., Rickards, K. J., Werling, D., Page, C. P. and Cunningham, F. M. (2010). Evaluation of the effect of phosphodiesterase on equine platelet activation and the effect of antigen challenge on platelet phosphodiesterase activity in horses with recurrent airway obstruction. *American Journal of Veterinary Research* **71**(5), 534–540.

Duvivier, D. H., Bayly, W. M., Votion, D., Vandenput, S., Art, T., Farnir, F. and Lekeux, P. (1999). Effects of inhaled dry powder ipratropium bromide on recovery from exercise of horses with COPD. *Equine Veterinary Journal* **31**(1), 20–24.

Eder, C., Crameri, R., Mayer, C., Eicher, R., Straub, R., Gerber, H., Lazary, S. and Marti, E. (2000). Allergen-specific IgE levels against crude mould and storage mite extracts and recombinant mould allergens in sera from horses affected with chronic bronchitis. *Veterinary Immunology and Immunopathology* **73**(3–4), 241–253.

Eder, C., Curik, I., Brem, G., Crameri, R., Bodo, I., Habe, F., Lazary, S., Solkner, J. and Marti, E. (2001). Influence of environmental and genetic factors on allergen-specific immunoglobulin-E levels in sera from Lipizzan horses. *Equine Veterinary Journal* **33**(7), 714–720.

Edington, N., Bridges, C. G. and Huckle, A. (1985). Experimental reactivation of equid herpesvirus 1 (EHV 1) following the administration of corticosteroids. *Equine Veterinary Journal* **17**(5), 369–372.

Elia, J. B., Erb, H. N. and Houpt, K. A. (2010). Motivation for hay: effects of a pelleted diet on behavior and physiology of horses. *Physiology & Behavior* **101**(5), 623–627.

Erichsen, D. F., Aviad, A. D., Schultz, R. H. and Kennedy, T. J. (1994). Clinical efficacy and safety of clenbuterol HCl when administered to effect in horses with chronic obstructive pulmonary disease (COPD). *Equine Veterinary Journal* **26**(4), 331–336.

Eustace, R. A. and Redden, R. R. (1990). Iatrogenic laminitis. *Veterinary Record* **126**(23), 586.

Fairbairn, S. M., Page, C. P., Lees, P. and Cunningham, F. M. (1993). Early neutrophil but not eosinophil or platelet recruitment to the lungs of allergic horses following antigen exposure. *Clinical & Experimental Allergy* **23**(10), 821–828.

Fong, C. Y., Pang, L., Holland, E. and Knox, A. J. (2000). TGF-beta1 stimulates IL-8 release, COX-2 expression, and PGE(2) release in human airway smooth muscle cells. *American Journal of Physiology: Lung Cellular and Molecular* **279**(1), L201–207.

Fortier, G., Richard, E., Hue, E., Fortier, C., Pronost, S., Pottier, D., Lemaitre, L., Lekeux, P., Borchers, K. and Thiry, E. (2013). Long-lasting airway inflammation associated with equid herpesvirus-2 in experimentally challenged horses. *Veterinary Journal* **197**(2), 492–495.

Franchini, M., Gilli, U., Akens, M. K., Fellenberg, R. V. and Bracher, V. (1998). The role of neutrophil chemotactic cytokines in the pathogenesis of equine chronic obstructive pulmonary disease (COPD). *Veterinary Immunology and Immunopathology* **66**(1), 53–65.

Galey, F. D. (2001). Botulism in the horse. *Veterinary Clinics of North America: Equine Practice* **17**(3), 579–588.

George, L. W., Tanner, M. L., Roberson, E. L. and Burke, T. M. (1981). Chronic respiratory disease in a horse infected with Dictyocaulus arnfieldi. *Journal of the American Veterinary Medical Association* **179**(8), 820–822.

Gerber, H. (1973). Chronic pulmonary disease in the horse. *Equine Veterinary Journal* (5), 26–32.

Gerber, H. (1989). Sir Frederick Hobday memorial lecture. The genetic basis of some equine diseases. *Equine Veterinary Journal* **21**(4), 244–248.

Grunig, G., Hermann, M., Howald, B., Winder, C. and von Fellenberg, R. (1989). Partial divergence between airway inflammation and clinical signs in equine chronic pulmonary disease. *Equine Veterinary Journal* **21**(2), 145–148.

Halliwell, R. E., McGorum, B. C., Irving, P. and Dixon, P. M. (1993). Local and systemic antibody production in horses affected with chronic obstructive pulmonary disease. *Veterinary Immunology and Immunopathology* **38**(3–4), 201–215.

Halwani, R., Al-Muhsen, S. and Hamid, Q. (2013). T helper 17 cells in airway diseases: from laboratory bench to bedside. *Chest* **143**(2), 494–501.

Hare, J. E., Viel, L., O'Byrne, P. M. and Conlon, P. D. (1994). Effect of sodium cromoglycate on light racehorses with elevated metachromatic cell numbers on bronchoalveolar lavage and reduced exercise tolerance. *Journal of Veterinary Pharmacology and Therapeutics* **17**(3), 237–244.

Hare, J. E., Viel, L., Conlon, P. D. and Marshall, J. S. (1999). *In vitro* allergen-induced degranulation of pulmonary mast cells from horses with recurrent airway obstruction (heaves). *American Journal of Veterinary Research* **60**(7), 841–847.

He, S. H., Liu, Z. Q., Chen, X., Song, C. H., Zhou, L. F., Ma, W. J., Cheng, L., Du, Y., Tang, S. G. and Yang, P. C. (2011). IL-9(+) IL-10(+) T cells link immediate allergic response to late phase reaction. *Clinical & Experimental Immunology* **165**(1), 29–37.

Hirsch, G., Lavoie-Lamoureux, A., Beauchamp, G. and Lavoie, J. P. (2012). Neutrophils are not less sensitive than other blood leukocytes to the genomic effects of glucocorticoids. *PLoS One* **7**(9), e44606.

Horohov, D. W., Beadle, R. E., Mouch, S. and Pourciau, S. S. (2005). Temporal regulation of cytokine mRNA expression in equine recurrent airway obstruction. *Veterinary Immunology and Immunopathology* **108**(1–2), 237–245.

Hotchkiss, J. W., Reid, S. W. and Christley, R. M. (2007). A survey of horse owners in Great Britain regarding horses in their care. Part 2: Risk factors for recurrent airway obstruction. *Equine Veterinary Journal* **39**(4), 301–308.

Jackson, K. A., Stott, J. L., Horohov, D. W. and Watson, J. L. (2004). IL-4 induced CD23 (FcepsilonRII) up-regulation in equine peripheral blood mononuclear cells and pulmonary alveolar macrophages. *Veterinary Immunology and Immunopathology* **101**(3–4), 243–250.

Jean, D., Vrins, A. and Lavoie, J. P. (1999). Monthly, daily, and circadian variations of measurements of pulmonary mechanics in horses with chronic obstructive pulmonary disease. *American Journal of Veterinary Research* **60**(11), 1341–1346.

Ji, X., Li, J., Xu, L., Wang, W., Luo, M., Luo, S., Ma, L., Li, K., Gong, S., He, L., Zhang, Z., Yang, P., Zhou, Z., Xiang, X. and Wang, C. Y. (2013). IL-4 and IL-17A provide a Th2/Th17-polarized inflammatory milieu in favor of TGF-beta1 to induce bronchial epithelial-mesenchymal transition (EMT). *International Journal of Clinical and Experimental Pathology* **6**(8), 1481–1492.

Jost, U., Klukowska-Rotzler, J., Dolf, G., Swinburne, J. E., Ramseyer, A., Bugno, M., Burger, D., Blott, S. and Gerber, V. (2007). A region on equine chromosome 13 is linked to recurrent airway obstruction in horses. *Equine Veterinary Journal* **39**(3), 236–241.

Joubert, P., Cordeau, M. E., Boyer, A., Silversides, D. W. and Lavoie, J. P. (2008). Cytokine expression by peripheral blood neutrophils from heaves-affected horses before and after allergen challenge. *Veterinary Journal* **178**(2), 227–232.

Joubert, P., Cordeau, M. E. and Lavoie, J. P. (2011). Cytokine mRNA expression of pulmonary macrophages varies with challenge but not with disease state in horses with heaves or in controls. *Veterinary Immunology and Immunopathology* **142**(3–4), 236–242.

Kaup, F. J., Drommer, W., Damsch, S. and Deegen, E. (1990). Ultrastructural findings in horses with chronic obstructive pulmonary disease (COPD). II: Pathomorphological changes of the terminal airways and the alveolar region. *Equine Veterinary Journal* **22**(5), 349–355.

Khan, Z. U., Misra, V. C. and Randhawa, H. S. (1985). Precipitating antibodies against Micropolyspora faeni in equines in north-western India. *Antonie Van Leeuwenhoek* **51**(3), 313–319.

Klebanoff, S. J. (2005). Myeloperoxidase: friend and foe. *Journal of Leukocyte Biology* **77**(5), 598–625.

Kleiber, C., McGorum, B. C., Horohov, D. W., Pirie, R. S., Zurbriggen, A. and Straub, R. (2005). Cytokine profiles of peripheral blood and airway CD4 and CD8T lymphocytes in horses with recurrent airway obstruction. *Veterinary Immunology and Immunopathology* **104** (1–2), 91–97.

Klukowska-Rotzler, J., Swinburne, J. E., Drogemuller, C., Dolf, G., Janda, J., Leeb, T. and Gerber, V. (2012a). The interleukin 4 receptor gene and its role in recurrent airway obstruction in Swiss Warmblood horses. *Animal Genetics* **43**(4), 450–453.

Klukowska-Rotzler, J., Marti, E., Lavoie, J. P., Ainsworth, D. M., Gerber, V., Zurbriggen, A. and Janda, J. (2012b). Expression of thymic stromal lymphopoietin in equine recurrent airway obstruction. *Veterinary Immunology and Immunopathology* **146**(1), 46–52.

Klukowska-Rotzler, J., Gerber, V. and Leeb, T. (2012c). Association analysis of SNPs in the IL21R gene with recurrent airway obstruction (RAO) in Swiss Warmblood horses. *Animal Genetics* **43**(4), 475–476.

Koblinger, K., Nicol, J., McDonald, K., Wasko, A., Logie, N., Weiss, M. and Leguillette, R. (2011). Endoscopic assessment of airway inflammation in horses. *Journal of Veterinary Internal Medicine* **25**(5), 1118–1126.

Koch, C., Straub, R., Ramseyer, A., Widmer, A., Robinson, N. E. and Gerber, V. (2007). Endoscopic scoring of the tracheal septum in horses and its clinical relevance for the evaluation of lower airway health in horses. *Equine Veterinary Journal* **39**(2), 107–112.

Kunzle, F., Gerber, V., Van Der Haegen, A., Wampfler, B., Straub, R. and Marti, E. (2007). IgE-bearing cells in bronchoalveolar lavage fluid and allergen-specific IgE levels in sera from RAO-affected horses. *Journal of Veterinary Medicine Series A-physiology Pathology Clinical Medicine* **54**(1), 40–47.

Laan, T.T., Westermann, C.M., Dijkstra, A.V., van Nieuwstadt, R.A. and Fink-Gremmels, J. (2004). Biological availability of inhaled fluticasone propionate in horses. *Veterinary Record* **155**(12), 361–364.

Laan, T.T., Bull, S., van Nieuwstadt, R.A. and Fink-Gremmels, J. (2006a). The effect of aerosolized and intravenously administered clenbuterol and aerosolized fluticasone propionate on horses challenged with Aspergillus fumigatus antigen. *Veterinary Research Communications* **30**(6), 623–635.

Laan, T.T., Bull, S., Pirie, R.S. and Fink-Gremmels, J. (2006b). The anti-inflammatory effects of IV administered clenbuterol in horses with recurrent airway obstruction. *Veterinary Journal* **171**(3), 429–437.

Larson, V.L. and Busch, R.H. (1985). Equine tracheobronchial lavage: comparison of lavage cytologic and pulmonary histopathologic findings. *American Journal of Veterinary Research* **46**(1), 144–146.

Lacasse, Y. and Cormier, Y. (2006). Hypersensitivity pneumonitis. *Orphanet Journal of Rare Diseases* **1**, 25.

Lavoie-Lamoureux, A., Moran, K., Beauchamp, G., Mauel, S., Steinbach, F., Lefebvre-Lavoie, J., Martin, J. G. and Lavoie, J. P. (2010). IL-4 activates equine neutrophils and induces a mixed inflammatory cytokine expression profile with enhanced neutrophil chemotactic mediator release *ex vivo*. *American Journal of Physiological Society Lung Cellular and Molecular Physiology* **299**(4), L472–482.

Lavoie-Lamoureux, A., Beauchamp, G., Quessy, S., Martin, J. G. and Lavoie, J. P. (2012a). Systemic inflammation and priming of peripheral blood leukocytes persist during clinical remission in horses with heaves. *Veterinary Immunology and Immunopathology* **146**(1); 35–45.

Lavoie-Lamoureux, A., Leclere, M., Lemos, K., Wagner, B. and Lavoie, J. P. (2012b). Markers of Systemic Inflammation in Horses with Heaves. *Journal of Veterinary Internal Medicine* **26**(6), 1419–1426.

Lavoie, J. P., Maghni, K., Desnoyers, M., Taha, R., Martin, J. G. and Hamid, Q. A. (2001). Neutrophilic Airway Inflammation in Horses with Heaves Is Characterized by a Th2-type Cytokine Profile. *American Journal of Respiratory and Critical Care Medicine* **164**(8), 1410–1413.

Lavoie, J. P., Leguillette, R., Pasloske, K., Charette, L., Sawyer, N., Guay, D., Murphy, T. and Hickey, G. J. (2002). Comparison of effects of dexamethasone and the leukotriene D4 receptor antagonist L-708,738 on lung function and airway cytologic findings in horses with recurrent airway obstruction. *American Journal of Veterinary Research* **63**(4), 579–585.

Lavoie, J. P., Dalle, S., Breton, L. and Helie, P. (2004). Bronchiectasis in three adult horses with heaves. *Journal of Veterinary Internal Medicine* **18**(5), 757–760.

Lavoie, J. P., Pasloske, K., Joubert, P., Cordeau, M. E., Mancini, J., Girard, Y., Friesen, R. W., Frenette, R., Blouin, M., Young, R. N. and Hickey, G. (2006). Lack of clinical efficacy of a phosphodiesterase-4 inhibitor for treatment of heaves in horses. *Journal of Veterinary Internal Medicine* **20**(1), 175–181.

Lavoie, J. P., Lefebvre-Lavoie, J., Leclere, M., Lavoie-Lamoureux, A., Chamberland, A., Laprise, C. and Lussier, J. (2012). Profiling of differentially expressed genes using suppression subtractive hybridization in an equine model of chronic asthma. *PLoS One* **7**(1), e29440.

Lawson, G. H., McPherson, E. A., Murphy, J. R., Nicholson, J. M., Wooding, P., Breeze, R. G. and Pirie, H. M. (1979). The presence of precipitating antibodies in the sera of horses with chronic obstructive pulmonary disease (COPD). *Equine Veterinary Journal* **11**(3), 172–176.

Leclere, M., Lavoie-Lamoureux, A., Gelinas-Lymburner, E., David, F., Martin, J. G. and Lavoie, J. P. (2011). Effect of antigenic exposure on airway smooth muscle remodeling in an equine model of chronic asthma. *American Journal of Respiratory Cell and Molecular Biology* **45**(1), 181–187.

Leclere, M., Lavoie-Lamoureux, A., Joubert, P., Relave, F., Setlakwe, E. L., Beauchamp, G., Couture, C., Martin, J. G. and Lavoie, J. P. (2012). Corticosteroids and antigen avoidance decrease airway smooth muscle mass in an equine asthma model. *American Journal of Respiratory Cell and Molecular Biology* **47**(5), 589–596.

Lecoq, L., Vincent, P., Lavoie-Lamoureux, A. and Lavoie, J. P. (2009). Genomic and non-genomic effects of dexamethasone on equine peripheral blood neutrophils. *Veterinary Immunology and Immunopathology* **128**(1–3), 126–131.

Leguillette, R. (2003). Recurrent airway obstruction--heaves. *Veterinary Clinics of North America: Equine Practice* **19**(1), 63–86, vi.

Lepage, O. M., Laverty, S., Marcoux, M. and Dumas, G. (1993). Serum osteocalcin concentration in horses treated with triamcinolone acetonide. *American Journal of Veterinary Research* **54**(8), 1209–1212.

Lorch, G., Hillier, A., Kwochka, K. W., Saville, W. J., Kohn, C. W. and Jose-Cunilleras, E. (2001). Results of intradermal tests in horses without atopy and horses with chronic obstructive pulmonary disease. *American Journal of Veterinary Research* **62**(3), 389–397.

Lowell, F. C. (1964). Observations on Heaves. An Asthma-Like Syndrome in the Horse. *Journal of Allergy and Clinical Immunology* **35**, 322–330.

Macdowell, A. L. and Peters, S. P. (2007). Neutrophils in asthma. *Current Allergy and Asthma Reports* **7**(6), 464–468.

MacKay, R. J. and Urquhart, K. A. (1979). An outbreak of eosinophilic bronchitis in horses possibly associated with Dictyocaulus arnfieldi infection. *Equine Veterinary Journal* **11**(2), 110–112.

Mair, T. S. (1996). Obstructive pulmonary disease in 18 horses at summer pasture. *Veterinary Record* **138**(4), 89–91.

Mair, T. S. and Brown, P. J. (1993). Clinical and pathological features of thoracic neoplasia in the horse. *Equine Veterinary Journal* **25**(3), 220–223.

Mansmann, R. A., Osburn, B. I., Wheat, J. D. and Frick, O. (1975). Chicken hypersensitivity pneumonitis in horses. *Journal of the American Veterinary Medical Association* **166**(7), 673–677.

Marr, K. A., Foster A. P., Lees, P., Cunningham, F. M. and Page, C. P. (1997). Effect of antigen challenge on the activation of peripheral blood neutrophils from horses with chronic obstructive pulmonary disease. *Research in Veterinary Science* **62**(3), 253–260.

Marti, E., Gerber, H., Essich, G., Oulehla, J. and Lazary, S. (1991). The genetic basis of equine allergic diseases. 1. Chronic hypersensitivity bronchitis. *Equine Veterinary Journal* **23**(6), 457–460.

McGorum, B. C., Dixon, P. M. and Halliwell, R. E. (1993a). Responses of horses affected with chronic obstructive pulmonary disease to inhalation challenges with mould antigens. *Equine Veterinary Journal* **25**(4), 261–267.

McGorum, B. C., Dixon, P. M. and Halliwell, R. E. (1993b). Quantification of histamine in plasma and pulmonary fluids from horses with chronic obstructive pulmonary disease, before and after 'natural (hay and straw) challenges'. *Veterinary Immunology and Immunopathology* **36**(3), 223–237.

McGorum, B. C., Dixon, P. M. and Halliwell, R. E. (1993c). Phenotypic analysis of peripheral blood and bronchoalveolar lavage fluid lymphocytes in control and chronic obstructive pulmonary disease affected horses, before and after 'natural (hay and straw) challenges'. *Veterinary Immunology and Immunopathology* **36**(3), 207–222.

McGorum, B. C., Nicholas, D. R., Foster, A. P., Shaw, D. J. and Pirie, R. S. (2013). Bronchodilator activity of the selective muscarinic antagonist revatropate in horses with heaves. *Veterinary Journal* **195**(1), 80–85.

Meyts, I., Vanoirbeek, J. A., Hens, G., Vanaudenaerde, B. M., Verbinnen, B., Bullens, D. M., Overbergh, L., Mathieu, C., Ceuppens, J. L. and Hellings, P. W. (2008). T-cell mediated late increase in bronchial tone after allergen provocation in a murine asthma model. *Clinical Immunology* **128**(2), 248–258.

Miskovic, M., Couetil, L. L. and Thompson, C. A. (2007). Lung function and airway cytologic profiles in horses with recurrent airway obstruction maintained in low-dust environments. *Journal of Veterinary Internal Medicine* **21**(5), 1060–1066.

Moran, G., H. Folch, O. Araya, R. Burgos and M. Barria (2010). Detection of reaginic antibodies against Faenia rectivirgula from the serum of horses affected with Recurrent Airway Obstruction by an in vitro bioassay. *Veterinary Research Communications* **34**(8): 719–726.

Moran, G., Folch, H., Henriquez, C., Ortloff, A. and Barria, M. (2012). Reaginic antibodies from horses with recurrent airway obstruction produce mast cell stimulation. *Veterinary Research Communications* **36**(4), 251–258.

Munoz, T., M. Leclere, D. Jean and J. P. Lavoie (2015). "Serum cortisol concentration in horses with heaves treated with fluticasone proprionate over a 1 year period." *Research in Veterinary Science* **98**: 112–114.

Nabe, T., Morishita, T., Matsuya, K., Ikedo, A., Fujii, M., Mizutani, N. and Yoshino, S. (2011). Complete dependence on CD4+ cells in late asthmatic response, but limited contribution of the cells to airway remodeling in sensitized mice. *Journal of Pharmacological Sciences* **116**(4), 373–383.

Nabe, T., Matsuya, K., Akamizu, K., Fujita. M., Nakagawa, T., Shioe, M., Kida, H., Takiguchi, A., Wakamori, H., Fujii, M., Ishihara, K., Akiba, S., Mizutani, N., Yoshino, S. and Chaplin, D. D. (2013). Roles of basophils and mast cells infiltrating the lung by multiple antigen challenges in asthmatic responses of mice. *British Journal of Pharmacology* **169**(2), 462–476.

Nakagome, K., Matsushita, S. and Nagata, M. (2012). Neutrophilic inflammation in severe asthma. *International Archives of Allergy and Immunology* **158**(Suppl 1), 96–102.

Nevalainen, M., Raulo, S. M., Brazil, T. J., Pirie, R. S., Sorsa, T., McGorum, B. C. and Maisi, P. (2002). Inhalation of organic dusts and lipopolysaccharide increases gelatinolytic matrix metalloproteinases (MMPs) in the lungs of heaves horses. *Equine Veterinary Journal* **34**(2), 150–155.

Noronha, L. E., Harman, R. M., Wagner, B. and Antczak, D. F. (2012). Generation and characterization of monoclonal antibodies to equine CD16. *Veterinary Immunology and Immunopathology* **146**(2), 135–142.

Olszewski, M. A., Robinson, N. E., Zhu, F. X., Zhang, X. Y. and Tithof, P. K. (1999). Mediators of anaphylaxis but not activated neutrophils augment cholinergic responses of equine small airways. *American Journal of Physiology* **276**(3, Part 1), L522–529.

Parbhakar, O. P., Duke, T., Townsend, H. G. and Singh, B. (2005). Depletion of pulmonary intravascular macrophages partially inhibits lipopolysaccharide-induced lung inflammation in horses. *Veterinary Research* **36**(4), 557–569.

Pastorello, E. A., Incorvaia, C., Ortolani, C., Bonini, S., Canonica, G. W., Romagnani, S., Tursi, A. and Zanussi, C. (1995). Studies on the relationship between the level of specific IgE antibodies and the clinical expression of allergy: I. Definition of levels distinguishing patients with symptomatic from patients with asymptomatic allergy to common aeroallergens. *Journal of Allergy and Clinical Immunology* **96**(5, Part 1), 580–587.

Pellegrini, A., Kalkinc, M., Hermann, M., Grunig, B., Winder, C. and Von Fellenberg, R. (1998). Equinins in equine neutrophils: quantification in tracheobronchial secretions as an aid in the diagnosis of chronic pulmonary disease. *Veterinary Journal* **155**(3), 257–262.

Picandet, V., Leguillette, R. and Lavoie, J. P. (2003). Comparison of efficacy and tolerability of isoflupredone and dexamethasone in the treatment of horses affected with recurrent airway obstruction (*heaves*). *Equine Veterinary Journal* **35**(4), 419–424.

Pirie, R. S., Dixon, P. M., Collie, D. D. and McGorum, B. C. (2001). Pulmonary and systemic effects of inhaled endotoxin in control and heaves horses. *Equine Veterinary Journal* **33**(3), 311–318.

Pirie, R. S., Collie, D. D., Dixon, P. M. and McGorum, B. C. (2002a). Evaluation of nebulised hay dust suspensions (HDS) for the diagnosis and investigation of heaves. 2: Effects of inhaled HDS on control and heaves horses. *Equine Veterinary Journal* **34**(4), 337–342.

Pirie, R. S., Dixon, P. M. and McGorum, B. C. (2002b). Evaluation of nebulised hay dust suspensions (HDS) for the diagnosis and investigation of heaves. 3: Effect of fractionation of HDS. *Equine Veterinary Journal* **34**(4), 343–347.

Pirie, R. S., Collie, D. D., Dixon, P. M. and McGorum, B. C. (2003). Inhaled endotoxin and organic dust particulates have synergistic proinflammatory effects in equine heaves (organic dust-induced asthma). *Clinical & Experimental Allergy* **33**(5), 676–683.

Pomorska, D., Larsson, L., Skorska, C., Sitkowska, J. and Dutkiewicz, J. (2007). Levels of bacterial endotoxin in air of animal houses determined with the use of gas chromatography-mass spectrometry and Limulus test. *Annals of Agricultural and Environmental Medicine* **14** (2), 291–298.

Racine, J., Gerber, V., Feutz, M. M., Riley, C. P., Adamec, J., Swinburne, J. E. and Couetil, L. L. (2011). Comparison of genomic and proteomic data in recurrent airway obstruction affected horses using Ingenuity Pathway Analysis(R). *BMC Veterinary Research* **7**, 48.

Ramseyer, A., Gaillard, C., Burger, D., Straub, R., Jost, U., Boog, C., Marti, E. and Gerber, V. (2007). Effects of genetic and environmental factors on chronic lower airway disease in horses. *Journal of Veterinary Internal Medicine* **21**(1), 149–156.

Read, J. R., Boston, R. C., Abraham, G., Bauquier, S. H., Soma, L. R. and Nolen-Walston, R. D. (2012). Effect of prolonged administration of clenbuterol on airway reactivity and sweating in horses with inflammatory airway disease. *American Journal of Veterinary Research* **73** (1), 140–145.

Rickards, K. J., Page, C. P., Lees, P. and Cunningham, F. M. (2001). Differential inhibition of equine neutrophil function by phosphodiesterase inhibitors. *Journal of Veterinary Pharmacology and Therapeutics* **24**(4), 275–281.

Rickards, K. J., Page, C. P., Lees, P., Gettinby, G. and Cunningham, F. M. (2003). *In vitro* and *ex vivo* effects of the phosphodiesterase 4 inhibitor, rolipram, on thromboxane production in equine blood. *Journal of Veterinary Pharmacology and Therapeutics* **26**(2), 123–130.

Riihimaki, M., Raine, A., Pourazar, J., Sandstrom, T., Art, T., Lekeux, P., Couetil, L. and Pringle, J. (2008). Epithelial expression of mRNA and protein for IL-6, IL-10 and TNF-alpha in endobronchial biopsies in horses with recurrent airway obstruction. *BMC Veterinary Research* **4**, 8.

Robinson, N. E., Derksen, F. J., Berney, C. and Goossens, L. (1993). The airway response of horses with recurrent airway obstruction (heaves) to aerosol administration of ipratropium bromide. *Equine Veterinary Journal* **25**(4), 299–303.

Robinson, N. E., Olszewski, M. A., Boehler, D., Berney, C., Hakala, J., Matson, C. and Derksen, F. J. (2000). Relationship between clinical signs and lung function in horses with recurrent airway obstruction (heaves) during a bronchodilator trial. *Equine Veterinary Journal* **32** (5), 393–400.

Robinson, N.E. (2001). International Workshop on Equine Chronic Airway Disease. Michigan State University 16–18 June 2000. *Equine Veterinary Journal* **33**, 5–19.

Rush, B. R., Flaminio, M. J., Matson, C. J. and Hakala, J. E. (1997). *Inhaled beclomethasone dipropionate for treatment of heaves.* The 15th Annual Comparative Respiratory Society Symposium, Liége.

Rush, B. R., Flaminio, M. J., Matson, C. J., Hakala, J. E. and Shuman, W. (1998a). Cytologic evaluation of bronchoalveolar lavage fluid from horses with recurrent airway obstruction after aerosol and parenteral administration of beclomethasone dipropionate and dexamethasone, respectively. *American Journal of Veterinary Research* **59**(8), 1033–1038.

Rush, B. R., Worster, A. A., Flaminio, M. J., Matson, C. J. and Hakala, J. E. (1998b). Alteration in adrenocortical function in horses with recurrent airway obstruction after aerosol and parenteral administration of beclomethasone dipropionate and dexamethasone, respectively. *American Journal of Veterinary Research* **59**(8), 1044–1047.

Ryu, S. H., Kim, B. S., Lee, C. W., Yoon, J. and Lee, Y. L. (2004). Glucocorticoid-induced laminitis with hepatopathy in a Thoroughbred filly. *Journal of Veterinary Science* **5**(3), 271–274.

Saluja, R., Delin, I., Nilsson, G. P. and Adner, M. (2012). Fc epsilonR1-mediated mast cell reactivity is amplified through prolonged Toll-like receptor-ligand treatment. *PLoS One* **7**(8), e43547.

Schmallenbach, K. H., Rahman, I., Sasse, H. H., Dixon, P. M., Halliwell, R. E., McGorum, B. C., Crameri, R. and Miller, H. R. (1998). Studies on pulmonary and systemic *Aspergillus fumigatus*-specific IgE and IgG antibodies in horses affected with chronic obstructive pulmonary disease (COPD). *Veterinary Immunology and Immunopathology* **66** (3–4), 245–256.

Seahorn, T. L. and Beadle, R. E. (1993). Summer pasture-associated obstructive pulmonary disease in horses: 21 cases (1983–1991). *Journal of the American Veterinary Medical Association* **202**(5), 779–782.

Seahorn, T. L., Beadle, R. E., McGorum, B. C. and Marley, C. L. (1997). Quantification of antigen-specific antibody concentrations in tracheal lavage fluid of horses with summer pasture-associated obstructive pulmonary disease. *American Journal of Veterinary Research* **58** (12), 1408–1411.

Shakhsi-Niaei, M., Klukowska-Rotzler, J., Drogemuller, C., Swinburne, J., Ehrmann, C., Saftic, D., Ramseyer, A., Gerber, V., Dolf, G. and Leeb, T. (2012). Replication and fine-mapping of a QTL for recurrent airway obstruction in European Warmblood horses. *Animal Genetics* **43**(5), 627–631.

Simonen-Jokinen, T., Pirie, R. S., McGorum, B. C. and Maisi, P. (2005). Effect of composition and different fractions of hay dust suspension on inflammation in lungs of heaves-affected horses: MMP-9 and MMP-2 as indicators of tissue destruction. *Equine Veterinary Journal* **37**(5), 412–417.

Singh Suri, S., Janardhan, K. S., Parbhakar, O., Caldwell, S., Appleyard, G. and Singh, B. (2006). Expression of toll-like receptor 4 and 2 in horse lungs. *Veterinary Research* **37**(4), 541–551.

Slack, J., Risdahl, J. M., Valberg, S. J., Murphy, M. J., Schram, B. R. and Lunn, D. P. (2000). Effects of dexamethasone on development of immunoglobulin G subclass responses following vaccination of horses. *American Journal of Veterinary Research* **61**(12), 1530–1533.

Soma, L. R., Beech, J. and Gerber, N. H., Jr. (1987). Effects of cromolyn in horses with chronic obstructive pulmonary disease. *Veterinary Research Communications* **11**(4), 339–351.

Sorrell, T. C. and Chen, S. C. (2009). Fungal-derived immune modulating molecules. *Advances in Experimental Medicine and Biology* **666**, 108–120.

Stamper, A. J., Rush, B. R., Wilkerson, M. J., Mitchell, K. E. and Shuman, W. (2002). *Glucocorticoid resistance in a horse with heaves.* Veterinary Comparative Respiratory Society Congress, Boston, Massachussets.

Swinburne, J. E., Bogle, H., Klukowska-Rotzler, J., Drogemuller, M., Leeb T., Temperton, E., Dolf, G. and Gerber, V. (2009). A whole-genome scan for recurrent airway obstruction in Warmblood sport horses indicates two positional candidate regions. *Mammalian Genome* **20**(8), 504–515.

Tahon, L., S. Baselgia, V. Gerber, M. G. Doherr, R. Straub, N. E. Robinson and E. Marti (2009). In vitro allergy tests compared to intradermal testing in horses with recurrent airway obstruction. *Veterinary Immunology and Immunopathology* **127** (1-2): 85–93.

Targowski, S. P. (1975). Effect of prednisolone on the leukocyte counts of ponies and on the reactivity of lymphocytes *In vitro* and in vivo. *Infection and Immunity* **11**(2), 252–256.

Thomson, J. R. and McPherson, E. A. (1981). Prophylactic effects of sodium cromoglycate on chronic obstructive pulmonary disease in the horse. *Equine Veterinary Journal* **13**(4), 243–246.

Thomson, J. R. and McPherson, E. A. (1983). Chronic obstructive pulmonary disease in the horse. 2: Therapy. *Equine Veterinary Journal* **15**(3), 207–210.

Thorsen, J., Willoughby, R. A., McDonell, W., Valli, V. E., Viel, L. and Bignell, W. (1983). Influenza hemagglutination inhibiting activity in respiratory mucus from horses with chronic obstructive pulmonary disorders (heaves syndrome). *Canadian Journal of Comparative Medicine* **47**(3), 332–335.

Thurlbeck, W.M. and Lowell, F.C. (1964). Heaves in horses. *American Review of Respiratory Diseases* **89**, 82–88.

Tremblay, G. M., Ferland, C., Lapointe, J. M., Vrins, A., Lavoie, J. P. and Cormier, Y. (1993). Effect of stabling on bronchoalveolar cells obtained from normal and COPD horses. *Equine Veterinary Journal* **25**(3), 194–197.

Turgut, K. and Sasse, H. H. (1989). Influence of clenbuterol on mucociliary transport in healthy horses and horses with chronic obstructive pulmonary disease. *Veterinary Record* **125**(21), 526–530.

Turlej, R. K., Fievez, L., Sandersen, C. F., Dogne, S., Kirschvink, N., Lekeux, P. and Bureau, F. (2001). Enhanced survival of lung granulocytes in an animal model of asthma: evidence for a role of GM-CSF activated STAT5 signalling pathway. *Thorax* **56**(9), 696–702.

Uzzaman, A. and Cho, S. H. (2012). Chapter 28: Classification of hypersensitivity reactions. *Allergy and Asthma Proceedings* Suppl 1, S96–99.

van der Haegen, A., Kunzle, F., Gerber, V., Welle, M., Robinson, N. E. and Marti, E. (2005). Mast cells and IgE-bearing cells in lungs of RAO-affected horses. *Veterinary Immunology and Immunopathology* **108**(3–4), 325–334.

Vandenput, S., Votion, D., Duvivier, D. H., Van Erck, E., Anciaux, N., Art, T. and Lekeux, P. (1998). Effect of a set stabled environmental control on pulmonary function and airway reactivity of COPD affected horses. *Veterinary Journal* **155**(2), 189–195.

Varin, A. and Gordon, S. (2009). Alternative activation of macrophages: immune function and cellular biology. *Immunobiology* **214**(7), 630–641.

Venugopal, C. S., Mendes, L. C., Peiro, J. R., Laborde, S. S., Stokes, A. M. and Moore, R. M. (2010). Transcriptional changes associated with recurrent airway obstruction in affected and unaffected horses. *American Journal of Veterinary Research* **71**(4), 476–482.

Venugopal, C., N. Mariappan, E. Holmes, M. Kearney and R. Beadle (2013). Effect of potential therapeutic agents in reducing oxidative stress in pulmonary tissues of recurrent airway obstruction-affected and clinically healthy horses. *Equine Veterinary Journal* **45** (1): 80–84.

Votion, D., Ghafir, Y., Vandenput, S., Duvivier, D. H., Art, T. and Lekeux, P. (1999a). Analysis of scintigraphical lung images before and after treatment of horses suffering from chronic pulmonary disease. *Veterinary Record* **144**(9), 232–236.

Votion, D. M., Vandenput, S. N., Duvivier, D. H., Lambert, P., van Erck, E., Art, T. and Lekeux, P. M. (1999b). Alveolar clearance in horses with chronic obstructive pulmonary disease. *American Journal of Veterinary Research* **60**(4), 495–500.

Wagner, B. (2009). IgE in horses: occurrence in health and disease. *Veterinary Immunology and Immunopathology* **132**(1), 21–30.

Watanabe, A., Mishima, H., Renzi, P. M., Xu, L. J., Hamid, Q. and Martin, J. G. (1995a). Transfer of allergic airway responses with antigen-primed CD4+ but not CD8+ T cells in brown Norway rats. *Journal of Clinical Investigation* **96**(3), 1303–1310.

Watanabe, A., Rossi, P., Renzi, P. M., Xu, L. J., Guttmann, R. D. and Martin, J. G. (1995b). Adoptive transfer of allergic airway responses with sensitized lymphocytes in BN rats. *American Journal of Respiratory and Critical Care Medicine* **152**(1), 64–70.

Watanabe, A., Mishima, H., Kotsimbos, T. C., Hojo, M., Renzi, P. M., Martin, J. G. and Hamid, Q. A. (1997). Adoptively transferred late allergic airway responses are associated with Th2-type cytokines in the rat. *American Journal of Respiratory Cell and Molecular Biology* **16**(1), 69–74.

Watson, J. L., Stott, J. L., Blanchard, M. T., Lavoie, J. P., Wilson, W. D., Gershwin, L. J. and Wilson, D. W. (1997). Phenotypic characterization of lymphocyte subpopulations in horses affected with chronic obstructive pulmonary disease and in normal controls. *Veterinary Pathology* **34**(2), 108–116.

Wenzel, S. E. (2012). Asthma phenotypes: the evolution from clinical to molecular approaches. *Nature Medicine* **18**(5), 716–725.

Williams, K. J., Maes, R., Del Piero, F., Lim, A., Wise, A., Bolin, D. C., Caswell, J., Jackson, C., Robinson, N. E., Derksen, F., Scott, M. A., Uhal, B. D., Li, X., Youssef, S. A. and Bolin, S. R. (2007). Equine multinodular pulmonary fibrosis: a newly recognized herpesvirus-associated fibrotic lung disease. *Veterinary Pathology* **44**(6), 849–862.

Winder, C. (2001). The toxicology of chlorine. *Environmental Research* **85**(2), 105–114.

Winder, N. C. and von Fellenberg, R. (1990). Mast cells in normal and pathological specimens of the equine lung. *Zentralbl Veterinarmed A* **37**(9), 641–650.

Wong, D. M., Belgrave, R. L., Williams, K. J., Del Piero, F., Alcott, C. J., Bolin, S. R., Marr, C. M., Nolen-Walston, R., Myers, R. K. and Wilkins, P. A. (2008). Multinodular pulmonary fibrosis in five horses. *Journal of the American Veterinary Medical Association* **232**(6), 898–905.

17 Inflammatory Airway Disease

Mathilde Leclère and Jean-Pierre Lavoie

17.1 Definition

Inflammatory airway disease (IAD) is a common condition of horses characterized by airway inflammation, alterations in pulmonary function, and the presence of one or more clinical signs of respiratory disease. In 2007, a panel of experts from the American College of Veterinary Internal Medicine proposed the use of the following criteria to define IAD in horses of any age:

1 poor performance, exercise intolerance, or coughing, with or without excess tracheal mucus;
2 non-septic airway inflammation detected by cytological examination of bronchoalveolar lavage fluid (BALF), or pulmonary dysfunction based on evidence of lower airway obstruction, airway hyper-responsiveness, or impaired blood gas exchange at rest or during exercise.

Horses with respiratory difficulty at rest (such as seen in heaves), or with evidence of systemic illness (fever, depression, abnormal blood work), are excluded from this definition (Couetil, 2007). The panel also elected to exclude from this definition horses with solely evidence of tracheal inflammation.

Take home message

IAD is defined by (as per the American College of Veterinary Internal Medicine consensus statement of 2007):
- poor performance, exercise intolerance, or coughing, with or without excess tracheal mucus; *and*
- non-septic inflammation detected by cytological examination of bronchoalveolar lavage fluid; *or* pulmonary dysfunction based on evidence of lower airway obstruction, airway hyper-responsiveness, or impaired blood gas exchange at rest or during exercise.

17.1.1 Terminology

A limiting factor to our understanding of IAD is the very loose use of the term in the literature. There is a large body of literature using the presence of tracheal inflammation (increased mucus or neutrophils) as evidence of IAD (summarized by Cardwell, 2011a), in part because tracheal endoscopy can easily be performed without sedation and with a one-meter endoscope. The use of *trIAD* and *brIAD* has been suggested to make explicit the

site of examination (tracheal versus bronchoalveolar) that led to a diagnosis (Cardwell, 2011a). This may help to clarify what leads to these conditions, and how they could be related.

The term *subclinical IAD* is also sometimes used to describe the presence of inflammation in BALF without concurrent clinical signs (Gerber, 2003). In this chapter, the term IAD will be used in line with the 2007 ACVIM consensus statement, the term *tracheal inflammation* will be used if tracheal visual examination or aspirate analysis was used to define IAD in an original publication, and *lower airway inflammation* will describe inflammatory BALF cytology without clinical signs.

17.2 Signalment and clinical signs

Clinical signs of IAD include cough, poor performance, prolonged recovery after exercise, and increased airway secretions. Cough may be observed only at the beginning of exercise, and is often overlooked by owners or trainers until it becomes more frequent. Thoracic auscultation may be unremarkable, but crackles and wheezes can be heard when using re-breathing maneuvers. Respiratory rate and efforts can be exaggerated during exercise, or shortly afterwards. Horses of any age and breed can be affected but, because clinical signs are relatively subtle, it is rarely a complaint in non-athletic horses. Tracheal inflammation (see 17.1.1 Terminology) is more prevalent in young racehorses, and decreases with age or time spent in training (Chapman, 2000; Newton, 2003; Wood, 2005a, 2005b).

17.3 Immunologic mechanisms and etiologic associations

Although it is labeled as a *disease*, IAD is probably better defined as a clinical syndrome with a likely multifactorial etiopathogenesis. Since chronic inflammation from any cause can lower the activation threshold of cough receptors, any disease defined by cough and inflammation has the potential to regroup processes from different etiologies. The main hypotheses could be

---

Equine Clinical Immunology, First Edition. Edited by M. Julia B. Felippe.
© 2016 John Wiley & Sons, Inc. Published 2016 by John Wiley & Sons, Inc.

summarized as follows: some data support the concept that IAD is merely an environmental disease, while others suggest that IAD is an early stage or milder phenotype of heaves. Still other observations support an infectious etiology with secondary lower airway inflammation. The latter mainly comes from studies using tracheal inflammation to define IAD. It is likely that different conditions have been regrouped under the same umbrella based on a common phenotype. Therefore, the relative contribution of the possible etiologies to the development of airway inflammation and respiratory dysfunction probably varies between subsets of IAD and individual horses. Our current understanding of the disease is also limited by the fact that most data are at the association or correlation level, and there is currently no experimental reproduction of IAD.

Take home message

Potential etiologies of IAD include:
- environmental disease;
- an early stage or milder phenotype of heaves;
- an infectious process with secondary lower airway inflammation.

17.3.1 Environmental factors

Airway inflammation induced by hay feeding and housing in conventional barns could play a role in the development of IAD. Bringing horses to indoor stabling induces neutrophilic airway inflammation in otherwise healthy animals (Tremblay, 1993; Gerber, 2001; Holcombe, 2001), and tracheal mucus is associated with recent introduction to the training environment (Cardwell, 2011b). Stabled horses are exposed to much higher concentrations of endotoxin (up to eight times higher) than horses maintained on pasture (Berndt, 2010), and respirable endotoxin levels correlate with neutrophilic inflammation in racehorses (Malikides, 2003a). Barn environments are also associated with exposure to molds, mites, organic dust particles, peptidoglycans, and noxious gases (May, 2012).

A longitudinal study on healthy stabled horses found an up-regulation of interleukin (IL)-6 in the winter, possibly due increased in respirable dust or beta-glucan, suggesting activation of innate immunity (Riihimaki, 2008). In a study looking specifically at stabled performance sport horses, with no current or past history of respiratory disease, all horses examined had evidence of inflammation based on BALF cytology (Gerber, 2003). This raises the question of why do not all stabled horses develop IAD, and why do some horses have lower airway inflammation without evidence of clinical signs or altered lung function.

Nevertheless, stabling is likely contributing to lower airway inflammation, and the ACVIM panel concluded that high burdens of aerosolized organic particles (including endotoxins, mite debris, and beta-glucan) and inorganic particles present in barns were probably involved in the pathophysiology of IAD without a clear evidence of an allergic-type response (Woods, 1993; McGorum, 1998; Malikides, 2003b; Cardwell, 2007; Couetil, 2007). The relative contribution of environment (indoor housing) versus hay feeding has not been clarified in the context of IAD.

17.3.2 Infectious agents

In the relatively narrow definition of IAD described above, active viral and bacterial infections are unlikely to play a central role in the pathogenesis of the disease. It is, however, possible that respiratory infections at an early age predispose to IAD later in life, although this has not been demonstrated so far. Conversely, when tracheal inflammation is used as main criteria for the diagnosis of "IAD" in young racehorses, there is more convincing evidence of the contribution of bacterial pathogens (Wood, 1993, 2005a; Burrell, 1996; Christley, 2001; Newton, 2003), even if there was no evidence of concurrent infections (from viruses, bacteria or mycoplasma) in a majority of horses with a cough in one study (Christley, 2001). The reduction of tracheal inflammation with age in racehorses can be interpreted as being the consequence of immunity, and may support an infectious etiology (Wood, 2005b).

There is evidence linking exercise intolerance, cough, and inflammation to high bacterial load in the distal trachea of young racehorses. More specifically, *Streptococcus zooepidemicus* is most consistently associated with tracheal inflammation (Wood, 1993, 2005a; Burrell, 1996; Chapman, 2000; Christley, 2001). One study also found than high bacterial count in BALF was associated with inflammation and exercise intolerance, although definite conclusions are difficult to draw, because more than 90% of these racehorses had positive cultures (Fogarty, 1991). The contribution of bacteria in IAD, as defined by the ACVIM panel, is much less clear and is not considered central to the disease (Couetil, 2007). It is, however, not uncommon to have increased bacterial colonization of the trachea in clinical cases of IAD, and antimicrobials are sometimes recommend as an adjunct therapy when bacteria are found in high numbers (more than 10^2 or 10^3 colony forming units/ml) (Christley, 2007; Slater, 2007).

Viral infections have been associated to tracheal inflammation in young racehorses, but only in a small percentage (approximately 5%) of episodes recorded in a longitudinal study. Those episodes were linked to seroconversion to Equine Herpes Virus (EHV)-1 and EHV-4, but not to influenza, equine rhinovirus and adenovirus (Wood, 2005a). In another study, EHV-2 DNA was significantly more common in horses with respiratory inflammation (regrouping IAD and tracheal inflammation) while EHV-1 and EHV-4 were found only in a small proportion of healthy and diseased horses (Fortier, 2009). The reported positive effect of interferon-α in horses with tracheal inflammation would also support a role of viral infections in at least some cases (Moore, 2004). To the author's knowledge, there is currently no study that specifically addresses the possible involvement of respiratory infections at a young age in the development of IAD later in life.

17.4 Types of bronchoalveolar lavage fluid inflammation and cytokine profile

Bronchoalveolar lavage fluid analysis can support the presence of pulmonary inflammation by showing a relative increase in neutrophils, eosinophils or mast cells (Couetil, 2007). High bronchoalveolar total cell count, increased lymphocytes or macrophages, and smaller proportion of CD4-positive cells and B cells, have also been observed in horses with tracheal inflammation (Moore, 1995; Christley, 2007), and high total cell count has been associated with lower arterial oxygen tension during exercise (McKane, 1995). Other non-specific markers of inflammation have been detected in the bronchoalveolar fluid of horses with tracheal inflammation, including increased proteins and procoagulant activity (Moore, 1997). In the same study, prostaglandins E_2 and $F_1\alpha$ were not elevated.

It has been hypothesized that different types of inflammation are related to different pathogenesis and predominant clinical signs. Neutrophilic and mastocytic inflammation types in BALF are associated with different cytokine profiles (Hughes, 2011; Lavoie, 2011; Beekman, 2012; Table 17.1). Neutrophils are more closely associated with cough while mastocytes are associated with airway hyperresponsiveness in some (Hoffman, 1998; Bedenice, 2008), but not all, studies (Nolen-Walston, 2013).

17.4.1 Neutrophils
In addition to indoor housing, as mentioned previously, a high percentage of neutrophils in BALF has been associated with cough and age (Bedenice, 2008; Lavoie, 2011), tracheal mucus, tracheal neutrophils, the use of round bales (Robinson, 2006), and low arterial oxygen tension during exercise (Couetil, 1999; Sanchez, 2005).

17.4.2 Mast cells and eosinophils
Among horses with poor performance and respiratory signs, horses with increased eosinophils or mast cells in their BALF tend to be younger, and are examined because of decreased performance, rather than cough (Bedenice, 2008; Lavoie, 2011). Increased pulmonary eosinophils and mast cells have been associated with altered baseline lung function, as well as hyper-reactivity to bronchoprovocation (Hare, 1998; Hoffman, 1998; Bedenice, 2008). The strong association between mast cell percentages and airway reactivity to histamine suggests that mast cell degranulation may contribute to bronchospasm, at least in this subset of horses with IAD (Hoffman, 1998). Interestingly, airway hyperresponsiveness to histamine bronchoprovocation is also associated with mast cells in apparently healthy horses (Mazan, 2001). Similarly, eosinophils are associated with increased respiratory resistance in horses without apparent clinical signs (Richard, 2009).

17.4.3 Cytokine profile
Studies have looked at the link between cytokine gene expression and different cell types observed in BALF of horses with IAD (Hughes, 2011; Lavoie, 2011; Beekman, 2012; Table 17.1). These studies measured the messenger RNA (mRNA) expression of bronchoalveolar cells by qPCR. Comparison between studies are difficult because, even when inclusion criteria are in

Table 17.1 Cytokine gene expression of bronchoalveolar lavage cells of horses with Inflammatory Airway Disease.

Study A (Lavoie, 2011)	
22 racehorses with IAD based on poor performance and BALF	
9 controls with poor performance and normal BALF	
Cytokines measured	**Cytokines upregulated**
IL-1β, IL-4, IL-8,	IL-4, IFN-γ TNFα
IFN-γ, TNFα	IL-4 and IFN-γ associated with mast cells
	IL-1β associated with neutrophils
Study B (Hughes, 2011)	
21 horses with IAD based on poor performance or respiratory signs and BALF	
17 controls with poor performance and normal BALF	
Cytokines measured	**Cytokines upregulated**
IL-1β, IL-2, IL-4,	IL-1β, TNFα, IL-23
IL-8, IL-13, IL-17,	
IL-23, IFN-γ, TNFα	
Study C (Beekman, 2012)	
17 horses with IAD based on clinical signs and BALF	
10 controls based on the absence of clinical signs and normal BALF	
Cytokines measured	**Cytokines upregulated**
IL-1β, IL-4, IL-5,	IL-1β, IL-5, IL-6, IL-8, IL-10,
IL-6, IL-8, IL-10,	In IAD *mast cells* only: IL-4 and IL-12p35
IL-12p35, IL-17, IFN-γ, eotaxin-2	In IAD *neutrophils* only: IL-17

IAD – inflammatory airway disease; BALF – bronchoalveolar lavage fluid; IL – interleukin; IFN – interferon; TNF – tumor necrosis factor.

line with ACVIM recommendations, populations studied vary, and only few markers of inflammation have been measured in more than one study. Among these, IL-1β was found to be up-regulated in three studies (out of three studies in which it was measured), TNFα in two (out of two), and IL-4 in two (out of three) in association with mast cells. In an *ex vivo* study, exposing bronchial epithelial cells to hay dust extract and endotoxin induced up-regulation of IL-8, IL-1β and CXCL2 (Ainsworth, 2012). Taken together, these studies suggest that innate inflammation is probably involved in IAD, and that a T helper-2 (Th-2) profile may predominate over Th-1 in IAD with increased mast cells.

17.5 Links between IAD and heaves

Heaves and IAD share some similarities, such as pulmonary inflammation (neutrophilic in heaves and in many cases of IAD), altered pulmonary function, cough and exercise intolerance. Horses with IAD also tend to show more clinical signs when housed indoors and fed hay, but a clear allergic-type reaction has not been demonstrated (Couetil, 2007). Most horses with heaves have a history of chronic mild clinical signs before they present respiratory difficulty at rest. Therefore, they are likely to fall into the definition of IAD at some point in the progression of the disease.

There are no clear data on the current prevalence of IAD in horses, but few clinicians will argue that it is largely above the prevalence of heaves. The main question is, therefore, do these *pre-heaves* IAD have a different type of inflammation, or are they similar to other horses with IAD but exposed to environmental (or other factors) that will make them progress to heaves? Currently, there are no diagnostic criteria predicting which horses with IAD will progress to become heaves-affected.

17.6 Links between IAD and EIPH

Exercise-induced pulmonary hemorrhage (EIPH) has been suggested to be a cause of IAD in athletic horses. Instillation of blood in the lungs of horses does induce pulmonary inflammation and alterations in pulmonary function (Aguilera-Tejero, 1995; McKane, 1999). Blood could induce neutrophils recruitment by promoting the release of IL-8 by bronchial epithelial cells (Ainsworth, 2012). Also, pulmonary inflammation increases the risk of developing EIPH (McKane, 2010). EIPH is highly prevalent in racehorses, and could contribute to neutrophilic airway inflammation in this population, but it is unlikely to be the main cause of IAD (otherwise, virtually all racehorses would be affected). It is also unlikely to be a significant factor in sport horses, or in horses with other types of IAD (eosinophils or mast cells).

17.7 Diagnostics

17.7.1 Clinical signs
Clinical signs, based on history and physical examination, are central to the diagnosis of IAD. As mentioned earlier, these include cough, nasal discharge and poor performance, in the absence of systemic signs of infection (fever, abnormal leukogram). These clinical signs may be subtle, sometimes variable in time, and not specific for IAD, or even for a respiratory problem (in the case of poor performance). Exclusion of other respiratory diseases and causes of impaired performance is, therefore, paramount to the diagnosis of IAD.

17.7.2 Bronchoalveolar lavage fluid and endoscopy
As mentioned above, analysis of BALF obtained from horses with IAD usually reveals high percentage of neutrophils, eosinophils or mast cells and, sometimes, high total nucleated cell counts (Figures 17.1 and 17.2). Total cell counts are affected by

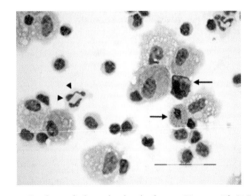

Figure 17.1 Cytology of a bronchoalveolar lavage. Horses with IAD can have increased mast cells (arrow, purple granules), eosinophils (arrow, red granules) or neutrophils (arrowheads). Cytospin stained with a modified Wright-Giemsa (M. Leclere, Université de Montréal).

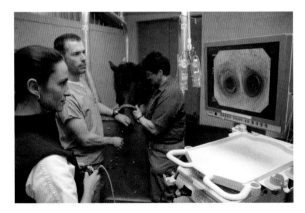

Figure 17.2 Bronchoalveolar lavage on a five year old Quarter Horse mare with exercise intolerance and intermittent cough. A videoendoscope is often used in referral centers but the procedure can also be done blindly with a cuffed tube (M. Leclere, Université de Montréal).

return volume and dilution effect, while percentages are inter-dependent. Therefore, an increase in one cell type may be hidden by a greater increase of another cell type. Reported reference ranges vary with populations studied, age, and method of collection and processing of BALF (Lapointe, 1994; Pickles, 2002), to the point where the appropriateness of using single "normal" values when interpreting bronchoalveolar fluid collected with various methods (catheter/endoscopes diameter, fluid type and volume) can be questioned.

Nevertheless, eosinophils and mast cells are generally considered abnormal above 1% and 2%, respectively, and the percentage of neutrophils considered abnormal varies between 5% and 10% (Couetil, 2007; Richard, 2009; Lavoie, 2011). Other cut-offs are sometimes used, and one should be aware of this when reviewing the literature. The current recommendations are that lower airway inflammation should be documented on the basis on BALF, and not tracheal aspirate, because the former is clearly linked to pulmonary dysfunction (Hoffman, 1998; Couetil, 1999, 2001; Sanchez, 2005) and exercise intolerance (Fogarty, 1991; Vrins, 1991; Moore, 1995). There is also poor agreement between tracheal and bronchoalveolar inflammation (Derksen, 1989; Hughes, 2003; Malikides, 2003c; Allen, 2006), despite a link between tracheal mucus and poor performance (Holcombe, 2006; Widmer, 2009).

Finally, abnormal BALF cytology, in the absence of clinical signs, should not be sufficient to diagnose IAD. This is illustrated by the fact that inflammation is frequent (up to 45% and 100%) in some populations of healthy, well performing horses (Gerber, 2003; Courouce-Malblanc, 2010). Finally, tracheal mucus, tracheal septum thickness, and airway collapse during BALF aspiration, are often observed in horses with BALF inflammation (Koblinger, 2011, 2013). However, tracheal septum thickness in itself is a poor predictor of lower airway inflammation (Koch, 2007).

17.7.3 Pulmonary function testing

Alterations in pulmonary function are more subtle than the ones observed in heaves and, therefore, are more difficult to measure. It is in part for this reason that this parameter was not included as a mandatory criterion for the diagnosis of IAD by the ACVIM. These alterations include: mild to moderate airflow limitation; airway hyperresponsiveness to exogenous broncho-constrictors; and impaired gas exchange during exercise (Hare, 1998; Hoffman, 1998; Bedenice, 2008). Airflow limitation can be detected by forced expiration method (Couetil, 2001), induced hyperventilation (Pirrone, 2007) or impulse oscillometry (Richard, 2009). Horses affected with IAD also show significant greater contribution of the thorax when hyperpnoea is induced (Haltmayer, 2013). Bronchoalveolar inflammation is also associated with impaired gas exchange during exercise in some (McKane, 1995; Couetil, 1999; Sanchez, 2005), but not all, studies (Nolen-Walston, 2013).

These measurements are not easily performed in field studies, because they require specialized equipment, sedation, or measurement of gas exchange during exercise. However, taken together, these findings suggest that IAD is associated with ventilation-perfusion mismatch, airflow limitation and airway hyperresponsiveness.

17.7.4 Other diagnostics

When investigating chronic respiratory problems, complete blood count and thoracic radiographs are used to rule out infectious, infiltrative or neoplastic processes. Horses with IAD can have bronchial or bronchointerstitial patterns on thoracic radiographs, but these findings have poor predictive value in the diagnosis of IAD (Mazan, 2005). Bacterial culture of tracheal aspirate has been used when investigating IAD in young horses or horses with a history of poor response to corticosteroids. High numbers of bacteria (in a horse suspected of IAD and without signs of systemic illness) suggest bacterial overgrowth in the distal trachea, which may contribute to perpetuating lower airway inflammation and cough. Serum surfactant protein D, a protein participating in innate pulmonary defenses, and synthesized by alveolar type II cells and non ciliated bronchiolar cells, is increased in horses with BALF inflammation (Richard, 2011). It is not specific for IAD, but supports the presence of pulmonary inflammation. It could, therefore, be useful in the diagnosis of IAD in horses with poor performance as primary complaint.

17.8 Treatment and prevention

Current treatment recommendations are directed at decreasing exposure to environmental dust particles (irritant and potential allergens), in conjunction with steroidal anti-inflammatory drugs and bronchodilators. These recommendations are extrapolated from treatments used to control clinical signs in heaves, and are based on presumptive shared aspects of pathogenesis, but there is limited evidence-based data regarding their efficacy. Common use is to recommend dust control measures (improving indoor ventilation, increasing turn outs, low-dust bedding) and limiting access to hay-associated inhaled antigens. This is achieved by using soaked, pasteurized or pelleted hay, which reduces molds and inhaled particles to different degrees (Woods, 1993; Moore-Colyer, 1996; McGorum, 1998; Earing, 2013). Grass pasture is also used when available. Systemic or inhaled corticosteroids and bronchodilators are often prescribed, in conjunction with dust-limiting measures.

Few studies have evaluated the effect of pharmacological interventions on clinical signs, airway inflammation and function of horses with IAD. Among them, one study showed that horses with increased mast cells in their bronchoalveolar fluid benefited from the administration of nebulized sodium cromoglycate, a mast cell stabilizer, in terms of clinical signs and respiratory score (Hare, 1994). Clenbuterol, a β2-adrecep-tor agonist, transiently increases mucociliary clearance (Barr, 2013) and reduces airway sensitivity to inhaled histamine, but tachyphylaxis was observed, with an increase in airway reactivity, after three weeks of treatment (Read, 2012).

Interferon alpha decreased total protein concentrations and procoagulant activity in BALF (Moore, 1997), and had a mild positive effect in young racehorses with tracheal inflammation (Moore, 2004). In a small number of horses with IAD, dexamethasone and fluticasone administered for 15 days did not change BALF neutrophil percentage or count (Beekman, 2011). This is also often observed with heaves, even when function improves significantly (Couetil, 2006; Leclere, 2012). Finally, in one study, albuterol did not improve performance in Standardbreds, but only a subset had BALF inflammation or airway hyperresponsiveness (Mazan, 2001).

17.9   Prognosis and clinical outcomes

IAD is considered a transient disease when diagnosed in young, athletic horses, and probably in a majority of older horses as well, although there is little data to support this statement. It is likely that horses that eventually develop heaves are initially diagnosed as having IAD and, although clinical signs can be controlled in most cases, there is no curative treatment. In one recent (unpublished) study, for a majority of pleasure and sport horses diagnosed with IAD, and for whom measures limiting exposure to hay and barn dust were implemented (alone or with corticosteroids and bronchodilators), there was improvement of clinical signs to the client's satisfaction (Pilon, 2013). This was based on subjective client evaluation, and there is a great need for prospective and standardized studies to evaluate the effect of different treatment approaches.

References

Aguilera-Tejero, E., Pascoe, J.R., Tyler, W.S. and Woliner, M.J. (1995). Autologous blood instillation alters respiratory mechanics in horses. *Equine Veterinary Journal* **27**(1), 46–50.

Ainsworth, D.M. and Reyner, C.L. (2012). Effects of in vitro exposure to autologous blood and serum on expression of interleukin-8, interleukin-1beta, and chemokine (C-X-C motif) ligand 2 in equine primary bronchial epithelial cell cultures. *American Journal of Veterinary Research* **73**(2), 296–301.

Allen, K.J., Tremaine, W.H. and Franklin, S.H. (2006). Prevalence of inflammatory airway disease in national hunt horses referred for investigation of poor athletic performance. *Equine Veterinary Journal Suppl* (**36**), 529–534.

Barr, C.A., Tomlinson, J., Boston, R., Soma, L. and Nolen-Walston, R.D. (2013). The effect of chronic clenbuterol administration on mucociliary clearance and repartitioning in adult horses. *Journal of Veterinary Internal Medicine* **27**(3), 668–669.

Bedenice, D., Mazan, M.R. and Hoffman, A.M. (2008). Association between cough and cytology of bronchoalveolar lavage fluid and pulmonary function in horses diagnosed with inflammatory airway disease. *Journal of Veterinary Internal Medicine* **22**(4), 1022–1028.

Beekman, L., Tohver, T., Dardari, R. and Léguillette, R. (2011). Evaluation of suitable reference genes for gene expression studies in bronchoalveolar lavage cells from horses with inflammatory airway disease. *BMC Molecular Biology* **12**, 5.

Beekman, L., Tohver, T. and Léguillette, R. (2012). Comparison of cytokine mRNA expression in the bronchoalveolar lavage fluid of horses with inflammatory airway disease and bronchoalveolar lavage mastocytosis or neutrophilia using REST software analysis. *Journal of Veterinary Internal Medicine* **26**(1), 153–161.

Berndt, A., Derksen, F.J. and Robinson, N.E. (2010). Endotoxin concentrations within the breathing zone of horses are higher in stables than on pasture. *Veterinary Journal*, **183**(1), 54–57.

Burrell, M.H., Wood, J.L., Whitwell, K.E., Chanter, N., Mackintosh, M.E. and Mumford, J.A. (1996). Respiratory disease in thoroughbred horses in training: the relationships between disease and viruses, bacteria and environment. *The Veterinary Record* **139**(13), 308–313.

Cardwell, J.M. (2007). An epidemiological study of inflammatory airway disease in National Hunt racehorses in the United Kingdom. Open University. PhD Thesis.

Cardwell, J.M., R.M. Christley, V. Gerber, N. Malikides, J.L. Wood, J.R. Newton, and J.L. Hodgson. (2011a). What's in a name? Inflammatory airway disease in racehorses in training. *Equine Veterinary Journal* **43** (6), 756–758.

Cardwell, J.M., Wood, J.L., Smith, K.C. and Newton, J.R. (2011b). Descriptive results from a longitudinal study of airway inflammation in British National Hunt racehorses. *Equine Veterinary Journal* **43**(6), 750–755.

Chapman, P.S., Green, C., Main, J.P., Taylor, P.M., Cunningham, F.M., Cook, A.J. and Marr, C.M. (2000). Retrospective study of the relationships between age, inflammation and the isolation of bacteria from the lower respiratory tract of thoroughbred horses. *The Veterinary Record* **146**(4), 91–95.

Christley, R.M., Hodgson, D.R., Rose, R.J., Wood, J.L., Reids, S.W., Whitear, K.G. and Hodgson, J.L. (2001). A case-control study of respiratory disease in Thoroughbred racehorses in Sydney, *Australia. Equine Veterinary Journal* **33**(3), 256–264.

Christley, R.M. and Rush, B.R. (2007). Inflammatory airway disease. In: McGorum, B., Dixon, P.M., Robinson, N.E. and Schomacher, J. (eds). *Equine respiratory medicine and surgery*, pp. 591–600. Philadelphia, Saunders Elsevier.

Couetil, L.L. and Denicola, D.B. (1999). Blood gas, plasma lactate and bronchoalveolar lavage cytology analyses in racehorses with respiratory disease. *Equine Veterinary Journal Suppl* **30**, 77–82.

Couetil, L.L., Rosenthal, F.S., DeNicola, D.B. and Chilcoat, C.D. (2001). Clinical signs, evaluation of bronchoalveolar lavage fluid, and assessment of pulmonary function in horses with inflammatory respiratory disease. *American Journal of Veterinary Research* **62**(4), 538–546.

Couetil, L.L., Art, T., de Moffarts, B., Becker, M., Mélotte, D., Jaspar, F., Bureau, F. and Lekeux, P. (2006). Effect of beclomethasone dipropionate and dexamethasone isonicotinate on lung function, bronchoalveolar lavage fluid cytology, and transcription factor expression in airways of horses with recurrent airway obstruction. *Journal of Veterinary Internal Medicine* **20**(2), 399–406.

Couetil, L.L., Hoffman, A.M., Hodgson, J., Buechner-Maxwell, V., Viel, L., Wood, J.L., Lavoie, J.P. (2007). Inflammatory airway disease of horses. *Journal of Veterinary Internal Medicine* **21**(2), 356–361.

Courouce-Malblanc, A., Deniau, V., Rossignol, F., Corde, R., Leleu, C., Maillard, K., Pitel, P.H., Pronost, S. and Fortier, G. (2010).

Physiological measurements and prevalence of lower airway diseases in Trotters with dorsal displacement of the soft palate. *Equine Veterinary Journal* **42** Suppl 38, 246–255.

Derksen, F.J., Brown, C.M., Sonea, I., Darien, B.J. and Robinson, N.E. (1989). Comparison of transtracheal aspirate and bronchoalveolar lavage cytology in 50 horses with chronic lung disease. *Equine Veterinary Journal* **21**(1), 23–26.

Earing, J.E., Hathaway, M.R., Sheaffer, C.C., Hetchler, B.P., Jacobson, L.D., Paulson, J.C. and Martinson, K.L. (2013). Effect of hay steaming on forage nutritive values and dry matter intake by horses. *Journal of Animal Science* **91**(12), 5813–5820.

Fogarty, U. and Buckley, T. (1991). Bronchoalveolar lavage findings in horses with exercise intolerance. *Equine Veterinary Journal* **23**(6), 434–437.

Fortier, G., van Erck, E., Fortier, C., Richard, E., Pottier, D., Pronost, S., Miszczak, F., Thiry, E. and Lekeux, P. (2009). Herpesviruses in respiratory liquids of horses: putative implication in airway inflammation and association with cytological features. *Veterinary Microbiology* **139**(1–2) 34–41.

Gerber, V., Robinson, N.E. and Luethi, E. (2001). *Comparison of airway inflammation and mucus between younger versus older stabled clinically healthy horses.* In World Equine Airways Symposium Conference Proceedings.

Gerber, V., Robinson, N.E., Luethi, S., Marti, E., Wampfler, B. and Straub, R. (2003). Airway inflammation and mucus in two age groups of asymptomatic well-performing sport horses. *Equine Veterinary Journal* **35**(5), 491–495.

Haltmayer, E., Reiser, S., Schramel, J.P. and van den Hoven, R. (2013). Breathing pattern and thoracoabdominal asynchrony in horses with chronic obstructive and inflammatory lung disease. *Research in Veterinary Science* **95**(2), 654–659.

Hare, J.E. and Viel, L. (1998). Pulmonary eosinophilia associated with increased airway responsiveness in young racing horses. *Journal of Veterinary Internal Medicine* **12**(3), 163–170.

Hare, J.E., Viel, L., O'Byrne, P.M. and Conlon, P.D. (1994). Effect of sodium cromoglycate on light racehorses with elevated metachromatic cell numbers on bronchoalveolar lavage and reduced exercise tolerance. *Journal of Veterinary Pharmacology and Therapeutics* **17**(3), 237–244.

Hoffman, A.M., Mazan, M.R. and Ellenberg, S. (1998). Association between bronchoalveolar lavage cytologic features and airway reactivity in horses with a history of exercise intolerance. *American Journal of Veterinary Research* **59**(2), 176–181.

Holcombe, S.J., Jackson, C., Gerber, V., Jefcoat, A., Berney, C., Eberhardt, S. and Robinson, N.E. (2001). Stabling is associated with airway inflammation in young Arabian horses. *Equine Veterinary Journal* **33**(3), 244–249.

Holcombe, S.J., Robinson, N.E., Derksen, F.J., Bertold, B., Genovese, R., Miller, R., de Feiter Rupp, H., Carr, E.A., Eberhart, S.W., Boruta, D. and Kaneene, J.B. (2006). Effect of tracheal mucus and tracheal cytology on racing performance in Thoroughbred racehorses. *Equine Veterinary Journal* **38**(4), 300–304.

Hughes, K.J., Malikides, N., Hodgson, D.R. and Hodgson, J.L. (2003). Comparison of tracheal aspirates and bronchoalveolar lavage in racehorses. 1. Evaluation of cytological stains and the percentage of mast cells and eosinophils. *Australian Veterinary Journal* **81**(11), 681–684.

Hughes, K.J., Nicolson, L., Da Costa, N., Franklin, S.H., Allen, K.J. and Dunham, S.P. (2011). Evaluation of cytokine mRNA expression in

bronchoalveolar lavage cells from horses with inflammatory airway disease. *Veterinary Immunology and Immunopathology*, **140**(1–2) 82–89.

Koblinger, K., Nicol, J., McDonald, K., Wasko, A., Logie, N., Weiss, M. and Léguillette, R. (2011). Endoscopic assessment of airway inflammation in horses. *Journal of Veterinary Internal Medicine* **25**(5), 1118–1126.

Koblinger, K., Hecker, K., Nicol, J., Wasko, A., Fernandez, N. and Léguillette, R. (2013). Bronchial collapse during bronchoalveolar lavage in horses is an indicator of lung inflammation. *Equine Veterinary Journal* **46**(1), 50–55.

Koch, C., Straub, R., Ramseyer, A., Widmer, A., Robinson, N.E. and Gerber, V. (2007). Endoscopic scoring of the tracheal septum in horses and its clinical relevance for the evaluation of lower airway health in horses. *Equine Veterinary Journal* **39**(2), 107–112.

Lapointe, J.M., Vrins, A. and Lavoie, J.P. (1994). Effects of centrifugation and specimen preparation technique on bronchoalveolar lavage analysis in horses. *Equine Veterinary Journal* **26**(3), 227–229.

Lavoie, J.P., Cesarini, C., Lavoie-Lamoureux, A., Moran, K., Lutz, S., Picandet, V., Jean, D. and Marcoux, M. (2011). Bronchoalveolar lavage fluid cytology and cytokine messenger ribonucleic acid expression of racehorses with exercise intolerance and lower airway inflammation. *Journal of Veterinary Internal Medicine* **25**(2), 322–329.

Leclere, M., Lavoie-Lamoureux, A., Joubert, P., Relave, F., Setlakwe, E.L., Beauchamp, G., Couture, C., Martin, J.G. and Lavoie, J.P. (2012). Corticosteroids and antigen avoidance decrease airway smooth muscle mass in an equine asthma model. *American Journal of Respiratory Cell and Molecular Biology* **47**(5), 589–596.

Malikides, N. and Christley, R.M. (2003a). *Effect of respirable and total endotoxin on neutrophilic inflammation of lower airways in young Thoroughbred racehorses in Sydney, Australia.* In International Symposia on Veterinary Epidemiology and Economics conference proceedings, Vina del Mar, Chile.

Malikides, N. (2003b). *The epidemiology of inflammatory airway disease in young Thoroughbred racehorses in Australia.* Veterinary Clinical Sciences, Camden, Australia, University of Sydney. PhD Thesis.

Malikides, N., Hughes, K.J., Hodgson, D.R. and Hodgson, J.L. (2003c). Comparison of tracheal aspirates and bronchoalveolar lavage in racehorses. 2. Evaluation of the diagnostic significance of neutrophil percentage. *Australian Veterinary Journal* **81**(11), 685–687.

May, S., Romberger, D.J. and Poole, J.A. (2012). Respiratory health effects of large animal farming environments. *Journal of Toxicology and Environmental Health Part B Critical Reviews* **15**(8), 524–541.

Mazan, M.R. and Hoffman, A.M. (2001). Effects of aerosolized albuterol on physiologic responses to exercise in Standardbreds. *American Journal of Veterinary Research* **62**(11), 1812–1817.

Mazan, M.R., Vin, R. and Hoffman, A.M. (2005). Radiographic scoring lacks predictive value in inflammatory airway disease. *Equine Veterinary Journal* **37**(6), 541–545.

McGorum, B.C., Ellison, J. and Cullen, R.T. (1998). Total and respirable airborne dust endotoxin concentrations in three equine management systems. *Equine Veterinary Journal* **30**(5), 430–434.

McKane, S.A., Rose, R.J. and Evans, D.L. (1995). Comparison of bronchoalveolar lavage findings and measurements of gas exchange during exercise in horses with poor racing performance. *New Zealand Veterinary Journal* **43**(5), 179–182.

McKane, S.A. and Slocombe, R.F. (1999). Sequential changes in bronchoalveolar cytology after autologous blood inoculation. *Equine Veterinary Journal Suppl* (**30**), 126–130.

McKane, S.A. and Slocombe, R.F. (2010). Experimental mild pulmonary inflammation promotes the development of exercise-induced pulmonary haemorrhage. *Equine Veterinary Journal Suppl* (**38**), 235–239.

Moore, B.R., Krakowka, S., Robertson, J.T. and Cummins, J.M. (1995). Cytologic evaluation of bronchoalveolar lavage fluid obtained from Standardbred racehorses with inflammatory airway disease. *American Journal of Veterinary Research* **56**(5), 562–567.

Moore, B.R., Krakowka, S., Mcvey, D.S., Cummins, J.M. and Robertson, J.T. (1997). Inflammatory markers in bronchoalveolar lavage fluid of Standardbred racehorses with inflammatory airway disease: response to interferon-alpha. *Equine Veterinary Journal* **29**(2), 142–147.

Moore, I., Horney, B., Day, K., Lofstedt, J. and Cribb, A.E. (2004). Treatment of inflammatory airway disease in young standardbreds with interferon alpha. *Canadian Veterinary Journal* **45**(7), 594–601.

Moore-Colyer, M.J.S. (1996). Effects of soaking hay fodder for horses on dust and mineral content. *Animal Science* **63**(02), 337–342.

Newton, J.R., Wood, J.L. and Chanter, N. (2003). A case control study of factors and infections associated with clinically apparent respiratory disease in UK Thoroughbred racehorses. *Preventive Veterinary Medicine* **60**(1), 107–132.

Nolen-Walston, R.D., Harris, M., Agnew, M.E., Martin, B.B., Reef, V.B., Boston, R.C. and Davidson, E.J. (2013). Clinical and diagnostic features of inflammatory airway disease subtypes in horses examined because of poor performance: 98 cases (2004–2010). *Journal of the American Veterinary Medical Association* **242**(8), 1138–1145.

Pickles, K., Pirie, R.S., Rhind, S., Dixon, P.M. and McGorum, B.C. (2002). Cytological analysis of equine bronchoalveolar lavage fluid. Part 2: Comparison of smear and cytocentrifuged preparations. *Equine Veterinary Journal* **34**(3), 292–296.

Pilon, F. and Lavoie, J.P. (2013). *Treatment compliance and short-term outcome of inflammatory airway disease in pleasure and sport horses.* In World Equine Airway Symposium Conference Proceedings, Calgary, AB.

Pirrone, F., Albertini, M., Clement, M.G. and Lafortuna, C.L. (2007). Respiratory mechanics in Standardbred horses with sub-clinical inflammatory airway disease and poor athletic performance. *Veterinary Journal* **173**(1), 144–150.

Read, J.R., Boston, R.C., Abraham, G., Bauquier, S.H., Soma, L.R. and Nolen-Walston, R.D. (2012). Effect of prolonged administration of clenbuterol on airway reactivity and sweating in horses with inflammatory airway disease. *American Journal of Veterinary Research* **73**(1), 140–145.

Richard, E.A., Fortier, G.D., Denoix, J.M., Art, T., Lekeux, P.M. and Van Erck, E. (2009). Influence of subclinical inflammatory airway disease on equine respiratory function evaluated by impulse oscillometry. *Equine Veterinary Journal* **41**(4), 384–389.

Richard, E.A., Pitel, P.H., Christmann, U., Lekeux, P., Fortier, G. and Pronost, S. (2011). Serum concentration of surfactant protein D in horses with lower airway inflammation. *Equine Veterinary Journal* **44**(3), 277–281.

Riihimaki, M., Raine, A., Elfman, L. and Pringle, J. (2008). Markers of respiratory inflammation in horses in relation to seasonal changes in air quality in a conventional racing stable. *Canadian Journal of Veterinary Research* **72**(5), 432–439.

Robinson, N.E., Karmaus, W., Holcombe, S.J., Carr, E.A. and Derksen, F.J. (2006). Airway inflammation in Michigan pleasure horses: prevalence and risk factors. *Equine Veterinary Journal* **38**(4), 293–299.

Sanchez, A., Couetil, L.L., Ward, M.P. and Clark, S.P. (2005). Effect of airway disease on blood gas exchange in racehorses. *Journal of Veterinary Internal Medicine* **19**(1), 87–92.

Slater, J. (2007). Bacterial Infections of the Equine Respiratory Tract. In: McGorum, B., Dixon, P.M., Robinson, N.E. and Schomacher, J. (eds). *Equine Respiratory Medicine and Surgery*, pp. 327–340. Philadelphia, Saunders Elsevier.

Tremblay, G.M., Ferland, C., Lapointe, J.M., Vrins, A., Lavoie, J.P. and Cormier, Y. (1993). Effect of stabling on bronchoalveolar cells obtained from normal and COPD horses. *Equine Veterinary Journal* **25**(3), 194–197.

Vrins, A., Doucet, M. and Nunez-Ochoa, L. (1991). A retrospective study of bronchoalveolar lavage cytology in horses with clinical findings of small airway disease. *Zentralblatt für Veterinärmedizin Reihe A* **38**(6), 472–479.

Widmer, A., Doherr, M.G., Tessier, C., Koch, C., Ramseyer, A., Straub, R. and Gerber, V. (2009). Association of increased tracheal mucus accumulation with poor willingness to perform in show-jumpers and dressage horses. *Veterinary Journal* **182**(3), 430–435.

Wood, J.L., Burrell, M.H., Roberts, C.A., Chanter, N. and Shaw, Y. (1993). Streptococci and Pasteurella spp. associated with disease of the equine lower respiratory tract. *Equine Veterinary Journal* **25**(4), 314–318.

Wood, J.L., Newton, J.R., Chanter, N. and Mumford, J.A. (2005a). Association between respiratory disease and bacterial and viral infections in British racehorses. *Journal of Clinical Microbiology* **43**(1), 120–126.

Wood, J.L., Newton, J.R., Chanter, N. and Mumford, J.A. (2005b). Inflammatory airway disease, nasal discharge and respiratory infections in young British racehorses. *Equine Veterinary Journal* **37**(3), 236–242.

Woods, P.S., Robinson, N.E., Swanson, M.C., Reed, C.E., Broadstone, R.V. and Derksen, F.J. (1993). Airborne dust and aeroallergen concentration in a horse stable under two different management systems. *Equine Veterinary Journal* **25**(3), 208–213.

18

Inflammation, Endotoxemia and Systemic Inflammatory Response Syndrome

Erin L. McConachie and Kelsey A. Hart

18.1 Definition

Horses suffer from a long list of diseases in which inflammation is central to the pathogenesis of the primary disease process and plays a key role in undesirable, and often fatal, secondary complications of organ failure. Therefore, an understanding of how the immune system orchestrates acute inflammation, and the role it plays in the inflammatory syndromes, is critical for guiding clinical decisions regarding diagnostic testing, therapeutic management, assessment of disease progression, and prognosis.

Inflammation is the normal physiologic response to tissue damage. The immune system is at the core of all inflammatory processes, and it plays the vital role of containing and overcoming infection and tissue damage. Damage to tissues can occur from mechanical, environmental (heat, solar), toxic, chemical or pathogenic insults. Any one or number of these insults will result in an inflammatory reaction by way of a chain of interactions between the damaged tissues, the immune system, and the inflammatory mediators released by both immune and non-immune cells. Specifically, inflammatory mediators generated by the innate immune system ultimately produce the clinically recognized cardinal signs of inflammation: *rubor* (redness), *tumor* (swelling), *calor* (heat), *dolor* (pain), and loss of function.

The overarching purpose of the inflammatory response is to eliminate pathogens and restore damaged tissue. The ideal outcome is *focused damage control* at the affected site, in order to contain the insult, prevent further injury, remove pathogens and damaged tissue, and initiate tissue repair. When the inflammatory response extends beyond the local injured tissues, widespread systemic inflammation ensues and can generate the clinical syndrome known as the *systemic inflammatory response syndrome (SIRS)*. SIRS is a non-specific term used to describe the physiologic response to widespread inflammation.

The clinical criteria for SIRS are well-defined in human patients, and include tachycardia, tachypnea, hypothermia or fever, and leukogram derangements (leukocytosis, leukopenia, or increased band neutrophils) (Bone, 1992). These criteria, derived from human critical care, are often extrapolated and modified to describe this state in the horse and neonatal foal (Table 18.1), but universally accepted equine SIRS criteria have not been defined to date (Corley, 2005; Epstein, 2011; Hart, 2013).

In SIRS, the same inflammatory mediators that are critical to the amelioration of a local insult are produced in massive quantities in multiple sites, circulate throughout the body, and can damage tissues at sites far removed from the initial inflammatory insult. If prolonged and severe, SIRS can result in *multiple organ dysfunction syndrome* (MODS) and multi-organ failure. MODS occurs when two or more organ systems are simultaneously dysfunctional due to reversible organ injury, and it is detected through routine monitoring of hematologic and serum biochemical parameters. Multi-organ failure results when organ damage in MODS is severe enough to produce irreversible organ dysfunction. Equine MODS is typically manifested by some combination of renal damage, gastrointestinal (GI) dysfunction, laminitis, coagulopathy, or cardiovascular dysfunction, though other organs can also be affected.

Sepsis (previously referred to as *septicemia*), as best defined by Bone *et al.* (1992), and updated by Levy *et al.* (2003), is essentially SIRS with a confirmed or strongly suspected infectious etiology. *Bacteremia*, or confirmed bacterial infection in circulation, is not synonymous with sepsis, as bacteremia can, but does not always, result in clinical sepsis.

In human medicine, sepsis is further stratified by severity. *Severe sepsis* is sepsis with the addition of dysfunction in one or more organs, evidence of hypoperfusion (lactic acidosis, oliguria, altered mentation), or hypotension. *Septic shock* is severe sepsis (sepsis with organ dysfunction or evidence of hypoperfusion) with concurrent hypotension that is not responsive to fluid resuscitation. These definitions may seem arbitrary, but they are vital for clear definition of sepsis criteria in clinical studies, and for initiation of *early goal-directed therapy*, which has dramatically improved sepsis survival in human critical care (Rivers, 2008). Similar sepsis syndromes are certainly recognized clinically in horses and neonatal foals, but diagnostic criteria for sepsis, severe sepsis and septic shock in equine medicine are not yet clearly defined.

Endotoxemia is literally the presence of endotoxin in the circulation, but the term is often used interchangeably to

Equine Clinical Immunology, First Edition. Edited by M. Julia B. Felippe.
© 2016 John Wiley & Sons, Inc. Published 2016 by John Wiley & Sons, Inc.

Table 18.1 Criteria for systemic inflammatory response syndrome in horses with organ dysfunction.

Adult SIRS criteria (two or more of the following)	
Core body temperature	< 98°F or > 101.5°F
Tachycardia	> 60 beats/min
Tachypnea	> 30 breaths/min or PaCO$_2$ < 32 mm Hg
Peripheral leukocyte count	< 4000/μL or > 12,500/μL or ≥ 10% band cells
Neonatal SIRS criteria (two or more of the following)	
Core body temperature	< 99°F or > 102.5°F
Tachycardia	> 120 beats/minute
Tachypnea	> 50 breaths/minute
Peripheral leukocyte count	< 4000/μL or > 12,500/μL or ≥ 10% band cells

describe the clinical signs of SIRS that can be induced by circulating endotoxin in the horse. Endotoxin (synonymous with lipopolysaccharide, LPS) is a molecule embedded in the outer leaflet of the cell membrane of Gram-negative bacteria. During bacterial death or reproduction, portions of the cell membrane are released into circulation, and the liberated endotoxin interacts with specific soluble proteins and cell associated receptors. Endotoxin is composed of three regions:

1 a lipid A molecule that is integrated into the outer leaflet of the outer membrane;
2 a polysaccharide core; and
3 a variable O antigen region that extends from the cell membrane into the immediate microenvironment.

The lipid A portion is responsible for inciting the immune response.

The environment that horses inhabit, and the horse's own GI tract, provide readily available sources of endotoxin. Thus, it is not surprising that many naturally-occurring disease processes in the horse implicate a systemic inflammatory reaction triggered by endotoxin in their pathogenesis. Classic examples include colitis, pleuropneumonia, metritis and neonatal sepsis. It is critically important to understand, however, that:

1 endotoxin is not always detected in the circulation of horses with clinical signs of SIRS;
2 many other bacterial and host components besides endotoxin can induce SIRS (e.g., flagellin, lipoteichoic acid, cpgDNA, heat shock proteins); and
3 SIRS/clinical signs of endotoxemia represent clinical manifestations of disease, and are not themselves a diagnosis.

When there is clinical evidence of SIRS or endotoxemia, diagnostics to identify the underlying disease process should be employed, because treatment of the underlying disease when, and if, possible is a key component of therapy.

18.2 Signalment and clinical signs

Horses of any age, breed, sex or discipline that have incurred either a sterile or infectious inflammatory insult are at risk for SIRS. The disease states that are triggered by inflammation exist on a continuum and, therefore, at presentation, the patient may have clinical signs that vary widely in severity and are reflective of a varied time course.

A specific signalment for inflammation, SIRS or endotoxemia does not exist. Factors that play a role in the severity of the clinical signs include virulence of the involved pathogen(s), duration of illness, and the horses' individual response to inflammation, which may be affected by age and co-morbidities. Neonatal foals, horses with endocrine disorders (Equine Metabolic Syndrome, Pituitary Pars Intermedia Dysfunction), and older horses, may have altered responses to inflammatory stimuli, specifically in regard to cytokine expression (Merant, 2009; Tadros, 2013; McFarlane, 2008; Adams, 2008, 2009).

Historical or clinical evidence of a primary infection or traumatic injury is a prerequisite, as SIRS, sepsis and endotoxemia are *never* primary conditions. In adult horses, the initial inflammatory response is often triggered by ischemic or infectious GI disease (intestinal strangulation, colitis, enteritis), though other etiologies (pneumonia, metritis), trauma, surgery, neoplasia, toxins, hemorrhage, or burns can also induce SIRS or sepsis in horses. In neonatal foals, bacteremia occurring secondary to failure of transfer of immunoglobulins at birth, or overwhelming local bacterial infection (e.g., umbilical remnant infection, diarrhea, pneumonia), is the most common trigger of SIRS or sepsis (Table 18.2). Thus, localizing clinical signs related to the primary insult can differ significantly and might be obvious on initial exam (e.g., nasogastric reflux, trauma, external hemorrhage), or may be more elusive (e.g., intra-abdominal hemorrhage, peracute colitis, hepatic failure), necessitating clinicopathologic testing and advanced diagnostic imaging.

Table 18.2 Possible etiologies for SIRS or sepsis in horses and foals.

Infectious	Sterile
Endocarditis	Hemorrhage
Pneumonia/pleuropneumonia	Hemoperitoneum/hemothorax
Metritis	Trauma
Enterocolitis	Surgery
Proximal enteritis	Ischemic gastrointestinal injury
Bacteremia	Neoplasia
Viremia	End-stage organ failure
Fungemia	Toxins
Local fungal infection	Immune mediated
Clostridial myositis	Smoke inhalation
Septic pericarditis	Burns
Cholangiohepatitis	
Peritonitis	
Meningitis (bacterial, viral)	
Hemotropic parasites	
Septic arthritis/tenosynovitis	
Umbilical remnant infection	
Pyelonephritis	**Miscellaneous**
Septic thrombophlebitis	Envenomation

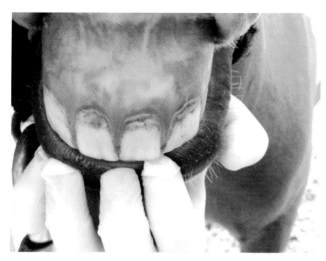

Figure 18.1 The *toxic line* is a clinical sign of endotoxemia/SIRS in horses, and manifests as a hyperemic or purple rim just above the gingival line on the upper incisors, with pallor of the mucosa dorsal to the line. It represents severe vasoconstriction with concomitant stasis of blood in the capillaries.

Clinical signs in horses with systemic inflammation vary greatly with the severity, stage and inciting cause of the underlying disease. Horses with SIRS due to any cause will have clinical evidence of an inflammatory response and related global perfusion derangements. Signs of pain associated with the primary disease process (e.g., an ischemic intestinal lesion or laminitis) are frequently observed. Animals with severe sepsis or septic shock often have clinical signs associated with hypotension, coagulopathy, and organ system dysfunction. Careful and complete physical examination is critical in patients with suspected SIRS or sepsis, in order to determine the severity of disease, to identify the underlying cause, and to detect secondary complications as early as possible.

Clinical indications of inflammation and global perfusion derangements in horses and foals with SIRS include fever or hypothermia, tachycardia, tachypnea, hyperemic or injected mucous membrane color with or without a *toxic line*, rapid or prolonged capillary refill time (CRT), cool distal extremities, poor peripheral pulse quality, or delayed jugular filling. The so-called *toxic line* (Figure 18.1) is somewhat unique to the horse, and manifests clinically as a hyperemic or purple rim just above the gingival line on the upper incisors, with pallor of the mucosa dorsal to the line. This represents severe vasoconstriction with concomitant sludging/stasis of blood in the capillaries, and it has long been considered a clinical hallmark of endotoxemia/SIRS in horses. A rapid CRT is sometimes recognized with the initial phase of inflammation, characterized by marked peripheral vasoconstriction, increased cardiac output and resultant hyperperfusion, while a prolonged CRT is present with severe vasodilation, dehydration or hypovolemia in later stages of SIRS and sepsis.

Discoloration, recognized when evaluating oral mucous membranes, other mucocutaneous junctions, the inner pinnae of foals and the sclera, occurs with SIRS and sepsis-associated perfusion derangements in horses. Hyperemia is a result of vasodilation of the peripheral capillary beds, and it usually occurs secondary to the initial phase of inflammation and response to endotoxin, in which there is a transient vasoconstrictive period, mediated by endothelin. Petechiation or ecchymoses may represent capillary damage from inflammatory cells, platelet dysfunction or secondary coagulopathy. In addition, the presence of pitting edema of the distal limbs, ventral abdomen, and/or prepuce/udder provides clinical evidence of increased vascular permeability or vasculitis associated with SIRS or sepsis.

The perfusion derangements that are seen in horses with SIRS, endotoxemia and sepsis are dynamic and can change rapidly, depending on the integrity of the vasomotor control and vascular permeability in individual tissue beds. The blood volume is likely to be maldistributed, with blood pooling in some tissue beds, while severe vasoconstriction exists in others. In some cases, it may prove useful to employ more objective hemodynamic monitoring methods in order to better assess perfusion (see Section 18.5).

Painful behaviors in horses with SIRS or sepsis are similar to those seen in other conditions and can include weight shifting, muscle fasciculation, avoidance behaviors, restlessness, agitation, lethargy, depression, recumbency, rolling, flank watching, and kicking. Scoring systems for evaluating abdominal pain in the horse post-celiotomy that are likely to be applicable to horses with SIRS or sepsis have been published (Pritchett, 2003; Graubner, 2011). Early detection of pain and provision of adequate targeted analgesia is a major consideration in humans with SIRS/sepsis conditions, as increased sympathetic tone associated with the pain response is in itself pro-inflammatory, and perpetuates morbidity in patients (Mizock, 2009; Dunser, 2009).

Evidence of SIRS-induced organ dysfunction on physical examination varies depending on the organ system involved, and often requires clinicopathologic testing, advanced diagnostic imaging, or both, to verify the dysfunction and to serially monitor the patient for response to treatment.

In any horse presenting with signs of SIRS or sepsis, clinical aberrations solely provide evidence that there is a disseminated inflammatory response, but this does not elucidate the underlying etiology. A thorough physical examination and case-appropriate diagnostics are key next steps to determining the underlying cause.

18.3 Immunologic mechanisms and etiologic associations

The innate immune system is integral to the pathogenesis of the clinically recognized acute inflammatory disorders of SIRS, endotoxemia and sepsis syndromes. Without the innate immune system, these often harmful inflammatory syndromes would not exist. Instead, the host would quickly succumb to overwhelming infection, and would not be able to repair tissues appropriately after trauma. In the past 10–15 years, intricate and complex innate signaling pathways have been uncovered, and these are now recognized as the vital link between innate and adaptive immunity (O'Neill, 2013). These pathways have also provided myriad potential targets for therapeutic intervention.

In essence, clinical inflammation results from the following events:

1 Innate immune cells recognize a threat to the host.
2 Inflammatory mediators are up-regulated and released in response to receptor-mediated intracellular signaling.
3 Local and circulating mediators elicit local and systemic inflammatory reactions by the host, be it beneficial or harmful.

18.3.1 Recognition of a threat

It is the responsibility of the innate immune system to alert the immune system to, and defend the host against, microorganisms, and to initiate tissue repair when damage occurs. Beyond and interspersed within the defensive barriers (skin, mucosal surfaces) are a subset of immune cells that play the part of "watchdogs" for danger and tissue damage. These *sentinel cells* include macrophages, mast cells and dendritic cells, and they are stationed throughout the body. Along with neutrophils and the complement system, they make up the majority of the innate response, which functions to alert other immune cells that a threat – a pathogen, damaged tissue, or toxin – is present.

The cells of the innate immune system employ a conservative, yet ingenious technique to detect danger: they express *pattern recognition receptors* (PRR). PRRs recognize highly conserved molecular motifs that represent a vital functional or structural component of bacterial, viral, fungal, protozoal, or parasitic organisms, aptly named *pathogen associated molecular patterns* (PAMPs).

The prototypical PRRs are the Toll-like receptors (TLRs), which are a closely related family of germline-encoded proteins. Each TLR has a domain responsible for the reaction with its specific ligand. It also has a domain that, through interactions with adaptor proteins (e.g., MyD88, TRIF, TRAM), initiates downstream signaling, which typically culminates in the translocation of the transcription factor nuclear factor kappa B (NF-kappa B) to the promoter region of genes encoding pro-inflammatory cytokines (Kawai, 2010). In addition to TLRs, other families of pattern recognition receptors exist, including Nod-like receptors (NLR) and receptors for advanced glycation end-products (RAGE). However, to date, their ligands and signaling pathways are less well described in horses, compared with the TLR family.

PRRs are expressed by nearly every cell in the body, though the specific location can vary among PRRs: some span the cell membrane with an extracellular domain that is essential for recognition of extracellular pathogens; others are stationed in the cytosol, or on the membranous surface of various intracellular organelles, with the role of recognizing internalized pathogens or defunct endogenous cellular components. Others are soluble and circulate in plasma, particularly those that activate the complement family of proteins. TLRs 2–9 have been described in horses (Table 18.3).

Despite some redundancy, each TLR tends to recognize a specific ligand, including bacterial components (e.g., endotoxin in Gram-negative bacteria, lipoteichoic acid in Gram-positive bacteria, mycobacterial glycolipids, and bacterial CpG-DNA),

Table 18.3 Partial list of pattern recognition receptors (PRRs) and damage-associated molecular patterns (DAMPs).

Toll-like receptors	Primary cellular location	PAMPs	DAMPs
TLR-2 (TLR-2/1, ILR-2/6)	extracellular	lipoprotein peptidoglycan N-acetyl glucosamine lipoteichoic acid zymosan lipoaribinomannan (mycobacteria)	HMGB1 HSP 60 and 70
TLR-4	extracellular	LPS (endotoxin)	HMGB1 S-100 proteins fibrinogen HSP 60 and 70
TLR-3	intracellular	viral dsRNA	HSPs
TLR-5	extracellular	flagellin	
TLR-7	intracellular	viral ssRNA	
TLR-8	intracellular	viral ssRNA	
TLR-9	intracellular	CpG-DNA	HMGB1
Other PRRs			
RAGE	extracellular	LPS	HMGB-1, S-100 proteins SAA AGE
NOD-like receptors (NLR)	intracellular	peptidoglycan polymers- receptor mediated phagocytosis and lysosomal degradation	

LPS – lipopolysaccharide; RAGE – receptor for advanced glycation end-products; NOD – nucleotide-binding oligomerization domain-containing protein; HSP – heat shock proteins, HMGB1 – high mobility group box 1; SAA – serum amyloid A; CpG-DNA – unmethylated DNA (viral, bacterial, fungal origin); TLR-2/1 – TLR-2 heterodimer with TLR-1; TLR-2/6 – TLR-2 heterodimer with TLR-6; AGE – advanced glycation end products viral RNA, and mannans of yeast. Hence, PRRs (including TLRs) recognize specifically their respective ligands (PAMPS) expressed on microorganisms and toxins. In addition, subsets of endogenously derived ligands released from host cells during cell damage or death represent the status of danger, and are recognized by PRRs. These molecules are referred to as *damage-associated molecular patterns* (DAMPs).

18.3.2 Release of inflammatory mediators

Following a successful interaction between a PRR on an innate immune cell and a PAMP or DAMP, intracellular signaling pathways are stimulated, and the ultimate result is the release of inflammatory mediators (e.g., cytokines, eicosanoids) in the local environment and, often, into the systemic circulation. These inflammatory mediators directly stimulate innate immune cells to home to the site of infection/tissue damage, to direct pathogen clearance and tissue repair, and they serve as the link between the innate and adaptive immune system.

The type of inflammatory mediators produced and released is dependent on a variety of factors, including:
1 The specific PRR-PAMP/DAMP interaction.
2 The cell type that is being stimulated (i.e., peripheral blood mononuclear cell vs. cardiomyocyte).
3 The immediate biochemical microenvironment.
4 The influence of cytokine signaling from adjacent cells.

In general, signaling through PRRs involves a variety of intracellular adaptor molecules (such as MyD88, TRIF/TRAM, ERK, and mitogen-activated protein kinase (MAPK)) and activation of corresponding transcription factors that induce gene transcription of pro-inflammatory cytokines.

Cytokines are small proteins, released primarily by cells of the innate immune system, that function to modulate the immune response. The aforementioned transcription factor, NF-kappa B, is a key regulatory factor that controls production of inflammatory cytokines, although other transcription factors may be involved, depending on the cell type and receptor being stimulated. The quintessential cytokine profile of acute inflammation includes up-regulation in the production and release of the potent pro-inflammatory cytokines tumor necrosis factor-alpha (TNF-alpha) and interleukin (IL) 1-beta, which then promote the production of IL-6, IL-8, and the anti-inflammatory cytokine IL-10. This cytokine profile is reliably produced in *in vivo* experimental studies utilizing intravenous endotoxin infusions (Barton, 1997a; Nieto, 2009).

In a study investigating intracellular signaling pathways in equine monocytes, prototypical ligands for equine TLR-4 and TLR-2 differentially activated MyD88, resulting in expression of TNF-alpha, IL-1-beta, IL-6 and IL-10, while TLR-3 ligation resulted in signaling through an alternate pathway, with expression of unique cytokine genes (Barton, 1997b; Figueiredo, 2009). TLR binding illustrates the complexity, specificity and redundancy of the innate immune system. Diversity in inflammatory mediators also exists as they are up-regulated by a variety of PAMPs and DAMPs, on a variety of cell types, in diverse cellular locations, all of which differentially influence gene transcription by utilizing specific intracellular signaling pathways and transcription factors (Kaczorowski, 2010; Chao, 2009; Figueiredo, 2009).

While the clinical signs of SIRS are generally similar regardless of the PAMP, PRR, and signaling pathways involved, varied cytokine profiles can exact subtle differences in the clinical presentation or severity of SIRS/sepsis and, more importantly, impact the effectiveness of the adaptive immune response and subsequent resolution of disease. Furthermore, an understanding of the specific receptors and intracellular pathways stimulated by a certain pathogen or molecule becomes critically important as these mediators are potential targets for immune modulation and therapeutic intervention in SIRS or sepsis. For instance, a patient with SIRS secondary to the release of endotoxin from a Gram-negative infection would likely respond favorably to a drug that interferes with endotoxin binding to TLR-4, while an animal that has SIRS or sepsis secondary to a Gram-positive bacterial infection mediated via lipoteichoic acid binding to TLR-2 would not benefit from such therapy. However, if the therapeutic target is a key intermediate of an overlapping/common intracellular signaling pathway, a uniform anti-inflammatory therapy may provide benefit, irrespective of the initiating PAMP/DAMP.

18.4 Multi-systemic response triggered by inflammatory mediators

A highly coordinated, targeted inflammatory response at the site of infection is induced by PRR signaling and the resultant local up-regulation of *pro-inflammatory cytokines*. Through autocrine and paracrine actions, these cytokines influence first responder cells (mononuclear phagocytes, neutrophils) to become activated and, subsequently, to liberate a milieu of inflammatory cytokines, such as interferon-gamma (IFN-gamma). IFN-gamma and other cytokines then serve to link the innate and adaptive immune responses systems, and stimulate tissue defenses and repair by impacting the function of both immune and non-immune cells.

Inflammatory cytokines have many additional biologic roles that extend beyond their paracrine and autocrine influence on neighboring immune cells. For example, some cytokines directly influence the central nervous system to create the typical clinical picture of illness, as depicted by lethargy, fever, and anorexia. IL-1-beta directly induces muscle catabolism, resulting in myalgia, common to many viral and bacterial infections. Individual cytokine effects on their prototypical target cells, as well as their physiologic effects, are listed in Table 18.4.

In addition to their role as cellular messengers, many cytokines also act as *chemokines*, most notably IL-8 and monocyte chemoattractant protein-1 (MCP-1). The activity of a chemokine differs from cytokine activity, in that chemokines direct

Table 18.4 Cellular and physiologic effects of key cytokine mediators in SIRS/sepsis*.

Cytokine	Main source	Main function	Influence on other mediators
TNF-alpha	Innate and adaptive immune cells (macrophages and lymphocytes); fibroblasts	Induce release of other pro-inflammatory cytokines, coagulation, fever, cachexia, apoptosis	Promotes downstream upregulation of pro-inflammatory cytokines
IL-1beta		Promotes coagulation, fever, hematopoiesis, leukocyte diapedesis, muscle catabolism (myalgia)	Promotes downstream upregulation of pro-inflammatory cytokines
IL-6		B and T lymphocyte proliferation mediates acute phase reaction, fever	Inhibits release of TNF-alpha and IL-1; promotes release of anti-inflammatory cytokine TGF-beta
IL-8	Macrophages; endothelial cells	Chemokine	Neutrophil influx
IL-12	Monocyte/macrophages, neutrophils, dendritic cells	Promotes cell mediated immune response, Th1 lymphocytes	Induces release of IFN-gamma
IFN-gamma	NK cells, Th1 and CD8$^+$ cytotoxic T cells	Antiviral activity; potential role for reversal of immunoparalysis in sepsis	Increased levels in sepsis
Anti-inflammatory			
IL-10	Immune cells of innate and adaptive immune response	Immunosuppression impaired antigen presentation and phagocytosis	Suppresses release of pro-inflammatory cytokines and promotes sTNFR and IL-1Ra
IL-4	Th2 lymphocytes, eosinophils, basophils	Promotes humoral immune response through differentiation of Th0 to Th2 T lymphocyte	Induces release of IL-4 and IL-13
TGF-beta	Macrophages; smooth muscle cells	Tissue repair, fibrosis, sepsis induced immunosuppression	Suppresses release of pro-inflammatory cytokines and promotes sTNFR and IL-1Ra

*Modified from Schulte (2013).
sTNFR – soluble TNF receptor; IL-1a IL-1 receptor antagonist; NK – natural killer.

inflammatory cells to influx and home to tissues. IL-8 is a potent chemoattractant for neutrophil influx, and promotes expression of adhesion molecules, which first slow the neutrophils racing through the bloodstream, causing them to roll and interact with the endothelium, they then become *tethered* and, ultimately enter into the adjacent tissues via diapedesis. This margination of neutrophils and influx into affected tissues contributes to the often-profound neutropenia documented in horses with SIRS, endotoxemia, and sepsis (Young, 1990; Hedges, 2001).

Many pro-inflammatory cytokines also up-regulate the enzymes responsible for generating lipid-derived inflammatory mediators (eicosanoids), activate the coagulation cascade primarily through tissue factor, and up-regulate the production of reactive oxygen species and nitric oxide at sites of infection or tissue damage. *Eicosanoids* include a variety of inflammatory mediators derived from cellular phospholipid membranes (i.e., the leukotrienes and prostanoids). These molecules are products of the enzymatic activity of lipoxygenases (LOX) or cyclooxygenases (COX) on arachadonic acid, which is cleaved from membrane phospholipids by the enzyme phospholipase A2 (PLA2).

Together, cytokines, chemokines and eicosanoids cause the cardinal signs of inflammation (redness, swelling, heat, pain and loss of function), which correspond to their vasodilatory, increased microvascular permeability, and central and peripheral nervous tissue effects. Some eicosanoids are also directly pyrogenic through effects on thermoregulatory neurons in the hypothalamus (Blatteis, 2007).

At sites of active inflammation, neutrophils, macrophages and endothelial cells are stimulated by cytokines, PAMPs and opsonized pathogens to release *reactive oxygen species* (ROS). ROS are chemically reactive molecules that contain oxygen, including oxygen ions and hydrogen peroxide, and they directly destroy cell membranes of pathogens and damaged host cells to aid in clearance of infectious organisms and damaged cells. In addition, they induce NF-kappa B to stimulate production of additional inflammatory mediators and further perpetuate the inflammatory response. The ROS superoxide anion can also react with nitric oxide (NO), a reactive nitrogen species (RNS) produced by endothelial cells via cytokine-mediated induction of inducible nitric oxide synthase (iNOS). The resulting reactive peroxynitrite radicals are cytotoxic, and aid in the clearance of microbes and damaged tissue.

18.4.1 Endotoxin-induced SIRS: from start to finish

In the horse, endotoxin contributes to the pathogenesis of a variety of equine disease states, including neonatal sepsis and acute GI disease in the adult horse. When horses are administered endotoxin intravenously or intraperitoneally, clinical signs of SIRS (fever, tachycardia, tachypnea and leukopenia), with the addition of hypotension and abdominal pain, are consistently produced.

Healthy horses challenged with an endotoxin infusion were shown to have cytokine gene expression of TNF-alpha, IL-1beta and IL-8 peak at 60 minutes post-infusion, while gene expression of IL-6 peaked at 90 minutes post-infusion (Nieto, 2009).

These cytokines mediate SIRS and sepsis syndromes in humans and other species (Schulte, 2013; Andaluz-Ojeda, 2012). In essence, experimental endotoxemia is clinically manifested as severe SIRS.

In naturally occurring endotoxin-induced SIRS, horses are exposed to endotoxin or Gram-negative bacteria through a number of ways, including inhalation, GI translocation, infected wounds, or from direct intravenous administration of contaminated injectable medications. Once endotoxin has breached the defensive barriers, a number of key proteins and accessory molecules are critical to the development of an inflammatory response. LPS first interacts with LPS-binding protein (LBP), a plasma acute-phase protein, and this interaction facilitates subsequent binding to the soluble or cell-associated co-receptor CD14. The LPS/LBP/CD14 complex recruits and activates TLR-4 on mononuclear phagocytes, neutrophils, endothelial cells, and dendritic cells. Finally, the new complex recruits an accessory component, MD-2, necessary for intracellular signaling.

On ligation of TLR-4, the conserved intracellular domain of the receptor initiates multiple downstream pathways that culminate in translocation to the nucleus of the inducible transcription factor NF-kappa B. NF-kappa B binds to consensus sequences on the promoter or enhancer regions of an array of genes, modulating the production of inflammatory molecules, including proinflammatory cytokines (TNF-alpha, IL-1beta, IL-6, IL-8, IL-12, IL-18), chemokines (IL-8), pro-coagulants, adhesion molecules, immunoreceptors (TNF receptors), enzymes (elastase), and acute phase proteins (fibrinogen). Two of the cytokines secreted by macrophages, IL-12 and IL-18, stimulate IFN-gamma synthesis and secretion from natural killer (NK) and T cells (Schroder, 2004). Because IFN-gamma is a potent stimulator of both innate and acquired immune responses, it is considered to be a principal link between the two systems.

Simultaneously with the cellular activation, endotoxin interacts with soluble PRRs normally present in plasma. Of particular importance, endotoxin binds to complement proteins to initiate the lectin-dependent and alternative pathways of complement activation. It also activates coagulation factor XII (Hageman factor) to activate the contact system of intravascular coagulation.

The initial production of inflammatory mediators concurrent with activation of the complement and coagulation systems by endotoxin has been described as a *cytokine storm*, during which there is flooding of inflammatory, procoagulant, and vasoactive mediators throughout the body. The net effects of these mediators promote microvascular injury and hypotension.

In addition, they promote the expression of selectins on endothelial cells and neutrophils for *tethering* the neutrophil to the endothelial surface, which results in progressive *rolling* along and attachment to the endothelial surface, and diapedesis between adjacent cells.

Sequestration of neutrophils on activated endothelium in affected tissues (particularly in areas of low shear force (i.e., postcapillary venules in the laminae and GI tract), and in

pulmonary capillaries) accounts for the neutropenia found in most horses exposed to endotoxin. These neutrophil-endothelial conjugates, formed during sepsis, seal off microscopic pockets between the juxtaposed cells, into which cytotoxic products such as ROS and RNS can be concentrated. Digital laminae of horses may be particularly vulnerable to the effects of ROS, because of low content of the endogenous oxidant scavenger superoxide dismutase (Loftus, 2007).

In addition, to direct damage caused by membrane lipid peroxidation, ROS and RNS indirectly stimulate the expression of additional inflammatory, procoagulant, and vasoactive mediators via activation of NF-kappa B in both neutrophils and endothelial cells (Bosmann, 2012). These mediators, such as bradykinin, platelet activating factor, complement proteins, leukotrienes, and eicosanoids, directly increase vascular permeability by promoting active retraction of endothelial cells via phosphorylation of the light chain of nonmuscle myosin. Vascular leak then facilitates the movement of these potentially harmful substances into tissues, eventually causing organ damage. Poor perfusion pressure, direct microvascular injury, thrombosis, and increased vascular permeability, induced by the endotoxin-TLR-4 mediated pathway, lead to ischemia and tissue hypoxia which, if persistent, results in organ injury and failure (Belknap, 2007).

18.4.2 Transition from appropriate inflammation to SIRS, sepsis, and septic shock

Several events dictate whether a patient develops a normal and beneficial immune response as opposed to a dysfunctional and disproportionate inflammatory response:

1 The virulence or pathogenicity of the microorganism.
2 The magnitude of the exposure to the microorganism or the magnitude of tissue damage.
3 The state of the host's immune system, including other diseases, nutritional deficiency, stress, iatrogenic corticosteroids, immunosuppressant therapy.
4 Genetic polymorphisms of molecules of the inflammatory response (receptor, signaling pathway protein, cytokine, target cell).

While genetic polymorphisms have been detected in equine TLR-4, they have not been shown to alter the downstream response to ligation with LPS (Werners, 2006). However, in humans, genetic polymorphisms in pattern recognition receptors, signaling pathways and cytokines are gaining attention, as they appear clinically significant, either as predictors for the risk of sepsis after trauma, or as a prognostic indicator for those with confirmed sepsis (Dong, 2013; Shimada, 2011; Thompson, 2013). Each one of these factors probably plays some role in whether or not the insult is contained, or if inflammation ensues on a global scale.

Another factor that governs the intensity of the immune/ inflammatory response is that of two *hits* on the host. For example, in a horse with a large colon volvulus, intestinal strangulation and the resultant tissue ischemia and cellular necrosis leads to the release of DAMPS, representing the first (non-infectious) hit, which stimulates a systemic inflammatory response. After surgical correction of the volvulus, return of the blood supply can result in both reperfusion injury and mural translocation of bacteria across a compromised mucosal barrier. This is the *second hit* to the already activated immune system, which can result in transformation of a beneficial, regulated inflammatory response, that aids in tissue repair, to a detrimental overzealous systemic inflammatory response that can perpetuate tissue damage and cause multi-organ failure.

If inflammatory stimuli persist, such as in the face of severe or virulent bacterial infection, severe sepsis and septic shock develop, resulting in altered perfusion and widespread microvascular and mitochondrial injury, which then decreases oxygen delivery and use at the cell, tissue, and organ levels (Bosmann, 2012; Galley, 2010; Rocha, 2012).

Indeed, the fundamental event in severe sepsis induced by endotoxin and other PAMPs is the development of global tissue hypoxia, perhaps also complicated by *dysoxia* (impaired oxygen utility) (Castellheim, 2009). Activation of local and systemic inflammatory responses results in production of ROS and RNS, as described above, which can directly and irreversibly damage cells and inhibit normal cellular activity. In health, ROS and RNS production is tightly regulated by inducible antioxidant enzymes, but these enzymes are impaired by excessive ROS and RNS production, resulting in an overall pro-oxidant environment. Mitochondria are a key source of ROS and RNS, but they are also very sensitive to oxidative injury. Mitochondrial dysfunction and oxidative stress are both well described in sepsis and SIRS, and can result in tissue dysoxia and organ failure. This further stimulates inflammatory responses and NF-kappa B activation, creating the vicious cycle characteristic of severe sepsis and MODS.

Prolonged or severe inflammation can actually result in an inappropriate anti-inflammatory response and undesirable immunosuppression. Horses and humans develop *immunotolerance* to endotoxin, which is characterized *in vitro* by a significant reduction of TNF-alpha production and a progressive decline in IL-12 production (Frellstedt, 2012). IL-12 serves to mediate Th1 responses, particularly to intracellular bacteria. Increased IL-12 levels can be detrimental and exacerbate inflammation, so this cytokine must be tightly controlled to convey a benefit to the host. Immunosuppression from apoptosis of lymphocytes also commonly occurs in the later phases of severe sepsis and septic shock, which is particularly unfortunate if the initial pathogen has not yet been cleared, if tissue destruction is ongoing, or should a second hit (e.g., exposure to another nosocomial pathogen) occur. Therefore, in addition to the detrimental effects of an inappropriately robust and widespread pro-inflammatory response, inappropriate immunologic exhaustion, or an untimely anti-inflammatory cytokine profile, is just as integral to understanding and preventing mortality in SIRS and sepsis syndromes.

18.5 Diagnostics

A clinical diagnosis of SIRS is simply made from physical examination of the patient (see Section 18.2) and a complete blood count with a differential cell count. In SIRS and sepsis, there is often early and profound leukopenia caused by neutropenia, usually accompanied by left shift and toxic appearance of stained cells. Lymphopenia (< 1000 cells/μL) is found in the most severe cases, and is likely to reflect sepsis-induced apoptosis and immunosuppression. Adapted diagnostic criteria for SIRS in horses, based on clinical signs and leukogram parameters, are outlined in Table 18.1, although such criteria have not been systematically defined or universally accepted for horses or foals. Similar criteria defined for people have been criticized as being too non-specific and simplistic. Nevertheless, when two or more of the SIRS criteria are met, the clinician should be on alert because, in many cases, SIRS precedes the development of multiple organ dysfunction or failure (Alberti, 2005; Mizock, 2009).

Under SIRS, confirmed or suspected infection defines sepsis, so therefore, blood, wound, or fluid cultures, and advanced imaging, are used to try to identify sites of infection. Sometimes, infection cannot be confirmed, due to poor growth of organisms in culture or the need to initiate antimicrobial therapy prior to sampling. In foals, such difficulty has led to the development of sepsis scoring systems to predict the likelihood of bacterial sepsis (Brewer, 1988).

In general, a minimum database in a horse or foal that meets SIRS criteria on physical examination and CBC should include: a plasma biochemistry profile to assess organ function; coagulation testing to evaluate for disordered hemostasis; and thoracic and abdominal ultrasonography, to disclose a site of infection that might not be clearly apparent on physical examination. Potential sites of infection should be sampled for bacterial culture and sensitivity to guide therapy.

Biochemical abnormalities are common in horses with SIRS and sepsis. Adult horses often are hyperglycemic at presentation, whereas neonates with sepsis are usually hypoglycemic. Based on parallels drawn between human diabetic complications and sepsis, hyperglycemia is not only detrimental to the vascular endothelium but is, in itself, pro-inflammatory (Mortuza, 2013). However, hypoglycemia is also possible in adult horses in cases with severe septic effusions, such as septic peritonitis secondary to GI strangulation or rupture, or those with MODS that develop hepatic failure. This highlights the need for serial glucose monitoring in equine patients, to detect persistent blood glucose derangements for interventions to restore glucose homeostasis, and to prevent other metabolic disorders.

Other common abnormalities typically reflect altered tissue perfusion and organ dysfunction, such as azotemia which persists despite rehydration, increased liver enzyme activity and serum bile acids concentration, and electrolyte derangements in animals with GI disease, renal dysfunction, or inappetance (Groover, 2006; Underwood, 2010).

Calcium and magnesium derangements (in particular hypocalcemia and hypomagnesemia) are also common in horses and foals with sepsis or SIRS, and these electrolytes play important roles in inflammatory and coagulant pathways. Pro-inflammatory cytokines IL-1 and IL-6 impair equine parathyroid cell function, and are likely to be involved in the pathogenesis of hypocalcemia in critically ill horses (Toribio, 2005, 2011). Endotoxin also has a depressive effect on the parathyroid gland. Prolonged hypocalcemia can result in ileus and coagulopathy, and may contribute to organ dysfunction in some cases.

Hypomagnesemia at admission was documented in a retrospective study of hospitalized horses (Johansson, 2003). Although not directly associated with increased mortality, it was associated with gastrointestinal disease, infectious respiratory disease and multiorgan disease in adults, sepsis in foals, and a longer period of hospitalization. Magnesium has protective roles against neurotoxicity, cardiotoxicity and free radical damage. Hypomagnesemia occurs commonly with systemic inflammation, in conjunction with an increase of pro-inflammatory cytokines and endotoxin in circulation (Stewart 2011a). Because of the essential role that magnesium plays in cellular function, ionized plasma magnesium concentrations should be measured in equine patients with SIRS/sepsis to determine if supplementation is indicated.

Abnormalities in serum or plasma iron concentrations are also common in animals with SIRS or sepsis, and provide an early sensitive, albeit non-specific, indication of systemic inflammation. Iron sequestration is one mechanism that the host uses to limit bacterial growth, and it occurs rapidly after the induction of inflammatory cytokines by pathogens and endotoxin. A decrease in plasma iron has been purported to provide a more sensitive indication of acute systemic inflammation than plasma fibrinogen concentration (Borges, 2007).

Coagulopathies are likely to exist in patients with moderate to severe systemic inflammation or endotoxemia, with variable clinicopathologic evidence of disordered hemostasis. Results can include any to all of the following: reduction in the circulating platelet count ($< 100,000/\mu L$); reduction in plasma fibrinogen concentration; prolongation of the activated partial thromboplastin, prothrombin, or thrombin time; increased activity of plasminogen activator inhibitor-1 (PAI-1); increased concentration of fibrin degradation products; and evidence of hyper- or hypocoagulability on viscoelastic coagulation testing (e.g., thromboelastography) (Epstein, 2011; Dunkel, 2010). Careful monitoring of hemostasis will result in more accurate decisions for treatment than a uniform approach.

Inflammatory biomarkers and markers of organ injury, such as procalcitonin, C-reactive protein, blood lactate, and cardiac troponin I are widely utilized in human critical care settings with the intention of predicting bacterial sepsis, organ dysfunction and mortality (Mehta, 2004; Hoffman, 2005; Anderson, 2010; Pierrakos, 2010). However, according to the 2012 Surviving Sepsis Campaign, there is no current evidence for the use of such biomarkers to differentiate between bacterial infection and severe systemic inflammation of non-infectious origin (Dellinger, 2012). Lactate and cardiac troponin I, easily measured in the plasma and/or serum, have been studied in association with mortality or disease severity in horses and foals with gastrointestinal diseases or sepsis, respectively (Corley, 2005; Tennent-Brown, 2010; Radcliffe, 2012; Nath, 2012). Thus far, changes in concentrations or activity of these molecules over time have proven more predictive than a single point in time measurement, but there remains a large overlap between values in survivors and non-survivors, in most cases. No single biomarker or set of biomarkers is currently available to definitively predict sepsis and survival in horses or foals.

Measurement of blood lactate as a marker of tissue hypoxia in septic animals and people has, in particular, garnered attention in the setting of the intensive care unit. As described above, impaired tissue oxygen utilization occurs in SIRS or sepsis as a result of altered perfusion, metabolic derangements, and mitochondrial dysfunction (cytopathic hypoxia). Serum or plasma lactate concentration correlates to increased tissue anaerobic metabolism, which may be indicative of global perfusion deficits and decreased oxygen delivery to tissues. Increased plasma lactate concentrations at admission, and over time, do correlate with poorer prognoses in some studies in horses with SIRS and septic foals, but no one cut-off value can reliably predict survival in these populations.

There are many other causes of hyperlactatemia besides sepsis-related tissue hypoxia, which include: ischemic tissues (strangulated bowel); abnormal cellular metabolism (cytopathic hypoxia); decreased oxygen carrying capacity subsequent to severe anemia, hemorrhage, or toxins; decreased lactate clearance by the liver; increase in aerobic glycolysis due to sympathetic stimulation and resultant increase in $Na^+K^+ATPase$ activity; and altered metabolism in hyperglycemic states (Michaeli, 2012; Green, 2012). Thus, while the measurement of plasma lactate in animals with suspected SIRS or sepsis can serve as a valuable adjunct parameter for serially assessing cellular function, tissue perfusion and tissue oxygen delivery, it should be considered in light of other clinical and clinicopathologic findings. It should not be used as a surrogate for appropriate hemodynamic monitoring, or as a sole predictor of the animal's disease severity and prognosis.

Finally, demonstration of circulating endotoxin is definitive proof of endotoxemia in clinical cases with SIRS that is suspected to be associated with endotoxin (e.g., Gram-negative bacterial infection). Approximately 12–29% of horses with acute gastrointestinal disease have detectable plasma endotoxin. However, measurement of plasma endotoxin requires specialized methodology that is not currently available for use in clinical settings (Barton, 1999; Senior, 2011). Tests for other microbial PAMPs or DAMPs that could play a role in equine SIRS/sepsis (e.g., staphylococcal toxins, flagellin, high-mobility group protein B1 (HMGB1)) are also currently unavailable, or limited to research settings.

18.6 Treatment

A variety of different diseases, pathogens, and immune stimuli can initiate a systemic inflammatory response. Therefore, it should not be a surprise that a single universally-effective therapy for horses with SIRS, sepsis and endotoxemia does not exist. Instead, a multimodal therapeutic approach with a variety of supportive and anti-inflammatory strategies (or therapies) are employed, as one silver-bullet therapy for SIRS is unlikely ever to be available.

This multimodal approach to therapy is largely based upon amelioration of the cardiovascular and inflammatory derangements that occur as a consequence of the immune response to PAMPS and DAMPS. Support of the cardiovascular system provides the cornerstone for clinical treatment of SIRS and endotoxemia. There are also integral therapeutic considerations, such as: elimination of the underlying disease process; neutralization of endotoxin or inflammatory mediators; amelioration of systemic inflammation; prevention of laminitis and other organ failure; and supportive nursing care.

18.6.1 Cardiovascular support

The cardiovascular system is dynamically, and often profoundly, affected in all stages of SIRS. The clinical signs of SIRS or sepsis in people and horses, including dull mentation, a rapid hypokinetic pulse with cool distal extremities, profuse sweating, and mucous membrane discoloration, reflect a state of hypotension and hypoperfusion that can progress to irreversible ischemic and hypoxic organ damage. The mainstay for cardiovascular resuscitation for both human and equine patients with SIRS or sepsis is intravenous crystalloid replacement fluids.

In human intensive care units, patients are initially administered crystalloid fluids with the addition of an inotrope, vasopressor and/or packed red blood cells as necessary to meet a set of physiologically-derived cardiovascular endpoints within the first 6 hours of hospitalization. This practice, coined *early goal directed therapy* by Rivers in 2001 was shown to reduce mortality rates in humans with septic shock by as much as 16%, and is considered the most vital immediate intervention. Interestingly, a laboratory animal model of shock induced by septic peritonitis demonstrated immunomodulatory and metabolic benefits, in addition to amelioration of circulatory failure, with low volume 7.2% hypertonic saline administration (Shih, 2012). Similar endpoints have not yet been defined for SIRS or sepsis therapy in horses but, owing to their large vascular space, the logistics of achieving similar cardiovascular endpoints with crystalloids alone may prove challenging.

Various studies using the endotoxin challenge model failed to find a significant difference in hemodynamics under general anesthesia when administration of intravenous hypertonic saline and 6% hydroxyethyl starch were compared to intravenous crystalloid fluids (Pantaleon, 2006). No matter what fluid therapy is decided upon, the ultimate goal is to improve cardiac output, thereby improving tissue perfusion and microcirculatory function. In the horse, a reduction in heart rate and plasma lactate concentration, along with improved peripheral pulse quality, mentation and urination, would suggest clinical improvement in the hemodynamic status.

In horses with colitis, pleuropneumonia and strangulating gastrointestinal lesions, there is a likelihood of plasma protein loss in the underlying disease process. In cases of severe hypoproteinemia, aggressive crystalloid fluid resuscitation may be detrimental, with resultant large fluid losses into the interstitial space of skin, third spaces (pleural, pericardial, peritoneal) and parenchymatous organs, and such edema could worsen hemodynamic disturbances and potentiate organ dysfunction. Crystalloid fluids must be used judiciously in these situations, and be accompanied by an appropriate oncotic agent.

18.6.2 Management of the underlying disease process and antimicrobials

General principles for clinical management include removing the source of infection or inflammation whenever possible, and the use of targeted antimicrobial therapy, based on location and pathogens that are most likely to be recovered when justified. Trauma, toxins, neoplasia, and many gastrointestinal diseases (e.g., ischemic intestinal lesions) often result in SIRS and septic shock-like syndromes in adult horses, yet they are not the direct result of a pathogen. In adult horses with signs of SIRS, antimicrobial therapy should be reserved for cases where:

1 bacteremia is likely playing a direct role in the pathogenesis of the disease (e.g., endocarditis, cholangiohepatitis, septic jugular thrombophlebitis); or

2 when there is an identifiable source of bacterial or fungal infection (e.g., bronchopneumonia, pleuropneumonia, septic peritonitis, metritis).

Samples for microbial cultures should be obtained whenever possible, and quantitative antibacterial or antifungal susceptibility panels should be used to guide therapy.

In contrast, the approach to antimicrobial use in neonatal foals is considerably different than in adult horses. Neonates that present in a state of hypovolemic shock with signs of SIRS are likely to have bacterial sepsis as an underlying disease process. As such, early intervention with broad-spectrum systemic antimicrobials in neonates with signs of SIRS is critical to a positive outcome.

18.6.3 Neutralizing circulating endotoxin
18.6.3.1 Hyperimmune plasma and serum

An antiserum (Endoserum; Immvac Inc., Columbia, MO), and several hyperimmune plasma products (e.g., Equiplas-J, Plasvacc) produced by immunization of horses against rough mutant endotoxins, are used in equine patients with suspected endotoxemia (in some cases, with off-label use).

As with experimental studies of human and small animals, the use of cross-reactive endotoxin antibodies in horses with either experimentally or naturally acquired endotoxemia has yielded conflicting results. In several studies, there was an impressive reduction of mortality rate or improvement in clinical signs when antiendotoxin serum or plasma was given to horses. However, in other studies, no improvement was demonstrated (Garner, 1988; Peek, 2006; Morris, 1986, 1987; Spier, 1989). Pretreatment of foals with antiserum was associated in one report with significant worsening of clinical response to intravenous administered endotoxin compared with foals that received no pretreatment (Durando, 1994). These disparate results probably reflect, at least in part, variation in the quality of antisera and experimental conditions. Therefore, no blanket recommendation can be made as to the clinical use of such products.

As evidence of the potential general value of hyperimmune plasma, there is one masked, well-controlled study at a single hospital showing reduction in mortality achieved when anti-endotoxin plasma raised against the *E. coli* mutant J5 was given to bacteremic humans (39% for controls versus 22% for those give antiendotoxin plasma) (Ziegler, 1982). In contrast, subsequent large multicenter studies of two different antiendotoxin products failed to show beneficial effects (Ziegler, 1991; Angus, 2000). A recent equine study demonstrated no effect of hyperimmune plasma on clinical parameters or peak plasma TNF-alpha concentrations in horses undergoing an experimental low-dose endotoxin challenge, although peak plasma TNF-alpha bioactivity was reduced in horses receiving plasma, when compared to controls (Forbes, 2012). This suggests that hyperimmune plasma may contain factors, such as soluble TNF-alpha receptor, that could limit the activity of endotoxin-induced inflammatory cytokines. Hyperimmune plasmas (raised against any antigens) also contain colloid, anticoagulant, and increased amounts of substances such as acute-phase proteins, which might have a non-specific beneficial effect in the setting of endotoxemia and sepsis. Therefore, the use of 10–40 mL of hyperimmune plasma (of any specificity) per kilogram can be justified in treatment of endotoxemia, SIRS or sepsis in horses.

18.6.3.2 Polymixin

Polymyxin B is a broad-spectrum cyclic peptide antibiotic with potent endotoxin-binding activity. Potentially lethal side-effects of respiratory paralysis and nephrotoxicity have precluded use of this agent as a systemic antimicrobial drug, but polymyxin B retains endotoxin-neutralizing capacity at nontoxic dosages. Pretreatment of foals with polymyxin B at a dosage rate of 6000 U/kg significantly suppressed clinical and cytokine responses to intravenous endotoxin without causing toxic side effects (Durando, 1994). Repeated administration to ponies of 15,000 U/kg also produced no sign of toxicity (Raisbeck, 1989). At a dose of 5000 U/kg, polymyxin B protected even when given 30 minutes after the start of LPS infusion (Barton, 2004).

The results of a pharmacokinetic and pharmacodynamic study of polymyxin B in horses suggested that the drug could safely be given at 6000 U/kg every eight hours to maintain continuous endotoxin neutralization (Morresey, 2006). Lower doses also appear to have anti-TNF-alpha effects, though for shorter time periods (Parviainen, 2001; Barton, 2004). Thus, in horses with moderate or severe endotoxemia, consideration should be given to the cautious use of polymyxin B given intravenously BID or TID at a dosage rate of 5000–6000 U/kg. Each treatment should be diluted in saline and given over at least 15 minutes.

While polymyxin B and the nontoxic polymyxin B-dextran 70 conjugate PMX622 safely prevented signs of endotoxemia when given before LPS to otherwise healthy horses, the drug has not advanced beyond Phase 1 trials in human patients, because experimental studies showed that it did not protect mice if given after intraperitoneal endotoxin (Mackay, 1999; Lake, 2004; Barton, 2004; Morresey, 2006).

18.6.4 Inhibition of endotoxin-induced inflammation and related sequelae
18.6.4.1 Non-steroidal anti-inflammatory drugs
Non-steroidal anti-inflammatory medications have been a clinical mainstay for the treatment of endotoxemia and SIRS for over 25 years (Shuster, 1997). Through inhibition of cyclo-oxygenase (COX), NSAIDs reduce the formation of prostanoid metabolites (e.g., thromboxanes and prostaglandins) from arachidonic acid, and attenuate much of the adverse effect of endotoxin. Flunixin meglumine, phenylbutazone, ketoprofen, carprofen, meloxicam, firocoxib, and aspirin are examples of this class of drugs used in horses. When flunixin meglumine is administered at 0.25 mg/kg every 6–8 hours in horses, endotoxin-induced prostanoid production is prevented, and maximal anti-endotoxic effects are produced in experimental situations without obscuring the signs of colic or risking toxic side-effects of the drug (Semrad, 1987). However, flunixin does not reduce endotoxin-induced leukopenia. Aspirin does not prevent endotoxin-induced aggregation of equine platelets and, consequently, there appears to be no rationale for adding aspirin to the NSAID regimen (Jarvis, 1994).

Most NSAIDs inhibit constitutive COX-1 activity (in addition to endotoxin-induced COX-2 activity), so there is some morbidity associated with their use. There may be gastric ulceration, right dorsal colitis, renal papillary necrosis and, possibly, impairment of intestinal motility (Blikskager, 1997; van Hoogmoed, 1999). Furthermore, flunixin meglumine has been shown to slow mucosal healing and increase mucosal permeability to LPS in ischemic-injured equine jejunum, though similar inhibition of mucosal barrier function does not appear to occur in the equine colon (Cook, 2009; Tomlinson, 2004; Morton, 2011). However, concurrent administration of misoprostol (a prostaglandin-E1 analogue), or a lidocaine constant rate infusion, ameliorated these effects in an equine model, suggesting that these drug combinations might be more appropriate for horses with endotoxemia due to intestinal ischemia than flunixin alone.

In the light of this toxic potential of equine NSAID use, it has also been suggested that the use of COX-2 selective drugs may minimize side-effects while maintaining efficacy. Three NSAIDs with documented analgesic effect in horses (e.g., firocoxib, carprofen and meloxicam) have been shown to be COX-2-selective in horses (Beretta, 2005; Kvaternick, 2007). Etodolac, a COX-2-specific drug in dogs and humans, is not COX-2 selective in horses when used at analgesic doses (23 mg/kg PO SID or BID) (Davis, 2007). Firocoxib and meloxicam do not appear to retard small intestinal mucosal healing or increase LPS permeability in ischemic-injured equine jejunum as flunixin can, which suggests that these agents could be better suited for provision of analgesic, anti-inflammatory, and anti-endotoxic effects in horses after intestinal ischemia (Little, 2007; Cook, 2009).

COX-2 activity may also have potentially beneficial effects in horses with sepsis, as COX-2 products (e.g., prostaglandin-E2 and prostaglandin-I2) mediate epithelial restitution in damaged equine colon, and are thought to be important in maintaining the antithrombotic phenotype of normal endothelium. However, NSAIDs in the coxib class (COX-2 specific) have also been shown to increase the risk of atherosclerotic cardiovascular disease in humans (Blikslager, 1997; Fosslein, 2005). Similar risks for coxibs in horses have not been described but, at present, firocoxib is the only drug in this class labeled for equine use.

Although various NSAIDs have been shown to effectively prevent the clinical and molecular sequelae of equine endotoxemia in experimental models, there is no convincing study that shows NSAIDs actually save lives in human or equine patients with naturally-occurring SIRS/sepsis (Moore, 1981; Ewert, 1985; Olson, 1985; Moore, 1986; Semrad, 1987; Baskett, 1997; Bryant, 2003; Daels, 1991; Mackay, 2000). A large, multi-center, controlled, masked, prospective study of ibuprofen in humans with sepsis syndrome showed no effect of this drug on the development of shock or acute respiratory distress syndrome, and no improvement in survival (Bernard, 1997). Similar studies have not been conducted in horses to date.

18.6.4.2 Methyl xanthine derivatives

Inflammatory cytokine production by macrophages is suppressed in dose-dependent fashion by methyl xanthine derivatives. This effect appears to be caused by phosphodiesterase inhibition and consequent elevation of intracellular cyclic adenonsine monophosphate (cAMP).

Pentoxifylline, a hemorheologic agent used in human patients, has also been shown to increase red blood cell deformability in horses (Weiss, 1994). Pentoxifylline also inhibits TNF production in horse blood and in cultured equine macrophages, while increasing secretion of prostacyclin (Barton, 1994, 1997). Studies in other species suggest that pentoxifylline stimulates production of the anti-inflammatory cytokine IL-10, suppresses neutrophil activation, and inhibits activation of NF-kappa B (Coimbra, 2005). A pharmacokinetic study in horses has indicated that administration at 10 mg/kg PO BID provides serum concentrations equivalent to those used therapeutically in humans (Liska, 2006). Finally, intravenous pentoxifylline partially reduced adverse signs in horses given LPS (Barton, 1997). Pentoxifylline alone increased white blood cell counts in horses, though this effect is prevented by flunixin (Barton, 1994, 1997).

Thus, there may be a conceptual and potential beneficial effect of pentoxifylline therapy (7.5–10 mg/kg PO BID) in endotoxic horses, though any effect could be partially neutralized by concurrent NSAID administration.

18.6.4.3 Beta-2 adrenergic agonist

Pre-challenge oral clenbuterol administration was investigated in a low-dose endotoxin model, and was shown to significantly decrease leukocyte activation and TNF-alpha production (Cudmore, 2013). The proposed mechanism of action for clenbuterol, a beta-2 adrenergic agonist, is activation of leukocytes, with increased intracellular cAMP and resulting anti-inflammatory effects. At this time, it is not known whether or not this medication would have similar effects in clinical cases of endotoxemia/SIRS/sepsis in horses.

18.6.4.4 Corticosteroids

Corticosteroids, theoretically, have many useful actions for fighting inflammation in endotoxemia, SIRS, and sepsis. These include reduced production of cytokines, inhibition of TNF-alpha production by macrophages, stabilization of cell membranes, and prevention of neutrophil activation. It is surprising, however, that neutral or negative effects of moderate or high-dose steroid use were found in large, multicenter studies of humans with Gram-negative sepsis, most likely related to immunosuppressive effects at these doses (Minneci, 2004). Corticosteroids also are believed to increase susceptibility to laminitis in endotoxemic horses, perhaps by increasing the sensitivity of digital vessels to the constrictive actions of circulating catecholamines or by inducing insulin resistance and hyperglycemia (Bailey, 2010). Therefore, the use of high-dose corticosteroids is currently contraindicated in the treatment of endotoxemia or sepsis in people and horses.

Some human patients with sepsis appear to respond favorably to low, *physiologic* doses of hydrocortisone (synthetic cortisol) (Annane, 2002; Aneja, 2007; Fernandez, 2009; Marik, 2009). Most of these patients have higher baseline cortisol concentrations than healthy people, but are thought to be in a state of adrenal insufficiency termed Critical Illness-Related Corticosteroid Insufficiency (CIRCI), in which the cortisol response is inadequate for the current degree of severe illness. CIRCI also appears to occur in septic neonatal foals, and in horses with systemic illness and SIRS (Hurcombe, 2008; Hart, 2009; Wong, 2009; Stewart, 2011b).

Low-dose hydrocortisone is associated with reduced vasopressor use and lower mortality rates in people with septic shock in a number of reports, though other studies have not demonstrated a beneficial effect (Keh, 2004; Marik, 2003, 2008; Sprung, 2008). At present, low-dose hydrocortisone therapy is recommended for septic people meeting criteria for CIRCI but not universally for all septic patients (Marik, 2008). The use of low-dose hydrocortisone therapy has not yet been reported in septic equine patients, but a 3.5 day tapering low-dose hydrocortisone regimen (1.3 mg/kg/day divided every four hours IV), administered to healthy neonatal foals, was recently shown to ameliorate LPS-induced inflammatory cytokine production from peripheral blood leukocytes, without impairment of neutrophil function, in an *ex vivo* model (Hart, 2011).

18.6.4.5 Heparin

The use of heparin in horses with endotoxemia is somewhat controversial. It prevents microvascular thrombosis, principally by promoting the anticoagulant activity of antithrombin III (AT-III). Unfortunately, heparin cannot reverse existing thrombosis and, because AT-III is consumed during severe coagulopathy, it may not prevent additional intravascular coagulation in such cases. Fresh and fresh-frozen plasma are good sources of AT-III, but also provide clotting factors that could potentiate intravascular coagulation. When given at the recommended intravenous or subcutaneous dose of 40 U/kg TID or 150 U/kg BID, respectively, unfractionated heparin causes intravascular agglutination of equine red blood cells (Moore, 1987). Therefore, it could be argued that the use of heparin might actually exacerbate intravascular cellular plugging, which is theorized to play a role in some cases of laminitis in equine sepsis. This side-effect can be avoided by using *low-molecular-weight* heparin (LMWH), which is non-agglutinating but retains anticoagulant activity, principally via inhibition of factor Xa (Monreal, 1995).

Two clinical studies have suggested that LMWH may have benefits over unfractionated heparin for the prevention of jugular thrombosis or laminitis in some equine colic patients, though this is not universally accepted (de la Rebiere de Pouvade, 2009; Feige, 2003). The use of heparin should be considered in horses with sepsis that are at high risk for laminitis (e.g., duodenitis-proximal jejunitis, colitis, grain overload), or that have evidence of hypercoagulation (e.g., spontaneous venous thrombosis). For the latter setting, unfractionated heparin may be given at a dose of 40 U/kg IV or SC TID or LMWH at 50–100 U/kg SC SID. Either formulation of heparin should be administered along with plasma (10–40 mL/kg). Foals at risk for thrombosis may require a higher dose of LMWH in the range of 100 U/kg SC SID (Armengou, 2010).

18.6.4.6 Lidocaine

Lidocaine hydrochloride (2%), an amide anesthetic agent, is routinely used in equine practice for local and regional analgesia. Systemically administered lidocaine therapy also has benefits, as a component of balanced general anesthesia, for the treatment of post-operative ileus and as an anti-arrhythmic therapy (Cook, 2008, Torfs, 2009; Doherty, 2010; Valverde, 2013). While the mechanism for these systemic applications of lidocaine are incompletely understood, both sodium channel blocking action and anti-inflammatory action via down-regulation of COX-2 are purported to play a role (Cook, 2008; Lee, 2008). Lidocaine administration is reported to result in reduced neutrophil invasion of tissues via decrease of chemoattractant factors, and reduced local and somatic

pain. A decrease in post-operative ileus and improved likelihood of survival have been attributed to the systemic effects of lidocaine (Torfs, 2009).

18.6.4.7 Scavengers of reactive oxygen species

Reactive oxygen species (ROS) are thought to cause corrosive tissue damage during endotoxemia, and potentiate the production of inflammatory cytokines via further activation of NF-kappa B. Ischemia-reperfusion injury, which may contribute to the development of SIRS in many types of equine GI disease, generates ROS from epithelial xanthine oxidase. Ironically, life-saving fluid resuscitation in horses with hypovolemic shock may lead to whole-body ischemia-reperfusion injury and systemic release of ROS. Despite these key associations between oxidant stress and sepsis, little effort has been made to intervene therapeutically at this level.

There is some evidence that allopurinol, a hydroxyl radical scavenger and inhibitor of xanthine oxidase activity, has positive clinical effect during sub-lethal experimental endotoxin infusion in horses (Lochner, 1989). A recommended dose for allopurinol is 5 mg/kg IV, though this has not been evaluated clinically. Because dimethyl sulfoxide (DMSO) has been shown to be a potent scavenger of hydroxyl radicals, with efficacy in rodent sepsis models, it has been considered for use in the treatment of equine endotoxemia despite variable efficacy in experimental models (Chang, 2001).

DMSO is typically administered via intravenous infusion (or by nasogastric tube) as a 10% solution in saline at dose of 0.02–1 g/kg BID. However, intravenous infusion of DMSO at the low and high ends of this dose range was recently shown to have little to no effect on clinical signs (with the exception of fever at the high dose), clinicopathologic abnormalities, and TNF-alpha production after endotoxin infusion in horses (Kelmer, 2008). DMSO may also reduce intestinal mucosal injury after ischemia-reperfusion although, to date, evidence for efficacy in this setting in horses is also mixed.

18.6.4.8 Ethyl pyruvate

Ethyl pyruvate, a stable analog of pyruvate with antioxidant effect, has been shown to have protective efficacy in a variety of models of septic and non-septic shock in rodents and other species (Das, 2006). Additionally, ethyl pyruvate prevented NF-kappa B binding to its nuclear receptor, thus interfering with pro-inflammatory cytokine transcription (Han, 2005; Fink, 2007). A final potential benefit comes from the prevention of bacterial translocation and promotion of barrier function in a rat model of thermal injury (Karabeyoglu, 2008). Because this agent is inexpensive and can be given in intravenous crystalloid fluids, it could have potential for the treatment of endotoxemia and sepsis in horses. Recent reports in equine experimental endotoxemia support this theory, demonstrating beneficial effects on clinical manifestations of endotoxemia (except fever) and suppression of pro-inflammatory gene expression (Cook, 2011;

Schroeder, 2011; Jacobs, 2012). The use of ethyl pyruvate in clinical cases of equine sepsis or endotoxemia has not been described to date, and other antioxidants that have shown benefit in rodent sepsis models (e.g., vitamin C, vitamin E, and *N*-acetylcysteine) have not yet been evaluated in horses with endotoxemia or SIRS/sepsis.

18.6.5 Supportive care

Impeccable supportive care, including nutritional support and adequate analgesia, is of paramount importance in horses and foals with SIRS or sepsis. Excellent reviews on nutritional support and pain management for the critical equine patient are available (McKenzie, 2009; Magdesian, 2003; Muir, 2010). An important consideration when formulating an analgesic plan is that, while the low dose of flunixin meglumine (0.25 mg/kg), as described above, does efficiently block production of key prostanoid inflammatory mediators, it should not be expected to provide adequate visceral analgesia at this dose. Thus, additional analgesic therapy with a higher dose of flunixin meglumine or other agents should be considered.

A unique consideration for supportive care in adult horses with endotoxemia, SIRS or sepsis is laminitis prophylaxis. Our understanding of the best way to prevent this uniquely equine manifestation of MODS is woefully lacking, but current recommendations include distal limb cryotherapy and frog support, along with maintenance of blood volume and tissue perfusion, and non-steroidal anti-inflammatory drugs.

Finally, gastric ulceration is common in septic human patients, resulting in the routine administration of gastric acid reducers (Dellinger, 2013). With the knowledge that adult horses held off feed also develop gastric ulcers rapidly, gastric ulcer prophylaxis should be considered in horses that cannot, or will not, eat (Murray, 1996). However, the pathogenesis of gastric ulceration in neonatal foals appears to be different, and reduction of gastric acidity may in fact be counter-productive, as gastric acid provides an important first-line defensive barrier against Gram-negative enteric bacteria transmissible via the oral route. In one report, critically ill neonatal foals treated routinely with gastric ulcer prophylaxis actually had an increased incidence of diarrhea (Furr, 2012).

18.7 Prognosis and clinical outcome

The clinical outcome of horses and foals with SIRS and sepsis is largely dependent on the ability to identify and correct the underlying disease process before extensive organ damage occurs (Parsons, 2007; Dallap Schaer, 2009; Southwood, 2009; Orsini, 2010). Early recognition of a systemic inflammatory disturbance allows the clinician to provide support of the cardiovascular system, which is essential, irrespective of the underlying disease.

Providing an accurate, early prognosis in these cases remains challenging. Perfusion parameters, such as plasma lactate concentration, have proven useful when measured serially (Tennent-Brown, 2010). In horses with surgical or inflammatory GI lesions, cardiac troponin I has been investigated as a biomarker that might predict survival. Similarly to lactate, it tends to provide an estimate of disease severity, though single time-point measurements are not useful for predicting mortality and should not be used alone to provide a prognosis (Radcliffe, 2012).

Horses that recover from severe SIRS and sepsis are not necessarily at risk to have recurrent episodes of disease. However, inflammation-related end-organ damage might predispose them to organ failure or related complications in the future. In addition, some clinical complications of SIRS and sepsis in horses (e.g., laminitis) can have long-lasting effects on performance, quality of life, and survival, even after resolution of SIRS/sepsis and the underlying cause.

References

Adams, A.A., Breathnach, C.C., Katepalli, M.P., Kohler, K. and Horohov, D.W. (2008). Advanced age in horses affects divisional history of T cells and inflammatory cytokine production. *Mechanisms of Ageing and Development* **129**, 656–664.

Adams, A.A., Katepalli, M.P., Kohler, K., Reedy, S.E., Stilz, J.P., Vick, M.M., Fitzgerald, B.P., Lawrence, L.M. and Horohov, D.W. (2009). Effect of body condition, body weight and adiposity on inflammatory cytokine responses in old horses. *Veterinary Immunology and Immunopathology* **127**, 286–294.

Alberti, C., Brun-Buisson, C., Chevret, S., Antonelli, M., Goodman, S.V. and Martin, C. (2005). Systemic inflammatory response and progression to severe sepsis in critically ill infected patients. *American Journal of Respiratory and Critical Care Medicine* **171**, 461–468.

Andaluz-Ojeda, D., Bobillo, F., Iglesias, V., Almansa, R., Rico, L., Gandia, F., Resino, S., Tamayo, E., de Lejarazu, R.O. and Bermejo-Martin, J.F. (2012). A combined score of pro- and anti-inflammatory interleukins improves mortality prediction in severe sepsis. *Cytokine* **57**, 332–336.

Anderson, R. and Schmidt, R. (2010). Clinical biomarkers in sepsis. *Frontiers in Bioscience (Elite edition)* **2**, 504–520.

Aneja, R. and Carcillo, J. (2007). What is the rationale for hydrocortisone treatment in children with infection-related adrenal insufficiency and septic shock. *Archives of Disease in Childhood* **92**, 165–169.

Angus, P. D., Birmingham, M., Balk, R., Scannon, P.J., Collins, D., Kruse, J.A., Graham, D.R., Dedhia, H.V., Homann, S. and MacIntyre, M. (2000). E5 murine monoclonal antiendotoxin antibody in gram-negative sepsis: a randomized controlled trial. E5 Study Investigators. *JAMA* **283**, 1723–1730.

Annane, D., Sebille, V., Charpentier, C., Bollaert, P.E., Francois, B., Korach, J.M., Capellier, G., Cohen, Y., Azoulay, E., Troche, G., Chaumet-Riffaud, P. and Bellissant, E. (2002). Effect of treatment with low doses of hydrocortisone and fludrocortisone on mortality in patients with septic shock. *JAMA* **288**(7), 862–871.

Armengou, L., Monreal, L., Delgado, M., Rios, J., Cesarini, C. and Jose-Cullineras, E. (2010). Low-molecular weight heparin dosage in newborn foals. *Journal of Veterinary Internal Medicine* **24**, 1190–1195.

Bailey, S. (2010). Corticosteroid-associated laminitis. *Veterinary Clinics of North America: Equine Practice* **26**, 277–285.

Barton, M. and Collators, C. (1999). Tumor necrosis factor and interleukin-6 activity and endotoxin concentration in peritoneal fluid and blood of horses with acute abdominal disease. *Journal of Veterinary Internal Medicine* **13**, 457–464.

Barton, M. and Moore, J. (1994). Pentoxifylline inhibits mediator synthesis in an equine *in vitro* whole blood model of endotoxemia. *Circulatory Shock* **44**, 216–220.

Barton, M., Ferguson, D., Davis, P. and Moore, J.N. (1997a). The effects of pentoxifylline infusion on plasma 6-keto-prostaglandin F1 alpha and *ex vivo* endotoxin-induced tumour necrosis factor activity in horses. *Journal of Veterinary Pharmacology and Therapeutics* **20**, 487–492.

Barton, M., Moore, J. and Norton, N. (1997b). Effects of pentoxifylline infusion on response of horses to *in vivo* challenge of exposure with endotoxin. *American Journal of Veterinary Research* **58**, 1300–1307.

Barton, M.H., Williamson, L., Jacks, S. and Norton, N. (2003). Effects on plasma endotoxin and eicosanoid concentrations and serum cytokine activities in horses competing in a 48-,83- or 159-km endurance ride under similar terrain and weather conditions. *American Journal of Veterinary Research* **64**, 754–761.

Barton, M., Parviainen, A. and Norton, N. (2004). Polymyxin B protects horses against induced endotoxaemia *in vivo*. *Equine Veterinary Journal* **36**, 397–401.

Baskett, A., Barton, M., Norton, N., Anders, B. and Moore, J.N. (1997). Effect of pentoxifylline, flunixin meglumine, and their combination on a model of endotoxemia in horses. *American Journal of Veterinary Research* **58**, 1291–1299.

Belknap, J., Giguere, S., Pettigrew, A., Cochran, A.M., Van Eps, A.W. and Pollitt, C.C. (2007). Lamellar pro-inflammatory cytokine expression patterns in lamintiis at the developmental stage and at the onset of lameness: innate vs. adaptive immune response. *Equine Veterinary Journal* **39**, 42–47.

Beretta, C., Garavaglia, G. and Cavalli, M. (2005). COX-1 and COX-2 inhibition in horse blood by phenylbutazone, flunixin, carpofen, and meloxicam: an *in vitro* analysis. *Pharmacological Research* **52**, 302–306.

Bernard, G., Wheeler, S., Russell, J., Schein, R., Summer, W.R., Steinberg, K.P., Fulkerson, W., Wright, P., Dupont, W.D. and Swindell, B.B. (1997). The effects of ibuprofen on the physiology and survival of patients with sepsis. The ibuprofen in Sepsis Study Group. *New England Journal of Medicine* **336**, 912–918.

Blatteis, C.M. (2007). The onset of fever: new insights into its mechanism. *Progress in Brain Research* **162**, 3–14.

Blikslager, A. and Roberts, M. (1997). Mechanisms of intestinal mucosal repair. *Journal of the American Veterinary Medical Association* **211**, 1437–1441.

Bone, R.C., Balk, R.A., Cerra, F.B., Dellinger, R.P., Fein, A.M., Knaus, W.A., Schein, R.M., and Sibbald, W.J. (1992). Definitions for sepsis and organ failure and guidelines for the use of innovative therapies in sepsis. The ACCP/SCCM Consensus Conference Committee. *Chest* **101**, 1644–1655.

Borges, A.S., Divers, T.J., Stokol, T. and Mohammed, H. (2007). Serum iron and plasma fibrinogen concentrations as indicators of systemic inflammatory diseases in horses. *Journal of Veterinary Internal Medicine* **21**, 489–494.

Bosmann, M. and Ward, P. (2012). The inflammatory response in sepsis. *Trends in Immunology* **34**, 129–136.

Breuhaus, B.A. and DeGraves, F.J. (1993). Plasma endotoxin concentrations in clinically normal and potentially septic equine neonates. *Journal of Veterinary Internal Medicine* **7**, 296–302.

Brewer, B.D. and Koterba, A.M. (1988). Development of a scoring system for the early diagnosis of equine neonatal sepsis. *Equine Veterinary Journal* **20**, 18–22.

Bryant, C., Farnfield, B. and Janicke, H. (2003). Evaluation of the ability of carprofen and flunixin meglumine to inhibit activation of nuclear factor kappa B. *American Journal of Veterinary Research* **64**, 211–215.

Castellheim, A., Brekke, O.L., Espeviks, T., Harboe, M. and Mollnes, T.E. (2009). Innate immune responses to danger signals in systemic inflammatory response syndrome and sepsis. *Scandinavian Journal of Immunology* **69**, 479–491.

Chang, C., Albarillo, M. and Schumer, W. (2001). Therapeutic effect of dimethyl sulfoxide on ICAM-1 gene expression and activation of NF-kappaB and AP-1 in septic rats. *Journal of Surgical Research* **95**, 181–187.

Chao, W. (2009). Toll-like receptor signaling: a critical modulator of cell survival and ischemic injury in the heart. *American Journal of Physiology – Heart and Circulatory Physiology* **296**, H1–12.

Chaumet-Riffaut, P. and Bellissant, E. (2002). Effect of treatment with low dose hydrocortisone and fludrocortisone on mortality in patients with septic shock. *JAMA* **288**, 862–871.

Coimbra, R., Melbostad, H., Loomis, W., Tobar, M. and Hout, D.B. (2005). Phosphodiesterase inhibition decreases nuclear factor-kabba B activation and shifts the cytokine response toward anti-inflammatory activity in acute endotoxemia. *Journal of Trauma* **59**, 575–582.

Cook, V., Jones Shults, J., McDowell, M., Campell, N.B., Davis, J.L. and Blikslager, A.T. (2008). Attenuation of ischaemic injury in the equine jejunum by administration of systemic lidocaine. *Equine Veterinary Journal* **40**, 353–357.

Cook, V.L. and Blikslager, A.T. (2008). Use of systemically administered lidocaine in horses with gastrointestinal tract disease. *Journal of the American Veterinary Medical Association* **232**, 1144–1148.

Cook, V., Meyer, C., Campbell, N. and Blikslager, A.T. (2009). Effect of firocoxib or flunixin meglumine on recovery of ischemic-injured equine jejunum. *American Journal of Veterinary Research* **70**, 992–1000.

Cook, V., Holcombe, S., Gandy, J., Cori, C.M. and Sordillo, L.M. (2011). Ethyl pyruvate decreases proinflammatory gene expression in lipopolysaccharide-stimulated equine monocytes. *Veterinary Immunology and Immunopathology* **141**, 92–99.

Corley, K.T., Donaldson, L.L. and Furr, M.O. (2005). Arterial lactate concentration, hospital survival, sepsis and SIRS in critically ill neonatal foals. *Equine Veterinary Journal* **37**, 53–59.

Cudmore, L.A., Muurlink, T., Whittem, T. and Bailey, S.R. (2013). Effects of oral clenbuterol on the clinical and inflammatory response to endotoxaemia in the horse. *Research in Veterinary Science* **94**, 682–686.

Daels, P., Stabenfeldt, G., Hughes, J., Odensvik, K. and Kindahl, H. (1991). Effects of flunixin meglumine on endotoxin-induced prostaglandin F2 alpha secretion during early pregnancy in mares. *American Journal of Veterinary Research* **52**, 276–281.

Dallap Schaer, B.L., Bentz, A.I., Boston, R.C., Palmer, J.E. and Wilkins, P.A. (2009). Comparison of viscoelastic coagulation analysis and standard coagulation profiles in critically ill neonatal foals to outcome. *Journal of Veterinary Emergency and Critical Care (San Antonio)* **19**, 88–95.

Das, U. (2006). Pyruvate is an endogenous anti-inflammatory and anti-oxidant molecule. *Medical Science Monitor* **12**, RA79–84.

Davis, J., Papich, M.G., Morton, A., Gayle, J., Blikslager, A.T. and Campbell, N.B. (2007). Pharmacokinetics of etodolac in the horse following oral and intravenous administrationq. *Journal of Veterinary Pharmacology and Therapeutics* **30**, 43–48.

de la Rebiere de Pouvade, G., Grulke, S., Detilleux, J., Salciccia, A., Verwilghen, D.R., Caudron, I., Gangl, M. and Serteyn, D.D. (2009). Evaluation of low-molecular-weight heparin for the prevention of equine laminitis after colic surgery. *Journal of Veterinary Emergency and Critical Care* **19**, 113–119.

Dellinger, R.P., Levy, M.M., Rhodes, A., Annane, D., Gerlach, H., Opal, S.M., Sevransky, J.E., Sprung, C.L., Douglas, I.S., Jaeschke, R., Osborn, T.M., Nunnally, M.E., Townsend, S.R., Reinhart, K., Kleinpell, R.M., Angus, D.C., Deutschman, C.S., Machado, F.R., Rubenfeld, G.D., Webb, S.A., Beale, R.J., Vincent, J.L., Moreno, R., SSCG Committee, and Pediatric Subgroup. (2012). Surviving Sepsis Campaign: international guidelines for management of severe sepsis and septic shock: 2012. *Critical Care Medicine* **41**, 580–637.

Dellinger, R.P., Levy, M.M., Rhodes, A., Annane, D., Gerlach, H., Opal, S.M., Sevransky, J.E., Sprung, C.L., Douglas, I.S., Jaeschke, R., Osborn, T.M., Nunnally, M.E., Townsend, S.R., Reinhart, K., Kleinpell, R.M., Angus, D.C., Deutschman, C.S., Machado, F.R., Rubenfeld, G.D., Webb, S.A., Beale, R.J., Vincent, J.L., Moreno, R., SSCG Committee, and Pediatric Subgroup. (2013). Surviving Sepsis Campaign: international guidelines for management of severe sepsis and septic shock, 2012. *Intensive Care Medicine* **39**, 165–228.

Doherty, T.J. and Seddighi, M.R. (2010). Local anesthetics as pain therapy in horses. *Veterinary Clinics of North America: Equine Practice* **26**, 533–549.

Dong, G.H., Gong, J.P., Li, J.Z., Luo, Y.H., Li, Z.D., Li, P.Z. and He, K. (2013). Association between gene polymorphisms of irak-m and the susceptibility of sepsis. *Inflammation* **36**, 1087–2576.

Dunkel, B., Chan, D.L., Boston, R. and Monreal, L. (2010). Association between hypercoagulability and decreased survival in horses with ischemic or inflammatory gastrointestinal disease. *Journal of Veterinary Internal Medicine* **24**, 1467–1474.

Dunser, M.W. and Hasibeder, W.R. (2009). Sympathetic overstimulation during critical illness: adverse effects of adrenergic stress. *Journal of Intensive Care Medicine* **24**, 293–316.

Durando, M., Mackay, R., Linda, S. and Skelley, L.A. (1994). Effects of polymixin B and salmonella typimurium antiseum on horses given endotoxin intravenously. *American Journal of Veterinary Research* **55**, 921–927.

Epstein, K.L., Brainard, B.M., Gomez-Ibanez, S.E., Lopes, M.A., Barton, M.H. and Moore, J.N. (2011). Thrombelastography in horses with acute gastrointestinal disease. *Journal of Veterinary Internal Medicine* **25**, 307–314.

Ewert, K., Fessler, J., Templeton, C., Bottoms, G.D., Latshaw, H.S. and Jonson, M.A. (1985). Endotoxin-induced hematologic and blood chemical changes in ponies: effects of flunixine meglumine, dexamethasone, and prednisolone. *American Journal of Veterinary Research* **46**, 24–30.

Feige, K., Schwarzwald, C. and Bombeli, T. (2003). Comparison of unfractionated and low-molecular-weight heparin for prophylaxis of coagulopathies in 52 horses with colic: a randomised double-blind clinical trial. *Equine Veterinary Journal* **35**, 506–513.

Fernandez, E. and Watterberg, K. (2009). Relative adrenal insufficiency in the preterm and term infant. *Journal of Perinatology* **29**, S44–S49.

Figueiredo, M.D., Vandenplas, M.L., Hurley, D.J. and Moore, J.N. (2009). Differential induction of MyD88- and TRIF-dependent pathways in equine monocytes by Toll-like receptor agonists. *Veterinary Immunology and Immunopathology* **127**, 125–134.

Fink, M.P. (2007). Ethyl pyruvate: a novel treatment for sepsis. *Current Drug Targets* **8**, 515–518.

Forbes, G., Savage, C.J. and Bailey, S.R. (2012). Effects of hyperimmune plasma on clinical and cellular responses in a low-dose endotoxaemia model in horses. *Research in Veterinary Science* **92**, 40–44.

Fosslein, E. (2005). Cardiovascular complications of non-steroidal anti-inflammatory drugs. *Annals of Clinical & Laboratory Science* **35**, 347–385.

Frellstedt, L., McKenzie, H.C., Barrett, J.G. and Furr, M.O. (2012). Induction and characterization of endotoxin tolerance in equine peripheral blood mononuclear cells *in vitro*. *Veterinary Immunology and Immunopathology* **149**, 97–102.

Furr, M., Cohen, N.D., Axon, J.E., Sanchez, L.C., Pantaleon, L., Haggett, E., Campbell, R. and Tennent-Brown, B. (2012). Treatment with histamine-type 2 receptor antagonists and omeprazole increase the risk of diarrhoea in neonatal foals treated in intensive care units. *Equine Veterinary Journal Supplement* **44**, 80–86.

Galley, H. (2010). Bench-to-bedside review: targeting antioxidants to mitochondria in sepsis. *Critical Care* **14**, 230.

Garner, H., Sprouse, R. and Lager, K. (1988). Cross protection of ponies from sublethal Escherichia coli endotoxemia by *Salmonella typhimurium* antiserum. *Equine Practice* **10**, 10.

Graubner, C., Gerber, V., Doherr, M. and Spadavecchia, C. (2011). Clinical application and reliability of a post abdominal surgery pain assessment scale (PASPAS) in horses. *Veterinary Journal* **188**, 178–183.

Green, J.P., Berger, T., Garg, N., Horeczko, T., Suarez, A., Radeos, M.S., Hagar, Y. and Panacek, E.A. (2012). Hyperlactatemia affects the association of hyperglycemia with mortality in nondiabetic adults with sepsis. *Academic Emergency Medicine* **19**, 1268–1275.

Groover, E.S., Woolums, A.R., Cole, C.J. and LeRoy, B.E. (2006). Risk factors associated with renal insufficiency in horses with primary gastrointestinal disease: 26 cases (2000–2003). *Journal of the American Veterinary Medical Association* **228**, 572–577.

Han, Y., Englert, J.A., Yang, R., Delude, R.L. and Fink, M.P. (2005). Ethyl pyruvate inhibits nuclear factor-kappaB-dependent signaling by directly targeting p65. *Journal of Pharmacology and Experimental Therapeutics* **312**, 1097–1105.

Hart, K., Slovis, N. and Barton, M. (2009). Hypothalamic-pituitary-adrenal axis dysfunction in hospitalized neonatal foals. *Journal of Veterinary Internal Medicine* **23**, 901–912.

Hart, K., Barton, M., Vandenplas, M. and Hurley, D.J. (2011). Effects of low-dose hydrocortisone therapy on immune function in neonatal horses. *Pediatric Research* **70**, 72–77.

Hart, K.A. and MacKay, R.J. (2013). Endotoxemia. In: Smith, B.P. (ed.) *Large Animal Internal Medicine, fifth edition*. St. Louis, Elsevier-Mosby.

Hedges, J.F., Demaula, C.D., Moore, B.D., Mclaughlin, B.E., Simon, S.I. and Maclachlan, J. (2001). Characterization of equine E-selectin. *Immunology* **103**, 498–504.

Hoffmann, U., Brueckmann, M., Bertsch, T., Wiessner, M., Liebetrau, C. and Lang, S. (2005). Increased plasma levels of NT-proANP and

NT-proBNP as markers of cardiac dysfunction in septic patients. *Clinical Laboratory* **51**, 373–379.

Hurcombe, S., Toribio, R., Slovis, N., Kohn, C.W., Refsal, K., Saville, W. and Mudge, M.C. (2008). Blood arginine vasopressin, adrenocorticotropin hormone, and cortisol concentrations at admission in septic and critically ill foals and their association with survival. *Journal of Veterinary Internal Medicine* **22**, 639–647.

Jacobs, C., Holcombe, S., Cook, V., Gandy, J.C., Hauptman, J.G. and Sordillo, L.M. (2012). Ethyl pyruvate diminishes the inflammatory response to lipopolysaccharide infusion in horses. *Equine Veterinary Journal* **45**, 333–339.

Jarvis, G. and Evans, R. (1994). Endotoxin-induced platelet aggregation in heparinised equine whole blood *in vitro*. *Research in Veterinary Science* **7**, 317–324.

Johansson, A.M., Gardner, S.Y., Jones, S.L., Fuquay, L.R., Reagan, V.H. and Levine, J.F. (2003). Hypomagnesemia in hospitalized horses. *Journal of Veterinary Internal Medicine* **17**, 860–867.

Kaczorowski, D.J., Afrazi, A., Scott, M.J., Kwak, J.H., Gill, R., Edmonds, R.D., Liu, Y., Fan, J. and Billiar, T.R. (2010). Pivotal advance: The pattern recognition receptor ligands lipopolysaccharide and polyinosine-polycytidylic acid stimulate factor B synthesis by the macrophage through distinct but overlapping mechanisms. *Journal of Leukocyte Biology* **88**, 609–618.

Karabeyoglu, M., Unal, B., Bozkurt, B., Delapici, I., Bilgihian, A., Kakrabeyoglu, I. and Cengiz, O. (2008). The effect of ethyl pyruvate on oxidative stress in intestine and bacterial translocation after thermal injury. *Journal of Surgical Research* **144**, 59–63.

Kawai, T. and Akira, S. (2010). The role of pattern-recognition receptors in innate immunity: update on Toll-like receptors. *Nature Immunology* **11**, 373–384.

Keh, D. and Sprung, C. (2004). Use of corticosteroid therapy in patients with sepsis and septic shock: an evidence-based review. *Critical Care Medicine* **32**, S527–S533.

Kelmer, G., Doherty, T., Elliott, S., Saxton, A., Fry, M.M. and Andrews, F.M. (2008). Evaluation of dimethyl sulphoxide effects on initial response to endotoxin in the horse. *Equine Veterinary Journal* **40**, 358–363.

Kvaternick, V., Pollmeier, M., Fischer, J. and Hanson, P.D. (2007). Pharmacokinetics and metabolism of orally administered firocoxib, a novel second generation coxib, in horses. *Journal of Veterinary Pharmacology and Therapeutics* **30**, 208–217.

Lake, P., DeLeo, J., Cerasoli, F., Logdberg, L., Weetall, M. and Handley, D. (2004). Pharmacodynamic evaluation of the neutralization of endotoxin by PMX622 in mice. *Antimicrobial Agents and Chemotherapy* **48**, 2987–2992.

Lee, P.Y., Tsai, P.S., Huang, Y.H. and Huang, C.J. (2008). Inhibition of toll-like receptor-4, nuclear factor-kappaB and mitogen-activated protein kinase by lignocaine may involve voltage-sensitive sodium channels. *Clinical and Experimental Pharmacology and Physiology* **35**, 1052–1058.

Leentjens, J., Kox, M., Koch, R.M., Preijers, F., Joosten, L.A., van der Hoeven, J.G., Netea, M.G. and Pickkers, P. (2012). Reversal of immunoparalysis in humans *in vivo*: a double-blind, placebo-controlled, randomized pilot study. *American Journal of Respiratory and Critical Care Medicine* **186**, 838–845.

Liska, D., Akucewich, L.H., Marsella, R., Maxwell, L.K., Barbara, J.E. and Cole, C.A. (2006). Pharmacokinetics of pentoxifylline and its 5-hydroxyhexyl metabolite after oral and intravenous administration

of pentoxifylline to healthy adult horses. *American Journal of Veterinary Research* **67**, 1621–1627.

Little, D., Brown, S., Campbell, N., Moeser, A.J., Davis, J.L. and Blikslager, A.T. (2007). Effects of the cyclooxygenase inhibitor meloxicam on recovery of ischemia-injured equine jejunum. *American Journal of Veterinary Research* **68**, 614–624.

Lochner, F., Sangiah, S., Burrows, G., Shawley, R., McNew, R. and Wlaker, J. (1989). Effects of allopurinol in experimental endotoxin shock in horses. *Research in Veterinary Science* **47**, 178–184.

Loftus, J., Belknap, J., Stankiewicz, K. and Black, S.J. (2007). Laminar xanthine oxidase, superoxide dismutase and catalase activities in the prodromal stage of black-walnut induced equine laminitis. *Equine Veterinary Journal* **39**, 48–53.

Mackay, R., Clark, C., Logdberg, L. and Lake, P. (1999). Effect of a conjugate of polymyxin B-dextran 70 in horses with experimentally induced endotoxemia. *American Journal of Veterinary Research* **60**, 68–75.

Mackay, R., Daniels, C., Bleyaert, H., Bailey, J.E., Gillis. K.D., Merritt. A.M., Katz. T.L., Johnson, J.C. and Thompson. K.C. (2000). Effect of eltenac in horses with induced endotoxemia. *Equine Veterinary Journal Supplement* **32**, 26–31.

Magdesian, K.G. (2003). Nutrition for critical gastrointestinal illness: feeding horses with diarrhea or colic. *Veterinary Clinics of North America: Equine Practice* **19**, 617–644.

Marik, P. (2009). Critical illness-related corticosteroid insufficiency. *Chest* **135**, 181–193.

Marik, P. and Zaloga, G. (2003). Adrenal insufficiency during septic shock. *Critical Care Medicine* **31**, 141–145.

Marik, P., Pastores, S., Annane, D., Umberto Meduri, G., Sprung, C.L., Arlt, W., Keh, D., Briegel, J., Beishuizen, A., Dimopoulou, I., Tsagarakis, S., Singer, M., Chrousos, G.P., Zaloga, G., Bokhari, F. and Vogeser, M. (2008). Recommendations for the diagnosis and management of corticosteroid insufficiency in critically ill adult patients: consensus statements from an international task force by the American College of Critical Care Medicine. *Critical Care Medicine* **36**, 1937–1949.

McFarlane, D. and Holbrook, T.C. (2008). Cytokine dysregulation in aged horses and horses with pituitary pars intermedia dysfunction. *Journal of Veterinary Internal Medicine* **22**, 436–442.

McKenzie, H.C. 3rd. and Geor, R.J. (2009). Feeding management of sick neonatal foals. *Veterinary Clinics of North America: Equine Practice* **25**, 109–119, vii.

Mehta, N.J., Khan, I.A., Gupta, V., Jani, K., Gowda, R.M. and Smith, P.R. (2004). Cardiac troponin I predicts myocardial dysfunction and adverse outcome in septic shock. *International Journal of Cardiology* **95**, 13–17.

Merant, C., Breathnach, C.C., Kohler, K., Rashid, C., Van Meter, P. and Horohov, D.W. (2009). Young foal and adult horse monocyte-derived dendritic cells differ by their degree of phenotypic maturity. *Veterinary Immunology and Immunopathology* **131**, 1–8.

Michaeli, B., Martinez, A., Revelly, J.P., Cayeux, M.C., Chiolero, R.L., Tappy, L. and Berger, M.M. (2012). Effects of endotoxin on lactate metabolism in humans. *Critical Care* **16**, R139.

Minneci, P., Deans, K., Banks, S., Eichacker, P.Q. and Natason, C. (2004). Meta-analysis: the effect of steroids on survival and shock during sepsis depends on the dose. *Annals of Internal Medicine* **141**, 47–56.

Mizock, B.A. (2009). The multiple organ dysfunction syndrome. *Disease-A-Month* **55**, 476–526.

Monreal, L., Villatoro, A., Monreal, M., Espada, Y., Angles, A.M. and Ruiz-Gopegui, R. (1995). Comparison of the effects of low-molecular-weight and unfractionated heparin in horses. *American Journal of Veterinary Research* **56**, 1281–1285.

Moore, J., Garner, H., Shapland, J. and Hatfield, D.G. (1981). Prevention of endotoxin-induced arterial hypoxaemia and lactic acidosis with flunixin meglumine in the conscious pony. *Equine Veterinary Journal* **13**, 95–98.

Moore, J., Hardee, M. and Hardee, G. (1986). Modulation of arachidonic acid metabolism in endotoxic horses: comparison of flunixin meglumine, phenylbutazone, and a selective thromboxane synthetase inhibitor. *American Journal of Veterinary Research* **47**, 110–113.

Moore, J., Mahaffey, E. and Zboran, M. (1987). Heparin-induced agglutination of erythrocytes in horses. *American Journal of Veterinary Research* **48**, 68–71.

Morresey, P. and Mackay, R. (2006). Endotoxin-neutralizing activity of polymyxin B in blood after IV administration in horses. *American Journal of Veterinary Research* **67**, 642–747.

Morris, D., Whitlock, R. and Corbell, L. (1986). Endotoxemia in horses: protection provided by antiserum to core lipopolysaccharide. *American Journal of Veterinary Research* **47**, 544–550.

Morris, D. and Whitlock, R. (1987). Therapy of suspected septicemia in neonatal foals using plasma-containing antibodies to core lipopolysaccharide (LPS). *Journal of Veterinary Internal Medicine* **1**, 175–182.

Morton, A., Grosche, A., Matyjaszek, S., Polyak, M.M.R. and Freeman, D.E. (2011). Effects of flunixin meglumine on the recovery of ischaemic equine colonic muscoal in vitro. *Equine Veterinary Journal Supplement* **39**, 112–116.

Mortuza, R. and Chakrabarti, S. (2013). Glucose-induced cell signaling in the pathogenesis of diabetic cardiomyopathy. *Heart Failure Reviews* **19**, 75–86.

Muir, W.W. (2010). Pain: mechanisms and management in horses. *Veterinary Clinics of North America: Equine Practice* **26**, 467–480.

Murray, M.J. and Eichorn, E.S. (1996). Effects of intermittent feed deprivation, intermittent feed deprivation with ranitidine administration, and stall confinement with *ad libitum* access to hay on gastric ulceration in horses. *American Journal of Veterinary Research* **57**, 1599–1603.

Nath, L.C., Anderson, G.A., Hinchcliff, K.W. and Savage, C.J. (2012). Clinicopathologic evidence of myocardial injury in horses with acute abdominal disease. *Journal of the American Veterinary Medical Association* **241**, 1202–1208.

Nieto, J.E., MacDonald, M.H., Braim, A.E. and Aleman, M. (2009). Effect of lipopolysaccharide infusion on gene expression of inflammatory cytokines in normal horses *in vivo*. *Equine Veterinary Journal* **41**, 717–719.

Olson, N., Meyer, R. and Anderson, D. (1985). Effects of flunixin meglumine on cardiopulmonary responses to endotoxin in ponies. *Journal of Applied Physiology* **59**, 1464–1471.

O'Neill, L.A., Golenbock, D. and Bowie, A.G. (2013). The history of Toll-like receptors - redefining innate immunity. *Nature Reviews Immunology* **13**, 453–460.

Orsini, J.A., Parsons, C.S., Capewell, L. and Smith, G. (2010). Prognostic indicators of poor outcome in horses with laminitis at a tertiary care hospital. *Canadian Veterinary Journal* **51**, 623–628.

Pantaleon, L.G., Furr, M.O., McKenzie, H.C. 2nd. and Donaldson, L. (2006). Cardiovascular and pulmonary effects of hetastarch plus hypertonic saline solutions during experimental endotoxemia in anesthetized horses. *Journal of Veterinary Internal Medicine* **20**, 1422–1428.

Parsons, C.S., Orsini, J.A., Krafty, R., Capewell, L. and Boston, R. (2007). Risk factors for development of acute laminitis in horses during hospitalization: 73 cases (1997–2004). *Journal of the American Veterinary Medical Association* **230**, 885–889.

Parviainen, A., Barton, M. and Norton, N. (2001). Evaluation of polymyxin B in an *ex vivo* model of endotoxemia in horses. *American Journal of Veterinary Research* **62**, 72–76.

Peek, S., Semrad, S., McGuirk, S., Riseberg, A., Slack, J.A., Marques, F., Coombs, D., Lien, L., Keuler, N. and Darien, B.J. (2006). Prognostic value of clinicopathologic variables obtained at adminission and effect of antiendotoxin plasma on survival in septic and critically ill foals. *Journal of Veterinary Internal Medicine* **20**, 569–574.

Pierrakos, C. and Vincent, J.L. (2010). Sepsis biomarkers: a review. *Critical Care* **14**, R15.

Pritchett, L.C., Ulibarri, C., Roberts, M.C., Schneider, R.K. and Sellon, D.C. (2003). Identification of potential physiological and behavioral indicators of postoperative pain in horses after exploratory celiotomy for colic. *Applied Animal Behaviour Science* **80**, 31–43.

Radcliffe, R.M., Divers, T.J., Fletcher, D.J., Mohammed, H. and Kraus, M.S. (2012). Evaluation of L-lactate and cardiac troponin I in horses undergoing emergency abdominal surgery. *Journal of Veterinary Emergency and Critical Care (San Antonio)* **22**, 313–319.

Raisbeck, M., Garner, H. and Osweiler, G. (1989). Effects if polymyxin B on selected features of equine carbohydrate overload. *Veterinary and Human Toxicology* **31**, 422–426.

Rivers, E.P., Coba, V. and Whitmill, M. (2008). Early goal-directed therapy in severe sepsis and septic shock: a contemporary review of the literature. *Current Opinion in Anaesthesiology* **21**, 128–140.

Rocha, M., Herance, R., Rovira, S., Hernandez-Mijares, A. and Victor, V.M. (2012). Mitochondrial dysfunction and anti-oxidant therapy in sepsis. *Infectious Disorders – Drug Targets* **12**, 161–178.

Schroder, K., Hertzog, P., Ravasi, T. and Hume, D.A. (2004). Interferon-gamma: an overview of signals, mechanisms, and functions. *Journal of Leukocyte Biology* **75**, 163–189.

Schroeder, E., Holcombe, S., Cook, V., James, M.D., Gandy, J.C., Hauptman, J.G. and Sordillo, L.M. (2011). Preliminary safety and biological efficacy studies of ethyl pyruvate in normal mature horses. *Equine Veterinary Journal* **43**, 341–347.

Schulte, W., Bernhagen, J. and Bucala, R. (2013). Cytokines in sepsis: potent immunoregulators and potential therapeutic targets – an updated view. *Mediators of Inflammation* **2013**, 165974.

Semrad, S., Hardee, G., Hardee, M. and Moore, J.N. (1987). Low dose flunixin meglumine: effects on eicosanoid production and clinical signs induced by experimental endotoxemia in horses. *Equine Veterinary Journal* **19**, 201–206.

Semrad, S. and Moore, J. (1987). Effects of multiple low doses of flunixin meglumine on repeated endotoxin challenge in the horse. *Prostaglandins, Leukotrienes, and Medicine* **27**, 169–181.

Senior, J.M., Proudman, C.J., Leuwer, M. and Carter, S.D. (2011). Plasma endotoxin in horses presented to an equine referral hospital: correlation to selected clinical parameters and outcomes. *Equine Veterinary Journal* **43**, 585–591.

Shih, C.C., Tsai, M.F., Chen, S.J., Tsao, C.M., Ka, S.M., Huang, H.C. and Wu, C.C. (2012). Effects of small-volume hypertonic saline on acid-base and electrolytes balance in rats with peritonitis-induced sepsis. *Shock* **38**, 649–655.

Shimada, T., Oda, S., Sadahiro, T., Nakamura, M., Hirayama, Y., Watanabe, E., Abe, R., Nakada, T., Tateishi, Y., Otani, S., Hirasawa, H., Tokuhisa, T. and Uno, H. (2011). Outcome prediction in sepsis combined use of genetic polymorphisms – A study in Japanese population. *Cytokine* **54**, 79–84.

Shuster, R., Traub-Dargatz J., and Baxter, G. (1997). Survey of diplomates of the American College of Veterinary Internal Medicine and the American College of Veterinary Surgeons regarding clinical aspects and treatment of endotoxemia in horses. *Journal of the American Veterinary Medical Association* **210**, 87–92.

Southwood, L.L., Dolente, B.A., Lindborg, S., Russell, G. and Boston, R. (2009). Short-term outcome of equine emergency admissions at a university referral hospital. *Equine Veterinary Journal* **41**, 459–464.

Spier, S., Lavoie, J., Cullor, J., Smith, B.P., Snyder, J.R. and Sischo, W.M. (1989). Protection against clinical endotoxemia in horses by using plasma containing antibody to an Rc mutant *E. coli* (J5). *Circulatory Shock* **28**, 235–248.

Sprung, C., Annane, D., Keh, D., Moreno, R., Singer, M., Freivogel, K., Weiss, Y.G., Benhenishty, J., Kalenka, A., Forst, H., Laterre, P.F., Reinhart, K., Cuthbertson, B.H., Payen, D. and Briegel, J. (2008). Hydrocortisone therapy for patients with septic shock. *New England Journal of Medicine* **358**, 111–124.

Stewart, A.J. (2011a). Magnesium disorders in horses. *Veterinary Clinics of North America: Equine Practice* **27**, 149–163.

Stewart, A., Hackett, E., Towns, T. *et al.* (2011b). *Identification of Critical Illness Related Corticosteroid Insufficiency in Critically Ill Horses*. Proceedings of the Annual Forum of the American College of Veterinary Internal Medicine Denver, CO.

Tadros, E.M., Frank, N. and Donnell, R.L. (2013). Effects of equine metabolic syndrome on inflammatory responses of horses to intravenous lipopolysaccharide infusion. *American Journal of Veterinary Research* **74**, 1010–1019.

Tennent-Brown, B.S., Wilkins, P.A., Lindborg, S., Russell, G. and Boston, R.C. (2010). Sequential plasma lactate concentrations as prognostic indicators in adult equine emergencies. *Journal of Veterinary Internal Medicine* **24**, 198–205.

Tennent-Brown, B.S. (2011). Lactate production and measurement in critically ill horses. *Compendium on Continuing Education for the Practicing Veterinarian* **33**, E5.

Thompson, C.M., Holden, T.D., Rona, G., Laxmanan, B., Black, R.A., O'Keefe, G.E. and Wurfel, M.M. (2013). Toll-like receptor 1 polymorphisms and associated outcomes in sepsis after traumatic injury: a candidate gene association study. *Annals of Surgery* **259**, 179–185.

Tomlinson, J. and Blikslager, A. (2004). Effects of ischaemia and the cyclooxygenase inhibitor flunixin on *in vitro* passage of lipopolysaccharide across equine jejunum. *American Journal of Veterinary Research* **65**, 1377–1383.

Tomlinson, J. and Blikslager, A.T. (2005). Effects of cyclooxygenase inhibitors flunixin and deracoxib on permeability of ischaemic-injured equine jejunum. *Equine Veterinary Journal* **37**, 75–80.

Torfs, S., Delesalle, C., Dewulf, J., Devisscher, J. and Depres, P. (2009). Risk factors for equine postoperative ileus and effectiveness of prophylactic lidocaine. *Journal of Veterinary Internal Medicine* **23**, 606–611.

Toribio, R.E., Kohn, C.W., Hardy, J. and Rosol, T.J. (2005). Alterations in serum parathyroid hormone and electrolyte concentrations and urinary excretion of electrolytes in horses with induced endotoxemia. *Journal of Veterinary Internal Medicine* **19**, 223–231.

Toribio, R.E. (2011). Endocrine dysregulation in critically ill foals and horses. *Veterinary Clinics of North America: Equine Practice* **27**, 35–47.

Underwood, C., Southwood, L.L., Walton, R.M. and Johnson, A.L. (2010). Hepatic and metabolic changes in surgical colic patients: a pilot study. *Journal of Veterinary Emergency and Critical Care (San Antonio)* **20**, 578–586.

Valverde, A. (2013). Balanced anesthesia and constant-rate infusions in horses. *Veterinary Clinics of North America: Equine Practice* **29**, 89–122.

Van Hoogmoed, L., Rakestraw, P., Snyder, J. and Harmon, F.A. (1999). *In vitro* effects of nonsteroidal anti-inflammatory agents and prostaglandins I2, E2, and F2alpha on contractility of taenia of the large colon of horses. *American Journal of Veterinary Research* **60**, 1004–1009.

Weiss, D., Evanson, O. and Geor, R. (1994). The effects of furosemide and pentoxyfylline on the flow properties of equine erythrocytes: *in vitro* studies. *Veterinary Research Communications* **18**, 373–381.

Werners, A.H., Bull, S., Vendrig, J.C., Smyth, T., Bosch, R.R., Fink-Gremmels, J. and Bryant, C.E. (2006). Genotyping of Toll-like receptor 4, myeloid differentiation factor 2 and CD-14 in the horse: an investigation into the influence of genetic polymorphisms on the LPS induced TNF-alpha response in equine whole blood. *Veterinary Immunology and Immunopathology* **111**, 165–173.

Wong, D., Vo, D., Alcott, C., Peterson, A.D., Sponseller, B.A. and Hsu, W.H. (2009). Baseline plasma cortisol and ACTH concentrations and response to low dose ACTH stimulation testing in ill foals. *Journal of the American Veterinary Medical Association* **234**, 126–132.

Young, S.K., Worthen, G.S., Haslett, C., Tonnesen, N.G. and Henson, P.M. (1990). Interaction between chemoattractants and bacterial lipopolysaccharide in the induction and enhancement of neutrophil adhesion. *American Journal of Respiratory Cell and Molecular Biology* **2**, 523–532.

Ziegler, E.J., McCutchan, J.A., Fierer, J., Glauser, M.P., Sadoff, J.C., Douglas, H. and Braude, A.I. (1982). Treatment of gram-negative bacteremia and shock with human antiserum to a mutant *Escherichia coli*. *New England Journal of Medicine* **307**(20), 1225–1230.

Ziegler, E., Fisher, C.J., Sprung, C., Straube, R.C., Sadoff, J.C., Foulke, G.E., Wortel, C.H., Fink, M.P., Dellinger, R.P. and Teng, N.N. (1991). Treatment of gram-negative bacteremia and septic shock with HA-1A human monoclonal antibody against endotoxin. A randomized, double-blind placebo-controlled trial. The HA-1A Sepsis Study Group. *New England Journal of Medicine* **324**, 429–436.

Ziegler, E., McCutchan, J., Fierer, J., Glauser, M.P., Sadoff, J.C., McFarlane, H. and Holbrook, T.C. (2008). Cytokine dysregulation in aged horses and horses with pituitary pars intermedia dysfunction. *Journal of Veterinary Internal Medicine* **22**, 436–442.

19 Leukemia

Tracy Stokol

19.1 Definition

Leukemia means that there are tumor cells of hematopoietic origin in the blood and/or the bone marrow. However, this simple term belies the complexity of the different types of leukemia that can arise. In small animal patients, the different leukemias display quite disparate biological behavior in terms of progression, treatment, and prognosis. In reality, most types of leukemia that arise in the horse have a poor prognosis. Horses usually present at an advanced stage of disease, and treatment of these large animals is costly. Also, many of the drugs used to treat leukemia in small animals are of unknown efficacy or toxicity in horses. Luckily for the horse, leukemias are quite uncommon. Indeed, most cases of leukemia are usually published as individual case reports, with only a few small case series.

19.2 Classification of leukemias

Leukemias are generally classified on the basis of two criteria:
1 *Cell of origin:* lymphoid or myeloid, determined by morphologic features and by the expression of lineage – specific markers on the neoplastic cells using specialized diagnostic techniques (immunophenotyping and cytochemistry, see below).
2 *Degree of differentiation:* acute or chronic, usually assessed by the morphologic appearance of the neoplastic cells in blood or bone marrow.

  Chronic leukemia (particularly that of lymphocytic origin) is considered a disorder of accumulation, where the neoplastic clone undergoes differentiation but increases to high numbers, because the cells fail to die. Since the neoplastic cells are differentiated, they can be recognized by their morphologic appearance.

  In contrast, acute leukemia is considered a disorder of proliferation, where the neoplastic clone has a growth advantage over normal cells, effectively replacing them. The neoplastic cells in acute leukemia also fail to differentiate completely, such that they have immature morphologic features and do not resemble

their normal counterparts (and are called *blasts*). Usually, however, they express markers that indicate which lineage they arose from or towards which they were differentiating. These markers are used to help identify the cells, and to classify them as lymphoid or myeloid and their respective subtypes (Table 19.1).

  Even though the terms "acute" and "chronic" usually indicate chronology, for leukemia they are used primarily to distinguish between cells that are immature (cannot be conclusively identified as to their lineage by appearance alone) or mature (can be identified by appearance alone). However, these terms also imply chronology, in that chronic leukemias are usually indolent and slowly progressive disorders, whereas acute leukemias are usually of acute onset and progression in small animal patients. This chronologic distinction is not as apparent in horses, for the reasons mentioned above.

  The reader may also come across other terms that are applied to leukemia in the literature, including "aleukemic" and "subleukemic". These two terms indicate that there are no or low numbers of neoplastic cells in peripheral blood, respectively. However, other than indicating that these cases could be a diagnostic challenge, these terms are of no relevance and are uninformative.

19.3 Specialized diagnostic techniques for leukemia

Two techniques are used to determine the cell of origin of leukemia: immunophenotyping and cytochemistry. These techniques are used primarily for acute leukemia, where neoplastic cells cannot be distinguished on the basis of morphologic features, but they are also used in chronic lymphocytic leukemia (CLL) to determine the phenotype (B or T cell) of the neoplastic lymphocytes. They are not routinely used for chronic myeloid leukemia, because the involved cell lineage can be identified based on morphologic features alone. The major limitations with these techniques are their relative unavailability (not

Equine Clinical Immunology, First Edition. Edited by M. Julia B. Felippe.
© 2016 John Wiley & Sons, Inc. Published 2016 by John Wiley & Sons, Inc.

Table 19.1 Classification and diagnosis of the different types of leukemia.

Lineage	Lymphoid		Myeloid	
Cell of origin	B cell, T cell, natural killer (NK) cell		granulocytes (neutrophils, eosinophils, basophils), monocytes, erythrocytes, megakaryocytes	
Degree of differentiation	**Acute** Immature	**Chronic** Mature	**Acute** Immature	**Chronic** Mature
Morphologic features	medium to large (*blasts*), euchromatin (fine chromatin), ± nucleoli	small to medium, heterochromatin (clumped), no nucleoli	medium to large (*blasts*), euchromatin, ± nucleoli	granulocytes, monocytes, platelets, erythrocytes
Subtypes	cell of origin, as determined by immunophenotyping		cell of origin as determined by immunophenotyping and cytochemistry[*]	cell of origin based on morphologic appearance[**]
Peripheral blood	bi/pancytopenia no to many *blasts*	lymphocytosis, ± cytopenias (depending on disease stage)	bi/pancytopenia no to many *blasts*	high cell numbers (e.g., neutrophilia, thrombocytosis, erythrocytosis), ± dysplasia
Bone marrow	> 25% *blasts* required (usually >80%), few normal hematopoietic cells	normal, ± infiltrate of lymphocytes	> 20% *blasts* required (usually > 80%), few normal hematopoietic cells, ± dysplasia	hyperplasia (e.g., granulocytic, megakaryocytic, erythroid hyperplasia), ± dysplasia
Identified in horse	B-ALL, T-ALL	B-CLL, T-CLL	myeloblastic, myelomonocytic, monocytic, possibly eosinophilic	chronic granulocytic leukemia

Note that there are rare acute leukemias that cannot be differentiated on the basis of markers (acute undifferentiated leukemia). Those that demonstrate more than one type of marker (mixed lineage or biphenotypic leukemia) are not depicted (these have not been identified to date in horses).
[*] Many different subtypes, depending on cell lineage (e.g., acute monoblastic leukemia, acute megakaryocytic leukemia).
[**] Subtypes include chronic granulocytic leukemia (involves neutrophils, eosinophils or basophils), essential thrombocythemia (chronic platelet leukemia), polycythemia vera (chronic erythroid leukemia) and chronic myeloid leukemia (multiple myeloid lineages involved).

routinely offered as diagnostic tests at diagnostic laboratories), and the paucity of equine-specific reagents.

19.3.1 Immunophenotyping

This technique involves the application of antibodies that have been raised against markers expressed on cells. The marker could be on the membrane, within the cytoplasm, or in the nucleus of the cell. In some cases, these markers are lineage-specific (e.g., CD4 is only present on helper or regulatory T cells in the horse) while, in others, they are expressed on more than one cell type (e.g., CD172a is expressed on neutrophils and monocytes).

The antibodies can be applied to cells in suspension or cells on slides. With suspended cells (e.g., venous blood or bone marrow aspirates), the antibodies that bind to the cell are detected with fluorescence-based techniques using flow cytometry. When the antibodies are applied to cells on cytologic or histologic slides (called immunocyto- and immunohistochemistry, respectively), they can be detected with colorimetric or fluorescent reagents, although colorimetric-based methods are more routinely used. Flow cytometry has advantages over slide-based techniques, because many more antibodies can be applied simultaneously to the sample. With cytology smears, the number of slides usually limits the numbers of antibodies that can be applied. Formalin fixation destroys many markers, and several antibodies cannot be used on formalin-fixed smears, which limits the phenotyping that can be done on routine histologic samples. Also, there are more available antibodies to detect lymphoid versus myeloid markers.

19.3.2 Cytochemistry

This technique involves the application of substrates to cells to detect enzyme activity within the cell (i.e., myeloperoxidase, alkaline phosphatase, and various esterases). Enzymes are mostly expressed in cells of myeloid origin and, therefore, this technique is most useful to diagnose acute leukemias that are myeloid in origin (particularly granulocytic and mono-cytic). They are less useful for lymphoid leukemia, because lymphoid cells usually lack these enzymes. Cytochemistry can only be done on cytologic specimens (venous blood, bone marrow, aspirates of body cavity fluid or solid organs), and not on formalin-fixed tissues, because formalin destroys enzyme activity. Cytochemistry has been mostly supplanted by immunophenotyping for classification of leukemias, but it is still useful to confirm an acute myeloid leukemia, since there are so few antibodies against myeloid markers of the horse.

19.4 Chronic leukemia

19.4.1 Definition

Chronic leukemia is a disorder of accumulation, in which the neoplastic cells fail to die and increase to high numbers in peripheral blood. Chronic leukemias can be lymphoid or myeloid in origin, and both types can be further subdivided on the basis of the specific cell type involved (Table 19.1). The neoplastic cells differentiate and can be readily recognized by their morphologic features, with many of them in blood. Thus, this type of leukemia is diagnosed by documenting high counts of the involved cell lineage in blood (e.g., a high hematocrit (HCT) with polycythemia vera (chronic erythroid leukemia), an absolute lymphocytosis with CLL). The increased numbers of cells should be persistent (i.e., present in several blood samples taken over several months). A bone marrow aspirate may not be helpful to confirm a diagnosis of chronic leukemia. In chronic myeloid leukemia, bone marrow aspirates usually only reveals hyperplasia of the involved cell lineage. With CLL, the genetic mutation in the lymphoid cells occurs in peripheral lymphoid tissue (spleen or lymph node), and the neoplastic cells may not infiltrate the bone marrow, although they usually do to some extent. In essence, the diagnosis of chronic leukemia is one of exclusion (see below).

All types of chronic leukemia are quite rare in the horse. There has only been one case of chronic granulocytic leukemia (Johansson, 2007) and nine cases of CLL (Dascanio, 1992; McClure, 2001; Rendle, 2007) reported in the veterinary literature. An additional case of chronic granulocytic leukemia was probably an acute myeloid leukemia with concurrent myelodysplasia (Searcy, 1981).

19.4.2 Chronic myeloid leukemia

19.4.2.1 Clinical signs and signalment

The one horse reported with chronic granulocytic leukemia was a four year old Warmblood gelding that presented with lethargy, fever and inflamed, slow-healing skin wounds. The horse was severely anemic (HCT, 11 L/L) and thrombocytopenic (15×10^9 platelets/L). It had a leukocytosis characterized by a neutrophilia with a left shift, consisting of more immature (metamyelocytes and promyelocytes) than band neutrophils, and a monocytosis. Mature and immature neutrophils were dysplastic.

19.4.2.2 Diagnosis

In the reported case, a bone marrow aspirate revealed a myeloid hyperplasia with an erythroid and megakaryocytic hypoplasia, and evidence of dysplasia in granulocyte precursors. The neoplastic cells infiltrated and effaced the submandibular lymph nodes. The diagnosis of chronic granulocytic leukemia was supported by the neutrophilia with a disproportionate left shift, granulocytic dysplasia (indicating abnormal maturation), concurrent severe cytopenias due to decreased bone marrow production, with fewer than 20% *blasts* in bone marrow, and infiltration of extramedullary tissues. The wound infections

suggested that the horse had a defect in neutrophil function, which is not surprising for neoplastic cells. The horse was submitted to euthanasia soon after diagnosis (Johansson, 2007).

The main differential diagnosis for a chronic myeloid leukemia is cytokine-driven hematopoiesis due to neoplasia (not leukemia) and inflammation. Paraneoplastic erythrocytosis has been reported with lymphoma, hepatocellular tumors, and carcinomas in horses (Cook, 1995; Lennox, 2000; Koch, 2006). A primary erythrocytosis was identified in a two year old Arabian gelding, although this was not confirmed to be a neoplastic process, and could have been due to a congenital defect (McFarlane, 1998). Furthermore, hypoxia can stimulate a persistent appropriate erythrocytosis (Belli, 2011). Splenic contraction can yield a transitory erythrocytosis. Inflammation can drive leukocytosis and thrombocytosis (Sellon, 1997), but the increases in the numbers of platelets or leukocytes are usually only mild to moderate ($< 400 \times 10^9$ platelets/L and $< 20 \times 10^9$ neutrophils/L).

A chronic myeloid leukemia should be considered in the horse if there is a marked increase in cell numbers, particularly if persistent and unexplained or if there is evidence of abnormal maturation or other non-responsive cytopenias.

19.4.3 Chronic lymphocytic leukemia

19.4.3.1 Clinical signs and signalment

Horses reported with CLL, including an additional case seen by the author, were older, with ages ranging from 10–20 years. Affected animals were of different breeds and both sexes, although most were males (eight of ten, usually geldings). However, there have been too few reported cases to confirm any sex predilection. Reported clinical signs were vague and nonspecific but most horses presented with edema of the ventrum, prepuce, and limbs. Other clinical signs were inappetance, weight loss, fever, poor body condition, mild colic, diarrhea, and solitary or multiple peripheral lymph node enlargement (including mandibular, preputial, inguinal lymph nodes). Affected horses had demonstrated clinical signs for two days to seven months.

19.4.3.2 Diagnosis

The diagnosis of CLL was based on markedly increased numbers of lymphocytes in peripheral blood, ranging from 26 to 208×10^9 cells/L. In most horses, the lymphocytes were small to intermediate. In one horse, approximately 50% of the lymphoid cells were large, suggesting a blast crisis (Rendle, 2007). In another horse, the cells were described as large (Rendle, 2007), which is not consistent with a CLL but more compatible with an acute lymphoid leukemia (ALL). Concurrent cytopenias were present in seven of the ten horses, one of which was pancytopenic (anemia, neutropenia and thrombocytopenia; the neoplastic cells in this horse were small). Cytopenias were usually mild, with the exception of thrombocytopenia, which was severe (4 and 19×10^9/L) in two horses. An inflammatory response was evident in eight horses, indicated by the presence of band

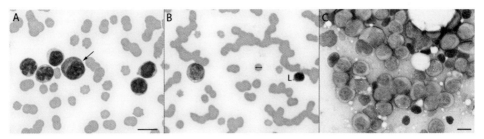

Figure 19.1 Representative photomicrographs of leukemia in the horse that have been seen by the author.
A: Chronic lymphocytic leukemia in a 14 year old Clydesdale mare. The horse had a lymphocyte count of 103.8 x 10^9/L consisting of small to intermediate lymphocytes. The cells had clumped chromatin (heterochromatin) and an indented nucleus that was smaller than a neutrophil (none seen in this image, as the mare was neutropenic). A single reactive-appearing large lymphocyte is also noted(arrow), which may not be part of the tumor population.
B: Acute lymphoid leukemia in a 2 year old Standardbred gelding. The horse was pancytopenic but rare "*blasts*" were identified on scanning the blood smear. These "*blasts*" were much larger than a small lymphocyte (L) and had fine chromatin (i.e. euchromatin, indicating active DNA synthesis) with no nucleoli. A bone marrow aspirate revealed more than 70% "*blasts*", which were positive for Pax-5 (a B cell marker) on immunohistochemical staining, indicating a B-ALL.
C: Bone marrow aspirate from an 8 year old Warmblood mare with pancytopenia. A few "*blasts*" were seen on scanning and a bone marrow aspirate revealed >70% "*blasts*". These were positive for CD172a (a marker of neutrophils and monocytes) on flow cytometry of the bone marrow, indicating a diagnosis of AML. (Wright's stain, scale bars = 10 um).

neutrophils or toxic change in neutrophils, or a high fibrinogen or serum amyloid A. The most consistent abnormalities on a biochemical panel were an increased total protein, due to increased globulins. Only two horses had evidence of organ dysfunction and were azotemic.

Serum protein electrophoresis was done on three horses, and revealed a monoclonal gammopathy in two animals. In one of these animals, the monoclonal protein was shown to be immunoglobulin G with a radial immunodiffusion assay. The third horse had a polyclonal gammopathy, with increases in both IgG and IgM.

A bone marrow aspirate was performed in six horses antemortem, and showed low (< 20%), moderate (35–45%) and high (> 75%) numbers of infiltrating lymphocytes in three, one, and two horses, respectively. The low level of infiltrates reinforces that bone marrow aspirates may not be useful to confirm the diagnosis of CLL.

The main differential diagnosis for CLL is a leukemic phase of a small cell lymphoma (Polkes, 1999; McClure, 2001; Meyer, 2006). These two disorders are very difficult to distinguish, and there is substantial overlap in presenting clinical signs, blood results and post-mortem findings. Indeed, distinguishing between these two neoplasms may be an academic exercise. Essentially, a diagnosis of CLL is favored if the lymphocytosis is marked and there is no, or only mild, lymphadenopathy or organomegaly. A diagnosis of lymphoma is favored if there is moderate to marked lymphadenopathy and organomegaly, and only a mild lymphocytosis, or if the lymphocytosis (even if marked) is preceded by a lymphadenopathy, as reported for one horse with lymphoma by McClure (2001). Indeed, two of the reported cases of CLL may actually have been a lymphoma that progressed to a leukemic phase. In one horse, the leukemia consisted of large lymphocytes, and only a few cells were found in the bone

marrow but neoplastic cells were present in lymph nodes (Rendle, 2007). The second horse had a documented submandibular lymphadenopathy of unknown cause for seven months before the diagnosis of leukemia (McClure, 2001).

Other differential diagnoses for a lymphocytosis include an epinephrine response and chronic antigenic stimulation, although these are quite rare and should only result in a mild lymphocytosis. Also, foals up to several months of age may have higher lymphocyte counts than adult animals, or reported reference intervals.

Immunophenotyping of the leukemia was performed in seven cases of CLL with flow cytometry (some supplemented with immunohistochemistry), and confirmed B cell leukemia in one horse and $CD4^+$ T cell leukemia in the remaining horses. This suggests that CLL usually involves T-helper or T-regulatory cells in the horse. The leukemia in the horse seen by the author (Figure 19.1) was phenotyped as a B-CLL and had a concurrent monoclonal B-CLL gammopathy. In six horses, lymphocyte blastogenesis assays revealed abnormal proliferation of the neoplastic B and T cells (Dascanio, 1992; Rendle, 2007), suggesting dysfunction of the neoplastic lymphocytes.

19.4.3.3 Treatment and prognosis
Two horses were treated with corticosteroids, but treatment was discontinued in one horse after three months, due to laminitis. Both horses were submitted to euthanasia after 11–12 months of diagnosis, one from displacement of the right colon, and the second from dyspnea. Three horses survived for 45 days, 60 days and five years after diagnosis, at which time they were submitted to euthanasia due to clinical disease progression or owner choice. In some horses, the lymphocytosis and cytopenias worsened over time. The remaining horses were submitted to euthanasia at, or shortly after, diagnosis (within one week), due to severe disease. Clinical and laboratory findings supportive of

severe disease were pyrexia, weight loss, poor body condition, fever, severe thrombocytopenia, and inflammatory leukogram (left shift and toxic change in neutrophils).

These findings suggest that acquired immunodeficiency may develop in advanced cases, and concurrent secondary infections are a poor prognostic indicator in horses with CLL. In contrast, prognosis was not related to the degree of lymphocytosis, with longer-term survivors having some of the highest lymphocyte counts (88.3 to 208.3×10^9 cells/L). On necropsy, infiltrates of lymphocytes were present in multiple organs, including lymph nodes, spleen, kidney, mammary glands, intestines, lung, heart, cornea, skin, and bone marrow.

19.5 Acute leukemia

19.5.1 Definition

The genetic mutation that gives rise to acute leukemia occurs within the hematopoietic stem cell in the bone marrow. The mutation usually allows the neoplastic clone to proliferate uncontrollably, and gives it a growth advantage over the normal cells in the bone marrow. The neoplasm effectively replaces the bone marrow, casing myelophthisis, preventing normal hematopoiesis from occurring, and resulting in cytopenias in peripheral blood, a characteristic feature of acute leukemia.

The diagnosis of acute leukemia requires the presence of greater than 20% (>25% for acute lymphocytic leukemia) immature neoplastic cells (*blasts*) in the bone marrow, irrespective of their presence in blood. Indeed, the neoplastic cells may not spill over into blood. In some cases, the genetic mutation may also result in abnormal maturation (dysplasia), which can be identified in differentiated cells in peripheral blood.

There are various types of acute leukemia that are distinguished by their expression of lineage-specific markers into acute lymphoid leukemia (ALL) or acute myeloid leukemia (AML). They can then be further sub-classified into more specific cell lineages (Table 19.1). In humans, this distinction can be useful, because ALL and AML are treated with different drugs and have a different prognosis (good for ALL and poor for AML). However, acute leukemia has a uniformly poor prognosis in horses, so this distinction is mostly academic, and both types of acute leukemias will be discussed together.

Acute leukemias consist of immature cells, which are usually nondescript. They are medium to large cells with fine or slightly clumped chromatin, and may or may not have nucleoli (Figure 19.1). They can display morphologic features that help determine their lineage (Burkhardt, 1984; Mori, 1991; Monteith, 1995; Clark, 1999). Concurrent abnormalities (dysplasia) in differentiating hematopoietic cells (neutrophils, red blood cells, platelets) may be seen in rare cases (Mori, 1991). Because immature cells lack features of differentiation, and look similar regardless of their lineage, they are referred to as *blasts*, and immunophenotyping and cytochemistry is required to determine the cell of origin. Note that dysplasia in differentiating hematopoietic cells supports a

diagnosis of AML or myelodysplasia (Durando, 1994), both of which are neoplastic or clonal disorders of myeloid cells. This is because dysplasia has not been reported in horses with ALL.

19.5.2 Clinical signs and signalment

In contrast to chronic leukemia, numerous cases of acute leukemia have been reported in horses (Roberts, 1977; Allen, 1984; Boudreaux, 1984; Burkhardt, 1984; Spier, 1986; Blue, 1987; Platt, 1988; Mori, 1991; Lester, 1993; Buechner-Maxwell, 1994; Monteith, 1995; Ringger, 1997; Clark, 1999; McClure, 2001). This is also the experience of the author, having seen one case of CLL and six cases of confirmed acute leukemia in horses since 1995 (with an additional two suspected cases from hemogram results). This suggests that acute leukemia may be more common in horses, but is still rare overall.

Affected horses were generally younger than those with CLL, ranging from 2–11 years old. Horses were of both sexes and various breeds, including Quarter Horse, Standardbred, Thoroughbred, Warmblood, and Belgian. As for CLL, clinical signs were vague and not specific. The most common reported signs were weight loss, inappetance, fever, edema (limbs, ventrum, prepuce), and lymphadenopathy (mandibular, mammary, inguinal, mesenteric), with a few horses also presenting depression, diarrhea, colic, and epistaxis. Some horses had infections that were unresponsive to analgesics or antibiotics. Clinical signs were present for a short time, ranging from two weeks to one month, with only a few cases having clinical signs for longer periods (2–4 months) (Burkhardt, 1984; Monteith, 1995).

19.5.3 Diagnosis

Hemogram findings are the first clue as to the possibility of leukemia. Since the tumor arises in, and usually effaces, the marrow, preventing normal hematopoiesis, affected horses usually have bi- or pancytopenia, which can be quite severe. The cytopenias are non-regenerative and persistent, indicating a bone marrow disorder. There may be a concurrent inflammatory leukogram, with immature and toxic neutrophils. However, in some horses, the immature neutrophils are part of the neoplasm (Clark, 1999). *Blasts* may be present in high numbers, facilitating a diagnosis from peripheral blood (Allen, 1984; Boudreaux, 1984; Burkhardt, 1984; Blue, 1987; Monteith, 1995).

Tumor cells can be present in low numbers, or not at all in peripheral blood, and these cases are more challenging to diagnose. In such cases, a bone marrow aspirate will be required to obtain a definitive diagnosis of acute leukemia, showing at least > 20% *blasts* (>25% for acute lymphocytic leukemia). Larger numbers of *blasts* (> 80%) are usually present on bone marrow aspirates or histopathologic assessment of bone marrow from necropsy, confirming the diagnosis.

As for CLL, the most common changes on a biochemical panel are high total protein, due to increased globulins, with observed increase in acute phase response proteins and polyclonal gammopathy when serum electrophoresis was performed. Unlike CLL, a monoclonal gammopathy has not been detected in affected horses. A few horses also have evidence of liver injury, based on increased activities of aspartate aminotransferase, sorbitol dehydrogenase, and gamma-glutamyl transferase (Mori, 1991; Lester, 1993; Buechner-Maxwell, 1994; Clark, 1999), which is probably secondary to tumor infiltrates in this organ.

Unresponsive pancytopenia is an unusual hemogram finding in horses, and should alert a clinician to the possibility of hematopoietic neoplasia. Only isolated cases of pancytopenia secondary to idiopathic aplastic anemia and myelofibrosis have been reported in horses (Lavoie, 1987; Angel, 1991). Horses with infectious agents, such as *Anaplasma phagocytophilum* and equine infectious anemia, can have single or multiple cytopenias, and testing for these infectious agents is advised in any horse with unexplained cytopenias. Tests for infectious agents have been uniformly negative in affected horses. If pancytopenia is detected in a hemogram from a horse, acute leukemia should be the primary differential diagnosis. In such cases, it would be worthwhile to have the blood smear reviewed by a clinical pathologist for any diagnostic clues, such as low numbers of *blasts*.

The main differential diagnosis for the presence of *blasts* in blood or the bone marrow is lymphoma, which can mimic an acute leukemia in presentation, clinical signs, and organ involvement (Platt, 1988; McClure, 2001). It is very difficult to distinguish between ALL and lymphoma. Indeed, in one case series of lymphoma, 16 horses had documented leukemia, with extensive bone marrow infiltration by the neoplastic cells (Meyer, 2006). Some of the horses in this case series (Meyer, 2006), and others diagnosed with lymphoma (Allen, 1984; Kelton, 2008), may actually have had acute leukemia. Since lymphoma infrequently infiltrates the marrow to the same extent as ALL and, subsequently, is not usually associated with severe cytopenias, a diagnosis of acute leukemia would be favored in a horse with bi- or pancytopenia and > 20-25% *blasts* in the bone marrow, despite the presence of lymphadenopathy.

Cytochemical staining has been traditionally performed to determine the cell lineage in acute leukemia in the horse (Burkhardt, 1984; Spier, 1986; Blue, 1987; Mori, 1991; Lester, 1993; Buechner-Maxwell, 1994; Monteith, 1995; Ringger, 1997; Clark, 1999; McClure, 2001), with only a few reports of immunophenotyping with flow cytometry or histochemistry (Buechner-Maxwell, 1994; McClure, 2001; Kelton, 2008). With the exception of the one case series of lymphoma, in which 16 cases of leukemia were identified (Meyer, 2006), most of the reported individual cases and small case series of acute leukemia in the horse have been of myeloid origin, particularly myelomonocytic leukemia (differentiating down both neutrophil and monocytic lineages). Neither cytochemistry nor immunophenotyping was performed on three cases of ALL (the diagnosis was based on morphology alone) (Roberts, 1977; Allen, 1984; Platt, 1988), and a few *blasts* were positive for chloroacetate esterase (a myeloid marker) in another case (with no immunophenotyping performed) (Lester, 1993). It is possible that all of these cases, and some of the unclassified leukemias in the case series of lymphoma (Meyer, 2006), were actually AML versus lymphoma or ALL.

Of the six confirmed cases seen by the author, three were classified as ALL (one B, one T, and one not phenotyped), two were classified as AML, and one expressed markers of both myeloid and lymphoid cells, based on cytochemical staining and immunophenotyping. T cell leukemia appears more common than B cell leukemia in horses (Meyer, 2006; Kelton, 2008). There has also been one case of a potential acute myeloid leukemia with eosinophilic differentiation in the horse (Morris, 1984).

Thorough immunologic assessments of affected horses have not been done, but horses may have defects in innate and acquired immunity. One horse with ALL was positive on Coombs testing, indicating an immune-mediated component to the horse's anemia (Lester, 1993). Due to severe neutropenia, horses can develop secondary bacterial infections, and some horses died or were submitted to euthanasia, due to complications of sepsis. Unlike horses with lymphoma or CLL, IgM deficiency has not been previously reported in horses with acute leukemia, but immunoglobulin testing was not performed on all cases. One of the ALL cases seen by the author did have a selective IgM deficiency. Some horses also suffer from secondary fungal infections with aspergillosis, suggesting an acquired cellular immunity defect against fungal agents (Blue, 1987; Buechner-Maxwell, 1994).

19.5.4 Treatment and prognosis

The prognosis of acute leukemia, regardless of phenotype, is uniformly poor. Horses with severe neutropenia are prone to secondary bacterial infection, and those with severe thrombocytopenia may bleed spontaneously (petechiae, epistaxis, prolonged bleeding after venipuncture). Few horses have been treated, with most being submitted to euthanasia within a few days of diagnosis. Treatment has only been attempted in a few horses. Three horses with AML were treated with cytosine arabinoside, a standard chemotherapeutic agent used for human and canine AML, and two other horses with AML were treated with prednisolone (Spier, 1986; Buechner-Maxwell, 1994; Clark, 1999; Ringger, 1997). Clinical signs and hematologic findings worsened after treatment, and horses were submitted to euthanasia within one day to four weeks of initiation of therapy.

Necropsies were done on most horses, and neoplastic cells were present in large numbers in the bone marrow, with infiltration in extramedullary tissues, including lymph nodes, spleen, liver, kidney, heart, testes, adrenal gland, gastrointestinal tract, skin, central nervous system, and lungs. Lymph nodes were frequently effaced by the tumor. In some cases, the neoplastic cells formed discrete masses, mimicking lymphoma. Interestingly, some horses had evidence of tissue necrosis with vascular thrombi, several of which were associated with cancer cells (Boudreaux, 1984; Spier, 1986; Buechner-Maxwell, 1994; Ringger, 1997). This suggests that the leukemia induced a hypercoagulable state but, unfortunately, this was not diagnosed ante-mortem, since coagulation profiles in most horses were normal.

References

Allen, B.V., Wannop, C.C. and Wright, I.M. (1984). Multicentric lymphosarcoma with lymphoblastic leukaemia in a young horse. *The Veterinary Record* **115**(6), 130–131.

Angel, K.L., Spano, J.S., Schumacher, J. and Kwapien, R.P. (1991). Myelophthisic pancytopenia in a pony mare. *Journal of the American Veterinary Medical Association* **198**(6), 1039–1042.

Belli, C.B., Baccarin, R.Y., Ida, K.K. and Fernandes, W.R. (2011). Appropriate secondary absolute erythrocytosis in a horse. *The Veterinary Record* **169**(23), 609.

Blue, J., Perdrizet, J. and Brown, E. (1987). Pulmonary aspergillosis in a horse with myelomonocytic leukemia. *Journal of the American Veterinary Medical Association* **190**(12), 1562–1564.

Boudreaux, M.K., Blue, J.T., Durham, S.K. and Vivrette, S.L. (1984). Intravascular leukostasis in a horse with myelomonocytic leukemia. *Veterinary Pathology* **21**(5), 544–546.

Buechner-Maxwell, V., Zhang, C., Robertson, J., Jain, N.C., Antczak, D.F., Feldman, B.F. and Murray, M.J. (1994). Intravascular leukostasis and systemic aspergillosis in a horse with subleukemic acute myelomonocytic leukemia. *Journal of Veterinary Internal Medicine* **8**(4), 258–263.

Burkhardt, E., von Saldern, F. and Huskamp, B. (1984). Monocytic leukemia in a horse. *Veterinary Pathology* **21**(4), 394–398.

Clark, P., Cornelisse, C.J., Schott, H.C., Swenson, C.L. and Bell, T.G. (1999). Myeloblastic leukaemia in a Morgan horse mare. *Equine Veterinary Journal* **31**(5), 446–448.

Cook, G., Divers, T.J. and Rowland, P.H. (1995). Hypercalcemia and erythrocytosis in a mare associated with a metastatic carcinoma. *Equine Veterinary Journal* **27**(4), 316–318.

Dascanio, J.J., Zhang, C.H., Antczack, D.F., Blue, J.T. and Simmons, T.R. (1992). Differentiation of chronic lymphocytic leukemia in the horse: A report of two cases. *Journal of Veterinary Internal Medicine* **6**(4), 225–229.

Durando, M.M., Alleman, A.R. and Harvey, J.W. (1994). Myelodysplastic syndrome in a Quarter Horse gelding. *Equine Veterinary Journal* **26**(1), 83–85.

Johansson, A.M., Skidell, J., Lilliehook, I. and Tvedten, H.W. (2007). Chronic granulocytic leukemia in a horse. *Journal of Veterinary Internal Medicine* **21**(5), 1126–1129.

Kelton, D.R., Holbrook, T.C., Gilliam, L.L., Rizzi, T.E., Brosnahan, M.M. and Confer, A.W. (2008). Bone marrow necrosis and myelophthisis: manifestations of T-cell lymphoma in a horse. *Veterinary Clinical Pathology* **37**(4), 403–408.

Koch, T.G., Wen, X. and Bienzle, D. (2006). Lymphoma, erythrocytosis, and tumor erythropoietin gene expression in a horse. *Journal of Veterinary Internal Medicine* **20**(5), 1251–1255.

Lavoie, J.P., Morris, D.D., Zinkl, J.G., Lloyd, K., Divers, T.J. (1987). Pancytopenia caused by bone marrow aplasia in a horse. *Journal of the American Veterinary Medical Association* **191**(11), 1462–1464.

Lennox, T.J., Wilson, J.H., Hayden, D.W., Bouljihad, M., Sage, A.M., Walser, M.M. and Manivet, J.C. (2000). Hepatoblastoma with erythrocytosis in a young female horse. *Journal of the American Veterinary Medical Association* **216**(5), 718–722.

Lester, G.D., Alleman, A.R., Raskin, R.E. and Meyer, J.C. (1993). Pancytopenia secondary to lymphoid leukemia in three horses. *Journal of Veterinary Internal Medicine* **7**(6), 360–363.

McClure, J.T., Young, K.M., Fiste, M., Sharkey, L.C. and Lunn, D.P. (2001). Immunophenotypic classification of leukemia in 3 horses. *Journal of Veterinary Internal Medicine* **15**(2), 144–152.

McFarlane, D., Sellon, D.C. and Parker, B. (1998). Primary erythrocytosis in a 2-year-old Arabian gelding. *Journal of Veterinary Internal Medicine* **12**(5), 384–388.

Meyer, J., Delay, J. and Bienzle, D. (2006). Clinical, laboratory, and histopathologic features of equine lymphoma. *Veterinary Pathology* **43**(6), 914–924.

Monteith, C.N. and Cole, D. (1995). Monocytic leukemia in a horse. *Canadian Veterinary Journal* **36**(12), 765–766.

Mori, T., Ishida, T., Washizu, T., Yamagami, T., Umeda, M., Sugiyama, M. and Motoyoshi, S. (1991). Acute myelomonocytic leukemia in a horse. *Veterinary Pathology* **28**(4), 344–346.

Morris, D.D., Bloom, J.C., Roby, K.A., Woods, K. and Tablin, F. (1984). Eosinophilic myeloproliferative disorder in a horse. *Journal of the American Veterinary Medical Association* **185**(9), 993–996.

Platt, H. (1988). Observations on the pathology of non-alimentary lymphomas in the horse. *Journal of Comparative Pathology* **98**(2), 177–194.

Polkes, A.C., Alleman, A.R., Lester, G.D., Beurgelt, C. and McSherry, L.J. (1999). B-cell lymphoma in a horse with associated Sezary-like cells in the peripheral blood. *Journal of Veterinary Internal Medicine* **13**(6), 620–624.

Rendle, D.I., Durham, A.E., Thompson, J.C., Archer, J., Mitchell, M., Saunders, K., Millere, J., Paillot, R., Smith, K.C. and Kydd, J.H. (2007). Clinical, immunophenotypic and functional characterisation of T-cell leukaemia in six horses. *Equine Veterinary Journal* **39**(6), 522–528.

Ringger, N.C., Edens, L., Bain, P., Raskin, R.E. and Larock, R. (1997). Acute myelogenous leukaemia in a mare. *Australian Veterinary Journal* **75**(5), 329–331.

Roberts, M.C. (1977). A case of primary lymphoid leukaemia in a horse. *Equine Veterinary Journal* **9**(4), 216–219.

Searcy, G.P. and Orr, J.P. (1981). Chronic granulocytic leukemia in a horse. *Canadian Veterinary Journal* **22**(5), 148–151.

Sellon, D.C., Levine, J.F., Palmer, K., Millikin, E., Grindem, C. and Covington, P. (1997). Thrombocytosis in 24 horses (1989–1994). *Journal of Veterinary Internal Medicine* **11**(1), 24–29.

Spier, S.J., Madewell, B.R., Zinkl, J.G. and Ryan, A.M. (1986). Acute myelomonocytic leukemia in a horse. *Journal of the American Veterinary Medical Association* **188**(8), 861–863.

20 Lymphoma

SallyAnne L. Ness

20.1 Definition

Lymphoma (used synonymously with lymphosarcoma and malignant lymphoma) is the most common hematopoietic neoplasm encountered in the horse, accounting for up to 3% of all equine neoplasias. Lymphoma represents a heterogeneous population of lymphoid-origin tumors affecting nearly every organ system of all ages and all breeds of horses. The majority of equine lymphomas can be categorized as multicentric, alimentary, mediastinal, or cutaneous. Leukemia in association with lymphoma is rare, but has been reported.

The clinical features of horses with lymphoma are often non-specific and dependent on the organ system affected. Common clinical signs include weight loss, lethargy, lymphadenopathy, and edema, while hematologic and serum biochemical abnormal findings include anemia, hyperfibrinogenemia, hyperproteinemia, hyperglobulinemia, and hypoalbuminemia. Ante-mortem diagnosis is pursued via histologic evaluation of biopsy tissues and/or cytologic examination of fine needle aspirates, imprint tissue smears, and fluid samples. At the present time, the prognosis for all forms of equine lymphoma is grave, but palliative therapies including surgical excision, radiation therapy, and chemotherapy are available and have been reported with varying degrees of success to improve quality of life and prolong survival time.

20.2 Signalment and clinical signs

The clinical features of horses with lymphoma are non-specific and vary greatly depending on the form (multicentric, alimentary, mediastinal, cutaneous) and the organ system affected. Neither breed nor sex predilection exist, although one retrospective study of 3351 cutaneous neoplasia biopsy samples found that Thoroughbreds were predisposed to cutaneous lymphoma when compared with other breeds (Schaffer, 2013). Most sources report mean ages of horses with lymphoma ranging from 5–10 years (Schneider, 2003; Meyer, 2006; Durham, 2013), although cases have been reported in aborted fetuses, foals, and horses of advanced age (Tomlinson, 1979; Dewes, 1980; Haley, 1983; Durham, 2013).

In a retrospective study of 37 horses with varying forms of lymphoma, 18 horses were less than five years old (Meyer, 2006). Frequently reported clinical signs for all forms of lymphoma include weight loss, lethargy, decreased appetite, edema (particularly along the ventral thorax and abdomen), and recurrent fevers (Schneider, 2003; Meyer, 2006; Taintor, 2011). Fever can result from tumor necrosis and infection, or may be mediated by tumor-produced lymphokines (e.g., IL-1, IL-6, TNFα) or reactive macrophages that release lymphokines in response to neoplastic tissues (Ogilvie, 1998; Axiak, 2012). Neoplasia should always be considered in an adult horse with recurrent bouts of inflammation and fever unresponsive to antimicrobial therapy.

Lymphadenopathy may occur in cases of multicentric and cutaneous lymphoma (Schneider, 2003; Meyer, 2006). Edema can develop secondary to hypoalbuminemia in cases of alimentary lymphoma, or as a result of space-occupying masses causing compression and impairment of venous and lymphatic circulation, such as in mediastinal lymphoma. Organ failure, attributable to invasion and destruction of normal tissue by neoplastic lymphocytes, may be measured in advanced stages of disease.

Paraneoplastic syndromes associated with equine lymphoma are uncommon, and are thought to be the result of soluble polypeptide hormones secreted by tumor cells. Reported paraneoplastic conditions in horses with lymphoma include: hypercalcemia and pseudohyperparathyroidism; immune-mediated anemia; immune-mediated thrombocytopenia; erythrocytosis; eosinophilia; hypoglycemia; hypertriglyceridemia; hypertrophic osteopathy; hypertrichosis; and polyuria/polydipsia (Marr, 1989; Mair, 1990; Ogilvie, 1998; Schneider, 2003; Koch, 2006; Meyer, 2006; Mitsui, 2007; McGovern, 2011; Taintor, 2011; Axiak, 2012).

Equine Clinical Immunology, First Edition. Edited by M. Julia B. Felippe.
© 2016 John Wiley & Sons, Inc. Published 2016 by John Wiley & Sons, Inc.

20.3 Forms of equine lymphoma

20.3.1 Multicentric

Multicentric or generalized lymphoma is the most common form of lymphoma in horses, and is characterized by variable involvement of nearly any organ system through metastasis of neoplastic lymphocytes. Commonly affected organs include the spleen, liver and kidneys. Less frequently reported sites include the heart, reproductive and urogenital tracts, central nervous system, eye, and upper airway (Marr, 1989; Schneider, 2003; Koch, 2006; Schnabel, 2006; Mitsui, 2007; Germann, 2008; Kelton, 2008; Morrison, 2008; Montgomery, 2009; Schnoke, 2013; Greet, 2011; Madron, 2011; Taintor, 2011; Penrose, 2012; Rendle, 2012; Canisso, 2013; Trope, 2014). Lymphadenopathy is often present, with the most commonly affected peripheral lymph nodes being the mandibular, caudal cervical, retropharyngeal and superficial inguinal. The most commonly abdominal internal lymph nodes include the mesenteric, colonic, and deep iliac (Schneider, 2003). Large granular lymphocyte neoplasia is a rare variant of lymphoma, with reported cases of disseminated multi-organ infiltration with characteristic large granular lymphocytes thought to be related to natural killer (NK) cells (Grindem, 1989; Quist, 1994).

Clinical signs in horses with multicentric lymphoma are directly attributable to the organ system affected, and often include the generalized signs of malaise associated with all forms of lymphoma (Meyer, 2006; Taintor, 2011). Lymphoma involving the central nervous system (CNS) may cause neurologic deficits localizable to the affected region, with signs of ataxia, blindness, lameness, seizures, paresis, cranial nerve deficits, and Horner's Syndrome reported. Ataxia is often the result of spinal cord compression from extradural or leptomeningeal neoplastic infiltration (Adolf, 2001; Morrison, 2008).

Lymphoma of the eye or adnexa commonly involves the palpebral conjunctiva and eyelids and may present as exophthalmus, conjunctivitis, keratitis, uveitis, or chemosis (Schneider, 2003; Germann, 2008; Schnoke, 2013; Rendle, 2012; Trope, 2014). Tumors affecting the upper airways often induce stridor, airway obstruction, facial deformation, and nasal discharge. Lymphoma affecting the liver has been associated with hypoalbuminemia and hepatic encephalopathy (Meyer, 2006; Schnabel, 2006).

Lymphoma originating in the bone marrow may displace normal hematopoietic tissue (myelophthisis), leading to impaired cell production and peripheral blood pancytopenia (Kelton, 2008). Rarely, neoplastic cells produced in the bone marrow may be released into circulation, resulting in a lymphocytic leukemia (Rendle, 2007; Cian, 2013). In the latter scenario, blood lymphocyte counts may be decreased, normal, or elevated, and atypical lymphocytes displaying criteria of malignancy can be observed on cytologic examination of peripheral blood smear. Differentiating leukemic lymphoma from primary leukemia may be difficult in some cases (Cian, 2013).

20.3.2 Alimentary

Alimentary or intestinal lymphoma is characterized by diffuse or segmental infiltration of the gastrointestinal (GI) tract with neoplastic lymphocytes. While one retrospective study found a mean age of 16 years for horses with alimentary lymphoma (Taylor, 2006), it often affects young horses less than five years old (Schneider, 2003). Any portion of the alimentary tract may be involved, with the small intestine being the most commonly affected section (Taylor, 2006). Lesions may be focal and mass-like or, more commonly, diffuse and infiltrative in nature.

In cases with diffuse neoplastic infiltration of the small intestine, local tissue destruction results in loss of absorptive capabilities and protein-losing enteropathy. These horses are often clinically indistinguishable from cases of inflammatory bowel disease or other protein-losing enteropathies, and frequently present with weight loss despite a vigorous appetite, hypoalbuminemia, reduced oral glucose absorption efficiency, and variably increased small intestinal wall thickness on abdominal ultrasound (Schneider, 2003; Taylor, 2006; Sanz, 2010; Mair, 2011). Ventral edema and peritoneal effusion, when present, results from low plasma oncotic pressure.

The author has observed alimentary lymphoma cases in which tissue samples obtained via duodenoscopy and rectal biopsy revealed only lymphocytic-plasmacytic enterocolitis (LPE), without evidence of neoplasia. In these cases, medical management for presumptive inflammatory bowel disease with immunosuppressants and diet modification was unrewarding or only transiently effective, and lymphoma was subsequently diagnosed on post-mortem examination. Distinguishing LPE from intestinal lymphosarcoma by histologic examination alone is reported to be difficult (Kleinschmidt, 2006; Fukushima, 2009), either due to sampling limitations or because alimentary lymphoma may manifest as LPE-like during its development.

Horses with lymphoma involving the large colon may present as diarrhea and colitis, and clinicians should keep lymphoma as a differential for refractory diarrhea cases in which more typical etiologies have been ruled out (Taylor, 2006; Sanz, 2010). Increased colonic wall thickness, diffusely or segmentally, may be observed on abdominal ultrasound. Horses with altered GI motility secondary to neoplastic infiltration of the bowel may show signs of colic (Taylor, 2006; Matsuda, 2013).

20.3.3 Mediastinal or thoracic

Mediastinal or thoracic lymphoma is the most common thoracic neoplasm in the horse, and it originates from lymphoid tissues in the thymus or mediastinal lymph nodes. This form of lymphoma generally affects adult horses (Mair, 1985, 1993; Schneider, 2003). Mediastinal tumors can grow large enough to cause compression of surrounding thoracic organs and impede venous return to the heart, resulting in clinical signs of tachycardia, dyspnea, distended jugular pulses, and ventral edema. Pleural effusion may result in muffled heart sounds, coughing and respiratory distress (Mair, 1985, 1993; Schneider, 2003; Marques, 2012). Compressive obstruction of the esophagus by a thoracic lymphoma mass

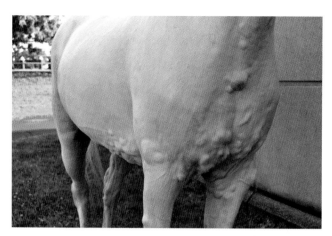

Figure 20.1 Cutaneous lymphoma: a 12-year-old Paint mare with cutaneous T cell-rich large B cell lymphoma (Sally Ness, Cornell University).

has been reported in horses presenting for dysphagia (Mair, 1985), and sudden death during training was attributed to thoracic lymphoma in a Standardbred racehorse (Lawn, 2005).

20.3.4 Cutaneous and subcutaneous

Cutaneous lymphoma is characterized by dermal or subdermal nodules, which can be found in nearly any location on the integument (Figure 20.1) The most commonly affected regions include the shoulder, axilla, perineum, and trunk, with a tendency for chain lesions to localize more ventrally (Schneider, 2003; Scott, 2003). Singular or multifocal nodules varying in size between 1–20 cm are generally well-circumscribed, firm, and non-painful. Nodules are usually smooth and covered by normal skin and hair, although alopecia and ulceration may occur secondary to trauma or necrosis.

Rare metastasis to internal lymph nodes or organs have been reported (Hermeyer, 2010), and the author has observed upper airway lesions involving the palate and pharyngeal wall in a horse with cutaneous lymphoma. The growth rate of cutaneous lymphoma lesions is highly variable; some lesions may appear suddenly and grow rapidly, while others will remain static for years with only intermittent periods of growth. Spontaneous regression and then reappearance of cutaneous nodules has been reported in pregnant mares, as well as a mare with a granulosa-theca cell tumor. This suggests that a relationship between steroid hormones such as progesterone and estrogen, and cutaneous lymphoma may exist in horses (Henson, 1998, 2000).

Epitheliotropic lymphoma, also termed mycoses fungoides, is a rare form of cutaneous lymphoma characterized by severe, generalized or multifocal exfoliative dermatitis with alopecia, scaling and crusting. This form is clinically unique and closely resembles other exfoliative dermatoses such as pemphigus foliaceus and sarcoidosis (Scott, 2003). *Borrelia*-associated cutaneous pseudolymphoma, a condition which histologically resembles T-cell rich large B-cell lymphoma or cutaneous

lymphoid hyperplasia, but which responds to treatment with tetracycline, has been reported in one horse, following removal of a tick from the masseter (Sears, 2012).

20.4 Immunologic mechanisms and etiologic associations

Equine lymphoma is currently thought to be a sporadic disease of unknown etiology. Viral association with lymphoid malignancies is well-recognized in other species, including Epstein-Barr and herpes virus-8 in humans, bovine leukemia virus (BLV) in cattle, and feline leukemia virus (FeLV) in cats (Alexander, 2007; Burton, 2010; Beatty, 2014; Castillo, 2014). Co-infection with immune-modulating viruses such as human immunodeficiency virus (HIV) and feline immunodeficiency virus (FIV) is also thought to have a contributory or synergistic role in the pathogenesis of lymphoma (Alexander, 2007; Beatty, 2014; Castillo, 2014). Although viral associations have been proposed in select equine case reports (Tomlinson, 1979; du Toit, 2012; Vander Werf, 2013), these findings have not had sufficient corroboration to confirm a viral etiology in equine lymphoma.

While there are currently no established risk factors for equine lymphoma, a great deal of research has been done to identify epidemiologic factors that may contribute to lymphoma in man. Numerous studies have examined proposed risk factors related to environment (pesticides, herbicides, occupational chemicals, radiation exposure), genetics, diet and lifestyle, and immune status (vaccination, comorbidities) (Alexander, 2007). The results of these studies suggest that the pathogenesis of lymphoma in humans is complex and multifactorial, and it is likely that the pathogenesis of equine lymphoma similarly involves a myriad of host, genetic, and environmental factors.

20.5 Diagnostics

The diagnostic work up of horses suspected of having lymphoma should include thorough physical examination with special attention paid to peripheral and internal lymph nodes, the latter via transrectal abdominal palpation. Abdominal and thoracic ultrasound examination may reveal effusions, masses, increased intestinal wall thickness, and/or abnormal organ architecture suggestive of neoplastic infiltration (Figure 20.2A, B; Marr, 1989; Chaffin, 1992; Garber, 1994; Taylor, 2006).

Definitive diagnosis of lymphoma can be obtained antemortem through identification of neoplastic lymphocytes in tissues, fluids, aspirates, or peripheral blood. Histology of biopsy samples is the most sensitive ante-mortem test, and also allows further characterization with immunophenotyping (see section below). In general, biopsies of masses or lymph nodes affected by lymphoma reveal invasion of normal tissue architecture by atypical or clonal lymphocytes (Figure 20.3).

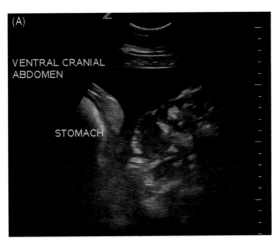
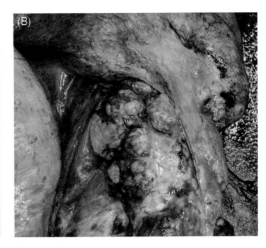

Figure 20.2 Intra-abdominal lymphoma.

(A) Abdominal ultrasound image obtained from a Thoroughbred gelding with splenic lymphoma. Note the irregular, mixed-echogenicity, nodular appearance of the spleen. Stomach is on the left of the screen, and appears normal. Cytologic examination of the peritoneal effusion seen in this image revealed neoplastic lymphocytes (not shown).

(B) Necropsy image from the gelding shown in Figure 20.3. B-cell lymphoma was identified diffusely throughout the spleen. Stomach is noted on the left of the photo, and is not affected. (Sally Ness, Cornell University).

The cytologic criteria for malignancy indicative of neoplastic transformation include: decreased nuclear chromatin condensation; increased cytoplasmic basophilia; mitotic figures; binucleation; and prominent nucleoli (Schneider, 2003; Harvey, 2012). Prior to placing biopsy specimens in formalin, the cut tissue surface may be pressed against a clean glass slide to create an imprint smear for cytologic examination. Aspirates of suspected lesions or masses may also be transferred to a clean glass slide for cytologic examination.

Fine needle aspirates from enlarged lymph nodes may be unrewarding for differentiating reactive lymphoid hyperplasia from lymphoma, and excisional biopsies are generally preferred whenever possible. Internal lesions may be sampled via fine needle aspirate or tru-cut biopsy, under ultrasound guidance (Madron, 2011; De Clercq, 2004). Biopsies of internal lesions may be obtained laparoscopically and/or endoscopically, depending on location (De Clercq, 2004; Pollock, 2006).

Figure 20.3 Cutaneous lymphoma histology. Photomicrographs of a T cell-rich large B cell lymphoma:

(A) Low magnification view illustrating a well demarcated, highly cellular mass of tightly packed round cells (H&E, 100 ×).

(B) High magnification view showing the tightly packed round cells with a prominent nucleus and scant cytoplasms intermingled with larger cells with more abundant cytoplasm (H&E 200 ×).

(C) CD3 immunohistochemistry, illustrating intense immunoreactivity in the smaller round cells, confirming them as T cells (200 ×).

(D) BSAP(PAX5) immunohistochemistry, showing the strong immunoreactivity in the larger tumoral cells, identifying them as B cells (200 ×) (courtesy Elizabeth Buckles, Cornell University).

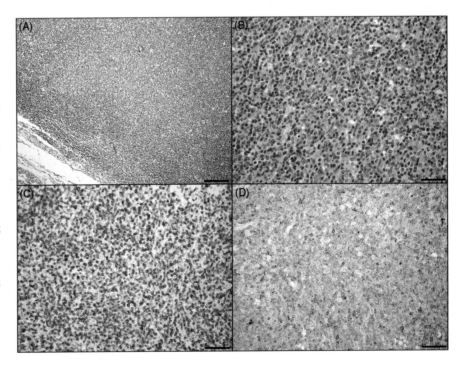

Although lymphoma tumors within the thorax and abdomen generally shed few neoplastic cells, cases in which effusions are identified should be sampled via thoracocentesis and/or abdomoninocentesis for cytologic examination (De Clerq, 2004; Taylor, 2006). In such cases, identification of serosanguinous fluid containing lymphoblasts and erythophagia, without evidence of organisms or sepsis, is highly suggestive of lymphoma. Identification of malignant lymphocytes in effusions provides a definitive diagnosis. Horses with pancytopenia on complete blood count, and/or atypical lymphocytes on peripheral blood smear, should have bone marrow aspiration or core biopsy performed to investigate bone marrow involvement (Kelton, 2008).

Cerebrospinal fluid analysis from horses with CNS lymphoma is variable, and may reveal no abnormalities, a lymphocytic pleocytosis or, less commonly, neoplastic lymphocytes (Adolf, 2001). Central nervous system lymphoma has a predilection for extradural structures (epidural space, leptomeninges), and can cause spinal cord compression without altering the composition of the CSF (Adolf, 2001). Cerebrospinal fluid should be obtained from the site closest to the suspected lesion whenever possible (e.g., atlanto-occipital centesis for a case with a suspected cerebral lesions).

Aqueocentesis and cytologic examination of aqueous humor revealed malignant lymphocytes in a horse with uveal lymphoma (Trope, 2014). Clinical signs of stridor or respiratory distress warrant upper airway endoscopy, skull radiographs, and thoracic ultrasound examination. If feasible, more advanced imaging modalities, such as computed tomography (CT) and magnetic resonance imaging (MRI), may be utilized to further characterize tumor extensity and plan for surgical intervention.

In horses with suspected alimentary lymphoma based on clinical signs and impaired absorption on glucose absorption test, biopsies may be obtained from the proximal duodenum using a transendoscopic biopsy device. The tissue samples retrieved from these devices are small and subject to crush injury, so obtaining 5–10 samples is recommended. In horses with signs of large colon involvement, such as diarrhea, rectal biopsies can be obtained using a uterine biopsy device. Horses undergoing exploratory laparotomy should have full-thickness intestinal biopsies obtained from several sites, as well as biopsies (tru-cut or excisional) from any other suspected lesions. These samples are more defining when questioning inflammatory versus neoplastic conditions (Kleinschmidt, 2006; Fukushima, 2009). For cases in which treatment options are pursued, thoracic radiographs are recommended in order to identify potential pulmonary metastases.

Complete blood count and serum biochemistry results are variable and often non-specific, but may include the following abnormalities:

1 *Anemia* – anemia of chronic inflammation, intravascular or extravascular immune-mediated hemolysis secondary to antibody binding to erythrocytes (positive Coombs' test); lack of production of erythrocytes, due to bone marrow dysfunction/myelophthisis; blood loss from GI ulceration or thrombocytopenia (McGovern, 2011; Taintor, 2011).

2 *Thrombocytopenia* – immune-mediated destruction, particularly with splenic involvement.

3 *Pancytopenia* – lack of production of hematopoietic cells, due to bone marrow dysfunction/myelopthisis (McGovern, 2011; Axiak, 2012).

4 *Lymphocytosis with atypical lymphocytes* – leukemic lymphoma.

5 *Neutrophilia* – systemic inflammatory response to tumor necrosis or infection.

6 *Eosinophilia* – rare paraneoplastic response to cytokines (e.g., IL-5 and GM-CSF) secreted by neoplastic cells (La Perle, 1998).

7 *Hyperglobulinemia* – systemic inflammatory response to tumor necrosis or infection (inflammatory globulins); humoral response to tumor antigens (polyclonal immunoglobulins); overproduction of immunoglobulins by clonal neoplastic B lymphocytes (monoclonal gammopathy).

8 *Hyperfibrinogenemia* – systemic inflammatory response to tumor necrosis, infection, or IL-6 production (Meyer, 2006; Axiak, 2012).

9 *Hypoalbuminemia* – negative acute phase response; chronic inflammation; protein-losing enteropathy and malabsorption in cases of alimentary lymphosarcoma; rarely, decreased production by the liver (Meyer, 2006).

10 *Hypogammaglobulinemia* – impaired production of immunoglobulins due to B cell lymphopenia or lack of B cell activation, secondary to the effects of the neoplastic cells. Consequently, some cases present low serum IgM concentrations, and serum IgM concentration $\leq 23\,\text{mg/dL}$ has 23% sensitivity and 88% specificity for the diagnosis of lymphoma in horses, with a low positive predictive value of 70% (Perkins, 2003).

11 *Hypercalcemia* – pseudohyperparathyroidism paraneoplastic syndrome, resulting from parathyroid (PTH)-like hormone secretion by neoplastic lymphocytes, production of osteoclastic activating factor 1,25-dihydroxy-vitamin D, and prostaglandin (Marr, 1989; Axiak, 2012); attention to the effect of hypoalbuminemia on total calcium values, which could be misleadingly low or normal.

20.6 Classification of lymphomas

20.6.1 Immunophenotyping

Immunophenotyping is a technique in which conjugated antibodies directed against specific lymphocyte surface antigens (termed cluster of differentiation (CD) molecules) or intracellular molecules are used to classify lymphomas, based on their predominant cell lineage (i.e., B cell versus T cell). Markers commonly used to identify B cell lymphomas include the intracellular B cell lineage-specific activator protein (BSAP or

PAX5), the transmembrane enzyme CD45-B220, and the cell surface CD19. Markers specific to T cell lymphomas include cell surface CD3, CD4, and CD8 (Kelley, 1998; McClure, 2001; de Bruijn, 2007; Durham, 2013; Harvey, 2012). Imprint smears or concentrated cell solutions on glass slides may be used for immunophenotyping. In addition, freshly frozen tissues offer more options for immunophenotyping than formalin-fixed tissues, due to reagent performance.

In a recent retrospective study classifying 203 cases of equine lymphoma according to the World Health Organization (WHO) criteria, the most common immunophenotype was T cell-rich large B cell (TCRLBC) lymphoma, which is characterized by a majority population of reactive T cell lymphocytes among a smaller percentage of malignant B cells (Durham, 2013). In this study, TCRLBC lymphomas comprised 43% (87/203) of the total equine study population (Durham, 2013). When equine lymphomas are grouped by location, multicentric lymphoma is usually either TCRLBC or peripheral T cell lymphoma, while mediastinal tumors are generally T cell in origin (Kelley, 1998; Durham, 2013). The predominant immunophenotype of cutaneous lymphoma is debated between reports; two studies found cutaneous lymphoma to be largely TCRLBC lymphoma (Kelley, 1998; Durham, 2013), while another study reported cutaneous lymphoma cases to be primarily T cell in origin (de Bruijn, 2007).

Immunophenotyping of lymphoma in human medicine is used to provide information regarding tumor behavior, progression, treatment choices, and prognosis. Although similar correlations have not yet been corroborated in equine medicine, performing immunophenotyping on cases of equine lymphoma and expanding the currently body of data, may yield similar clinical and prognostic guidelines in the future.

Estrogen and progesterone receptor expressions by lymphoma tumors have been investigated in response to several reports of equine cutaneous lymphoma regressing or even disappearing completely in response to pregnancy, progesterone therapy, or following removal of a granulosa-theca cell tumor (Henson, 1998, 2000). In a study of 29 cases of equine lymphoma, 55% were found to be positive for progesterone receptors, while none were found to express estrogen receptors (Henson, 2000). The clinical relevance of these findings has not been substantiated, but anecdotal evidence suggests a relationship between steroid hormones and cutaneous lymphoma in horses.

More detailed information regarding immunologic testing in horses is provided elsewhere, and clinicians are advised to contact their immunology reference laboratory prior to collecting samples in order to ensure proper handling and preparation.

20.7 Prognosis and treatment

The prognosis for all forms of equine lymphoma is grave. Clinical progression and survival time is variable and depends on the form of lymphoma, the extent of organ involvement, and the overall health of the patient. Many cases are end-stage at the time of diagnosis, and euthanasia is often recommended. Most forms of lymphoma are characterized by a steady decline in health progressing to multi-organ failure and death, although some cases of cutaneous lymphoma may remain stable for years, with slow progression and minimal effects on the overall health of the patient, even in the absence of any therapeutic intervention.

For veterinarians and owners wishing to pursue palliative treatment, there are a number of therapeutic options available, including surgical excision, chemotherapy, and radiation therapy. These modalities may be used alone or in combination – for example, surgical debulking of a tumor, followed by intralesional injection of a chemotherapeutic agent. With the exception of complete surgical excision of a solitary tumor, all currently available treatment modalities should be considered palliative, with the goal being to temporarily improve quality of life and extend survival time, rather than achieve complete remission or cure. Response to palliative treatment is highly variable, and whether cases that are diagnosed early in the course of disease respond more favorably to therapy is not currently known.

20.7.1 Surgical excision

There are a number of reports describing surgical tumor reduction or removal in cases of equine lymphoma involving the eye, colon, upper airway, and skin (Madron, 2011; Schnoke, 2013; Matsuda, 2013). Some of these cases experienced favorable outcomes with extended periods of survival, while others presented recurrence of the original tumor or developed multicentric lymphoma following surgery. As with all types of malignant neoplasia, the success of surgical excision is dependent on the ability to achieve adequate tissue margins surrounding the tumor and the presence of additional lesions and/or metastases at the time of surgery (Schnoke, 2013). Splenectomy has been reported with success and no recurrence of lymphoma at seven months post-operatively in a mule diagnosed with splenic lymphoma (Madron, 2011). Surgical debulking of non-excisable tumors may be performed in conjunction with other treatment modalities, such as radiation and chemotherapy (Doyle, 2013).

20.7.2 Radiation therapy

Two techniques are available for administering radiation therapy to horses with lymphoma: brachytherapy and teletherapy. Brachytherapy, also known as internal radiotherapy, is a form of radiation therapy in which a source of radiation, usually a platinum-coated iridium-192 "seed" or wire, is surgically implanted inside or adjacent to the area requiring treatment. Brachytherapy has the benefit of delivering high doses of targeted radiation with minimal systemic side-effects, and has been reported with success for the treatment of sarcoids, squamous cell carcinoma, and hemangiosarcoma in horses (Theon, 1995; Byam-Cook, 2006; Burks, 2009).

Teletherapy, also known as external beam radiotherapy, requires specialized equipment, facilities, and personnel. Teletherapy is administered via a linear accelerator, and delivers a focused beam of radiation to the area of interest. General anesthesia or heavy sedation is required, and the total radiation dose is divided over several sessions, in order to minimize injury to surrounding normal tissues. Teletherapy has been used successfully to treat three horses with solitary cutaneous lymphoma tumors and one horse with nasal lymphoma, all of which had no tumor regrowth at follow-up (Henson, 2004). Teletherapy has also been used for palliative treatment of nasal and paranasal sinus B cell lymphoma in a pony (Gerard, 2010). Surgical debulking of tumors is often performed prior to radiation therapy, in order to reduce the gross tumor volume and decrease the total radiation dose required.

20.7.3 Chemotherapy and immunosuppressive therapy

Chemotherapeutic protocols exist for intralesional and systemic administration. The goal of any chemotherapeutic protocol should be to maximize neoplastic cell death while minimizing local and systemic side-effects, toxicity, and drug exposure to personnel (Burns, 2009). Protocols in veterinary medicine offer lower doses and longer intervals between treatments than in human oncology, as the goal is to improve and prolong life rather than to achieve a cure (Burns, 2009).

Similar to the aforementioned treatment modalities, chemotherapy for cases of equine lymphoma is considered palliative, rather than curative. The exception to this rule would be intralesional therapy of a solitary mass; intralesional injection of cisplatin suspended in sesame oil has a reported cure rate (defined as no tumor regrowth at four years post-treatment) of 96% for cutaneous lymphoma tumors (Theon, 2007). Systemic chemotherapeutic protocols often utilize multiple drugs to minimize the development of acquired drug resistance of tumor cells (Schneider, 2003; Saulez, 2004; Burns, 2009; Taintor, 2011). When designing a multi-drug protocol, those with different mechanisms of action and non-overlapping toxicities are preferred. Alternatively, doxorubicin, L-Asparaginase, cyclophosphamide, and vincristine can all be utilized individually as single-agent therapies, depending on the clinician's preference, the treatment goal, and financial constraints (Burns, 2009). Lomustine (CCNU), a nitrosourea alkylating agent used to treat canine cutaneous lymphoma, was recently reported in a successful treatment of cutaneous lymphoma of a 12 year old gelding. This patient also received prednisolone and surgical debulking (Doyle, 2013).

Corticosteroid therapy is affordable, and may provide temporary palliative improvement by reducing inflammation, increasing appetite, inducing apoptosis of lymphoid cells, and mitigating paraneoplastic and immune-mediated syndromes (Burns, 2009). Prednisolone has excellent bioavailability when administered orally to horses, and may be used alone or as part of a multi-drug chemotherapy protocol. In contrast, oral prednisone is poorly absorbed in horses, and fails to be converted to its active metabolite prednisolone (Peroni, 2002). In humans, dexamethasone has been shown to be 5–6 times more cytotoxic to leukemia lymphoblasts when compared to prednisolone. However, it is also more potent at inducing deleterious metabolic side-effects, such as altered body mass index, insulin resistance, hyperglycemia, and myopathy, particularly when administered in the long term. For this reason, prednisolone is more commonly prescribed for lymphoma and leukemia in humans (Mitchell, 2005; Zheng, 2010).

Whether or not the two corticosteroids have similar physiologic behavior in horses with lymphoma and leukemia is unknown. The recommended dose for prednisolone in horses with lymphoma is 1–2.2 mg/kg PO q24–48 hours (Taintor, 2011), while the recommend dose for dexamethasone in horses with lymphoma is 0.02–0.2 mg/kg IV, IM, or PO q24 hours (Schneider, 2003). Horses receiving long-term treatment with corticosteroids may be at increased risk of developing gastric ulcers and right dorsal ulcerative colitis, and the concurrent administration of gastroprotectants, as well as avoidance of other non-steroidal anti-inflammatory drugs (NSAIDs), is highly recommended. The corticosteroid dose should be reduced with time and tailored to the patient according to side-effects and therapeutic response.

Chemotherapeutic drugs used in the treatment of equine lymphoma, as reported by Taintor (2011), are provided in Tables 20.1 and 20.2.

Chemotherapeutic drugs are dosed according to body surface area which, in horses, can be calculated using the formula below (Taintor, 2011). Using this formula, a 450 kg horse would have an approximate body surface area of $5\,m^2$:

$$\text{Body surface area}\,(m^2) = \text{weight}\,(g^{2/3}) \times 10.5/10^4$$

Examples of lymphoma chemotherapy protocols reported in the literature are provided below. The reader is encouraged to seek the primary reference for further information.

20.7.4 Example Protocol 1 (Burns, 2009)

This CAP protocol consists of three drugs: cyclophosphamide (an alkylating agent; 1 g per treatment for a 450 kg horse, IV), cytosine arabinoside (an antimetabolite; 1.0–1.5 g per treatment, IV or SQ), and prednisolone (a corticosteroid; 1 mg/kg PO). The cyclophosphamide and cytosine arabinoside are administered on an alternating basis at intervals of 1–2 weeks, and the prednisolone is given daily or every other day throughout the treatment period. Partial or complete remission usually occurs within 2–4 weeks after initiating therapy. This induction protocol is continued for 2–4 months, at which point the cyclophosphamide and cytosine arabinoside intervals can be lengthened, one week at a time, as long as the patient is stable and in

Table 20.1 Chemotherapeutic drugs used in treatment of equine lymphoma: mechanisms of action and toxicity.

Agent type	Drug	Mechanism of action	Toxicity
Alkylating agent	Cyclophosphamide	Inhibits DNA, RNA and protein synthesis	Bone marrow suppression, bladder irritation (in canine)
	Chlorambucil		Bone marrow suppression
Antimetabolides	Cytosine arabinoside (Cytarabine)	Kills cell in S-phase and blocks progression from G_1 to S phase of DNA synthesis	Thrombocytopenia, neutropenia
Antibiotics	Doxorubicin	Inhibition of protein synthesis, free radical formation	Cardiotoxic, nephrotoxic, potent vesicant
Antitublin	Vincristine	Inhibition of intracellular microtubules thus disrupting the cell cycle	Perivascular tissue reaction, hepatotoxic
Hormone	Prednisolone	Inhibits DNA synthesis	Laminitis
Miscellaneous	L-asparagfnase	Deprive cells of amino acid thus inhibit protein synthesis	Hypersensitivity reaction
	Cisplatin	Binds DNA strands preventing protein synthesis	Can be nephrotoxic in dogs

Source: Taintor (2011).

Table 20.2 Chemotherapeutic drugs used in treatment of equine lymphoma: protocols and dosages.

Protocol	Drug	Dosage	Route	Treatment regime
CAP	Cyclophosphamide	200 mg/m^2	i.v. (catheter)	Every 2 weeks
	Cytosine arabinoside	1.0–1.5 g/treatment	i.m. or subcut	alternating basis
	Prednisolone	1 mg/kg bwt	per os	daily
COP	Cytosine arabinoside	200–300 mg/m^2	sub cut/i.m.	q. 7–14 days
	Chlorambucil or	20 mg/m^2	per os i.v.	q. 14 days
	cyclophosphamide	200 mg/m^2	(catheter)	q. 14-21 days
	Prednisolone	1.1–2.2 mg/kg bwt	per os	q. 48 h
	Vincristine (can be added if no response initially)	0.5 mg/m^2	i.v. (catheter)	q. 7 days
Single agent therapy	L-asparaginase	10,000–40,000 iu/m^2	i.m.	q. 2–3 weeks
	Cyclophosphamide	200 mg/m^2	i.v. (catheter)	q. 2–3 weeks
	or vincristine	0.5 mg/m^2	i.v. (catheter)	
Combo chemotherapeutic	Cyclophosphamide	300 mg/m^2	i.v. (catheter)	Given Days 1 and 36
with autologous vaccine	Autologous tumour vaccine	2 ml injected at 4 sites	i.m.	Days 4, 21 and 39
Single drugs	Doxorubicin	30–65 mg/m^2	i.v. (catheter)	q. 3 weeks
	Cisplatin (1 ml of 10 mg/ml cisplatin and 2 ml sesame oil)	1 mg cisplatin/cm^3 of tumour spaced ~1 cm plane	Intraleslonal	q. 2 weeks

Source: Taintor (2011).

remission. This maintenance schedule can continue until the lymphoma relapses, or clinical deterioration occurs. Most patients are reported to remain in remission for 6–8 months on this particular protocol.

20.7.5 Example Protocol 2 (Schneider, 2003)

This COP protocol consists of three drugs: chlorambucil (20 mg/m^2 PO), cytosine arabinoside (200–300 mg/m^2 IM or SQ), and prednisolone (1–2 mg/kg PO). The chlorambucil and cytosine arabinoside are administered on an alternating basis at intervals of 1–2 weeks, and the prednisolone is given daily or every other day throughout the treatment period. Response should occur in 2–4 weeks. If no response is observed, vincristine (a cell cycle disruptor; 0.5 mg/m^2 IV once a week) may be added to the protocol. This induction protocol is continued for 2–3 months,

and then is switched to a maintenance protocol, in which the intervals between chlorambucil and cytosine arabinoside are lengthened one week at a time, as long as the patient is stable and in remission.

20.7.6 Example Protocol 3 (Theon, 2013a, 2013b)

Doxorubicin may be used as single-agent therapy and appears to have excellent efficacy against lymphoma in horses. In a recent study, doxorubicin was well tolerated and had a 100% response rate in horses with lymphoma at a dosage of 70 mg/m^2 administered at three-week intervals for 4–6 treatments. Despite its documented cardiotoxic effects in other species, no deleterious cardiac effects were reported in this group of horses, but clinical signs and markers of cardiotoxicity should be monitored during therapy. Adjunctive treatment with antihistamines and non-steroidal anti-inflammatory drugs were recommended to control hypersensitivity.

20.7.7 Example Protocol 4 (Schneider, 2003)

L-asparaginase (10,000–40,000 IU/m^2 IM once every 2–3 weeks).

20.8 Monitoring

Monitoring for deleterious side-effects and adjusting treatment schedules accordingly is crucial for managing horses undergoing chemotherapy. Horses should receive thorough physical examination and complete blood count prior to each treatment, and the treatment delayed if evidence of bone marrow suppression (usually evident as neutropenia), cardiotoxicity, nephrotoxicity, and/or sepsis are present. Systemic side-effects vary by drug, and may include: general malaise; inappetence; lethargy; bone marrow suppression; neutropenia; thrombocytopenia; cardiotoxicity (doxorubicin); nephrotoxicity; laminitis; and hypersensitivity reactions with repeated dosing (L-asparaginase, doxorubicin). Local side-effects of injectable chemotherapeutics include severe perivascular tissue reaction, necrosis and thrombophlebitis, and therefore it is strongly advised that intravenous chemotherapy drugs should only be administered through an intravenous catheter or long-term vascular access port.

Response to chemotherapy is highly variable, with some horses displaying dramatic improvement within 2–4 months of initiating induction protocols and remaining in remission for several months, while others show only modest or no response, regardless of treatment protocol. Regular progress checks for horses undergoing chemotherapy should include palpation per rectum, as well as abdominal and thoracic ultrasound examination, in order to assess response to treatment and monitor for progression, metastases or recurrence of lymphoma. Although a portion of horses may initially improve markedly, relapse typically occurs following discontinuation of therapy (Burns, 2009).

References

Adolf, J.E., Perkins, G.P., Ainsworth, D.A. and de Lahunta, A. (2001). Lymphoma of the central nervous system in horses. *Compendium* **23**(2), 194–201.

Alexander, D.D., Mink, P.J., Adami, H.O., Chang, E.T., Cole, P., Mandel, J.S. and Trichopoulos, D. (2007). The non-Hodgkin lymphomas: A review of the epidemiologic literature. *International Journal of Cancer* 120 Suppl 12, 1–39.

Axiak, S. and Johnson, P.J. (2012). Paraneoplastic manifestations of cancer in horses. *Equine Veterinary Education* **24**(7), 367–376.

Beatty, J. (2014). *Viral causes of feline lymphoma: Retroviruses and beyond. Veterinary Journal* **201**(2), 174–180.

Burks, B.S., Leonard, J.M., Orsini, J.A. and Trombetta, M. (2009). Interstitial brachytherapy in the management of haemangiosarcoma

of the rostrum of the horse: Case report and review of the literature. *Equine Veterinary Education* **21**(9), 487–493.

Burns, T.A and Couto, C.G. (2009). Systemic Chemotherapy for Oncologic Diseases. In: Robinson, N.E. and Sprayberry, K. (eds). *Current Therapies in Equine Medicine*, sixth edition, pp. 15–18. St Louis, Saunders Elsevier.

Burton, A.J., Nydam, D.V., Long, E.D. and Divers, T.J. (2010). Signalment and clinical complaints initiating hospital admission, methods of diagnosis, and pathological findings associated with bovine lymphosarcoma (112 cases). *Journal of Veterinary Internal Medicine* **24**(4), 960–964.

Byam-Cook, K.L., Henson, F.M. and Slater, J.D. (2006). Treatment of periocular and non-ocular sarcoids in 18 horses by interstitial brachytherapy with iridium-192. *The Veterinary Record* **159**(11), 337–341.

Canisso, I.F., Pinn, T.L., Gerdin, J.A., Ollivett, T.L., Buckles, E.L., Schweizer, C.M. and Ainsworth, D.M. (2013). B-cell multicentric lymphoma as a probable cause of abortion in a quarter horse broodmare. *The Canadian Veterinary Journal* **54**(3), 288–291.

Castillo, J.J., Reagan, J.L., Bishop, K.D. and Apor, E. (2014). Viral lymphomagenesis: From pathophysiology to the rationale for novel therapies. *British Journal of Haematology* **165**(3), 300–315.

Chaffin, M.K., Schmitz, D.G., Brumbaugh, G.W. and Hall, D.G. (1992). Ultrasonographic characteristics of splenic and hepatic lymphosarcoma in three horses. *Journal of the American Veterinary Medical Association* **201**(5), 743–747.

Cian, F., Tyner, G., Martini, V., Comazzi, S. and Archer, J. (2013). Leukemic small cell lymphoma or chronic lymphocytic leukemia in a horse. *Veterinary Clinical Pathology* **42**(3), 301–306.

de Bruijn, C.M., Veenman, J.N., Rutten, V.P., Teske, E., van Nieuwstadt, R.A. and van den Ingh, T.S. (2007). Clinical, histopathological and immunophenotypical findings in five horses with cutaneous malignant lymphoma. *Research in Veterinary Science* **83**(1), 63–72.

De Clercq, D., van Loon, G., Lefere, L. and Deprez, P. (2004). Ultrasound-guided biopsy as a diagnostic aid in three horses with a cranial mediastinal lymphosarcoma. *The Veterinary Record* **154**(23), 722–726.

Dewes, H.F. and Blakeley, J.A. (1980). Lymphosarcoma in a thoroughbred filly. *New Zealand Veterinary Journal* **28**(4), 82.

Doyle, A.J., MacDonald, V.S. and Bourque, A. (2013). Use of lomustine (CCNU) in a case of cutaneous equine lymphoma. *The Canadian Veterinary Journal* **54**(12), 1137–1141.

du Toit, N., Genovese, L.M., Dalziel, R.G. and Smith, S.H. (2012). Pulmonary angiocentric lymphoma (lymphomatoid granulomatosis) in a donkey. *Journal of Comparative Pathology* **146**(1), 24–29.

Durham, A.C., Pillitteri, C.A., San Myint, M. and Valli, V.E. (2013). Two hundred three cases of equine lymphoma classified according to the world health organization (WHO) classification criteria. *Veterinary Pathology* **50**(1), 86–93.

Fukushima, K., Ohno, K., Koshino-Goto, Y., Uchida, K., Nomura, K., Takahashi, M., Nakashima, K., Fujino, Y. and Tsujimoto, H. (2009). Sensitivity for the detection of a clonally rearranged antigen receptor gene in endoscopically obtained biopsy specimens from canine alimentary lymphoma. *The Journal of Veterinary Medical Science* **71**(12), 1673–1676.

Garber, J.L., Reef, V.B. and Reimer, J.M. (1994). Sonographic findings in horses with mediastinal lymphosarcoma: 13 cases (1985–1992).

Journal of the American Veterinary Medical Association **205**(10), 1432–1436.

Gerard, M., Pruitt, A. and Thrall, D.E. (2010). Radiation therapy communication: Nasal passage and paranasal sinus lymphoma in a pony. *Veterinary Radiology & Ultrasound* **51**(1), 97–101.

Germann, S.E., Richter, M., Schwarzwald, C.C., Wimmershoff, J. and Spiess, B.M. (2008). Ocular and multicentric lymphoma in a young racehorse. *Veterinary Ophthalmology* **11**, 51–56.

Greet, T.R., Boys Smith, S.J., Foote, A.K. and Steven, W.N. (2011). Mandibular lymphoma in a three-year-old thoroughbred filly. *The Veterinary Record* **168**(3), 80.

Grindem, C.B., Roberts, M.C., McEntee, M.F. and Dillman, R.C. (1989). Large granular lymphocyte tumor in a horse. *Veterinary Pathology* **26**(1), 86–88.

Haley, P.J. and Spraker, T. (1983). Lymphosarcoma in an aborted equine fetus. *Veterinary Pathology* **20**(5), 647–649.

Harvey, J.W. (2012). Disorders of Bone Marrow. In: *Veterinary Hematology: A Diagnostic Guide and Color Atlas*, pp. 261–327. St Louis, Saunders Elsevier.

Henson, F.M.D. and Dobson, J.M. (2004). The use of radiation therapy in the treatment of equine neoplasia. *Equine Veterinary Education* **16**(6), 315–318.

Henson, K.L., Alleman, A.R., Cutler, T.J., Ginn, P.E. and Kelley, L.C. (1998). Regression of subcutaneous lymphoma following removal of an ovarian granulosatheca cell tumor in a horse. *Journal of the American Veterinary Medical Association* **212**(9), 1419–1422.

Henson, K.L., Alleman, A.R., Kelley, L.C. and Mahaffey, E.A. (2000). Immunohistochemical characterization of estrogen and progesterone receptors in lymphoma of horses. *Veterinary Clinical Pathology* **29**(2), 40–46.

Hermeyer, K., Seehusen, F., Gehlen, H., Peters, M. and Wohlsein, P. (2010). Cutaneous T-cell-rich B-cell lymphoma in a horse. *Berliner Und Munchener Tierarztliche Wochenschrift* **123**(9–10), 422–424.

Kelley, L.C. and Mahaffey, E.A. (1998). Equine malignant lymphomas: Morphologic and immunohistochemical classification. *Veterinary Pathology* **35**(4), 241–252.

Kelton, D.R., Holbrook, T.C., Gilliam, L.L., Rizzi, T.E., Brosnahan, M.M. and Confer, A.W. (2008). Bone marrow necrosis and myelophthisis: Manifestations of T-cell lymphoma in a horse. *Veterinary Clinical Pathology* **37**(4), 403–408.

Kleinschmidt, S., Meneses, F., Nolte, I. and Hewicker-Trautwein, M. (2006). Retrospective study on the diagnostic value of full-thickness biopsies from the stomach and intestines of dogs with chronic gastrointestinal disease symptoms. *Veterinary Pathology* **43**(6), 1000–1003.

Koch, T.G., Wen, X. and Bienzle, D. (2006). Lymphoma, erythrocytosis, and tumor erythropoietin gene expression in a horse. *Journal of Veterinary Internal Medicine* **20**(5), 1251–1255.

La Perle, K.M., Piercy, R.J., Long, J.F. and Blomme, E.A. (1998). Multisystemic, eosinophilic, epitheliotropic disease with intestinal lymphosarcoma in a horse. *Veterinary Pathology* **35**(2), 144–146.

Lawn, K. (2005). Sudden death due to thoracic lymphoma in a standardbred racing horse. *The Canadian Veterinary Journal.La Revue Veterinaire Canadienne* **46**(6), 528–529.

Madron, M.S., Caston, S.S., Reinertson, E.L., Tracey, A.K. and Hostetter, J.M. (2011). Diagnosis and treatment of a primary splenic lymphoma in a mule. *Equine Veterinary Education* **23**(12), 606–611.

Mair, T.S., Lane, J.G. and Lucke, V.M. (1985). Clinicopathological features of lymphosarcoma involving the thoracic cavity in the horse. *Equine Veterinary Journal* **17**(6), 428–433.

Mair, T.S., Yeo, S.P. and Lucke, V.M. (1990). Hypercalcaemia and soft tissue mineralisation associated with lymphosarcoma in two horses. *The Veterinary Record* **126**(5), 99–101.

Mair, T.S. and Brown, P.J. (1993). Clinical and pathological features of thoracic neoplasia in the horse. *Equine Veterinary Journal* **25**(3), 220–223.

Mair, T.S., Pearson, G.R. and Scase, T.J. (2011). Multiple small intestinal pseudodiverticula associated with lymphoma in three horses. *Equine Veterinary Journal Supplement* (39) 128–132.

Marques, F.J., Hehenberger, E., Dickinson, R., Wojnarowicz, C. and Lohmann, K. (2012). Respiratory distress due to retropharyngeal and neck swelling in a horse with mediastinal lymphosarcoma. *Compendium* **34**(5), E5.

Marr, C.M., Love, S. and Pirie, H.M. (1989). Clinical, ultrasonographic and pathological findings in a horse with splenic lymphosarcoma and pseudohyperparathyroidism. *Equine Veterinary Journal* **21**(3), 221–226.

Matsuda, K., Shimada, T., Kawamura, Y., Sakaguchi, K., Tagami, M. and Taniyama, H. (2013). Jejunal intussusception associated with lymphoma in a horse. *The Journal of Veterinary Medical Science* **75**(9), 1253–1256.

McClure, J.T., Young, K.M., Fiste, M., Sharkey, L.C. and Lunn, D.P. (2001). Immunophenotypic classification of leukemia in 3 horses. *Journal of Veterinary Internal Medicine* **15**(2), 144–152.

McGovern, K.F., Lascola, K.M., Davis, E., Fredrickson, R.L. and Tan, R. (2011). T-cell lymphoma with immune-mediated anemia and thrombocytopenia in a horse. *Journal of Veterinary Internal Medicine* **25**(5), 1181–1185.

Meyer, J., Delay, J. and Bienzle, D. (2006). Clinical, laboratory, and histopathologic features of equine lymphoma. *Veterinary Pathology* **43**(6), 914–924.

Mitchell, C.D., Richards, S.M., Kinsey, S.E., Lilleyman, J., Vora, A., Eden, T.O. and Medical Research Council Childhood Leukaemia Working Party. (2005). Benefit of dexamethasone compared with prednisolone for childhood acute lymphoblastic leukaemia: Results of the UK medical research council ALL97 randomized trial. *British Journal of Haematology* **129**(6), 734–745.

Mitsui, I., Jackson, L.P., Couetil, L.L., Lin, T.L. and Ramos Vara, J.A (2007). Hypertrichosis in a horse with alimentary T-cell lymphoma and pituitary involvement. *Journal of Veterinary Diagnostic Investigation* **19**(1), 128–132.

Montgomery, J.B., Duckett, W.M. and Bourque, A.C. (2009). Pelvic lymphoma as a cause of urethral compression in a mare. *The Canadian Veterinary Journal* **50**(7), 751–754.

Morrison, L.R., Freel, K., Henderson, I., Hahn, C. and Smith, S.H. (2008). Lymphoproliferative disease with features of lymphoma in the central nervous system of a horse. *Journal of Comparative Pathology* **139**(4), 256–261.

Ogilvie, G.K. (1998). Paraneoplastic syndromes. *The Veterinary Clinics of North America Equine Practice* **14**(3), 439–449, v.

Penrose, L.C., Brower, A., Kirk, G., Bowen, I.M. and Hallowell, G.D. (2012). Primary cardiac lymphoma in a 10-year-old equine gelding. *The Veterinary Record* **171**(1), 20.

Perkins, G.A., Nydam, D.V., Flaminio, M.J. and Ainsworth, D.M. (2003). Serum IgM concentrations in normal, fit horses and horses with lymphoma or other medical conditions. *Journal of Veterinary Internal Medicine* **17**(3), 337–342.

Peroni, D.L., Stanley, S., Kollias-Baker, C. and Robinson, N.E. (2002). Prednisone per os is likely to have limited efficacy in horses. *Equine Veterinary Journal* **34**(3), 283–287.

Pollock, P.J., and Russell, T. (2006). Standing thoracoscopy in the diagnosis of lymphosarcoma in a horse. *The Veterinary Record* **159**(11), 354–356.

Quist, C.F., Harmon, B.G., Mahaffey, E.A. and Collatos, C. (1994). Large granular lymphocyte neoplasia in an aged mare. *Journal of Veterinary Diagnostic Investigation* **6**(1), 11111–11113.

Rendle, D.I., Durham, A.E., Thompson, J.C., Archer, J., Mitchell, M., Saunders, K., Millere, J., Paillot, R., Smith, K.C. and Kydd, J.H. (2007). Clinical, immunophenotypic and functional characterisation of T-cell leukaemia in six horses. *Equine Veterinary Journal* **39**(6), 522–528.

Rendle, D.I., Hughes, K.J., Farish, C. and Kessell, A. (2012). Multicentric T-cell lymphoma presenting as inferior palpebral swelling in a standardbred mare. *Australian Veterinary Journal* **90**(12), 485–489.

Sanz, M.G., Sellon, D.C. and Potter, K.A. (2010). Primary epitheliotropic intestinal T-cell lymphoma as a cause of diarrhea in a horse. *The Canadian Veterinary Journal* **51**(5), 522–524.

Saulez, M.N., Schlipf, J.W. Jr, Cebra, C.K., McDonough, S.P. and Bird, K.E. (2004). Use of chemotherapy for treatment of a mixed-cell thoracic lymphoma in a horse. *Journal of the American Veterinary Medical Association* **224**(5), 733–738, 699.

Schaffer, P.A., Wobeser, B., Martin, L.E., Dennis, M.M. and Duncan, C.G. (2013). Cutaneous neoplastic lesions of equids in the central United States and Canada: 3,351 biopsy specimens from 3,272 equids (2000–2010). *Journal of the American Veterinary Medical Association* **242**(1), 99–104.

Schnabel, L.V., Njaa, B.L., Gold, J.R. and Meseck, E.K. (2006). Primary alimentary lymphoma with metastasis to the liver causing encephalopathy in a horse. *Journal of Veterinary Internal Medicine* **20**(1), 204–206.

Schneider, D.A. (2003). Lymphoproliferative and Myeloproliferative Disorders. In: Robinson, N.E. (ed) *Current Therapies in Equine Medicine*, fifth edition, pp. 359–362. St Louis, Saunders Elsevier.

Schnoke, A.T., Brooks, D.E., Wilkie, D.A., Dwyer, A.E., Matthews, A.G., Gilger, B.C., Hendrix, D.V., Pickett, P., Grauwels, M., Monroe, C. and Plummer, C.E. (2013). Extraocular lymphoma in the horse. *Veterinary Ophthalmology* **16**(1), 35–42.

Scott, D.W. and Miller, W.H. (2003). Neoplastic and Non-Neoplastic Tumors. In: *Equine Dermatology*, pp. 699–795. St Louis, Saunders Elsevier.

Sears, K.P., Divers, T.J., Neff, R.T., Miller, W.H. Jr. and McDonough, S.P. (2012). A case of borrelia-associated cutaneous pseudolymphoma in a horse. *Veterinary Dermatology* **23**(2), 153–156.

Taintor, J. and Schleis, S. (2011). Equine lymphoma. *Equine Veterinary Education* **23**(4), 205–213.

Taylor, S.D., Pusterla, N., Vaughan, B., Whitcomb, M.B. and Wilson, W.D. (2006). Intestinal neoplasia in horses. *Journal of Veterinary Internal Medicine* **20**(6), 1429–1436.

Theon, A.P. and Pascoe, J.R. (1995). Iridium-192 interstitial brachytherapy for equine periocular tumours: Treatment results and prognostic factors in 115 horses. *Equine Veterinary Journal* **27**(2), 117–121.

Theon, A.P., Wilson, W.D., Magdesian, K.G., Pusterla, N., Snyder, J.R. and Galuppo, L.D. (2007). Long-term outcome associated with intratumoral chemotherapy with cisplatin for cutaneous tumors in equidae, 573 cases (1995–2004). *Journal of the American Veterinary Medical Association* **230**(10), 1506–1513.

Theon, A.P., Pusterla, N., Magdesian K.G., and Wilson, W.D. (2013a). Phase I dose escalation of doxorubicin chemotherapy in tumor-bearing equidae. *Journal of Veterinary Internal Medicine* **27**(5), 1209–1217.

Theon, A.P., Pusterla, N., Magdesian, K.G., Wittenburg, L., Marmulak, T. and Wilson, W.D. (2013b). A pilot phase II study of the efficacy and biosafety of doxorubicin chemotherapy in tumor-bearing equidae. *Journal of Veterinary Internal Medicine* **27**(6), 1581–1588.

Tomlinson, M.J., Doster, A.R. and Wright, E.R. (1979). Lymphosarcoma with virus-like particles in a neonatal foal. *Veterinary Pathology* **16**(5), 629–631.

Trope, G.D., McCowan, C.I., Tyrrell, D., Lording, P.M. and Maggs, D.J. (2014). Solitary (primary) uveal T-cell lymphoma in a horse. *Veterinary Ophthalmology* **17**(2), 139–145.

Vander Werf, K. and Davis, E. (2013). Disease remission in a horse with EHV-5-associated lymphoma. *Journal of Veterinary Internal Medicine* **27**(2), 387–389.

Zheng, C., Liu, X., Wu, J., Cai, X., Zhu, W. and Sun, Z. (2010). Which steroids should we choose for the treatment of adult acute lymphoblastic leukemia? *American Journal of Hematology* **85**(10), 817–818.

21 Immunodeficiencies

M. Julia B. Felippe

21.1 Definition

Immunodeficiency is a rare disorder of the immune system that results in failure to build protection against pathogens and, consequently, in a predisposition to recurrent or fatal infections.

Clinical manifestation of recurrent fevers and infections should alert for the possibility of an immunodeficiency disorder. In general, clinical signs are similar (fever, inflammatory blood work, system-related inflammatory signs), independent of the cause of the immunodeficiency. However, susceptibility to infections with bacteria is most common; the patient often responds to antibiotic therapy because pathogens tend to be opportunistic, but clinical signs return after treatment is discontinued. Indeed, clinical signs that should raise the suspicion of immunodeficiency include:

(a) two or more episodes of pneumonia within one year;
(b) two or more episodes of sinus infection within one year;
(c) multiple sites of infection (e.g., pneumonia plus sinusitis);
(d) recurrent pyodermatitis, deep skin or organ abscesses;
(e) a single episode of meningitis or osteomyelitis;
(f) two or more months on antibiotic therapy;
(g) infection with opportunistic organisms;
(h) failure to gain weight or grow normally;
(i) familial history of primary immunodeficiency.

In addition, autoimmunity and neoplasia may accompany immunodeficiency, reflecting imbalance of the immune system.

An immunodeficiency condition can affect an element of the immune system, with no or mild clinical consequences (e.g., selective IgA deficiency). In these cases, the condition may remain unknown and undiagnosed for years or for the whole lifetime, when the defect is compensated by different defenses of the immune system. Nevertheless, the lack or delay in the diagnosis of immunodeficiency often happens even when clinical signs are present and obvious, due to the low incidence of this type of disorder or poor understanding of clinical signs and types of immunodeficiencies. In any case, immunodeficiency does not make to the differential diagnosis list.

The presence of infections and fevers is essential for the diagnosis of immunodeficiency, and recurrent episodes are supportive. When there is failure to detect an infectious organism, other signs that indicate infection (e.g., fever, neutrophilia or neutropenia with or without a left shift, lymphopenia or lymphocytosis) should be investigated. In the absence of an infectious agent, fevers and abnormal blood work (e.g., an "*ain't doing right*", or ADR case), immunodeficiency is unlikely to be the cause of illness.

Every effort should be in place to identify the pathogen because the type of organism (i.e., bacterium, virus, fungus; encapsulated bacterium; opportunistic or highly virulent; intracellular versus extracellular) may suggest what area of the immune system is impaired. When asking what type of immunity is required for a specific organism, that is the area of the immune system that should be first investigated with existing immunologic testing.

In equine neonates and weanlings, the clinical recognition of underlying primary immunodeficiency may not be obvious because of the common presentation of disease at this age, often involving failure of transfer of immunoglobulins through colostrum, and the physiologic, gradual development of the immune system (i.e., immune population expansion), which creates windows of susceptibility to infections. Independent of the etiology, foals with immunodeficiency present recurrent infections (pneumonia, diarrhea, osteomyelitis, meningitis) for several weeks or months, or infections with opportunistic organisms. In some cases (but, surprisingly, not all), they fail to gain weight and grow properly. In addition, some types of immunodeficiencies are self-limited or transitory.

Management of horses with immunodeficiency can be complicated, and weighs on the decision of euthanasia. Affected horses should be routinely evaluated for the development of infections via routine physical examination and blood work. Special attention should be taken of the respiratory tract, and septicemia can lead to liver disease and meningitis, which often manifests with depression. Some patients are managed with continuous or intermittent antibiotic therapy for months or years. The addition of antifungal drugs may be necessary (e.g., in the presence of candidiasis or aspergillosis).

In the case of humoral deficiencies, administration of plasma transfusions when serum IgG is below 500 mg/dL may help the patient through a life-threatening infectious phase but it is

Equine Clinical Immunology, First Edition. Edited by M. Julia B. Felippe.
© 2016 John Wiley & Sons, Inc. Published 2016 by John Wiley & Sons, Inc.

unrealistic for routine management of adult horses (i.e., monthly administration, indefinitely). However, intravenous plasma therapy is beneficial to foals in transient immunodeficiencies. Vaccination of affected horses with modified-live or live vaccines should be avoided, but performed with inactivated vaccines because other elements of the immune system besides the faulty one can elaborate partial immunity.

21.2 Classification of immunodeficiencies

Immunodeficiencies may be transient or lasting; primary or secondary; and affect one or more cells/mechanisms of the immune system. A broad defective mechanism in the immune system leads to poorer quality of life and prognosis.

Primary immunodeficiencies are congenital processes associated with a genetic hereditary defect. Therefore, the manifestation of these disorders is more frequently observed in young rather than in adult horses but it does not exclude the latter. Single recessive genes may result in autosomal recessive inheritance. Defective genes in the X chromosome would show manifestation in males, while other disorders may not have a clear pattern of inheritance but may be found in several individuals in a family. A few primary conditions are transient or developmental, and improve with age.

Secondary immunodeficiencies are acquired disruptions in the immune function that reduce the ability of the system to fight against opportunistic and/or pathogenic organisms. They can manifest in any phase of life. Conditions that may predispose to secondary immunodeficiencies include: immunosuppressive treatment (e.g., glucocorticoids); infectious diseases; cancer (e.g., lymphoma/lymphosarcoma); metabolic/endocrine diseases (e.g., pituitary pars intermedia dysfunction); age; and nutritional deficiencies.

Immunodeficiencies can be grouped according to the components of the immune system affected:
1 humoral disorders (B cell deficiency);
2 cytotoxic and helper cell deficiencies (T cell deficiency);
3 combined B and T cell deficiencies;
4 phagocytic deficiency; and
5 complement deficiency.

Sometimes, deficiency in one cell type (e.g., CD4$^+$ helper T cell) may result in dysfunction of another cell type (e.g., B cell) because the latter is dependent on the former for its activity.

Many different types of immunodeficiencies have been described in the horse, with humoral deficiencies being the most prevalent, most likely because of the accessibility to diagnostics (e.g., measuring serum immunoglobulin concentrations) (Table 21.1).

21.2.1 Humoral immunodeficiencies

Antibody deficiency is characterized by intrinsic causes of failure of B cell development or differentiation, or B cell dysfunction. In addition, CD4$^+$ helper T cell dysfunction may result in failure to provide survival signals to B cells during their development in the lymphoid tissues. The consequence of lack of B cells, or dysfunctional B cells, is inadequate production of immunoglobulins affecting one or more isotypes (e.g., IgG, IgM, IgA, IgE).

In general, lack of IgG is the most significant humoral deficiency because its role in neutralization and opsonization. Other isotype-selective deficiencies (with normal IgG) may be asymptomatic. The lack of IgG leads to susceptibility to bacterial infections, particularly encapsulate bacteria (e.g., *Streptococcus* spp., *Staphylococcus* spp., *Klebsiella* spp.) because these organisms require both antibody and complement for effective opsonization and phagocytosis. Therefore, respiratory clinical signs are the most common, followed by sinusitis, sepsis, meningitis, osteomyelitis, hepato- or splenomegaly, dermatitis, oral candidiasis, and failure to grow.

21.2.1.1 Transient hypogammaglobulinemia of the young

Transient hypogammaglobulinemia results from a delay in endogenous immunoglobulin production by the foal, which brings a risk of bacterial infection. This condition has been described in foals with recurrent infections at the time when circulating maternally-derived antibody levels decrease, around 2–3 months old (or earlier, if transfer of antibodies at birth was low) (McGuire, 1975). The transient hypogammaglobunemic condition may last a few months (e.g., 5–10 months old) or several months (e.g., 18–24 months old) (Felippe, personal observation). Most foals maintain normal development when treated with antibiotics. The most challenging pathogens are encapsulated bacteria, as they require both immunoglobulin and complement for effective opsonization and phagocytic function, including *Staphylococcus aureus*, *Streptococcus zooepidemicus*, *Klebsiella* ssp, and *Actinobacillus equuli*.

It is not common practice to measure serum IgG and IgM concentrations in foals beyond the first month of life, so this condition may be more frequent than reported. Healthy foals (with no clinical signs of infection) produce antigen-specific antibodies immediately after birth, and serum IgG concentration around 500 mg/dL, and serum IgM concentration of at least 50 mg/dL are often measured at around 3–5 months old. While low, these IgG values do not necessarily indicate failure or delay in the production of immunoglobulins but a transition phase in which endogenous production is still rising to protective values. Values higher than 800 mg/dL are usually measured beyond 6–8 months of age.

In foals with delayed antibody production, though, clinical signs of recurrent bacterial infection are present and require antibiotic therapy. Serum IgG concentration is below protective levels (< 500 mg/dL), and IgM levels are often decreased (< 50 mg/dL). Because colostrum has low levels of IgM, and colostrum-derived IgM has a short half-life (around ten days), serum IgM concentration more clearly reflects endogenous production in a context that can still have circulating colostrum-derived IgG antibodies.

Table 21.1 Immunodeficiencies described in the horse.

Immunological condition	Age onset of clinical signs	Prognosis	Affected breed	Peripheral blood lymphocyte counts	B cell distribution	T cell distribution	Serum IgM	Serum IgG	Serum IgA
Total or partial failure of transfer of colostral immunoglobulins	< 3 weeks	Transient condition	All	Normal	Present functional	Present functional	Low to normal	Low* (< 800 mg/dL)	Low
Transient hypogammaglobulinemia of the young	2–18 months	Transient condition	All	Normal	Present poor response	Present functional	Low (< 50 mg/dL)	Low*	Low
Agammaglobulinemia	2–3 months (only males)	Fatal (< 18 months)	Thoroughbred Standardbred Quarter Horse	Normal or low	Absent no response	Present functional	Undetectable	Undetectable*	Undetectable
Juvenile selective IgM deficiency	2–18 months	Poor prognosis or transient condition	All	Normal	Present poor response	Present poor response low MHC class II	Undetectable (< 25 mg/dL)	Normal	Normal
Foal immunodeficiency syndrome (FIS)	< 2 months	Fatal (< 2 months)	Fell Pony Dale	Moderate lymphopenia	Present at birth Absent by 5 weeks no response	Present Questionable function low MHC class II	Undetectable (< 25 mg/dL)	Normal* to low	Low* to undetectable
Common variable immunodeficiency (CVID)	> 2 years (possible in younger age)	Fatal	All	Low normal or low (< 1,500 cells/uL)	Absent no response	Present functional	Low (< 25 mg/dL)	Low (< 800 mg/dL)	Normal to low
Transient CD4+ T cell lymphopenia of the young	2–18 months	Transient condition	All	Normal to mild lymphopenia	Present functional	Low CD4+ T cells Low CD4: CD8 ratio	Normal to low	Normal to low	Normal to low
Severe combined immunodeficiency (SCID)	< 2 months	Fatal (< 2 months)	Arabian Arabian crossbreeds	Severe lymphopenia	Absent no response	Absent no response	Undetectable (< 25 mg/dL)	Normal* to undetectable	Low* to undetectable

*In foals < 3 months old, serum IgG values may be low or normal at clinical onset due to colostral-derived immunoglobulins.

In general, peripheral blood B and T lymphocyte counts and distribution are normal in these foals. However, many cases have decreased $CD4^+$ T cell distribution ($< 50\%$), with a low CD4 : CD8 ratio (< 2.0) (Felippe, personal observation). T cell proliferation response to mitogen *in vivo* (skin) and *in vitro* has been reported normal (McGuire, 1975). Although foals present a physiologic age-dependent increase in the expression of major histocompatibility (MHC) class II in lymphocytes, affected foals tend to maintain low levels of expression ($< 50\%$) during this transient period, even after stimulation of lymphocytes *in vitro*. Therefore, the expression of MHC class II in peripheral blood lymphocytes should be monitored, as it can be used to evaluate lymphocyte maturation in this transitory condition (Lunn, 1993; Felippe, personal observation).

It is uncertain if the etiology for delayed humoral response also involves a delay in cellular function, and at what level such impairment would be. It is also unclear whether all cases of transient hypogammaglobulinemia involve the same faulty immunologic mechanism, or if the outcome (delayed immuno-globulin production) results from different dysfunctional immune processes. Perhaps it involves inadequate interaction and activation of antigen-presenting cells and lymphocytes in secondary lymphoid tissues for the proper expansion and function of the adapted immune system, including humoral response. Although a progressive increase in serum IgG and IgM concentrations may be measured in some foals during the recovery phase, others show little or no improvement in immunologic parameters for months until, suddenly, they start showing evidence of sustained antibody production (Felippe, personal observation).

The affected foals are managed with continuous or intermittent antibiotic therapy and routine physical examination and blood work to monitor infections. Immunologic testing, based on lymphocyte immunophenotyping ($CD4^+$ and $CD8^+$ T cells, B cells, MHC class II expression) and serum IgG and IgM concentrations every two months can be used to determine progress in immunologic competence, and guidance for the need of antibiotic therapy (e.g., when serum IgG concentration reaches values above 800 mg/dL, antibiotic therapy may be discontinued). Appropriate antibiotic therapy often protects foals during the period of abnormal immunoglobulin production, and plasma transfusion can also be used if infection is severe or refractory to antibiotic therapy. In this case, treatment confounds monitoring of endogenous IgG production.

In affected foals, the response to vaccines is unknown. At this time, a full vaccination program with boosters after the transient hypogammaglobulimia would be recommended to ensure proper long-lived immunization.

21.2.1.2 Agammaglobulinemia

Agammaglobulinemia is a very rare and fatal immuno-deficiency caused by failure in B lymphopoiesis and subsequent impaired endogenous immunoglobulin production, which has been reported in young male horses of different breeds (McGuire, 1976; Perryman, 1983). Serum IgM and IgA concentrations are undetectable, although circulating colostrum-derived IgG may be detected at low levels in foals younger than three months; in these cases, serum IgG values do not increase with age. These foals lack B cells, plasma cells and lymphoid follicles already at birth, and affected patients fail to produce antibodies upon vaccination (Deem, 1979). T lymphocytes are present in normal counts, and they proliferate in response to mitogenic stimulation *in vitro* and *in vivo* (Perryman, 1980).

Colts with this condition develop fevers, bacterial infections of the respiratory and/or gastrointestinal systems and skin. Peripheral lymphadenopathy is common, foals appear unthrifty and with poor development and, while infections are temporarily responsive to antibiotic and plasma therapies, complications lead to death or euthanasia before 18 months (Banks, 1976; McGuire, 1976; Deem, 1979).

The syndrome in male horses presents many features of the X-linked agammaglobulinemia (XLA) described in male human patients and xid-mutant mice (Vetrie, 1993). These patients carry a mutation of the *btk* gene, located in the X chromosome, which encodes the Bruton tyrosine kinase. The absence of this protein affects sustained signaling in response to B cell receptor engagement, leading to defects in B cell differentiation and proliferation.

Typical XLA patients present with recurrent bacterial respiratory infections, absence of B cells and plasma cells in blood and lymphoid tissues, and hypo- or agammaglobulinemia in early in life. Female carriers are healthy, although they may display non-random X-chromosome inactivation in their B cells. The involvement of the *btk* gene in equine agamma-globulinemia has not been confirmed to date, and no new cases have been reported in more than three decades. An important differential diagnosis is common variable immunodeficiency (CVID), although this condition has not been yet diagnosed in horses younger than two years.

21.2.1.3 Selective immunoglobulin deficiencies

In selective immunoglobulin deficiencies, serum immuno-globulin concentration is significantly below normal reference intervals for one immunoglobulin isotype.

Selective IgM deficiency has been reported in foals with chronic infections when serum IgM concentrations were more than two standard deviations below the normal mean, and IgG and IgA were within normal reference range for the age group (Perryman, 1977). Peripheral blood lymphocyte counts, B and T cell distribution, and response to mitogens *in vitro* were reported normal (Weldon, 1992).

The onset of clinical signs were reported to occur between 2–10 months of age, and both males and females of different breeds were affected. Two reported cases had a common sire and great-grandsire (Perryman, 1977). The clinical signs included recurrent fevers, bronchopneumonia, arthritis, enteritis, dermatitis, and lymph node pyogranulomatous response (Perryman,

2000; McGuire, 1983; Boy, 1992). Microorganisms isolated from the respiratory tract of affected foals included *Staphylococcus aureus, Streptococcus zooepidemicus, Actinobacillus equuli, Klebsiella* ssp, and *E. coli*.

In the foal, it is uncertain if selective IgM deficiency is an independent condition, or reflects transient hypogammaglobulinemia of the young, as some of the reported foals recovered IgM and IgG productions when yearlings (Perryman, 1980; Crisman, 1987). Serum IgM concentrations are quite specific for B cell function in foals, as IgM production occurs already *in utero* and colostrum-derived IgM has a short half-life of 5–16 days (Lavoie, 1989; Tallmadge, 2009). Serum IgM and IgG concentrations should be monitored to evaluate for persistence or change in values with age.

Selective IgM deficiency has also been reported in adult horses of both genders and different breeds, without association with susceptibility to infections. In these reports, serum IgM concentrations were more than two standard deviations below the mean normal value of age-matched controls. Serum concentrations for IgG, IgG(T), and IgA were described as normal in the adult horses. Peripheral blood lymphocyte count, B and T cell distribution, and response to mitogens were all reported within normal reference values. Conditions in adult horses may be secondary to lymphosarcoma, prolonged immunosuppressive therapy or stress. Caution should be used when interpreting low serum IgM concentrations: persistent serum IgM concentrations lower than 25 mg/dL better define deficiency (Perkins, 2003). The positive predicted value of serum IgM concentration < 25 mg/dL for the diagnosis of lymphoma or lymphosarcoma is not reliable, and these conditions should be investigated using more effective and definitive diagnostic tests (e.g., lymph node biopsy, cytology and histology).

The definition and pathogenesis of selective IgM deficiency are unclear and intriguing. All naive B cells must express IgM on the cell surface during development, and IgM is produced readily in response to foreign antigen after brief interaction of B and CD4$^+$ T cells, whereas other immunoglobulin isotypes require further robust interaction and selection with activated T cells for isotype switching in the germinal centers. In human patients with selective IgM deficiency, the most common clinical signs are recurrent rhinosinusitis, otitis and pneumonia. In addition, serum IgE concentration is often increased, and there is a high prevalence of allergies (e.g., asthma, rhinitis) and autoimmune diseases. Association with a chromosome deletion and familial cases have been proposed (Louis, 2014).

Selective IgA deficiency is the most prevalent primary immunodeficiency in human patients, and the incidence varies according to geographical region (Singh, 2014). In most patients, there is no association with increased susceptibility to infections (asymptomatic), whereas increased incidence of recurrent bacterial infections or autoimmune diseases has been reported in a small proportion of patients. Selective IgA deficiency has not been systematically studied in the horse. One

report suggested clinically relevant selective IgA deficiency in a cohort of endurance horses (Krick, 2002).

21.2.1.4 Foal immunodeficiency syndrome

Foal immunodeficiency syndrome (FIS) is an inheritable and fatal condition characterized by profound anemia and septicemia described in the Fell Pony, Dales and, potentially, other breeds that include common ancestors (Scholes, 1998; Jelinek, 2006; Dixon, 2000; Richards, 2000; Fox-Clipsham, 2009). Affected foals are born apparently healthy but illness develops within one month of life, and death occurs generally soon after. The foals present weight loss and dullness, and signs of infection, including enterocolitis, bronchopneumonia, and glossal hyperkeratosis, often caused by opportunistic infectious organisms (e.g., *Escherichia coli, Cryptosporidium* spp., and adenovirus) (Bell, 2001; Thomas, 2003; Butler, 2006). Management of infections and subsequent septicemia may be temporarily possible with antibiotic and supportive therapy. The severe, progressive anemia is fatal.

At birth, hemoglobin and hematocrit values may be measured within the low normal reference range, and peripheral blood B cell distribution may be equivalent to that of healthy unaffected foals (Gardner, 2006; Tallmadge, 2012). After a few weeks of life, however, profound anemia and B cell lymphopenia develop. The severe, progressive anemia results from lack of erythrocyte production in the bone marrow (non-regenerative), and it is not associated with hemorrhage or hemolysis. Bone marrow cytology in samples collected prospectively from newborns has shown that affected foals are born with erythroid precursors, but these rapidly evolve to erythrocyte hypoplasia (Figure 21.1; Tallmadge, 2012). At this period, cytologic evaluation of the marrow reveals differentiating myeloid precursors, megakaryocytes, and/or paucity of hematopoietic precursors. When present, proerythroblasts have been described to be binucleate, and a concomitant mild myeloid dysplasia questions the involvement of further types of cells.

Absolute lymphopenia in affected foals likely reflects poor lymphocyte development in primary and secondary lymphoid tissues, and failure of lymphocyte population expansion with age (Tallmadge, 2012). The B lymphopenia limits the ability of affected foals to produce immunoglobulins. Nevertheless, serum IgG concentration is often normal when clinical signs are detected within the first month of life, due to the presence of circulating colostrum-derived antibodies. Septicemia may develop despite normal serum IgG concentrations. Serum IgM concentrations (a parameter not confounded by maternally-derived antibodies at this age) are low in affected foals, and strongly suggest impaired primary humoral immune response.

The CD4$^+$ and CD8$^+$ T cell distribution has been reported normal in affected foals. However, T cell dysfunction is suggested by the small thymus, and opportunistic infections with cryptosporidia and adenovirus (McDonald, 1994). In addition, the expression of major histocompatibility complex class II (MHC class II) molecule in peripheral blood lymphocytes

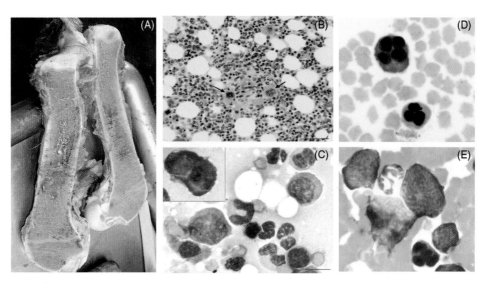

Figure 21.1 Foal immunodeficiency syndrome (FIS).

(A) Bone marrow of a FIS-affected Fell Pony at two months old; note the lack of red marrow.

(B) Photomicrographs of hematoxylin-eosin stained formalin-fixed bone marrow inprint smears, showing the majority of the cells being myeloid precursors, with some megakaryocytes (arrows), and rare erythroblasts (scale bar 50 µm).

Photomicrographs of Wright's-stained smears of a bone marrow aspirate collected from a FIS-affected Fell Pony foal at three weeks old.

(C) Most of the cells are differentiating myeloid precursors with rare erythroblasts, some of which are binucleate (insert, scale bar 10 µm).

(D) Abnormal nuclear shapes (lobulation, blebbing) in metarubricytes.

(Julia Felippe and Tracy Stokol, Cornell University).

(E) Binucleate prorubricyte.

may be decreased, and/or fail to increase with age in affected foals, when compared to healthy foals, also supporting abnormal lymphocyte development (Tallmadge, 2012). Nevertheless, when stimulated *in vitro*, the peripheral blood lymphocytes of affected foals respond normally to mitogens (Gardner, 2006).

In post-mortem, abnormal gross findings include generalized tissue pallor, thymic hypoplasia, inflammation, and lymphadenopathy associated with infections of many organs (e.g., necrotizing enteritis, pyogranulomatous bronchopneumonia, pancreatitis, myocarditis) (Figure 21.1). The medullary cavities of bones often do not contain red marrow, and instead are filled with pale or tan fatty tissue, a striking finding in early age. Histopathology reveals severe erythroid hypoplasia, with small numbers or absent late erythroid precursors in the bone marrow, and a high myeloid: erythroid ratio. Despite lymphadenopathy, there is severe lymphocytic hypoplasia and lack of secondary lymphoid follicles in the lymphoid organs; in addition, plasma cells are absent.

Immunohistochemical staining detects no B lymphocytes in the bone marrow, and rare or few B cells in the lymph nodes and spleen, dispersed in the tissues without forming germinal centers. In addition, peripheral ganglionopathy, characterized by neuronal chromatolysis involving trigeminal, cranial mesenteric and dorsal root ganglia, has been reported (Figure 21.2; Bell, 2001; Thomas, 2003).

The presence of erythrocytes and B cells in peripheral blood at birth suggests a limited hematopoiesis during fetal life, which is not sustained after birth. B lymphocytes and erythrocytes are the most severely affected cell populations in FIS, and both undergo critical developmental stages in the bone marrow. The condition may be caused by independent or common genetic abnormalities that affect both cell lines or the bone marrow environment.

Figure 21.2 Foal Immunodeficiency Syndrome (FIS). Immunohistochemical staining of microsections from tissues collected at necropsy of a FIS-affected foal at two months old. The presence of B cells was tested using a monoclonal antibody against the CD19 molecule and 3-amino-9-ethylcarbazole, AEC reagent, which indicates; positive cells in red. Note the paucity of B cells in the spleen, and the absence of B cells in the bone marrow and lymph node (Julia Felippe, Cornell University).

BONE MARROW   LYMPH NODE   SPLEEN

CD19+
B CELL

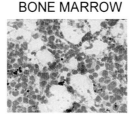
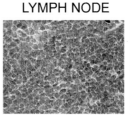
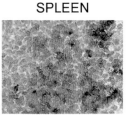

A genome-wide study identified a mutation in the gene SLC5A3 on chromosome ECA26, associated with the syndrome (Fox-Clipsham, 2011a, 2011b). The mechanistic implications of this mutation have not been fully resolved, and a causal relationship between the SLC5A3 mutation and FIS requires further studies to date. The presence of other mutations in that genomic region has not been ruled out as responsible for the phenotype of the immunodeficiency syndrome.

The Fell Pony breed experienced loss of genetic diversity due to the small numbers of animals and overuse of prominent stallions. Pedigree analysis of the Fell Pony breed suggests that FIS may have an autosomal recessive inheritance, with normal carriers (Butler, 2006; Thomas, 2005). The DNA-based test was developed by the Animal Health Trust, Newmarket, UK, and it offers powerful herd management planning to avoid the mating of two carriers with the genetic defect. The test, therefore, should be performed in all Fell Pony and Fell Pony-crossbred horses used in reproduction. The appropriate planning of breeding of carriers prevents the outcome of affected foals and decreases the incidence of the mutant gene in the population.

21.2.1.5 Common variable immunodeficiency

Common variable immunodeficiency (CVID) in the horse is a rare late-onset fatal immunologic disorder of B cell depletion and inadequate antibody production, due to impaired B cell differentiation in the bone marrow (Freestone, 1987; MacLeay, 1997; Flaminio, 2002a, 2009). Clinical signs manifest in adulthood (average age ten years, range 2–23 years), although the disease can potentially present in young age. Affected patients are unrelated adult horses of both sexes, different breeds (Thoroughbred, Quarter Horse, Arabian, Warmblood, Paint, Pony), and living in distinct geographic areas. To date, only isolated cases in a herd or location have been diagnosed.

B cell lymphopenia or depletion leads to hypogammaglobulinemia that predisposes to recurrent infections and fevers, with the most common presentations being pneumonia, sinusitis, meningitis, abnormal gait (ataxia), peritonitis, gingivitis, sinusitis, hepatitis, diarrhea, susceptibility to gastrointestinal parasites, uveitis, conjunctivitis, and/or skin abscesses (Flaminio, 2002a, 2009; Pellegrini-Masini, 2005; Tennent-Brown, 2010). Meningitis may clinically present with marked depression, alternating with periods of normal appetite. Weight loss and/or muscle atrophy are common.

The most common pathogens involved in infections are *Staphylococcus* spp., *Streptococcus* spp., *Actinobacillus* spp., and *Klebsiella* spp., which require opsonization with both antibody and complement for effective phagocytosis and bacterial killing.

Neutrophilia and hyperfibrinogenemia are present accordingly during active infections. Transient lymphopenia (< 1200 cells/uL) is common, although, during the period when infections respond to antibiotic therapy, both neutrophil and lymphocyte counts may be within normal reference intervals. An important feature is the presence of low-normal or low globulin levels, despite severe bacterial infections and hyperfibrinogenemia. The hypoglobulinemia reflects hypogammaglobulinemia but it should be confirmed by testing specifically serum IgG concentrations. Abnormal liver enzymes may also be measured when there is septicemia. In the case of meningitis, spinal fluid analysis reveals increased protein values and pleocytosis, potentially nondegenerate neutrophils, lymphocyte and monocytes. Blood culture has not been routinely performed in these patients but has resulted in bacterial growth in some cases; a culture of spinal fluid may or not result in bacterial growth.

The parameter that definitively indicates a humoral dysfunction is low serum IgG concentration (< 800 mg/dL) in all affected horses. Serum IgM concentrations are markedly reduced (< 25 mg/dL) in all patients, suggesting the inability to elaborate primary immune response (Thomas, 2005). Serum IgA concentrations may be within low normal values (approximately 60 mg/dL) in early diagnosis, but levels reduce with progression of clinical disease, severity of clinical condition, and proximity to euthanasia. Affected horses do not respond to tetanus toxoid vaccination with an increase in serum antibody titers, and pre-vaccination values are often low or undetectable.

Peripheral blood lymphocyte immunophenotyping reveals persistent, severe B cell lymphopenia (less than 2%) in all patients. A relative increase in the percentage of circulating CD8$^+$ T cells and CD4$^+$ T cells has been observed in most patients. T lymphocyte function and capacity to stimulate B cells during differentiation in lymphoid tissues seems intact, based on normal response to mitogenic stimulation *in vitro*, and the expression of IFN-gamma and CD40-ligand in stimulated cells when compared with healthy horses. A portion of CVID-affected horses may present a concomitant CD4$^+$ T cell lymphopenia, leading to a low CD4 : CD8 ratio (< 2.0), sometimes induced by inadvertent glucocorticoid therapy. In these cases, infection with intracellular organisms (fungi *Aspergillus* spp, *Bipolaris* spp., *Pneumocystis jiroveci*, or intracellular *Rhodococcus equi*) is observed. The *in vitro* phagocytosis and oxidative burst activity are normal or increased in these patients, reflecting *in vivo* activation in response to pathogenic challenge.

Horse patients may be managed for a few weeks or a few years with continuous or intermittent antimicrobial therapy (e.g., trimethoprim-sulfa) for mild to moderate infections, but episodes of more severe infection (i.e., including meningitis) may require intravenous antibiotic therapy and supportive care. Commercial equine plasma is the current available source of immunoglobulin for clinical use, and its low concentration prevents it from being a costly effective treatment or prophylactic management in adult horses. Monthly immunoglobulin replacement therapy in human patients is possible due to the availability of concentrated IgG products, which improves quality of life. Hematopoietic stem cell transplantation has been attempted in a horse with common variable immunodeficiency, but no replacement of B cell population and function has been successful to date, as the costs involved with the procedure may discourage clinical application (Felippe, unpublished).

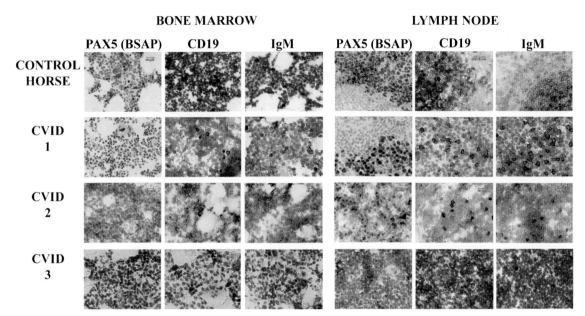

Figure 21.3 Common variable immunodeficiency (CVID). Immunohistochemical staining of microsections from tissues collected at necropsy of a control horse and different CVID-affected horses (1, 2 and 3). The presence of B cells was tested using monoclonal antibodies against BSPA-PAX5, CD19 and IgM, and 3-amino-9-ethylcarbazole, AEC reagent, which indicates positive cells in red. Note the paucity of B cells in primary (bone marrow) and secondary (lymph node) lymphoid tissues, and the absence of germinal centers in the lymph nodes of affected horses. The B cell depletion is thought to be progressive, and CVID-affected horses 1, 2 and 3 show differences in their B cell population distribution (1, clusters of B cells; 2, occasional B cells; 3, no B cells).

(Julia Felippe, Cornell University – Reprinted from Tallmadge (2012), p. 175. Copyright (2012), with permission from Elsevier).

Affected horses are submitted to euthanasia due to financial reasons or poor quality of life, often within six months of the diagnosis.

Necropsy findings include organ lesions according to the infectious processes. Histopathology confirms the lack of germinal cells in the lymph nodes, which affects the typical cortical-paracortical distribution, and the primary and secondary follicles in the cortex. In general, lymph nodes are small. In addition, there is absence of plasma cells in various lymphoid and mucosal tissues. Immunohistochemical analysis may identify occasional positive B cells disperse or in small clusters in the lymph nodes, but often absent B cells in the bone marrow and spleen (Figure 21.3).

The clinical history indicates no previous susceptibility in life until the late-onset recurrent infections develop. Nevertheless, failure of B cell development in the bone marrow is likely to be progressive, and leads to total B cell depletion in the body, including bone marrow, secondary lymphoid tissues and blood. B cells must be continuously generated over an individual's lifetime from hematopoietic stem cells in the bone marrow, to maintain adequate population and humoral function in the lymphoid tissues (Hao, 2001).

B cell differentiation and development is regulated by a network of transcription factors and demethylation of dinucleotides at promoter or regulatory sites (Hagman, 2006; Cobaleda, 2007). In the bone marrow of affected horses, the expression of key early B cell commitment genes, including *E2A* and *PAX5*, is significantly decreased in comparison with healthy horses. In addition, *PAX5* downstream target genes are also significantly reduced in CVID-affected horses, including *CD19*, *IGHM*, *IGHD* (Tallmadge, 2012).

The *PAX5* gene encodes the B cell-lineage specific activator protein (BSAP), a B cell signature transcription factor. Upstream, E2A transcription factor (an E-box binding protein, and also known as factor 3, TCF3) triggers B cell differentiation and the expression of *PAX5* for B cell lineage commitment. Immunohistochemical studies confirm the absence of PAX5-BSAP protein in the bone marrow of affected horses. Hence, CVID in horses may be caused by impairment of B cell development in the bone marrow at the transition between pre-pro-B cells and pro-B cells. Current studies are investigating epigenetic mechanisms that lead to gene silencing during that B cell differentiation stage (Tallmadge, 2015).

A differential diagnosis is lymphoma because some forms of this type of cancer may alter lymphocyte distribution and function, including B cell lymphopenia and hypogammaglobulinemia. If the disease manifests in young age (before the yearling phase), differential diagnoses would include X-linked agammaglobulinemia.

21.2.2 Cellular immunodeficiencies

Cellular immunodeficiencies are more difficult to diagnose and are, therefore, apparently less prevalent in the horse. Peripheral blood lymphocyte counts and subpopulation distributions reflect lymphoid tissue activity, as lymphocytes constantly circulate throughout the body. Cellular immune disorders may affect CD4[+] T cells, with implications both to cytotoxic and/or humoral functions, depending on the underlying mechanism. Cellular dysfunction may also be induced by upstream events of immunity, through dysfunctional antigen presentation and signaling, and consequent failure to activate T lymphocytes.

In general, persistent absolute lymphopenia suggests poor lymphocyte population proliferation and activation in lymphoid tissues and, potentially, lymphoid hypoplasia. In both healthy horses and foals, the reference interval of CD4 : CD8 ratio of peripheral blood lymphocytes is 2.5 and 4.5, and values above or below suggest immune imbalance secondary to lymphoid tissue activity. Of importance, a decreased CD4 : CD8 ratio of less than 2.0 predisposes to intracellular organism infections, which is often accompanied by lymphopenia. Such a result, however, may also be a consequence of infection with certain pathogens, making it difficult to determine a cause and effect.

In healthy foals, transient but marked lymphocytosis (4500–6000 cells/uL) is expected in the first few months of life and indicates adequate response to environmental antigenic stimuli. In addition, age-dependent increase in lymphocyte subpopulations (CD4$^+$ and CD8$^+$ T cells, and B cells) occurs (Flaminio, 1998, 1999, 2000). In some cases, foals show a delay in the lymphocyte population expansion (no lymphocytosis documented), and also in achieving CD4$^+$ lymphocyte distribution (< 50%) in peripheral blood, with consequent low CD4 : CD8 ratios (< 2.0). Commonly, failure to increase the expression of major histocompatibility complex (MHC) class II in lymphocytes (but not monocytes) is observed in this condition (Flaminio, personal observation).

In general, lymphocyte proliferation response *in vitro* upon mitogenic stimulation, serum immunoglobulin concentrations, and B cell distribution are normal in these foals. However, in some cases, these values are abnormal, and it is uncertain if these findings are associated with transient hypogammaglobulinemia of the young. Similarly, long-term antibiotic therapy (e.g., trimethoprim-sulfadiazine) may be necessary during this transition period. These foals should be monitored periodically with leukograms, thoracic ultrasound and radiographs, and immunologic testing to determine the need of treatment, and documented improvement of clinical and immunologic values.

Infections with intracellular pathogens (intracellular bacteria, viruses, fungi) suggest cellular immunodeficiency, and recurrent, pyogenic infections are similar to those of humoral immunodeficiencies. *Pneumocystis jiroveci* has been associated with several reports of respiratory disease in 3–4 month old foals, and one reported case confirmed transient marked CD4$^+$ and CD8$^+$ T cell lymphopenia (Tanaka, 1994; Flaminio, 1998, 1999). In another affected foal, an immunodeficiency was not identified, but the outcome was fatal (Perron, 1999).

Other cellular immunodeficiencies not recognized in the horse, but described in human patients, include defects in the expression or function of cell surface activation molecules (e.g., CD40L in lymphocytes; MHC class II, CD40 or Toll-like receptors in antigen presenting cells), and their cell-signaling components. Improved diagnostic immunologic assays for these conditions are under development for horses.

21.2.3 Combined immunodeficiencies
21.2.3.1 Severe combined immunodeficiency
Severe combined immunodeficiency (SCID) is an autosomal recessive hereditary condition that affects the development of B and T cells in affected Arabian foals (McGuire, 1973; Perryman, 1980). There is one published report of SCID in a two month old Appaloosa filly, which may reflect the inheritance of the disease from Arabian ancestors in the pedigree (Perryman, 1984).

Both humoral and cellular immunity are impaired in these patients (Lew, 1980). Consequently, SCID manifests clinically in both male and female foals around two months of life with bronchopneumonia non-responsive to antibiotic therapy. In addition to bacterial infections, these foals commonly present *Pneumocystis jiroveci* pneumonia, and adenovirus inclusions in the lungs and pancreas. Diarrhea is present in a few cases, and it has been associated with *Cryptosporidium parvum* and coronavirus (Clark, 1978; Mair, 1990).

The lymphoid tissues in SCID foals are hypoplastic for both B and T cells. The thymus has a paucity of lymphocytes, and is infiltrated by adipose tissue instead. Nevertheless, occasional CD8$^+$ cells have been reported in the thymus of SCID foals (Wyatt, 1987; Lunn, 1995). The secondary lymphoid tissues lack germinal centers (lymph nodes) and periarteriolar lymphocytic sheaths (spleen). These foals present severe peripheral blood lymphopenia (< 1000 cells/uL), IgM (< 23 mg/dL) and IgA deficiency. Although the production is impaired, serum IgG concentration is often low, and reflects colostrum-derived antibodies. The few recognized lymphocytes are not functional, for the affected foals fail to respond to vaccination with antibody production, do not respond to mitogenic stimulation, and are susceptible to organisms that require B and T cell function.

Treatment of SCID foals is challenging, due to severe respiratory infections with opportunistic organisms, including intracellular pathogens (Thompson, 1976; Perryman, 1978). Antibiotic therapy and intravenous plasma transfusion provide limited control of disease, and death occurs before five months of life. Successful experimental replacement of B and T cells in SCID foals has been accomplished with bone marrow and thymus transplantation (Bue, 1986). Using histocompatible cells from a healthy full sibling, a functional immune system was established in an affected foal, characterized by normal number of circulating lymphocytes, humoral response to immunization, and cell proliferation response to intradermal phytolectin stimulation.

In contrast, SCID foals are susceptible to graft versus host disease (GvHD) when given hepatic, thymic or peripheral blood from nonrelated horses (Ardans, 1977; Perryman, 1980). One-way mixed lymphocyte cultures revealed failure of SCID mononuclear cells to respond to allogenic stimulation. SCID foals develop prolonged parasitemia and persistent infection of visceral tissues after experimental infection with *Sarcocystis neurona*.

Curiously, and in contrast to immunocompetent foals, infected SCID foals do not develop neurologic signs (Sellon, 2004).

The defective B and T cell development is caused by a faulty V(D)J recombination during B and T cell receptor formation that affects coding and signal end joining. A frame-shift mutation in the gene encoding DNA-dependent protein kinase catalytic subunit (DNA-PKc) results in complete absence of this protein in affected Arabian foals (Wiler, 1995; Shin, 1997). Therefore, DNA repair during gene recombination of the variable region of the receptors is not achieved, B and T cell receptors do not develop, and B and T cell lymphopoiesis is blocked. The gene must be disrupted in both chromosome alleles in the affected foal and, therefore, the mutation must be present in one allele of each parent. Carrier horses are heterozygous for the defective gene and are immunocompetent. The breeding of two affected horses will produce an affected foal in 25% of the offspring.

Fortunately, the definitive diagnosis of carriers and affected foals can be done by a DNA test (VetGen, Veterinary Genetic Services, Michigan, USA) of whole blood or cheek swab samples (Shin, 1997). The test should be performed in all Arabian and Arabian-crossbred horses used in reproduction. The appropriate planning of breeding of carriers prevents the outcome of affected foals, and decreases the incidence of the mutant gene in the population.

21.2.4 Phagocytic deficiencies

Inherited forms of neutrophil dysfunction have not been described in the horse, but should be suspected in cases of recurrent infection (dermatitis, cutaneous or intracavitary abscesses, cellulitis, periodontal diseases) not associated with humoral immunodeficiency, and caused by *Staphylococcus*, *Pseudomonas*, *Serratia*, *Klebsiella*, or fungi (*Aspergillus*, *Candida*).

In the neonate foal, acquired neutrophil dysfunction has been reported during sepsis. Although healthy foals are born with competent neutrophil function, septic foals demonstrate a transient decrease in phagocytosis and oxidative burst activity that improves with control of infection during the hospitalization period (Gardner, 2007).

Pelger-Huët anomaly of neutrophils has been identified in the horse (Felippe, unpublished data; Wilkerson, personal communication). Pelger-Huët cell neutrophilic function is normal (i.e., they capably phagocytose and kill microorganisms), and no clinical signs of immunodeficiency are observed. Therefore, the diagnosis is incidental, during the evaluation of blood smears. Pelger-Huët cells present dumbbell-shaped bilobed nuclei, and a reduced number of nuclear segments. In humans, Pelger-Huët anomaly is a benign, dominantly inherited defect of terminal neutrophil differentiation, secondary to mutations in the lamin B receptor (*LBR*) gene.

Some of the diseases associated with phagocytic disorders described in other species include leukocyte adhesion deficiency (failure to express the CD18 integrin), chronic granulomatous disease (inability to produce oxygen reactive species), cyclic neutrophil hematopoiesis (cyclic changes in blood neutrophil), and Chediak-Higashi syndrome (giant granules in neutrophils).

21.2.5 Complement component deficiencies

Primary diseases of the complement components are rare, and have not been described in the horse. The foal is born with low serum complement activity, and colostrum is not a significant source of complement. Therefore, foals are transiently deficient in serum opsonic capacity, and rely on their own production of complement after birth (Gröndahl, 2001; Flaminio, 2002b). In sepsis, serum complement C3 components are rapidly consumed, which delays the physiological age-dependent increase that is normally observed in healthy foals (Gardner, 2007).

Deficiencies of complement components have been described in human patients and other domestic species. Some of the diseases associated with complement component disorders include:

(a) deficiencies of early components of complement C1q, C1r, C1s, C4 and C2 (e.g., systemic lupus erythematosus-like signs, glomerulonephritis);

(b) deficiencies of late components of complement C5, C6, C7, C8, and C9 (e.g., recurrent disseminated *Neisseria* spp. infections);

(c) deficiencies of C3 component, factor D, I and H (pyogenic infections);

(d) deficiencies of C1 inhibitor (hereditary angioedema or lymphoproliferative disorders); and

(e) properdin deficiency (meningococcemia).

References

Ardans, A.A., Trommershausen-Smith, A., Osburn, B.I., Mayhew, I.G., Trees, C., Park, M.I., Sawyer, M. and Stabenfeldt, G.H. (1977). Immunotherapy in two foals with combined immunodeficiency, resulting in graft versus host reaction. *Journal of American Veterinary Medical Association* **170**, 167–175.

Banks, K.L., McGuire, T.C. and Jerrells, T.R. (1976). Absence of B lymphocytes in a horse with primary agammaglobulinemia. *Clinical Immunology and Immunopathology* **5**(2), 282–290.

Bell, S.C., Savidge, C., Taylor, P., Knottenbelt, D.C. and Carter, S.D. (2001). An immunodeficiency in Fell ponies: a preliminary study into cellular responses. *Equine Veterinary Journal* **33**(7), 687–692.

Boy, M.G., Zhang, C., Antczak, D.F., Hamir, A.N. and Whitlock, R.H. (1992). Unusual selective immunoglobulin deficiency in an Arabian foal. *Journal of Veterinary Internal Medicine* **6**(4), 201–205.

Bue, C.M., Davis, W.C., Magnuson, N.S., Mottironi, V.D., Ochs, H.D., Wyatt, C.R. and Perryman, L.E. (1986). Correction of equine severe combined immunodeficiency by bone marrow transplantation. *Transplantation* **42**, 14–19.

Butler, C.M., Westermann, C.M., Koeman, J.P. and Sloet van Oldruitenborgh-Oosterbaan, M.M. (2006). The Fell pony immunodeficiency syndrome also occurs in the Netherlands: a review and six cases. *Tijdschr Diergeneeskd* **131**, 114–118.

Clark, E.G., Turner, A.S., Boysen, B.G. and Rouse, B.T. (1978). Listeriosis in an Arabian foal with combined immunodeficiency. *Journal of American Veterinary Medical Association* **172**, 363–366.

Cobaleda, C., Schebesta, A., Delogu, A. and Busslinger, M. (2007). Pax5: the guardian of B cell identity and function. *Nature Immunology* **8**, 463–470.

Crisman, M.V. (1987). *Selective immunoglobulin M deficiency in the horse.* In: Proceedings of the 33rd American Association of Equine Practitioners, New Orleans, LA.

Deem, D.A., Traver, D.S., Thacker, H.L. and Perryman, L.E. (1979). Agammaglobulinemia in a horse. *Journal of American Veterinary Medical Association* **175**(5), 469–472.

Dixon, J.B., Savage, M., Wattret, A., Taylor, P., Ross, G., Carter, S.D., Kelly, D.F., Haywood, S., Phythian, C., Macintyre, A.R., Bell, S.C., Knottenbelt, D.C. and Green, J.R. (2000). Discriminant and multiple regression analysis of anemia and opportunistic infection in Fell pony foals. *Veterinary Clinical Pathology* **29**(3), 84–86.

Flaminio, M.J., Rush, B.R., Cox, J.H. and Moore, W.E. (1998). CD4+ and CD8+ T-lymphocytopenia in a filly with *Pneumocystis carinii* pneumonia. *Australian Veterinary Journal* **76**(6), 399–402.

Flaminio, M.J., Rush, B.R. and Shuman, W. (1999). Peripheral blood lymphocyte subpopulations and immunoglobulin concentrations in healthy foals and foals with *Rhodococcus equi* pneumonia. *Journal of Veterinary Internal Medicine* **13**(3), 206–212.

Flaminio, M.J., Rush, B.R. and Shuman, W. (2000). Characterization of peripheral blood and pulmonary leukocyte function in healthy foals. *Veterinary Immunology and Immunopathology* **73**(3–4), 267–285.

Flaminio, M.J., LaCombe, V., Kohn, C.W. and Antczak, D.F. (2002a). Common variable immunodeficiency in a horse. *Journal of American Veterinary Medical Association* **22**, 1296–1302.

Flaminio, M.J., Rush, B.R., Davis, E.G., Hennessy, K., Shuman, W. and Wilkerson, M.J. (2002b). Simultaneous flow cytometric analysis of phagocytosis and oxidative burst activity in equine leukocytes. *Veterinary Research Communication* **26**(2), 85–92.

Flaminio, M.J., Tallmadge, R., Salles-Gomes, C.M. and Matychak, M.B. (2009). Common variable immunodeficiency in horses is characterized by B cell depletion in primary and secondary lymphoid tissues. *Journal of Clinical Immunology* **29**(1), 107–116.

Fox-Clipsham, L.Y., Swinburne, J.E., Papoula-Pereira, R.I., Blunden, A.S., Malalana, F., Knottenbelt, D.C. and Carter, S.D. (2009). Immunodeficiency/anaemia syndrome in a Dales pony. *Veterinary Record* **165**, 289–290.

Fox-Clipsham, L.Y., Brown, E.E., Carter, S.D. and Swinburne, J.E. (2011a). Identification of a mutation associated with fatal foal immunodeficiency syndrome in the Fell and Dales Pony. *PLoS Genetics* **7**, e1002133.

Fox-Clipsham, L.Y., Carter, S.D., Goodhead, I., Hall, N., Knottenbelt, D.C., May, P.D.F., Ollier, W.E. and Swinburne, J.E. (2011b). Population screening of endangered horse breeds for the foal immunodeficiency syndrome mutation. *Veterinary Record* **169**, 655–658.

Freestone, J.F., Hietala, S., Moulton, J. and Vivrette, S. (1987). Acquired immunodeficiency in a seven-year-old horse. *Journal of American Veterinary Medical Association* **190**, 689–691.

Gardner, R.B., Hart, K.A., Stokol, T., Divers, T.J. and Flaminio, M.J. (2006). Fell Pony syndrome in a pony in North America. *Journal of Veterinary Internal Medicine* **20**(1), 198–203.

Gardner, R.B., Nydam, D.V., Luna, J.A., Bicalho, M.L., Matychak, M.B. and Flaminio, M.J. (2007). Serum opsonization capacity, phagocytosis, and oxidative burst activity in neonatal foals in the intensive care unit. *Journal of Veterinary Internal Medicine* **21**(4), 797–805.

Gröndahl, G., Sternberg, S., Jensen-Waern, M. and Johannisson, A. (2001). Opsonic capacity of foal serum for the two neonatal pathogens *Escherichia coli* and *Actinobacillus equuli. Equine Veterinary Journal* **33**(7), 670–5.

Hagman, J., and Lukin, K. (2006). Transcription factors drive B cell development. *Current Opinion in Immunology* **18**, 127–134.

Hao, Z., and Rajewsky, K. (2001). Homeostasis of peripheral B cells in the absence of B cell influx from the bone marrow. *Journal of Experimental Medicine* **194**, 1151–1164.

Jelinek, F., Faldyna, M. and Jasurkova-Mikutova, G. (2006). Severe combined immunodeficiency in a Fell pony foal. *Journal of Veterinary Medicine* **53**, 69–73.

Krick, K.E. (2002). *Exercise and Immunodeficiency Affect Immunoglobulins in Endurance Horses.* Master of Science. Digital Library and Archives, Virginia Tech, etd-07292002-143104.

Lavoie, J.P., Spensley, M.S., Smith, B.P. and Mihalyi, J. (1989). Absorption of bovine colostral immunoglobulins G and M in newborn foals. *American Journal of Veterinary Research* **50**(9), 1598–1603.

Lew, A.M., Hosking, C.S. and Studdert, M.J. (1980). Immunologic aspects of combined immunodeficiency disease in Arabian foals. *American Journal of Veterinary Research* **41**, 1161–1166.

Louis, A.G., and Gupta, S. (2014). Primary selective IgM deficiency: an ignored immunodeficiency. *Clinical Reviews in Allergy and Immunology* **46**(2), 104–111.

Lunn, D., Holmes, M. and Duffus, W. (1993). Equine T-lymphocyte MHC II expression: variation with age and subset. *Veterinary Immunology and Immunopathology* **35**, 225–238.

Lunn, D.P., McClure, J.T., Schobert, C.S. and Holmes, M.A. (1995). Abnormal patterns of equine leucocyte differentiation antigen expression in severe combined immunodeficiency foals suggests the phenotype of normal equine natural killer cells. *Immunology* **84**(3), 495–499.

MacLeay, J.M., Ames, T.R., Hayden, D.W. and Tumas, D.B. (1997). Acquired B lymphocyte deficiency and chronic enterocolitis in a 3-year-old quarter horse. *Veterinary Immunology and Immunopathology* **57**, 49–57.

Mair, T.S., Taylor, F.G., Harbour, D.A. and Pearson, G.R. (1990). Concurrent cryptosporidium and coronavirus infections in an Arabian foal with combined immunodeficiency syndrome. *Veterinary Record* **126**, 127–130.

McDonald, V., Robinson, H.A., Kelly, J.P. and Bancroft, G.H. (1994). Cryptosporidium muris in adult mice: adoptive transfer of immunity and protective roles of CD4 versus CD8 cells. *Infection and Immunity* **62**, 2289–2294.

McGuire, T.C., and Poppie, M.J. (1973). Hypogammaglobulinemia and thymic hypoplasia in horses: a primary combined immunodeficiency disorder. *Infection and Immunity* **8**(2), 272–277.

McGuire, T.C., Poppie, M.J. and Banks, K.L. (1975). Hypogammaglobulinemia predisposing to infection in foals. *Journal of American Veterinary Medical Association* **166**(1), 71–5.

McGuire, T.C., Banks, K.L., Evans, D.R. and Poppie, M.J. (1976). Agammaglobulinemia in a horse with evidence of functional T lymphocytes. *American Journal of Veterinary Research* **37**(1), 41–6.

McGuire, T.C., Perryman, L.E. and Davis, W.C. (1983). Analysis of serum and lymphocyte surface IgM of healthy and immunodeficient horses with monoclonal antibodies. *American Journal of Veterinary Research* **44**(7), 1284–8.

Pellegrini-Masini, A., Bentz, A.I., Johns, I.C., Parsons, C.S., Beech, J., Whitlock, R.H. and Flaminio, M.J. (2005). Common variable immunodeficiency in three horses with presumptive bacterial meningitis. *Journal of American Veterinary Medical Association* **227**, 114–122.

Perkins, G.A., Nydam, D.V., Flaminio, M.J.B.F. and Ainsworth, D.M. (2003). Serum IgM concentrations in normal, fit horses and horses with lymphoma or other medical conditions. *Journal of Veterinary Internal Medicine* **17**, 337–342.

Perryman, L.E. (2000). Primary immunodeficiencies of horses. *Veterinary Clinics of North America: Equine Practice* **16**(1), 105–116.

Perryman, L.E. and McGuire, T.C. (1978). Mixed lymphocyte culture responses in combined immunodeficiency of horses. *Transplantation* **25**, 50–52.

Perryman, L.E., and McGuire, T.C. (1980). Evaluation for immune system failures in horses and ponies. *Journal of American Veterinary Medical Association* **176**(12), 1374–1377.

Perryman, L.E., McGuire, T.C., and Hilbert, B.J. (1977). Selective immunoglobulin M deficiency in foals. *Journal of American Veterinary Medical Association* **170**(2), 212–15.

Perryman, L.E., McGuire, T.C. and Banks, K.L. (1983). Animal model of human disease. Infantile X-linked agammaglobulinemia. Agammaglobulinemia in horses. *American Journal of Pathology* **111**(1), 125–127.

Perryman, L.E., Boreson, C.R., Conaway, M.W. and Bartsch, R.C. (1984). Combined immunodeficiency in an Appaloosa foal. *Veterinary Pathology* **21**, 547–548.

Richards, A.J., Kelly, D.F., Knottenbelt, D.C., Cheeseman, M.T. and Dixon, J.B. (2000). Anaemia, diarrhoea and opportunistic infections in Fell ponies. *Equine Veterinary Journal* **32**(5), 386–91.

Scholes, S.F., Holliman, A., May, P.D. and Holmes, M.A. (1998). A syndrome of anaemia, immunodeficiency and peripheral ganglionopathy in Fell pony foals. *Veterinary Record* **142**(6), 128–134.

Sellon, D.C., Knowles, D.P., Greiner, E.C., Long, M.T., Hines, M.T., Hochstatter, T., Tibary, A. and Dame, J.B. (2004). Infection of immunodeficient horses with Sarcocystis neurona does not result in neurologic disease. *Clinical and Diagnostic Laboratory Immunology* **11**, 1134–1139.

Shin, E.K., Perryman, L.E. and Meek, K. (1997). Evaluation of a test for identification of Arabian horses heterozygous for the severe combined immunodeficiency trait. *Journal of American Veterinary Medical Association* **211**(10), 1268–1270.

Singh, K., Chang, C. and Gershwin, M.E. (2014). IgA deficiency and autoimmunity. *Autoimmunity Review* **13**(2), 163–177.

Tallmadge, R.L., McLaughlin, K., Secor, E., Ruano, D., Matychak, M.B. and Flaminio, M.J. (2009). Expression of essential B cell genes and immunoglobulin isotypes suggests active development and gene recombination during equine gestation. *Developmental and Comparative Immunology* **33**, 1027–1038.

Tallmadge, R.L., Such, K.A., Miller, K.C., Matcychak, M.B. and Felippe, M.J. (2012). Expression of essential B cell developmental genes in horses with common variable immunodeficiency. *Molecular Immunology* **51**(2), 169–176.

Tallmadge, R.L., Shen, L., Tseng, C.T., Miller, S.C., Barry, J., Felippe, M.J. (2015). Bone marrow transcriptome and epigenome profiles of equine common variable immunodeficiency patients unveil block of B lymphocyte differentiation. *Clinical Immunology* **160**, 261–276.

Tanaka, S., Kaji, Y., Taniyama, H., Matsukawa, K., Ochiai, K. and Itakura, C. (1994). Pneumocystis carinii pneumonia in a thoroughbred foal. *Journal of Veterinary Medical Science* **56**(1), 135–137.

Tennent-Brown, B.S., Navas de Solis, C., Foreman, J.H., Goetz, T.E., Fredrickson, R.L., Borst, L.B. and Flaminio, M.J.B.F. (2010). Common variable immunodeficiency in a horse with chronic peritonitis. *Equine Veterinary Education* **22** 393–399.

Thomas, G.W., Bell, S. C., Phythian, C., Taylor, P., Knottenbelt, D.C and Carter, S.D. (2003). Aid to the antemortem diagnosis of Fell pony foal syndrome by the analysis of B lymphocytes. *Veterinary Record* **152** (20), 618–621.

Thomas, G.W., Bell, S.C. and Carter, S.D. (2005). Immunoglobulin and peripheral B-lymphocyte concentrations in Fell pony foal syndrome. *Equine Veterinary Journal* **37**, 48–52.

Thompson, D.B., Spradborw, P.B. and Studdert, M. (1976). Isolation of an adenovirus from an Arab foal with a combined immunodeficiency disease. *Australian Veterinary Journal* **52**, 435–437.

Vetrie, D., Vořechovský, I., Sideras, P., Holland, J., Davies, A., Flinter, F., Hammarström, L., Kinnon, C., Levinsky, R., Bobrow, M., Smith, C.I. and Bentley, D.R. (1993). The gene involved in X-linked agammaglobulinaemia is a member of the src family of protein-tyrosine kinases. *Nature* **361**, 226–233.

Weldon, A.D., Zhang, C., Antczak, D.F. and Rebhun, W.C. (1992). Selective IgM deficiency and abnormal B-cell response in a foal. *Journal of American Veterinary Medical Association*, **201**(9), 1396–1398.

Wiler, R., Leber, R., Moore, B.B., VanDyk, L.F., Perryman, L.E. and Meek, K. (1995). Equine severe combined immunodeficiency: a defect in V(D)J recombination and DNA-dependent protein kinase activity. *Proceedings of the National Academy of Sciences of the United States of America* **92**(25), 11485–11489.

Wyatt, C.R., Magnuson, N.S. and Perryman, L.E. (1987). Defective thymocyte maturation in horses with severe combined immunodeficiency. *Journal of Immunology* **139**, 4072–4076.

22 Immunologic Testing

M. Julia B. Felippe

22.1 Definition

Immunologic testing for the diagnosis of immunodeficiency should follow clinical signs of recurrent infections and fevers and/or potential inheritance of primary immune disorders.

The type of pathogen causing the clinical diseases helps with identifying the faulty area of the immune system. The most common pathogens implicated in horse immunodeficiencies are encapsulated bacteria (e.g., *Staphylococcus aureus, Streptococcus zooepidemicus, Klebsiella* ssp, *Actinobacillus equuli*), as they require both immunoglobulin and complement for effective opsonization and phagocytic function. These are also common organisms that share mucosal tissues with normal flora and can readily invade, proliferate and cause disease. Therefore, conditions that affect B cell differentiation or function for the impairment of immunoglobulin production, complement deficiencies, or phagocytic dysfunction should be investigated.

Infections with intracellular organisms (e.g., *Rhodococcus equi, Pneumocystis jiroveci, Candida albicans, Aspergillus* spp, *Bipolaris* spp.) are suggestive of faulty cellular immune mechanisms, including: absolute lymphopenia; CD4$^+$ T cell or CD8$^+$ T cell lymphopenia; low CD4 : CD8 ratio in peripheral blood; inadequate function of antigen presenting cells (APCs) with low expression of major histocompatibility complex (MHC); co-stimulatory molecules (CD40, CD86) and interleukein-12 (IL-12) production; and low activation of T cells with low production of IFN-gamma and expression of co-stimulatory molecules (CD28, CD40L). In these outcomes, the expression of a variety of receptors, ligands, and activation of signaling pathways could be involved, making the choice of immunologic testing and diagnosis complex.

Infections with opportunistic organisms (e.g., *Pneumocystis joroveci, Cryptosporidium parvum*, adenovirus) are also suggestive of immunodeficiency, and some of these organisms may require a combination of immune mechanisms for protection (e.g., humoral and cellular immunity).

Immunologic testing in foals should be accompanied by age-matched and, when possible, breed-matched control samples from healthy foals to account for developmental changes in the immune system (Flaminio, 2000). The results should also be compared to confidence intervals determined by the laboratory.

Repeated tests may be performed to confirm a persistent versus a transient condition.

22.2 Types of immunologic testing

22.2.1 Clinical history

Clinical history and signalment are essential elements for interpretation of immunologic testing.

Evidence of *infection* must be present for the suspicion of immunodeficiency. Recurrent clinical signs of infection (e.g., pneumonia, chronic dermatitis, polysynovitis, osteomyelitis, meningitis), fever and/or blood work that indicates inflammation or infection, are supportive of immunodeficiency. The type of pathogen, as suggested above, also alerts for the possibility of dysfunctional immunity.

Young and elderly horses are particularly more predisposed to infections with inadequate immune responses, and immunologic testing may verify transient of persistent conditions. For primary immunodeficiencies, genetic mutations may be prevalent in certain breeds, or may affect only males (e.g., X-linked agammaglobulinemia), and familial history of recurrent infections could suggested an inherited condition.

22.2.2 Complete blood cell count, cytology and biochemistry

Complete blood cell count and cytology (blood smear) may diagnose infections when neutrophilia, toxic changes and bands are present; neutropenia can be observed in acute endotoxemia with Gram-negative bacteria infections. Lymphopenia may be intermittent in response to stress, or may indicate lymphoid tissue hypoplasia, when persistent. Anemia of chronic infection and thrombocytopenia secondary to sepsis are also possible.

Differential diagnoses for immunodeficiencies include leukemias and tumors (e.g., lymphosarcoma), which can affect the production of immune cells or their function.

22.2.3 Humoral immunity

Humoral function can be readily and precisely assessed by measuring serum immunoglobulin concentrations, as antibodies

Equine Clinical Immunology, First Edition. Edited by M. Julia B. Felippe.
© 2016 John Wiley & Sons, Inc. Published 2016 by John Wiley & Sons, Inc.

are the final products of humoral immunity. Therefore, blood should be collected in red top tubes. Some tests offer the option of whole blood test (e.g., samples collected in ethylenediaminetetra-acetic acid, EDTA).

An accurate method to measure serum IgG concentration is the quantitative automated immunoturbidimetric assay (Hitachi P-modular, Roche Diagnostics) offered in diagnostic centers, and results are available on the same day (McCue, 2007). Radial immunodiffusion (RID) tests for IgG are also quantitative, and have acceptable sensitivity and specificity (Triple J Farms), but require 24 hours for results.

A commercially-available semi-quantitative enzyme immunoassay (SNAP® Foal IgG Test, Idexx) for IgG is practical, and provides results in minutes, which is particularly useful for measuring humoral protection in foals for prophylaxis and treatment planning. However, results are reported in interval concentrations (i.e., < 400 mg/dL, 400–800 mg/dL, and > 800 mg/dL), which limits its use for developmental assessment in the first 6–12 months of life, or for adult horses that have normal reference intervals above 800 mg/dL (Pusterla, 2002; Metzger, 2006). Spectroscopy methodology for measuring IgG concentration has been tested in plasma samples, with favorable results (Hou, 2014).

Serum IgM concentration may be assessed by RID (Triple J Farms) or enzyme-linked immunoabsorbant assay (ELISA). Both are quantitative tests and require at least 24 hours for results, but are not widely available (McGuire, 1983). Serum values lower than 25 mg/dL suggest an underlying humoral dysfunction.

Serum IgA concentration can be measured by ELISA but tests are not widely available. In general, serum IgA concentration is not reflective of mucosal concentrations, although deficiencies can be diagnosed on the basis of serum results.

Serum IgG isotype concentrations (IgG_1, $IgG_{4/7}$, $IgG_{3/5}$) can be determined by ELISA and micro-bead multiplex assays, and they have been used in studies addressing developmental immunology and vaccinology, but their value in the context of immunodeficiencies in uncertain.

In foals less than 3–4 months old, serum IgG concentration interpretation should take into account circulating levels of colostrum-derived antibodies, which vary individually, depending on the initial amount of absorption (colostral IgG half-life is estimated at 28–32 days) (Lavoie, 1989). Therefore, serum IgM concentrations are more specific for B cell function in foals, as IgM production occurs already *in utero* and colostrum-derived IgM has a short half-life of 5–16 days.

Measuring antigen-specific antibody titers in response to vaccination (e.g., tetanus toxoid) is a useful strategy to evaluate *in vivo* immunoglobulin production. In general, if patients have been vaccinated previously with a tetanus toxoid, a 15–12 day interval between the pre-vaccination and post-vaccination samples is recommended. When using enzyme-linked immunosorbant assay (ELISA) to measure antibody concentrations, it is important that pre-vaccination and post-vaccination serum samples are run in the same test, because variable magnitude of results is often obtained between assays. This approach may not be useful in young foals without optimal vaccines for the age, or during the period of development of their immune system (i.e., before eight months old).

Evaluation of peripheral blood B cell distribution provides information about faulty humoral immunity. Peripheral blood immunophenotying is a laboratorial test that uses monoclonal antibodies against B cell markers (e.g., CD19, CD20, CD21, CD79a, IgM), conjugated with a fluorescent molecule (fluorophore) that is detected by a biomarker detector or flow cytometer (Figure 22.1; Flaminio, 2009). Distribution of B cells should be compared to reference or confidence intervals determined by the laboratory. Decreased distribution of B cells (< 5%) suggests impaired development and population expansion. B cells can also be stimulated *in vitro* with antigens and mitogens, in order to measure proliferation and immunoglobulin production capacity. These tests are not widely available, and are more often used in studies addressing developmental immunology and vaccinology. Humoral immunity disorders can also be secondary to cellular deficiencies, when $CD4^+$ T cells cannot co-stimulate and support B cell differentiation and survival.

22.2.4 Cellular immunity

Assessment of $CD4^+$ and $CD8^+$ T cell function is challenging, because disorders may be intrinsic to T cells or involve upstream events of immunity, due to dysfunctional antigen presentation and signaling required to activate T lymphocytes.

Assessment of cellular immunity requires whole blood (EDTA or heparin). Peripheral blood lymphocyte counts and subpopulation distributions reflect lymphoid tissue activity, as lymphocytes constantly circulate throughout the body. Persistent lymphopenia could reflect lymphoid tissue hypoplasia; generally, disease and stress also cause lymphopenia that resolves or improves with clinical recovery. Absolute lymphopenia contributes to decreased circulating T cell subpopulations.

The distribution of $CD4^+$ and $CD8^+$ T cells can be assessed in peripheral blood, using immunophenotyping and flow cytometry, and compared to reference or confidence intervals determined by the laboratory (Figure 22.1). Changes in the CD4 : CD8 ratio (< 2.5 or > 4.5) suggest immune imbalance, often secondary to the infection process and not necessarily an underlying immunodeficiency.

Lymphocyte proliferation in response to mitogens (e.g., phytohemagglutinin, PHA; pokeweed, PWM; concanavalin A, ConA; phorbol 12-myristate 13-acetate plus ionomycin, PMAi) have been used to partially assess T cell function *in vitro* or *in vivo* (PHA intradermal injection) (Figure 22.2). In general, proliferation is inadequate in primary T cell immunodeficiencies. However, in acquired immunodeficiencies or developmental immunodeficiencies, T cell proliferation can be slightly decreased or comparable to control normal cells. By adding the measure of cytokine production (e.g., IL-2, IFN-gamma, IL-10), and expression of activation molecules

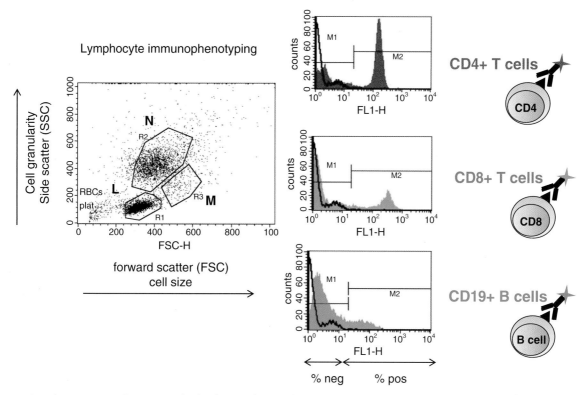

Figure 22.1 Lymphocyte immunophenotyping. The distribution of CD4 and CD8 T cells, and B cells, can be precisely measured by flow cytometry. In this technique, monoclonal antibodies against cell surface or intracellular markers conjugated with fluorescent molecules (fluorophores) are mixed with lymphocytes from blood or fluids. The reagents bind specifically to the target molecules in the cell. Once the cells go through a laser beam, the light emitted by the conjugated antibody is detected (FL1, fluorescence), revealing positive and negative cells. Negative (neg, M1) cells are dim, and positive (pos, M2) cells are brighter; appropriate negative controls are used to set up thresholds (black line). The more homogeneously a population expresses the amount of a marker in the cell, the narrower is the peak formed in a fluorescence histogram (e.g., CD4). Some populations have a heterogeneous amount of molecules in the cell, and distribute with broad histograms along the fluorescence axis (e.g., CD19). When reagents are not conjugated with fluorophores, a second step during cell labeling for adding the fluorescent reagent is necessary. Independently of the use of fluorescent markers, flow cytometry can distribute blood cells in a dot plot according to their granularity (side scatter, SSC) or size (forward scatter, FSC), revealing lymphocyte (L), neutrophil (N)and monocyte (M) populations that can be gated for analyses; in addition, smaller red blood cells (RBCs) and platelets (plat) can be identified.

(e.g., CD40L, MHC class II), other levels of impairment are then tested. The cellular response can also be assessed, by measuring cytokine production in serum (*in vivo* systemic condition, sometimes difficult to interpret), or in cell culture supernatant (after *in vitro* stimulation often uses a control to help with interpretation of results), using ELISA or Luminex® assays based on fluorescent bead technology (Cornell University Animal Health Diagnostic Center, Ithaca, NY).

In healthy foals, both absolute lymphocyte count and subpopulation (CD4$^+$ and CD8$^+$ T cells, and B cells) distribution increase in the first six months of life in response to environmental antigenic stimuli. In addition, there is an age-dependent increase in the expression of MHC class II and IFN-gamma. Therefore, tests should be run side by side with samples from age-matched, preferably breed-matched, control healthy foals. Immunologic testing in foals help with determining delayed development of the immune system and planning of treatment.

22.2.5 Phagocytic function

Phagocytosis and oxidative burst activity can be tested by flow cytometry, using opsonized inactivated fluorescence-conjugated bacteria (e.g., *Staphylococcus aureus, E. coli*) and an indicator of production of reactive oxygen species (e.g., oxidation of 123 dihydrorhodamine into fluorescent 123 rhodamine) (Figure 22.3 A, B; Flaminio, 2002). Phagocytes can also be tested for the expression of integrin CD18 (important in diapedesis), and for response to chemotaxis.

22.2.6 Complement component

Complement components in horses can be quantitatively measured using RID or ELISAs assays, or measured semi-quantitatively using hemolytic complement assays. However, these assays are not widely available for horses but used in research.

22.2.7 Genetic testing

For primary immunodeficiencies, genetic tests provide definitive diagnosis of disease in early age and the identification of

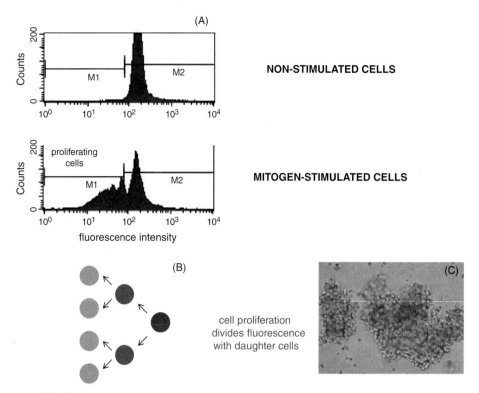

Figure 22.2 Lymphocyte proliferation assays.
The capacity of cell populations to respond to stimuli and become activated can be measured using lymphocyte proliferation *in vitro*. In this assay, isolated lymphocytes from blood or lymphoid tissues are labeled with a fluorescent molecule (carboxyfluorescein succinimidyl ester, CFSE), which binds to all amine groups of proteins in the cell. The cells are then stimulated unspecifically with mitogens (e.g., phytohemagglutinin, PHA; pokeweed mitogen, PWM; concanavalin A, ConA; or lipopolyssacharide, LPS) for 2–3 days. The changes in fluorescence intensity of the stimulated lymphocyte population is measured by flow cytometry and compared with non-stimulated cells (A). CFSE fluorescence progressively halves within daughter cells following each cell division, and the lower the mean fluorescence of a population, the more rounds of cell division have occurred (shift to the left on the fluorescence axis) (A, B). In addition, proliferation assays may be used to measure the up-regulation of activation molecules, including cytokines (IFN-gamma), and cell surface molecules (e.g., CD40L, MHC class II), using protein assays (flow cytometry, ELISA) or molecular assays (quantitative RT-PCR). In these cases, other stimulates can be used (e.g., phorbol 12-myristate 13-acetate, PMA, plus ionomycin). Lymphocyte proliferation *in vitro* is readily observed when cells for clonal clusters (C).

carriers. Genetic tests offer powerful herd management planning to avoid the mating of two or any carriers with the genetic defect, thus promoting progressive elimination of the defective gene in the population or breed.

DNA-based tests are available for Foal Immunodeficiency Syndrome (FIS, Animal Health Trust, Newmarket, UK) and Severe Combined Immunodeficiency Syndrome (SCID, VetGen, Veterinary Genetic Services, Michigan, USA) (Wiler, 1995; Shin, 1997; Fox-Clipsham, 2011). Whole blood samples, mucosal swabs, or hair pulled with root bulbs attached contain DNA for the analyses.

22.2.8 Immunologic testing and neoplasms
Clinical history, physical examination and basic blood work are also part of the diagnosis of neoplasms, as they characterize a clinical condition and identify abnormal function of organs and inflammation.

The use of peripheral blood immunophenotyping is limited in the diagnosis of neoplasms in the horse, unless there is associated-leukemia (i.e., the presence of tumoral cells circulating in the blood). Paraneoplastic effects of certain tumors that create imbalanced T and B cell distribution (e.g., type and stage of development of certain lymphoma cells may result in secretion of cytokines with autocrine, paracrine and endocrine effects on the immune system) may be detected in peripheral blood or tissues, but are not common, diagnostic or specific for neoplasms in general. Therefore, in the majority of neoplasm cases without leukemia studied by the author, the distribution of B and T cells are within the normal reference intervals, with mild abnormal findings. In two rare cases of chronic cutaneous lymphoma, however, B cell lymphopenia with consequent hypogammaglobulinemia was measured, and immunophenotyping was used to monitor the immunologic status of the patients throughout the years.

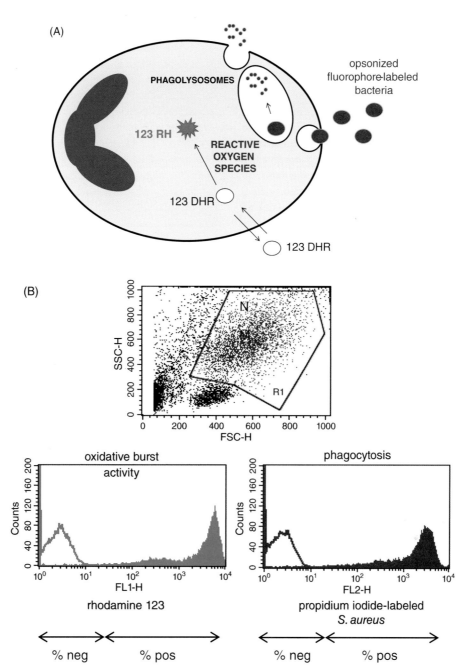

Figure 22.3 Phagocytosis and oxidative burst activity.

(**A**) The capacity of blood or fluid phagocytes to phagocytose and become activated with the production of reactive oxygen species can be measured by flow cytometry. Isolated neutrophils (N) and monocytes (M) are kept cold to prevent spontaneous activation, and opsonized fluorescent-labeled bacteria (e.g., propidium iodide-labeled inactivated *Staphylococcus aureus*) and membrane soluble non-fluorescent 123 dehydrorhodamine (123 DHR) are added to the cell solution. Once the cells become activated due to phagocytosis, 123 dehydrorhodamine is converted by oxidation (from oxidative reactive species) into fluorescent 123 rhodamine (123 RHO), and becomes entrapped into the cell.

(**B**) After 15 minutes of incubation at 37°C, and subsequent quenching of extracellular fluorescent bacteria, the cell population is analyzed by flow cytometry. A control sample is kept at 4°C (open lines). The fluorescence intensity for the intracellular bacteria indicates phagocytosis (filled red lines), and the production of reactive oxygen species is indicated by the 123 rhodamine fluorescence intensity (filled green lines). Results can also be provided as percent positive cells.

The most sensitive and specific diagnostic tests for neoplasms in horses are cytology and histopathology of bone marrow, masses, lymph nodes, cavitary fluid aspirates, and biopsies, respectively. The addition of cytochemistry, immunocytochemistry, and immunohistochemistry add information about the type and developmental stage of the tumoral cells. When using immunophenotyping in thoracocentesis and abdominocentesis fluids, or any other type of blood fluid, the presence and abundance of inflammatory cells (i.e., lymphocytes) is common. Consequently, the percentage distribution of subpopulations alone is not sufficient to characterize the type of tumoral cells, and an overlap of morphologic evaluation (such as in immunocytochemistry) would be required for a more precise analysis.

The staining of DNA content with fluorescent intercalating agents (e.g., propidium iodide) may show the presence of cells with aneuploidy, which is a common finding in tumoral cells. DNA ploidy measures the total DNA content of cells, The majority of cells (85%) with normal division group in the Go/G1 cell cycle phase, and about 15% cells are detected under DNA duplication (synthesis, S phase) or cell division (mitosis, G2/M phase) (Figure 22.4). Tumoral cells, in contrast, may have aberrant division and show aneuploidy, with DNA content of the Go/G1 phase that varies from the corresponding normal cells. Aneuploidy, therefore, indicates an inexact multiple of haploid chromosomal complement (i.e., extra or missing chromosome), characterizing an unbalanced genomic state. Limitations exist in the use of this technique for the diagnosis of neoplasms because some low-grade tumors do not present aneuploidy. However, detection of aneuploidy is helpful in cases of difficult access to cells, or tissues for more definitive cytologic and histologic tests.

Immunocytochemical, immunohistochemical and flow cytometric immunophenotyping of solid tumors and leukemic cells using cell lineage and malignancy markers should be attempted for their classification, in order to expand our knowledge and classification of the types of neoplasms in the horse, and to attempt, and test for, better treatment approaches.

Serum immunoglobulin concentrations can further investigate humoral status beyond results of hypoglobulinemia and hyperglobulinemia obtained from blood biochemistry tests. Lymphoid neoplasms may have no effect in the production of antibodies, or may cause hypogammaglobulinemia (e.g., poorly understood primary or secondary dysfunction of B cells) or hyperglobulinemia (e.g., immunoglobulin secretory cells in multiple myeloma, certain B cell lymphomas and leukemias). Altered humoral function can predispose these patients to infections, particularly when immunosuppressive therapy is used. Therefore, periodic physical examinations, routine blood work, monitoring of immunologic parameters, and antimicrobial coverage, are recommended when managing and monitoring these patients. Selective IgM deficiency has been associated with lymphomas in horses. However, the sensitivity of serum IgM concentration < 25 mg/dl to detect lymphoma has been calculated at 28%, and specificity 88%. In addition, a positive

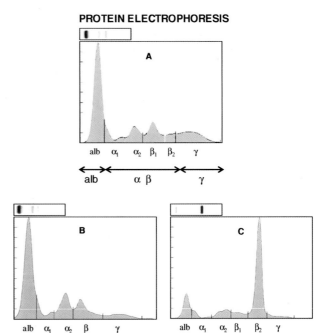

PROTEIN ELECTROPHORESIS

Figure 22.4 Serum protein electrophoresis.
(A) An electric current separates serum proteins into albumin (alb), alpha (α) and beta (β) acute inflammatory proteins, and gammaglobulins (γ). Regions may have different zones and interzones. Alpha-1 proteins include alpha-1-acid glycoprotein, antitrypsin, and antichymotrypsin. Alpha-2 proteins include alpha-2-macroglobulin and haptoglobulin. Beta-1 proteins include transferrin and beta lipoprotein. Beta-2 proteins include complement and C-reactive protein. Fibrinogen in plasma or not-well-clotted samples appears in the beta-2 region. Although the gamma region includes only immunoglobulins, some of these can also be found in the alpha and beta regions.
(B) A decrease in the gamma region indicates hypogammaglobulinemia.
(C) A narrow spike (*M-spike*) in the gamma region indicates monoclonal gammopathy; sometimes, a M-spike can be found in the beta regions.

predict value of 70% limits the use of this test to screen horses with lymphoma (Perkins, 2003).

Serum protein electrophoresis has been used to evaluate hyperglobulinemia and define monoclonal gammopathies (Figure 22.5). Hyperglobulinemia is commonly caused by inflammatory responses (production of alpha and beta globulins) and/or responses to infections (production of *polyclonal* gammaglobulins/immunoglobulins), but it can be also caused by hypergammaglobulinemia due to the production of *monoclonal* immunoglobulins in neoplasms (e.g., multiple myeloma, certain B cell lymphomas and leukemias). Serum protein electrophoresis can be diagnostic of hypogammaglobulinemia, but serum IgG and IgM concentrations should be used for this purpose, for their better concentration accuracy and longitudinal comparisons.

In the case of T and B cell lymphomas/lymphosarcoma and leukemias, the expansion of monoclonal tumoral populations can also be detected using polymerase chain reaction (PCR) for the antigen receptor rearrangement (PARR). This clonality

THORACIC ASPIRATE

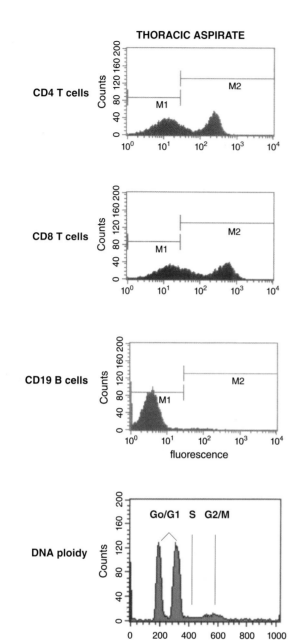

Figure 22.5 Lymphocyte immunophenotyping and total DNA content staining of cells, obtained via thoracocentesis from a patient with pleural fluid, revealed the presence of inflammatory and tumoral populations. Lymphocyte immunophenotyping in thoracic fluid measured comparable distribution of CD4$^+$ and CD8$^+$ T cells, and negligible B cells, without a predominant cell population. Note the wide distribution (broad peak) of cell marker expression. Nevertheless, when stained for DNA content with the fluorescent intercalating agent propidium iodide, aneuploidy was detected, based on the presence of non-overlapping Go/G1 peaks, indicating the presence of tumoral cells. This clinical case is an example of limitations of immunophenotypng alone in the diagnosis of lymphoma.

assay uses PCR primers that target genes flanking the hypervariable regions (VDJ genes) of the T cell receptor or B cell receptor. Therefore, the assay can not only identify clonality, but can also confirm a lymphoid origin. In contrast, inflammatory cells are not monoclonal.

SPECTRATYPING

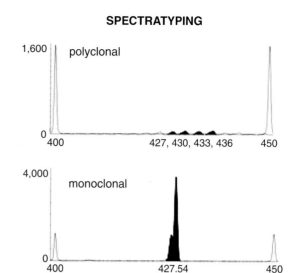

Figure 22.6 Immunoglobulin spectratyping. Immunoglobulin spectratyping offers a graphic representation of the cell immunoglobulin repertoire, based on the distribution of complementarity determining region 3 (hypervariable region CDR3) sequence lengths, using a genetic analyzer. Several small (polyclonal) peaks are detected in a normal blood leukocyte sample, whereas a sharp (monoclonal) peak is observed in a blood sample of B cell leukemia. Amplicon length(s) are labeled.

Specialized laboratories (e.g., University of California-Davis, Colorado State University, North Caroline State University) are now offering PARR testing for domestic species, and assays should be validated for each species. An additional molecular assay that measures clonality of B cells is spectratyping, which assesses the length of the complementarity determining region (CDR hypervariable region) of the immunoglobulin. The application of this assay was developed by Dr. Rebecca Tallmadge at Cornell University. Heterogeneous lengths are expected in normal polyclonal cells, whereas monoclonal cells have similar CDR length, which are represented by multiple or single peaks in a histogram, respectively (Figure 22.6).

22.2.9 Allergy tests
Allergy tests are addressed in Chapter 5.

References

Flaminio, M.J., Rush, B.R. and Shuman, W. (2000). Characterization of peripheral blood and pulmonary leukocyte function in healthy foals. *Veterinary Immunology and Immunopathology* **73**(3–4), 267–285.

Flaminio, M.J., Rush, B.R., Davis, E.G., Hennessy, K., Shuman, W. and Wilkerson, M.J. (2002). Simultaneous flow cytometric analysis of phagocytosis and oxidative burst activity in equine leukocytes. *Veterinary Research Communication* **26**(2), 85–92.

Flaminio, M.J., Tallmadge, R., Salles-Gomes, C.M. and Matychak, M.B. (2009). Common variable immunodeficiency in horses is characterized by B cell depletion in primary and secondary lymphoid tissues. *Journal of Clinical Immunology* **29**(1), 107–116.

Fox-Clipsham, L.Y., Brown, E.E., Carter, S.D. and Swinburne, J.E. (2011). Identification of a mutation associated with fatal foal immunodeficiency syndrome in the Fell and Dales Pony. *PLoS Genetics* **7**, e1002133.

Hou, S., McClure, J.T., Shaw, R.A. and Rilley, C.B. (2014). Immunoglobulin G measurement in blood plasma using infrared spectroscopy. *Applied Spectroscopy* **68**(4), 466–474.

Lavoie, J.P., Spensley, M.S., Smith, B.P. and Mihalyi, J. (1989). Absorption of bovine colostral immunoglobulins G and M in newborn foals. *American Journal of Veterinary Research* **50**, 1598–1603.

McCue, P.M. (2007). Evaluation of a turbidimetric immunoassay for measurement of plasma IgG concentration in foals. *American Journal of Veterinary Research* **68**(9), 1005–1009.

McGuire, T.C., Perryman, L.E. and Davis, W.C. (1983). Analysis of serum and lymphocyte surface IgM of healthy and immunodeficient horses with monoclonal antibodies. *American Journal of Veterinary Research* **44**(7), 1284–1288.

Metzger, N., Hinchcliff, K.W., Hardy, J., Schwarzwald, C.C. and Wittum, T. (2006). Usefulness of a commercial equine IgG test and serum protein concentration as indicators of failure of transfer of passive immunity in hospitalized foals. *Journal of Veterinary Internal Medicine* **20**(2), 382–7.

Perkins, G.A., Nydam, D.V., Flaminio, M.J.B.F. and Ainsworth, D.M. (2003). Serum IgM concentrations in normal, fit horses and horses with lymphoma or other medical conditions. *Journal of Veterinary Internal Medicine* **17**, 337–342.

Pusterla, N., Pusterla, J.B., Spier, S.J., Puget, B. and Watson, J.L. (2002). Evaluation of the SNAP foal IgG test for the semiquantitative measurement of immunoglobulin G in foals. *Veterinary Record* **151**(9), 258–60.

Shin, E.K., Perryman, L.E. and Meek, K. (1997). Evaluation of a test for identification of Arabian horses heterozygous for the severe combined immunodeficiency trait. *Journal of American Veterinary Medical Association* **211**(10), 1268–1270.

Wiler, R., Leber, R., Moore, B.B., VanDyk, L.F., Perryman, L.E. and Meek, K. (1995). Equine severe combined immunodeficiency: a defect in V(D)J recombination and DNA-dependent protein kinase activity. *Proceedings of the National Academy of Sciences of the United States of America* **92**(25), 11485–11489.

23 Non-steroidal Anti-inflammatories

Michelle H. Barton

23.1 Definition

There are numerous drugs that can directly or indirectly reduce inflammation. However, compared to other species, cost, efficacy, toxicity, or lack of equine-specific pharmacokinetic information, renders relatively fewer available choices for anti-inflammatory drug use in horses.

23.2 Non-steroidal anti-inflammatory drugs

Non-steroidal anti-inflammatory drugs (NSAIDs) represent the largest class of anti-inflammatory agents available for use in horses. The basic mechanism of action is essentially the same for all NSAIDs – inhibition of the active binding site of cyclooxygenase (COX), also known as prostaglandin H synthase, a key enzyme involved in the formation of eicosanoids by oxidation of arachidonic acid (Figure 23.1).

Arachidonic acid is an essential omega-6 twenty-carbon polyunsaturated fatty acid contained in the phospholipid bilayer of cell membranes. Once freed by phospholipases, arachidonic acid can be further metabolized by lipoxygenase to form leukotrienes, or by COX to form the prostanoids. The final product(s) of COX depend on the specific and differential expression of downstream eicosanoid enzymes within any given tissue. Cyclooxygenase has two active sites: one that converts arachidonic acid into prostaglandin G_2, and a second site that converts prostaglandin G_2 into prostaglandin H_2 (PGH_2) by hydroperoxidation (Hinz, 2002).

23.2.1 Cyclooxygenase

At least two isoforms of COX exist (Hinz, 2002). *Cyclooxygenase 1* (COX1) is often referred to as the *housekeeping* isoform that is continuously expressed in fixed amounts in most tissues, notably including platelets, the gastrointestinal mucosa, and the kidney (Hinz, 2002). *Cyclooxygenase 2* (COX2) is also constitutively expressed in some tissues but, in contrast to COX1, the COX2 gene has a specific promoter site that enables regulation

and is inducible by other pro-inflammatory transcription signals, such as binding of nuclear factor kappa-B (NF-kappa B) (Hinz, 2002). Subtle differences in the amino acid sequence of the COX isoform binding sites account for differential binding of NSAIDs, which varies from irreversible to reversible, and the specificity of inhibition of COX1 versus COX2. The important discovery of COX isoforms not only provided explanation for the common gastrointestinal and renal side-effects of non-specific pharmacologic inhibition of COX1, it opened the door to exploration of an entirely new family of selective COX2 inhibitors (also known as COXIBs, or COX1-sparing drugs).

Once formed by COX activity, further metabolism of PGH_2 by tissue-specific downstream enzymes results in the formation of the prostanoids, including prostaglandins (PG), thromboxane, and prostacyclin (Hinz, 2002). Prostanoids are found in a wide variety of tissues, and play a role in both inflammation and regulation of normal physiologic functions. The half-life of prostanoids is relatively short and, therefore, they mostly act locally in the tissue of origin, having both autocrine and paracrine functions via specific prostanglandin G protein coupled receptors (Khanapure, 2007).

One such important prostanoid is prostaglandin E_2 (PGE_2), formed by the metabolism of PGH_2 by PGE_2 synthase (Figure 23.1). Similar to COX, there are also at least three isoforms of PGE_2 synthase (PGES) that control constitutive production of PGE_2 for regulation of physiologic functions (microsomal PGES2 and cytosolic PGES), or are upregulated during inflammation (microsomal PGES1) (Nakanishi, 2010). Constitutively expressed PGE_2 is found in numerous tissues, including the gastrointestinal tract, vascular endothelium, platelets, the lungs, and the uterus. The biological functions of PGE_2 depend on its receptor locations and types at the site of synthesis, and include: reduction of gastric acid secretion; stimulation of gastric mucus secretion; vasodilation; bronchodilation; smooth muscle contraction; inhibition of platelet aggregation; increased vascular permeability; angiogenesis, apoptosis; enhancement of pain perception; and increased body temperature (Khanapure, 2007).

Equine Clinical Immunology, First Edition. Edited by M. Julia B. Felippe.
© 2016 John Wiley & Sons, Inc. Published 2016 by John Wiley & Sons, Inc.

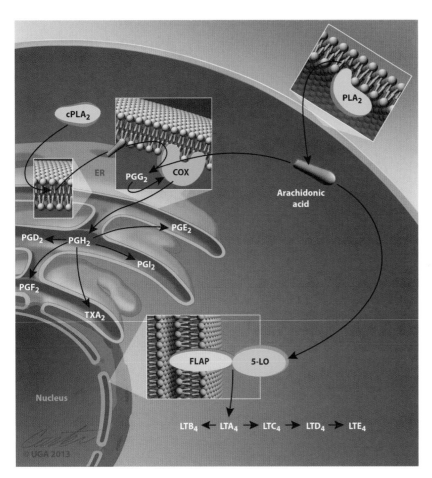

Figure 23.1 Eicosanoid metabolic pathway. The basic mechanism of action is essentially the same for all NSAIDs: inhibition of the active binding site of cyclooxygenase (COX), a key enzyme involved in the formation of eicosanoids by oxidation of arachidonic acid. Arachidonic acid is present in the cell membranes and, once freed by phospholipases, arachidonic acid can be further metabolized by lipoxygenase to form leukotrienes, or by COX to form the prostanoids. Cyclooxygenase has two active sites: one that converts arachidonic acid into prostaglandin G_2, and a second site that converts prostaglandin G_2 into prostaglandin H_2 (PGH_2). Further metabolism of PGH_2 results in the formation of prostaglandins (PGE_2), thromboxane (TXA_2), and prostacyclin (PGI_2).
PLA_2 – phospholipase A_2; COX – cyclooxygenase; PG – prostaglandin, LT – leukotriene; ER – endoplasmic reticulum; 5-LO – 5-lipoxygenase; FLAP – five lipoxygenase activating protein.

Inducible microsomal PGES1 is found in several tissues, notably leukocytes and chondrocytes (Farley, 2005). There is compelling evidence that COX2 and microsomal PGES1 regulation is coupled and, therefore, induction of COX2 during inflammatory states preferentially culminates in the production of PGE_2 (Nakanishi, 2010). Ultimately, up-regulation of inducible PGE_2 biosynthesis during the pro-inflammatory state explains the cardinal signs of inflammation, including rubor, heat, pain, and swelling.

When PGH_2 is metabolized by thromboxane synthase (Figure 23.1) primarily found in platelets, the product is thromboxane A_2 (TXA_2). Thromboxane A_2 is a potent vasoconstrictor and enables platelet aggregation (Khanapure, 2007). In contrast, when PGH_2 is metabolized by prostacyclin synthase located in endothelial cells, the product is PGI_2, which functions as a direct physiologic antagonist to TXA_2 (Khanapure, 2007).

Currently, there are literally dozens of NSAIDs on the market. Blockage of specific enzymes downstream from COX has been a target of more recent and novel NSAIDs, and adds an additional level of specificity of blockade. Pharmacokinetic and pharmacodynamic properties, dosage and COX selectivity can vary widely among species and, therefore, dose extrapolation for NSAIDs is imprudent.

23.2.2 Non-selective non-steroidal anti-inflammatory drugs
23.2.2.1 Phenylbutazone

Phenylbutazone (i.e., bute), an enolic acid derivative, is a non-selective COX inhibitor, first introduced into veterinary medicine in the 1950s (Soma, 2012). Its affordability and efficacy as an analgesic and anti-inflammatory drug for musculoskeletal disease make it one of the most widely used NSAIDS on the market today for horses. As is true for most NSAIDS, phenylbutazone is highly protein-bound in plasma (> 98%) and displaces other protein bound molecules. It is metabolized in the liver to its active metabolites, oxyphenbutazone and gamma hydroxyoxyphenbutazone, both excreted in the urine (Tobin, 1986).

Dose recommendations for phenylbutazone are the same for both intravenous and oral formulations, and have remained steadfast over time (Table 23.1). However, based on evidence of drug accumulation in the plasma after repeated doses, its narrow therapeutic index, and lack of improved efficacy in ameliorating lameness at higher doses, it is strongly recommended to achieve the lower maintenance dose levels as soon as possible (Gerring, 1981; Toutain, 1994; Soma, 2012).

Table 23.1 Non-steroidal anti-inflammatory drugs.

Drug	Recommended doses	Notes
Non-selective		
Phenylbutazone	4.4 mg/kg PO or IV BID as loading dose. 2.2 mg/kg PO or IV BID to SID as maintenance dose. It is highly recommended to achieve maintenance doses within 1–3 days.	Several trade names available. (Taylor, 1983; Soma, 2012)
Flunixin meglumine	1.1 mg/kg PO or IV BID as anti-inflammatory dose. 0.25 mg/kg PO or IV TID as anti-endotoxic dose.	Several trade names available. Original patent under the trade name of Banamine™, Merck Animal Health, Summit, NJ (Chay, 1982; Semrad, 1985)
Aspirin	12 mg/kg PO every other day to prolong bleeding time. 240 to 960 grains PO (package insert).	Several trade names available. VetOne Aspirin Bolus, MWI Veterinary Supply, Boise, ID. (Cambridge, 1991)
Ketoprofen	2.2 mg/kg IV SID for up to five days (package insert).	Approved for IV use in horses. Ketofen™, Zoetis, Florham Park, NJ.
Naproxen	5 mg/kg slow IV then 10 mg/kg PO BID to SID (package insert).	Approved oral and IV product for horses but not currently available in the United States. EquiproxenTM, Zoetis, Inc. (Soma, 1995)
Caprofen	0.7 mg/kg PO or IV SID.	Approved for use in dogs. (McKellar, 1991; Lees, 2002)
Meclofenamic acid	2.2 mg/kg PO or IV SID.	Approved for use in horses though currently not available in the United States. (Snow, 1981; Johansson, 1991)
Eltenac	0.5 mg/kg IV SID.	Approved for horses in Europe. (Dyke, 1998)
Vedaprofen	2 mg/kg PO or IV SID, then 1 mg/kg PO SID for up to 14 days (package insert).	Veterinary formulation available for horses in Canada and Europe.
COX2 selective		
Firocoxib	0.1 mg/kg PO or 0.09 mg/kg IV SID for up to 14 days.	Approved for use in the horse (Letendre, 2008; Kvaternick, 2007)
Meloxicam	0.6 mg/kg PO or IV SID.	Approved for use in small animals in the United States and for horses in Europe and other countries. (Lees, 1991; Toutain, 2004a, 2004b)
Deracoxib	2 mg/kg PO SID.	Approved for use in dogs. (Davis, 2011)
Etodolac	20–23 mg/kg PO or IV BID to SID.	Approved for use in dogs. (Morton, 2005; Symonds, 2006; Davis, 2007)

PO – *per os* or orally; IV – intravenously; SID – *semel in die* or once a day; BID – *bis in die* or twice a day; TID – *ter in die* or three times a day.

This concept was eloquently demonstrated in a combined pharmacokinetic/pharmacodynamic study using phenylbutazone in an experimentally induced model of arthritis (Toutain, 1994). The maximal effect on improvement in lameness was achieved at a dose of 2 mg/kg body weight. Effectiveness in reducing inflammation and lameness was not increased at higher doses, but the duration of action was prolonged from eight hours, when given at 2 mg/kg, to 24 hours, when dosed at 8 mg/kg (Toutain, 1994). Further clinical studies have also concluded that, in naturally-occurring cases of chronic lameness in horses, there is no further improvement in lameness at doses exceeding 4.4 mg/kg body weight SID (Hu, 2005).

Although available in intravenous preparations, the absorption of orally administered phenylbutazone is efficient, reaching peak plasma concentrations within six hours. The bioavailability of orally administered drug is unaffected by feeding. However, the time to peak plasma concentration will double to triple if hay is offered as a free choice (Tobin, 1986). It is suggested that the paste formulation is more slowly absorbed than other oral preparations.

The pharmacokinetics of phenylbutazone are dose-dependent, with plasma half-life increasing as the dosage increases (Tobin, 1986). In neonatal foals, the volume of distribution is larger, the half-life is longer, and the total clearance of phenylbutazone is lower, compared with similar values reported for adult horses (Wilcke, 1993). Mean total body clearance of phenylbutazone in donkeys is five times greater than in horses, so shorter intervals between doses may be appropriate in donkeys (Mealey, 1997). The therapeutic index for phenylbutazone is narrow and, in general, it is highly recommended not to exceed the recommended loading or maintenance doses.

Phenylbutazone has been most extensively used clinically to manage musculoskeletal inflammation and pain in horses, particularly those with osteoarthritis (Goodrich, 2006; Ross, 2011; Soma, 2012). Being a *mainstay* of treatment for musculoskeletal disease, phenylbutazone's efficacy has frequently been compared to newer NSAIDs as they have entered the market over the decades. The comparative efficacy of phenylbutazone to other NSAIDs varies depending on the model employed and the drug dose.

In general, phenylbutazone has performed well against other newer NSAIDs in lameness models. Flunixin meglumine and phenylbutazone appear to have similar analgesic effects in horses with navicular syndrome (Erkert, 2005). However, phenylbutazone was more effective than ketoprofen in duration of action and in reducing lameness, joint temperature, and synovial fluid volume in an experimentally induced model of acute synovitis (Owens, 1996). Only when given at 1.65 times its label dose was ketoprofen superior to phenylbutazone in alleviating lameness in horses with chronic laminitis (Owens, 1995a). Finally, in a large clinical study on 253 client owned horses with naturally occurring osteoarthritis, the efficacy of paste phenylbutazone was comparable to the paste formulation of the COX2 selective NSAID, firocoxib (Doucet, 2008).

Although phenylbutazone has been shown to reduce exercise-induced increases in cytokine gene expression (Lehnhard, 2010), it has not particularly been noted to be a performance-altering drug (Soma, 2012). Indeed, many sport horse events allow the use of phenylbutazone during competition, or have guidelines on acceptable levels of the drug in blood or urine. Nonetheless, in a recent review of 161 Thoroughbreds with musculoskeletal injuries that occurred during racing, the plasma concentrations of phenylbutazone and flunixin meglumine were higher in injured horses than in control horses (Dirikolu, 2009a). Although this study could not prove a direct cause-and-effect relationship, it has been suggested that NSAID use in horses may deter joint health (Goodrich, 2006), leading to further injury during exercise, or that NSAID use may mask subclinical injury that could not be contained during the additional stresses of high-intensity performance.

Despite its longevity, successful use for the management of musculoskeletal disease and desirable affordability, the well-described adverse side-effects of phenylbutazone have fueled the search for equal or superior NSAIDs with reduced toxicity. Although phenylbutazone can be used in horses at the recommended maintenance dose with no reported side-effects, some horses will develop signs of toxicity at recommended doses. Adverse effects include: anorexia; depression; gastric, right dorsal colon and urinary bladder ulceration; renal papillary necrosis; neutropenia; anemia; protein losing enteropathy; colitis; and death (Hough, 1999; McConnico, 2008; Aleman, 2011; Soma, 2012).

The development of renal papillary necrosis is more likely when phenylbutazone treatment is combined with water deprivation (Gunson, 1983). The increase in gastric permeability and formation of gastric ulcers appears to be the greatest for phenylbutazone, when compared to flunixin meglumine, ketoprofen, meloxicam, and firocoxib (MacAllister, 1993; D'Arcy-Moskwa, 2012; Soma, 2012). Concurrent use of phenylbutazone with flunixin meglumine increases the risk of gastric ulceration compared to phenylbutazone alone, so veterinarians should exercise caution in prescribing both drugs concurrently (Reed, 2006).

When higher doses or prolonged use of phenylbutazone is required, concurrent administration of sucralfate and antacids have been shown to reduce the severity of phenylbutazone-induced gastric ulceration (Geor, 1989). The likelihood of toxicity increases with increasing dosage and duration of use, so the strong recommendation is to use the lowest maintenance dose possible. Periodic monitoring of dehydration (blood hematocrit and total protein), serum creatinine and albumin concentrations may be beneficial in detecting early evidence of possible phenylbutazone toxicity.

23.2.2.2 Flunixin meglumine

Flunixin meglumine, a nicotinic acid derivative, was well received as a new NSAID for horses in the late 1970s because of its potent analgesic effect in controlling acute visceral pain. After intravenous injection at the recommended dose (Table 23.1), plasma levels peak within minutes, and then rapidly decline, with a short plasma half-life of about 1.6 hours, and a slower elimination phase best fitting a two-compartmental pharmacokinetic model (Chay, 1982). Despite its short time in the plasma, flunixin meglumine persists in inflammatory exudates, providing a clinical effect in the horse for more than 12 hours (Higgins, 1986).

The bioavailability of the drug is excellent, with peak plasma concentrations achieved within 30 minutes of oral administration (Chay, 1982). When the paste formulation is used, feeding does not affect the overall mean total absorption of the drug, but feeding may delay and reduce the peak plasma concentration, when compared to administration without feed access (Welsh, 1992). However, when the injectable preparation of flunixin meglumine is administered orally in fed horses, it is detected in plasma within 15 minutes of administration, and peak plasma concentrations are almost twice those reported for the paste formulation (Welsh, 1992), between 45–60 minutes (Pellegrini-Masini, 2004). Although it has label approval for use intramuscularly, rare reports of clostridial myositis after intramuscular injection in horses have deterred its use by that route (Anderson, 2013).

The mean residence time for flunixin meglumine is considerably shorter in healthy donkeys, compared to horses and mules, implying that the dosing interval for flunixin meglumine should be shorter in donkeys (Coakley, 1999). However, this observation was based on a single bolus injection protocol, and pharmacodynamic parameters were not included in that study, making it difficult to recommend a precise dosing interval for donkeys. The pharmacokinetics of flunixin meglumine in foals appear to be similar to adult horses, with the exception that the rate of elimination is slower in foals less than two days old, suggesting that a longer dosing interval should be used (Semrad, 1993). Likewise, the total body clearance and elimination rate constant are higher, and the half-life in the plasma is longer for horses older than nine years, compared to younger mature adult horses less than five years old (Jensen, 1990). These age-related differences should be kept in mind when considering drug withdrawal time prior to competition in sanctioned sports.

Training and exercise do not appear to affect elimination pharmacokinetics (Jensen, 1990; Colahan, 2002). The drug and its alkaline metabolites primarily undergo renal excretion, and are detectable for two to four days in urine after a single dose (Chay, 1982; Colahan, 2002).

The initial observation that flunixin meglumine was a potent analgesic for horses with visceral abdominal pain prompted a series of experimental studies in the 1980s, using endotoxin as a pro-inflammatory stimulus. When used intravenously at the marketed label dose of 1.1 mg/kg body weight, flunixin meglumine mitigated the deleterious effects of endotoxin on blood pressure, cardiac output, and pulmonary vascular endothelium in anesthetized ponies (Bottoms, 1981; Turek, 1985). Pre-treatment of horses with the label dose of flunixin meglumine was more effective in ameliorating endotoxin-induced clinical signs and prostanoid synthesis, when compared to pre-treatment with phenylbutazone or a selective thromboxane synthase inhibitor (Moore, 1986).

Subsequent studies in awake adult horses determined that, when given intravenously at approximately one fourth the label dose (0.25 mg/kg body weight) every eight hours, flunixin meglumine effectively suppressed serum thromboxane B_2 concentrations in clotted blood (Semrad, 1985). Furthermore, this reduced dose suppressed serum thromboxane, plasma prostacylin, and lactate concentrations in endotoxin challenged horses, while not significantly altering the associated clinical signs, such as tachycardia, tachypnea, fever, and abdominal discomfort (Semrad, 1987). Because it provided effective blockade of cyclooxygenase by reducing prostanoid synthesis, it did not mask valuable clinical signs used for monitoring clinical progression. This *quarter dose* of flunixin meglumine was, thus, popularized for treatment of horses with acute gastrointestinal disorders associated with endotoxemia.

As newer NSAIDs and COX1 sparing NSAIDs became available for use in horses, comparison studies to flunixin meglumine, especially in models of acute gastrointestinal disease and endotoxemia, entered the literature. In a small blinded field study on naturally occurring colic, flunixin meglumine and ketoprofen were both assessed to be effective analgesics for the treatment of mild to moderate equine colic pain when judged by the attending veterinarian (Betley, 1991). There were no significant differences between flunixin meglumine

and ketoprofen treatment groups in *in vitro* endotoxin-induced production of thromboxane B_2, PGE_2, 12-hydroxyeicosatetraenoic acid, tumor necrosis factor (TNF), or tissue factor in healthy horses (Jackman, 1994). Likewise, surgically implanted subcutaneous tissue cages stimulated by carrageenan were used to compare pharmacodynamic parameters of flunixin meglumine and ketoprofen in adult healthy horses.

Both drugs produced marked inhibition of serum thromboxane synthesis for up to 24 hours, whereas flunixin meglumine was a more potent inhibitor of exudate prostaglandin synthesis and bradykinin induced swelling (Landoni, 1995). Compared to newer COX2 selective inhibitors, such as etodolac, meloxicam, and firocoxib, flunixin meglumine appears to provide equivalent analgesia postoperatively in horses with experimentally induced jejunal strangulation (Tomlinson, 2004; Little, 2007; Cook, 2009a).

Although not frequently used as a first choice for the control of musculoskeletal pain, pharmacodynamic modeling in experimentally induced synovitis in horses predicts that flunixin meglumine at 1 mg/kg body weight will provide a near-maximum anti-inflammatory effect for up to 16 hours (Toutain, 1994). There was no significant difference in clinical parameters in horses with experimentally induced synovitis, treated with either eltenac or flunixin meglumine for four days (Hamm, 1997). In horses with naturally occurring navicular syndrome, daily flunixin meglumine (1.1 mg/kg body weight) provided analgesic effects that were similar to phenylbutazone (4.4 mg/kg body weight) (Erkert, 2005). Flunixin meglumine is effective in blocking exercise-induced increases in plasma thromboxane and prostacyclin levels, without altering performance parameters in healthy conditioned Thoroughbreds (Colahan, 2002).

Flunixin meglumine is generally well tolerated in adult horses when used at the label dose, with a wider therapeutic index than phenylbutazone (MacAllister, 1993). However, lesions typical of non-selective NSAIDs, including gastric ulceration and renal papillary necrosis, are reported when extra label doses are used (MacAllister, 1993). Concurrent use of phenylbutazone with flunixin meglumine increases the risk of gastric ulceration, compared with phenylbutazone alone, so veterinarians should exercise caution in prescribing both drugs concurrently (Reed, 2006). Flunixin meglumine is also reasonably well tolerated in neonatal foals, with no significant clinicopathological or histopathologic differences between healthy foals treated with the recommended dosage of flunixin meglumine twice daily for five days, and those treated with physiological saline (Carrick, 1989). However, once-daily dosing at 1.1 mg/kg body weight for 30 days in foals resulted in mild to moderate gastric ulceration (Traub-Dargatz, 1988).

Flunixin meglumine delays the recovery of intestinal barrier function after experimental induction of jejunal ischemic injury in horses (Tomlinson, 2005; Little, 2007; Cook, 2009a). However, it does not affect recovery of equine colonic mucosa following ischemic injury (Matyjaszek, 2009). The significance of the effect of flunixin meglumine on jejunal recovery in naturally occurring cases of ischemia is not known, and flunixin meglumine continues to be a mainstay of therapy for the postoperative colic patient.

23.2.2.3 Acetylsalicylic acid

Acetylsalicylic acid, or aspirin, was first manufactured around the start of the 20th century, making it the oldest NSAID on the market. Aspirin is a non-selective COX inhibitor by irreversible acetylation of the active site. Because of its extremely short half-life in plasma, following intravenous injection in horses (Lees, 1987), and subsequent rapid conversion to salicylate, it is not routinely used in horses as an anti-inflammatory drug. However, it is an effective antithrombotic agent, based on its unique ability to irreversibly bind COX in platelets, which preferentially express thromboxane synthase as a downstream enzyme to COX.

Although thromboxane is a potent agonist of platelet aggregation, it is not the only agent responsible for aggregation in horses, based on the observation that aspirin's ability to suppress thromboxane far exceeds its ability to inhibit platelet aggregation (Cambridge, 1991; Jarvis, 1994, 1996; Brainard, 2011). Furthermore, the ability of aspirin to inhibit platelet aggregation in the horse depends on the dose of aspirin used, and the agonist used to induce platelet aggregation. For example, 4 mg aspirin/kg body weight and 12 mg aspirin/kg body weight given orally to horses significantly prolonged bleeding time for four and 48 hours, respectively, despite successful concurrent suppression of platelet thromboxane synthesis for six days (Cambridge, 1991). Only the 12 mg aspirin/kg body weight dose was effective in inhibiting collagen induced platelet aggregation for 48 hours.

It has been suggested that higher aspirin doses are needed to provide an anti-inflammatory effect in horses, though there is insufficient clinical data to provide an accurate dose for routine use. Unless compounded, aspirin is only available in the United States as an oral preparation. A single rectal dose of aspirin of 20 mg/kg body weight in fasted horses results in higher peak plasma acetylsalicylic acid concentrations, and greater bio-availability, than the same dose given intragastrically to non-fasted horses (Broome, 2003).

23.2.2.4 Ketoprofen

Ketoprofen is a propionic acid derivative. Like carprofen, it is a chiral molecule that exits as two enantiomers. Ketoprofen is a non-selective COX inhibitor, with alleged assertion for dual inhibition of COX and lipoxygenase, although subsequent *ex vivo* and *in vivo* studies in horses have not been able to substantiate that claim (Jackman, 1994; Landoni, 1996; Owens, 1996). When it first entered the market, ketoprofen was considered to be a unique NSAID for use in horses, for its long duration of action and residual tissue levels, which enabled once-daily dosing, despite its short plasma half-life (Table 23.1). The oral bioavailability of ketoprofen is poor in horses. The package insert is only approved for intravenous use, though

intramuscular administration has been described in horses (Gregoricka, 1990; Anfossi, 1997).

The commercially available product is a 50:50 mixture of both enantiomers. The S isoform appears to be predominately responsible for COX inhibition. Similar to most NSAIDs, ketoprofen is highly protein-bound. When the racemic mixture is administered intravenously to horses, the S enantiomer predominates in the plasma and synovial fluid (Owens, 1995b), and is facilitated by one-way chiral inversion from the R to the S enantiomer (Landoni, 1996; Verde, 2001). Interestingly, chiral inversion is hindered by inflammation and, in severe inflammatory states, an increase in dose of the racemic mixture may be needed (Verde, 2001). Increasing the dose 1.5 times may be needed for foals less than 24 hours old, due to a larger volume of distribution and slower plasma clearance (Wilcke, 1998).

Ketoprofen's anti-inflammatory and analgesic efficacy has been compared to several other NSAIDs in horses, the results of which are dependent on the model. Ketoprofen was shown to have equivalent inhibition of COX and analgesia to flunixin meglumine in an *ex vivo* model of endotoxemia, and in naturally occurring cases of colic, respectively (Betley, 1991; Jackman, 1994). Compared to phenylbutazone, ketoprofen was a less effective analgesic in a carrageenan induced model of synovitis in horses (Owens, 1996), but it was more effective in reducing pain and lameness, when used at 1.65 times the recommended dose in horses with chronic laminitis (Owens, 1995a).

Being a non-selective COX inhibitor, the use of ketoprofen is not immune from potential adverse gastrointestinal and renal side-effects. However, in one study that compared the recommended dose of ketoprofen, flunixin meglumine, and phenylbutazone, each given three times daily for 12 days, there were no signs of renal toxicity at necropsy, and the gastric ulceration was least severe in horses receiving ketoprofen (MacAllister, 1993).

23.2.2.5 Naproxen

Structurally similar to ketoprofen and ibuprofen, naproxen is a member of the propionic acid subclass of NSAIDS. In equine studies, both *in vitro* and *ex vivo* characterized naproxen as a non-selective COX inhibitor (Cuniberti, 2012). There is little information about its relative clinical efficacy in horses, though there is one study indicating that naproxen was a more effective analgesic than phenylbutazone in myositis (Jones, 1978). The oral bioavailability is low at approximately 50%, and it may take several days before a beneficial effect is noted (Tobin, 1979).

23.2.2.6 Carprofen

Carprofen is a propionic acid derivative that exists in two stereoisomeric forms, though it is the R enantiomer that predominates in the plasma after dosing. At the recommended dose (Table 23.1), carprofen appears to have better analgesic than anti-inflammatory properties in the horse, being superior or approximately equivalent to flunixin meglumine, and superior to phenylbutazone in duration of analgesia (Schatzmann, 1990; Johnson, 1993; Lees, 1994). Although carprofen has been shown to preferentially inhibit COX2 in some species, this does not appear to be the case when used at the recommended dose in horses (Lees, 2002).

A unique feature of carprofen is its relatively long plasma half-life, ranging from 18–31 hours in ponies and horses, allowing once a day dosing, either orally or intravenously (McKellar, 1991; Lees, 1994). Based on sustained synovial fluid concentrations, antiprostaglandin and anticytokine effects, and stimulation of chondrocyte proteoglycan synthesis, carprofen may be a particularly useful drug for the treatment of osteo-arthritis in horses (Armstrong, 1999a, 1999b, 2002; Frean, 1999). The mean residence time of carprofen in donkeys is almost three times that in horses, suggesting that a longer dose interval should be considered (Mealey, 2004). Carprofen appears to be well tolerated in the horse, with no observable signs of toxicity when given at twice the recommended dose for 14 days (McKellar, 1991).

23.2.2.7 Meclofenamic acid

Meclofenamic acid is an anthranilic acid derivative and non-selective COX inhibitor that has been on the market since the 1980s. It is oxidized to two metabolites, one of which is bioactive. Currently, it is available only in an oral formulation for horses. The effect of feeding on absorption is inconsistent, with reports of either no effect to delayed absorption (Snow, 1981; Johansson, 1991). Because of its variable oral bioavailability and delayed onset of action (1.5–4 days), it is not commonly prescribed in the horse. Controlled clinical studies are scant, though it is reported to be effective in both acute and chronic laminitis (Lees, 1985). Interestingly, daily meclofenamate, given orally from nine days after ovulation, until seven days after embryo transfer, significantly improved pregnancy rates when recipients ovulated before donor's mares (Wilsher, 2006).

23.2.2.8 Eltenac

Eltenac is an acetic acid derivative that, when tested *in vitro* in horses, showed promise as a preferential COX2 inhibitor (Cuniberti, 2012). However subsequent *ex vivo* studies demonstrated that it actually is a non-selective COX inhibitor in horses (Cuniberti, 2012). When given intravenously at the recommended dose at 0.5 mg/kg body weight IV SID (Table 23.1) for five days, the drug does not accumulate (Dyke, 1998).

Clinical studies support its efficacy in horses. In an experimental model of synovitis, eltenac given at the recommended dose was equally as effective as flunixin meglumine in objective measures of carpal circumference, carpal flexion angle, stride length, carpal hyperthermia, and signs of carpal pain (Hamm, 1997). In an *in vivo* experimental model of endotoxemia, a single intravenous dose (0.5 mg/kg body weight) of eltenac ameliorated some of the clinical signs and clinicopathologic abnormalities of endotoxemia (MacKay, 2000). Lastly, in a blinded and placebo controlled clinical study involving 64 lame horses, eltenac significantly reduced pain scores after a single intravenous injection at 1 mg/kg body weight (Prugner, 1991). The

drug appears to be well tolerated, with no significant gastro-intestinal lesions or significant changes in clinical or clinico-pathologic data, when given at the recommended dose for 15 days (Goodrich, 1998). Eltenac is not available in the United States in a veterinary formulation.

23.2.2.9 Vedaprofen

Similar to ketoprofen and caprofen, vedaprofen is an arylpro-pionate derivative that is commercially available as a 50 : 50 mixture of enantiomers that requires only once daily dosing. Following intravenous injection, vedaprofen behaves identically to caprofen, in that the R isomer predominates in both plasma and tissue exudates, and there is no chiral inversion (Lees, 1999). In the horse, vedaprofen is highly COX1-selective. *In vivo* studies in the horse support its efficacy in several models by reducing subcutaneous carrageenan induced inflammation, ameliorating clinical signs of endotoxemia, and improving pregnancy rates in embryo recipient mares and mares with metritis (Lees, 1999; Renault, 2003; Koblischke, 2010; Rojer, 2010). In a recent clinical study in horses with naturally occur-ring lameness, vedaprofen did not perform as well the COX2-selective inhibitor, firocoxib (Koene, 2010). Vedaprofen is not currently available as a veterinary preparation in the United States.

23.2.3 Cyclooxygenase 2 selective inhibitors
23.2.3.1 Firocoxib

Firocoxib is a second generation COX2 inhibitor (Kvaternick, 2007) because of its high degree of selectivity of inhibition of COX2 relative to COX1. In horses, *in vitro* whole blood models have shown that firocoxib is approximately 265 times more COX2 selective relative to COX1 (McCann, 2002), making it approximately 10–70 times more COX2-selective, compared with deracoxib and meloxicam, respectively (Davis, 2011). It is the first COX2-selective inhibitor to be approved for both oral and intravenous use in horses in the United States.

Pharmacokinetic studies performed in horses indicate that, when given at the recommended dose (0.1 mg/kg body weight PO SID), firocoxib is readily absorbed following oral adminis-tration, even if hay is not withheld (Kvaternick, 2007). Its long half-life enables once-daily dosing. Whether administered intravenously or orally, the pharmacokinetic behavior of firocoxib is linear after multiple doses, and the plasma-to-urine ratio remains stable over time (Letendre, 2008). Ultimately, firocoxib is dealkylated and conjugated in the liver to inactive metabolites that are eliminated by urinary excretion (Kvaternick, 2007).

Following oral daily administration recommended dose, steady state plasma concentration is achieved by the seventh dose (Letendre, 2008). The mean plasma concentration of firocoxib at steady state concentration is 104 ng/ml, well above the concentration needed to inhibit 80% of COX2 activity (i.e., 67 ng/ml). The time to reach maximum plasma concentration after the first dose is considerably longer (approximately four hours) when compared to the seventh day of dosing, in which the maximal plasma concentration is reached within approximately 45 minutes (Letendre, 2008).

Although the plasma concentration of firocoxib following a single oral dose is only approximately half of that achieved at steady state, it is above the concentration needed to inhibit 50% of COX2 activity (i.e., 30 ng/ml). It has been shown that a single loading dose of 0.3 mg/kg body weight PO will achieve a maximum plasma concentration of 199 ng/ml, thus enabling achievement of a steady state plasma concentration (Cox, 2012). The approved canine chewable preparation given orally to horses, at the same dose as recommended for the approved equine paste formulation, achieves equivalent plasma concentrations of firocoxib, with equivalent pharmacodynamic properties (Barton, 2014). Although there are numerous reports of clinical use of the canine product in horses, such use is extra-label in the United States and, therefore, constitutes illegal activity, regulated by the Food and Drug Administration (Barton, 2014).

Several clinical trials investigating the use of the approved firocoxib paste formulation in horses with naturally occurring lameness due to osteoarthritis and navicular syndrome have shown significant improvement in lameness scores (Doucet, 2008; Back, 2009; Koene, 2010; Orsini, 2012). Compared to phenylbutazone (4.4 mg/kg body weight PO SID) given for 14 days to client-owned horses with naturally occurring osteoarthritis, the recommended dose of oral firocoxib was more effective in reducing pain scores on manipulation of the joint, joint circumference score, and improving range of motion, but was equally as effective as phenylbutazone, with improvement in overall lameness score and joint swelling score (Doucet, 2008). Likewise, 83% of firocoxib paste-treated horses with naturally occurring lameness improved clinically, compared to 65% of vedaprofen paste-treated horses (Koene, 2010).

In an experimentally induced low flow ischemia that results in up-regulation of COX2 gene expression in the jejunum of horses, the use of non-selective COX inhibitors, such as flunixin meglumine, delays recovery of intestinal barrier function after induction of the ischemic injury (Tomlinson, 2005; Little, 2007; Cook, 2009a). In that model, it has been shown that firocoxib was equally as effective as flunixin meglumine in providing postoperative analgesia, although firocoxib treatment did not delay mucosal recovery. This work suggests that treatment with firocoxib may be advantageous over non-selective COX inhibitors in horses recovering from ischemic intestinal injury (Cook, 2009a).

Finally, orally administered firocoxib paste penetrates the aqueous humor better than oral flunixin meglumine at label dosages, in the absence of ocular disease, suggesting that firocoxib should be considered for treatment of inflammatory ocular lesions in horses at risk of adverse effects from repeated administration of non-selective COX inhibitors (Hilton, 2011). The ability of firocoxib to provide an acceptable level of analgesia in horses with naturally occurring ocular disease remains to be proven.

Firocoxib appears to be well tolerated at the recommended dose given for 14 days (Doucet, 2008), as well as up to 42 days (Kunkle, 2010). Compared with the non-selective COX inhibitor phenylbutazone, gastric ulceration and tubulointerstitial nephropathy are significantly less likely to occur with firocoxib (Kunkle, 2010; Yamaga, 2012).

23.2.3.2 Meloxicam

Meloxicam is an enolic acid NSAID of the oxicam group that is structurally similar to piroxicam. As a strong COX2 selective inhibitor in other species, meloxicam became one of the first purported and proved COX2 selective inhibitors in the horse (Moses, 2001). *In vitro* studies in horses have shown that COX2 selectivity of meloxicam is 5–12 times that of flunixin meglumine or phenylbutazone (Beretta, 2005; Burns, 2010).

Meloxicam appears to be well tolerated in adult horses (Vander Werf, 2012). When given at the daily recommended dose (0.6 mg/kg body weight IV or PO SID) for up to 42 days, there were no significant changes in clinical signs, hematology, or serum biochemical parameters (D'Arcy-Moskwa, 2012; Noble, 2012). The plasma clearance of meloxicam in horses is at least twice as rapid as values reported for other species in which once-daily dosing of meloxicam is recommended (Sinclair, 2006). However, *in vivo* pharmacodynamic studies in horses support the concept that, despite its rapid plasma elimination, once-daily dosing should be sufficient (Lees, 1991; Toutain, 2004b).

Compared to horses, the plasma clearance of meloxican in foals and donkeys is more rapid, suggesting the need of more frequent administration of the drug (Sinclair, 2006). In foals less than six weeks old, meloxicam was evaluated at 0.6 mg/kg PO BID for up to 21 days without accumulation of the drug in the plasma (Raidal, 2013). Currently, it is impractical to use meloxicam in donkeys, without further evaluation of the dose and dosing interval in that species (Sinclair, 2006).

The oral formulation of meloxicam currently marketed for use in horses outside the United States is a suspension with excellent bioavailability that does not appear to be affected by feeding (Toutain, 2004a). A recent study in healthy adult horses evaluated the use of oral meloxicam tablets at 0.6 mg/kg body weight SID for 14 days. The tablets were crushed and mixed in molasses, and given within one hour of feeding. There was no significant difference between the maximum plasma concentration of the drug over the 14-day period, indicating lack of drug accumulation in the plasma (Vander Werf, 2012).

In vivo trials with meloxicam in horses have demonstrated positive effects of therapy. In a lipopolysaccharide-induced model of synovitis in horses, oral treatment with meloxicam at the recommended dose significantly reduced synovial fluid PGE_2, substance P, bradykinin, matrix metalloproteinase, glycosaminoglycans, and collagen fragment concentrations. Furthermore, clinical lameness scores were significantly improved, compared with placebo-treated horses (de Grauw, 2009).

When meloxicam was compared to flunixin meglumine in an experimentally induced model of acute strangulation of the small intestine, both drugs performed equally well in post-operative clinical parameters. However, compared to flunixin meglumine, intravenous meloxicam administration did not impede recovery of the ischemia-injured jejunum. The authors suggest that the COX2 selectivity of meloxicam allows for sufficient COX1 activity for prostaglandin mediated recovery of intestinal barrier function, while its COX2-sparing effects effectively mitigate the detrimental effects of induced prosta-glandins on clinical signs and intestinal repair (Little, 2007).

23.2.3.3 Deracoxib

Deracoxib is a diaryl-substituted pyrazole that is structurally related to celecoxib. In the United States, it is currently approved only for dogs as an oral preparation, so information is lacking on its clinical use in the horse. However, *ex vivo* pharmacodynamics studies in the horse confirm its preferen-tial COX2 selectivity, which appears to be approximately twice what is reported in dogs, and more than what is reported for meloxicam, but approximately ten times less than what is reported for firocoxib in horses (Davis, 2011). *In vitro*, dera-coxib appears to have the same beneficial effect on intestinal epithelial recovery following ischemic damage, as is reported for meloxacim and firocoxib (Tomlinson, 2005). Given orally at 2 mg/kg body weight, deracoxib was well absorbed in the horse, with a longer plasma half-life than that reported for small animals. In horses, sufficient plasma concentrations of the drug to sustain COX2 selectivity were maintained for 24 hours, suggesting that once-daily dosing might be sufficient for clinical use (Davis, 2011). There is no available safety data for horses at present.

23.2.3.4 Etodolac

Etodolac, an indole acetic acid derivative, is a chiral molecule that is approved for use in dogs as a racemic mixture. *In vitro*, the COX2 selectivity of etodolac in horses appears to be approximately equivalent to meloxicam (Beretta, 2005; Davis, 2007). The bioavailability following oral administration in horses is good (Davis, 2007). Clinical relevance and safety information on etodolac is sparse in horses. In a lipo-polysaccharide-induced model of synovitis, etodolac was as effective as phenylbutazone in reducing lameness, synovial fluid white blood cell counts, and PGE$_2$ concentrations. However, thromboxane B$_2$ concentrations were not reduced to the same degree as with phenylbutazone, demonstrating etodolac's COX2 selectivity (Morton, 2005).

In a clinical trial, enrolling 22 lame horses with chronic navicular syndrome, etodolac, at 23 mg/kg body weight PO SID for three days, was an effective analgesic (Symonds, 2006). Etodolac treatment in horses does not appear to have the same beneficial effects that meloxicam, deracoxib, and firocoxib have on recovery of intestinal barrier function in jejunal mucosa after ischemic damage (Tomlinson, 2004).

23.2.4 Topical non-steroidal anti-inflammatory drugs

23.2.4.1 Diclofenac

Diclofenac sodium is a phenylacetic acid derivative that pur-portedly inhibits both cyclooxygenase and lipoxygenase, although the later claim has not been substantiated in the horse. Diclofenate is available in oral, intravenous, as well as topical formulations for humans. However, when diclofenate was given orally to ponies, significant leukopenia and prolongation of prothrombin and activated partial thromboplastin times occurred (Azevedo, 2013). In contrast, in the same study, when a 7% sodium diclofenac ointment was applied topically over the tarsus, synovial fluid concentrations of the drug were greater than that achieved following oral administration, with-out development of hematologic abnormalities or coagulopathy. Thus, diclofenate is currently only available for topical use in the horse.

Experimental trials in horses have yielded mixed results on the efficacy of topical diclofenate as an anti-inflammatory agent (Caldwell, 2004; Villarino, 2006; Frisbie, 2007; Schleining, 2008). The conflicting reports may be due in part to differences in the models used to evoke inflammation, or due to differences in the diclofenate preparation, as it has been shown that absorption of topical diclofenate varies considerably, depending on the for-mulation (Andreeta, 2011).

Liposomal-based preparations appear to afford superior bio-availability, which is the formulation used in the currently approved product for horses. Use of the liposome cream prod-uct, in a model of arthroscopically induced carpal arthritis in horses, resulted in improvement of lameness, bone sclerosis, cartilage erosion, and total articular glycosaminoglycan content (Frisbie, 2007). Likewise, use of the liposomal formulation in a subcutaneous carrageenan injection model of inflammation in the horse significantly reduced local transudate concentrations of PGE$_2$ (Caldwell, 2004).

In contrast, in an amphotericin-induced carpal arthritis model, liposome-based topical diclofenac did not improve clinical lameness or biochemical markers of inflammation in synovial fluid (Schleining, 2008). Ultimately, there is only one report on the use of the liposomal diclofenate cream in a clinical setting (Lynn, 2004). In a blinded and placebo-controlled study involving 116 horses, use of the topical formulation twice daily for five days reduced lameness, as graded independently by both owners and veterinarians, regardless of the severity or chronicity of the clinical condition (Lynn, 2004).

23.2.4.2 Topical ophthalmic preparations

In the United States, there are two NSAID preparations that are available as approved ophthalmic solutions. One product con-tains 0.03% flurbiprofen, while the other contains 0.1% diclofen-ate; however, neither has a veterinary label. There are no experimental or clinical trials substantiating the use of either product in horses, although both preparations are widely used topically to control pain and inflammation in horses with various ocular diseases, such as keratitis and uveitis (Gilger, 2011).

23.2.5 Antihistamines

Histamine is a biogenic amine that is predominately located in mast cell and basophil granules, but is also located in platelets, enterochromaffin cells, and neurons. Histamine exerts its biological actions through four different G protein-coupled receptors, of which H1, H2, and H4 receptors are primarily responsible for immune mediated hypersensitivity reactions (Peters, 2009).

H1 receptors are located on smooth muscle cells, endothelium, and in neurons in the central nervous system. Occupation of the H1 receptor by histamine results in bronchoconstriction, vasodilation, increased vascular permeability, pruritis, pain, and inflammation. H2 receptors are located on the gastric parietal cells, vascular smooth muscle cells, basophils, neutrophils, and cardiac myocytes (Peters, 2009). H3 receptors are primarily located in the central nervous system, where they are involved in neurotransmission. The H4 receptors are located on mast cells, eosinophils, basophils, and T cells, and are involved in chemotaxis, and in cytokine and chemokine synthesis (Peters, 2009).

First generation antihistamines are H1 receptor antagonists that expert their action by competitive inhibition of H1 receptors; thus, they are most effective when given prior to the release of histamine (Peters, 2009). Because of the side-effect of sedation, the use of first generation antihistamines is banned in many equestrian sports, and is monitored by drug testing.

Second generation antihistamines are less likely to cross the blood brain barrier, limiting the adverse side effect of sedation. In horses, antihistamines are most commonly used for allergic mediated skin disease (Table 23.2). However, pharmacokinetic and pharmacodynamic information is sparse, and they have highly unpredictable clinical efficacy. Antihistamines offer limited value in treating anaphylactic shock in the horse (Eyre, 1982).

23.2.5.1 Hydroxyzine

Hydroxyzine is a first generation (H1 receptor antagonist) antihistamine, and is one of the antihistamines more commonly reported to be beneficial for the control of chronic urticaria in horses (Scott, 2011). Because antihistamines do not alter the release of histamine, their effect is not immediate. It has been suggested to withdraw hydroxyzine at least seven days prior to intradermal skin testing in horses (Petersen, 2009). There is no veterinary labeled product, though several generic human products are available.

23.2.5.2 Chlorpheniramine

Chlorpheniramine maleate is an alkylamine first generation antihistamine H1 receptor antagonist. It is a carbon chiral molecule, of which the S enantiomer (d-chlorpheniramine) is the more potent isoform, and there is only one published study on the pharmacokinetics and pharmacodynamics of chlorpheniramine in horses (Kuroda, 2013). When chlorpheniramine was given to horses intragastrically at 0.5 mg/kg body weight, the bioavailability was low at 38%. Histamine-induced intradermal wheal formation was reduced by 38% and 61%, thirty minutes after an intravenous dose of 0.1 mg/kg body weight and 0.5 mg/kg body weight, respectively. Maximal inhibition of histamine induced wheal formation was 39%, and occurred two hours after intragastric administration; it was less than 10% by 23 hours. Sedation was not reported following either intragastric or intravenous dosing.

Table 23.2 Antihistamines.

Drug	Class	Dose	Brand name
Hydroxyzine	First generation H1 receptor antagonist.	1–2 mg/kg PO TID to BID.	No approved veterinary preparation. (Scott, 2011)
Chlorpheniramine	First generation H1 receptor antagonist.	0.25–0.5 mg/kg PO BID.	No approved veterinary preparation. (Scott, 2011)
Diphenhydramine	First generation H1 receptor antagonist	1–2 mg/kg PO BID 0.67 to 1.5 mg/kg slow IV	No approved veterinary preparation for systemic use. Common human brand name Benadryl, Johnson and Johnson, New Brunswick, New Jersey. (Baird, 2006; Scott, 2011)
Pyrilamine	First generation H1 receptor antagonist.	Follow package insert recommendations. 0.52–0.66 mg/kg IV or PO.	Approved for use in horses as sole active ingredient or combined with pseudoephedrine or guaifenesin. (Dirikolu, 2009)
Doxepin	Tricyclic antidepressant.	0.5–0.75 mg/kg PO BID. 300–600 mg/500 kg BID.	No approved veterinary preparation. (White, 2005; Scott, 2011)
Cetirizine	Second generation H1 receptor antagonist.	0.2–0.4 mg/kg PO BID.	No approved veterinary preparation. Common human brand name is Zyrtec, Pfizer Labs, New York. (Olsen, 2008)

PO – *per os* or orally; IV – intravenously; SID – *semel in die* or once a day; BID – *bis in die* or twice a day; TID – *ter in die* or three times a day.

A pharmacokinetic/pharmacodynamic link model showed that chlorpheniramine in horses has lower efficacy, much lower potency, and slightly lower sensitivity, than other reported antihistamines (Kuroda, 2013). This may be due, in part, to the rapid disposition and rapid total clearance rate of the drug in horses. Thus, chlorpheniramine would need to be given intravenously at four-hour intervals, or larger doses given orally (1.3 mg/kg body weight) to be significantly beneficial to horses (Kuroda, 2013).

23.2.5.3 Diphenhydramine
Diphenhydramine is an ethanolamine derivative first generation antihistamine. Anecdotally, it is not clinically very effective in horses for the treatment of immune-mediated dermatopathies (Scott, 2011). It has been successful in some horses, for controlling or reversing idiosyncratic extrapyramidal excitation induced by fluphenazine (Baird, 2006). Diphenhydramine may cause paradoxical excitation when given rapidly intravenously.

23.2.5.4 Pyrilamine
Pyrilamine maleate is an ethylenediamine first generation antihistamine and is the only antihistamine with label approval for use in horses in the United States. It is available in an approved formulation, in combination with either pseudoephedrine or guaifenesin (Table 23.2). Pharmacokinetic studies in horses show that pyrilamine is poorly bioavailable orally (18%), and it can be detected by sensitive enzyme-linked immunosorbent assay tests in urine for up to one week after a single dose (Dirikolu, 2009b). There are no clinical trials on its efficacy in horses, though some authors report limited benefit in allergic-mediated skin diseases (Scott, 2011).

23.2.5.5 Doxepin
Doxepin is a dibenzoxazepine derivative tricyclic antidepressant with antihistamine, anticholinergic, and alpha-adrenergic blocking effects. Dopexin is a 5:1 mixture of trans and cis isomers. In veterinary medicine, it is used primarily as a sedative in psychogenic dermatoses. There is no approved veterinary preparation. There are no clinical studies in horses, other than information on the detection of both isomers in serum for up to 24 hours after a dose of 1 mg/kg body weight intravenously (Hagedorn, 2002). There are anecdotal reports of efficacy in some immune-mediated dermatoses in horses (Scott, 2011).

23.2.5.6 Cetirizine
Cetirizine dihydrochloride, a metabolite of hydroxyzine, is a non-sedative racemic second generation histamine H1 antagonist. It has also been shown to decrease eosinophil influx and down-regulate cytokine induction of NF-kappa B (Scott, 2011). In horses, cetirizine (0.2 mg/kg body weight PO BID, for three consecutive doses) was rapidly absorbed, and inhibited histamine induced wheal formation by approximately 45% (Olsen, 2008). With four additional administrations of the drug at 0.4 mg/kg body weight PO BID, wheal formation was inhibited

by 68%. It was possible to detect cetirizine in the plasma for 30 hours after the last dose was given. No adverse side-effects were reported. Pre-treatment of horses with ivermectin (0.2 mg/kg body weight), given orally 1.5 hour before cetirizine, did not affect its pharmacokinetics. However, ivermectin pre-treatment 12 hour before cetirizine increased the area under the plasma concentration time curve by 60%, which may be due to decreased renal secretion related to inhibition of P-glycoprotein in the proximal tubular cells of the kidney (Olsen, 2007).

There are two clinical studies on cetirizine in horses. In a randomized, placebo-controlled and double-blinded field study conducted in horses with insect bite hypersensitivity, cetirizine was given at 0.4 mg/kg body weight PO BID for three weeks. There was no difference in reduction in dermatitis between the treatment and placebo groups (Olsen, 2011). However, for eosinophilic keratitis, horses treated with cetirizine orally were less likely to have recurrence during the follow-up period (1 out of 13 horses, or 8%), relative to horses that were not treated (8 of 14 horses, or 57%) (Lassaline-Utter, 2014).

23.2.6 Miscellaneous anti-inflammatory agents
23.2.6.1 Dimethyl sulfoxide
Dimethyl sulfoxide (DMSO) is a by-product of the wood and paper industry, and has been widely used for its solvent properties. Since the 1960s, a myriad of potential medical uses have been proposed. The available electron pairs between the sulfur and oxygen terminals make the molecule dipolar, and a strong hygroscopic solvent, hydrogen bond acceptor, and free radical scavenger (Brayton, 1986). Other unique properties of DMSO include its rapid and nearly complete ability to penetrate skin, mucous and cell membranes, its ability to facilitate penetration of other substances across membranes, and its ability to inhibit or stimulate enzymes (Brayton, 1986). DMSO is also bacteriostatic or bacteriocidal, analgesic, and antithrombotic (Brayton, 1986).

However, despite decades of research on a seemingly endless list of inflammatory ailments, 5% DMSO is currently only approved for topical instillation in people with interstitial cystitis. Similarly, in horses, despite countless anecdotal proclamations for its use in topical, intravenous, intra-articular, and intrauterine applications, convincing clinical evidence of anti-inflammatory properties are sparse. The only current label approval for use of DMSO in horses is topically, to treat acute swelling due to trauma. Clinically, it is commonly used on the skin for several ailments, such as trauma, edema, cellulitis, insect bites, thrombophlebitis, and arthritis. It is also topically used on the cornea, and for intrauterine infusion. Hypothetically, its anti-inflammatory properties stem from its ability to scavenge free radicals, which are highly reactive and destructive by-products of inflammation. Dermal heat and vasodilation are generated by the strong exothermic reaction of DMSO with water, coupled with DMSO-induced histamine release (Brayton, 1986).

DMSO has been used topically in the equine eye, mostly as a carrier to facilitate corneal penetration of antifungal drugs. DMSO has minimal toxic effects on cellular morphology and proliferation of primary cultures of equine keratocytes (Mathes, 2010). Topical treatment of healthy horses with a 1% itraconazole/30% DMSO ointment QID for 28 treatments was well tolerated, and no gross or histopathological abnormalities of the cornea developed during the trial. Corneal tissue concentration of itraconazole was seven-fold higher in eyes treated with 1% itraconazole/30% DMSO ointment, compared with those treated with the 1% itraconazole ointment (Ball, 1997).

There are conflicting reports on the effects of intrauterine application of DMSO in mares, from no harmful histologic changes following instillation of up to a 30% DMSO solution (Ley, 1989), to dose-dependent epithelial ulceration and stromal inflammation (Frazer, 1988). Intrauterine DMSO did not improve pregnancy rates in barren mares (Ley, 1989).

There is one study in horses that evaluated the effect of topical 90% DMSO gel in an endotoxin-induced model of carpal synovitis. The gel was applied every 12 hours for 2.5 days, and resulted in lower synovial fluid total white blood cell counts when compared with untreated joints (Smith, 1998). Experimental data on intra-articular lavage or injection of DMSO are conflicting (Schleining, 2007a, 2007b). There is some evidence that intra-articular DMSO reduces synovial fluid superoxide production (Auer, 1990), synovial leukocyte counts, and histopathologic evidence of synovitis (Welch, 1991). However, adverse effects have also been reported. A 10% DMSO solution, applied to endotoxin-induced synovial membrane explants, reduced synovial cellularity and was associated with characteristics of synovial cell nuclear degeneration (Moses, 2001). Similarly, when evaluated *in vitro* using equine articular cartilage explants, DMSO in excess of 5% was found to have the detrimental effects of reducing proteoglycan synthesis, and suppressing articular cartilage matrix metabolism (Smith, 2000).

Although not approved for intravenous use in horses, clinically it has been commonly used for the treatment of reperfusion injury, endotoxemia, laminitis, acute neurological disorders and, basically, any acute systemic inflammatory disease. The pharmacokinetics of intravenous DMSO has been evaluated in horses, and showed a linear pattern. Twelve hours after the 1.0 gm/kg body weight and 0.1 gm/kg body weight doses were administered, 27% and 25% of the DMSO dose, respectively, was excreted unchanged into urine. Based on the half-life, DMSO should be administered BID (Blythe, 1986).

DMSO therapy appears to be well tolerated in horses at recommended dosages (Lin, 2004; Table 23.3). After repeated topical application, dermal hardening and desquamation have been reported (Brayton, 1986). The hydroscopic nature of DMSO necessitates dilution to at least 10% when given as an intravenous or oral solution, otherwise hemolysis will occur. The easily recognized and distinctive garlic-like smell that is rapidly emitted after topical or intravenous use is actually from its metabolite, dimethyl sulfide, which can be irritating and offensive to inhale (Brayton, 1986).

Teratogenic effects of DMSO are considered low at therapeutic levels, but it is not recommended to administer it during pregnancy (Brayton, 1986). One must be mindful of the efficient solvent properties of DMSO, and its ability to transfer other substances across the skin, mucous membranes, or cell membranes. These later properties may be beneficial to enhance drug absorption (e.g., by increasing oral bioavailability of ponazuril in horses) (Dirikolu, 2009c). However, its concurrent topical application with a mercuric blister was faulted as the cause of mercury toxicity in two horses (Schuh, 1988).

Other potential uses of DMSO's free radical scavenging properties are for the treatment of endotoxemia and reperfusion injury of the intestinal tract, following strangulation. In the solo experimental equine trial of induced endotoxemia, the benefit of DMSO treatment was limited to a modest reduction in fever

Table 23.3 Miscellaneous anti-inflammatory agents.

Drug	Mechanism of action	Dose	Notes
Dimethyl sulfoxide	Hygroscopic, free radical scavenger.	0.1 to 1 g/kg IV BID as a 10% solution.	Only approved for use topically in horses in the United States. (Blythe, 1986)
Pentoxifylline	Phosphodiesterase inhibitor.	10 mg/kg PO BID. up to 40 mg/kg PO SID for treatment of RAO. 8.5 mg/kg IV diluted in 1 liter saline BID to inhibit matrix metalloproteinase activity.	No approved veterinary formulation. Marketed under the trade name Trental™, Sofoni, France for human use. (Leguillette, 2002; Liska, 2006; Fugler, 2013)
Doxycycline	Inhibitor of matrix metalloproteinase.	5–10 mg/kg PO BID.	No approved sub-antimicrobial formulation for horses. (Watts, 2007; Fugler, 2013)
Omega-3 fatty Acids	Synthesis of anti-inflammatory 3 series prostanoids and 5 series leukotrienes.	Many.	Various supplements.
Lidocaine	Sodium channel blockade.	1.3 mg/kg IV slow bolus, followed by continuous infusion at 0.05 mg/kg/min.	(Malone, 2006; Mudge, 2007)

PO – *per os* or orally; IV – intravenously; SID – *semel in die* or once a day; BID – *bis in die* or twice a day.

(Kelmer, 2008). Several studies have investigated the use of intravenous DMSO in horses with experimentally-induced hemorrhagic strangulation obstruction, or ischemic strangulation of the small intestine or colon, with no demonstrable benefit of DMSO treatment when assessed by histology, immunohistochemistry, preservation of glutathione levels in the mucosa, or protection against free radical mediated damage (Arden, 1990; Reeves, 1990; Horne, 1994; Moore, 1995).

However, in a study that used 60 minutes of low flow jejunal ischemia, followed by 3.5 hours of reperfusion, DMSO at 20 mg/kg body weight IV QID reduced jejunal microvascular permeability, edema, and leukocyte infiltration when compared to horses treated with lactated Ringers solution (Dabareiner, 2005). The later dose of DMSO, given IV BID for ten days, was also shown to be effective at reducing the development of intestinal adhesions in weanlings with complete jejunal ischaemia followed by reperfusion (Sullins, 2004).

The proposed mechanisms for the potential beneficial effects of DMSO in acute central nervous system disorders, characterized by trauma, ischemia, edema, and inflammation, include its free radical scavenger, antithrombotic, and diuretic properties, and its ability to improve tissue perfusion and decrease intracranial pressure (Brayton, 1986; Morresey, 2006). Despite numerous trials in other species, conflicting reports of success have ended with no straightforward recommendation on its use for acute central nervous system disease (Brayton, 1986).

The same potential benefits of DMSO in central nervous system disease could apply to the treatment of laminitis. There are no well-controlled experimental or clinical trials on the use of DMSO for either acute central nervous system disease or laminitis in horses (Schleining, 2007a, 2007b). Nonetheless, DMSO is frequently given to horses with neurologic disease or laminitis, with anecdotal reports of success (Morresey, 2006; O'Grady, 2011).

23.2.6.2 Methylsulfonylmethane

Methylsulfonylmethane (MSM) is an organosulfur, $(CH_3)_2SO_2$, crystalline compound, related to DMSO, used as a dietary supplement. Review of randomized controlled trials on MSM in people provide positive, but not definitive, evidence that MSM is superior to placebo in the treatment of mild to moderate osteoarthritis (Brien, 2008). Although promoted as a beneficial nutriceutical for treatment of osteoarthritis, there are no approved medical uses for MSM in people. Likewise, MSM is available in numerous formulations as a dietary supplement for the treatment of osteoarthritis in horses. However, controlled experimental or clinical trials on its efficacy are lacking.

23.2.6.3 Pentoxifylline

Pentoxifylline is a synthetic derivative of theobromine originally marketed as a rheologic agent in people with chronic occlusive peripheral and cerebral arterial disease. Since its introduction almost 40 years ago, additional pharmacodynamic effects of pentoxifylline have been discovered. The hemorheologic

properties of pentoxifylline appear to be due to non-selective inhibition of membrane-bound phosphodiesterase, and by activation of protein kinase, thereby increasing intracellular cyclic adenosine monophosphate and decreasing intracellular calcium (Aviado, 1984; Sha, 2003). As a result, red blood cells are more flexible, and blood viscosity, platelet aggregation, fibrinogen concentrations, and thrombus formation are reduced. It was originally marketed in people for the treatment of intermittent claudication, resulting from obstructed arteries in the limbs and vascular dementia.

More recently, it has been discovered that pentoxifylline has anti-inflammatory properties, through its ability to inhibit TNF-alpha, interleukins, and interferon-gamma syntheses, inhibition of T cell and natural killer cell cytotoxicity and matrix metalloproteinase activity, and to reduce superoxide radical formation and granular release of enzymes by neutrophils (Weiss, 1992; Barton, 1994; Nagy, 1999; Gutierrez-Reyes, 2006; Fugler, 2013).

Along with its anti-inflammatory properties, inhibition of phosphodiesterase also induces bronchodilation, and may serve a role in the treatment of chronic inflammatory bronchoconstrictive diseases (Leguillette, 2002). Lastly, pentoxifylline has been shown to be a potent inhibitor of connective tissue and fibroblast growth factor, with the potential to deter the development of fibrosis in such diseases as alcoholic and non-alcoholic steatohepatitis, tubulointerstitial nephritis, Peyronie's disease, and radiation induced fibrosis (Goicoechea, 2012; Hamama, 2012; Larsen, 2012; Parker, 2013).

A recent pharmacokinetic study in horses suggest that at least 10 mg/kg body weight PO BID are needed to achieve therapeutic concentrations of pentoxifylline and its active 5-hydroxyhexyl metabolite (Liska, 2006; Table 23.3). Serum concentrations of pentoxifylline appear to decrease with repeated oral dosing; thus, it may be necessary to increase the dosage if clinical response diminishes with repeated administration (Liska, 2006).

In the last two decades, the attractive pharmacodynamic properties of pentoxifylline have prompted its study in equine patients in *in vitro*, *ex vivo* and *in vivo* experimental models of blood flow, blood viscosity, endotoxemia, neutrophil and platelet function, placentitis, and recurrent airway obstruction. Collectively, the *in vitro* equine studies demonstrated that pentoxifylline reduced endotoxin induced cytokine and thromboxane B_2 production in whole blood and macrophage cell line models (Milam, 1992; Barton, 1994), shortened onset time of collagen-induced platelet aggregation (Kornreich, 2010), suppressed neutrophil superoxide production (Weiss, 1992), and induced vasodilation of phenylephrine pre-contracted equine digital veins isolated from healthy horses (Kabbesh, 2010).

An *ex vivo* equine study showed that administration at 8.5 mg/kg body weight PO BID for 28 days resulted in increased red blood cell filterability, erythrocyte sedimentation rate, and decreased epinephrine induced changes in blood viscosity (Geor, 1992). Another *ex vivo* study in horses, using pentoxifylline at 7.5 mg/kg body weight IV bolus, followed by a continuous rate infusion of 1.5 mg/kg/hour, demonstrated significantly increased plasma 6-ketoprostaglandin F-1alpha concentrations and suppressed *ex vivo* endotoxin induced TNF activity in whole blood (Barton, 1997).

In equine endotoxin-challenge *in vivo* models, intravenous pentoxifylline produced some minimal benefits, including fever reduction and prolongation of whole blood recalcification time (Barton, 1997), but significant reduction of plasma matrix metalloproteinase 2 and 9 activities (Fugler, 2013). In an *in vivo* model of equine recurrent airway obstruction, pentoxifylline, at 30–40 mg/kg body weight PO BID for 14 days, significantly improved respiratory function determined by elastance and resistance values (Leguillette, 2002). Mares with experimentally-induced placentitis delivered more live foals when treated with a combination of oral pentoxifylline, trimethoprim sulfmethoxazole, and altrenogest when compared to untreated mares (Bailey, 2007).

In racing Thoroughbreds with naturally occurring exercise-induced pulmonary hemorrhage, oral pentoxifylline treatment, at 8.5 mg/kg body weight PO BID for seven days, significantly reduced the incidence and severity of pulmonary hemorrhage, compared with untreated cohorts (Semeco, 2006). Although pentoxifylline has been shown to be beneficial in human clinical trials of hepatic or renal disease (Goicoechea, 2012; Parker, 2013), there have been no controlled studies for hepatic or renal disease in horses. There is a report of positive outcomes in three yearlings with naturally acquired leptospirosis-induced acute renal failure, in which pentoxifylline was part of the therapy (Frellstedt, 2009).

23.2.6.4 Tetracyclines

In the 1980s, it was discovered that sub-antimicrobial doses of tetracycline inhibited matrix metalloproteinases (MMP), which are capable of destroying extracellular matrix proteins and several other biological molecules (Gu, 2012). Tetracyclines have also been shown to inhibit cytokine synthesis (Cazalis, 2008) and induce apotosis (Sagar, 2010). Sub-antimicrobial formulations of tetracycline approved for use in people have been used as adjunct therapy for the treatment of several diseases, including acne, rosacea, pemphigoid, rheumatoid arthritis, postmenopausal osteopenia, type II diabetes, cardiovascular diseases and lymphangioleiomyomatosis (Gu, 2012).

Although used clinically, there is sparse information on the use of tetracycline antimicrobials as anti-inflammatory agents in horses. In an *in vitro* study, chemically modified tetracyclines inhibited collagenase and gelatinase activity of tracheal epithelial lining fluid from horses with recurrent airway obstruction (Raulo, 2006). Similarly, 0.1% doxycycline, added to tear films obtained from horses with active ulcerative keratitis, inhibited 96% of total MMP2 and MMP9 activity (Ollivier, 2003).

In a recent *in vivo* experimentally induced model of endotoxemia in horses, pre-treatment with oxytetracycline (20 mg/kg body weight IV BID) was effective in inhibiting plasma MMP2 and MMP9 activity. In the same study, pre-treatment with doxycycline (10 mg/kg body weight intragastrically) was more effective in inhibiting plasma MMP2, compared with MMP9 (Fugler, 2013; Table 23.3). A sub-antimicrobial dose of doxycycline (5 mg/kg body weight intragastrically BID) achieved synovial fluid concentrations in healthy horses that should be sufficient to inhibit MMP3 and MMP13, with potential beneficial adjunct therapy for the treatment of osteoarthritis (Watts, 2007).

23.2.6.5 Omega-3 fatty acids

Alpha linolenic acid and linoleic acid are both essential fatty acids, and requirements can only be met by ingestion, because the mammalian host cannot synthesize these fatty acids. Alpha linolenic acid, the parent molecule of the omega-3 fatty acid family, is designated as such because the first carbon-to-carbon double bond occurs at the third carbon from the methyl (i.e., omega) end of the molecule (Logas, 1991). In contrast, linoleic acid is the parent molecule of the omega-6 fatty acid family, classified as such because the first carbon-to-carbon double bond is located at the sixth carbon from the omega end. Once ingested, small amounts of alpha linolenic acid are metabolized to eicosapentaenoic acid (EPA) and docosahexaenoic acid (DHA), both of which are found in abundant quantities in fish oil.

Omega-3 fatty acids are considered important natural anti-inflammatory molecules. As a 20-carbon fatty acid with five carbon-to-carbon double bonds, EPA essentially is the equivalent to arachidonic acid, a member of the omega-6 fatty acid family with 20 carbons and four carbon-to-carbon double bonds. Both EPA and arachidonic acid are metabolized in the same metabolic pathway, culminating in the formation of the prostanoids and leukotrienes (Figure 23.1). However, the fundamental difference is that when COX, lipoxygenase, and further downstream enzymes metabolize EPA, the products have different biological actions than do the metabolites of arachidonic acid. For example, thromboxane A_2, the 2 series metabolite of arachodonic acid, is vasoconstrictive and promotes platelet aggregation, whereas thromboxane A_3, the 3 series metabolite of EPA promotes vasodilation and inhibits platelet aggregation (Logas, 1991). The 4 series leukotriene metabolites of arachidonic acid are potent chemoattractants, where as the 5 series leukotriene metabolites of EPA are not.

As a member of the omega-6 fatty acid family, linoleic acid is metabolized to dihomo gamma linoleic acid, which can serve as a competitive inhibitor of arachidonic acid. However, dihomo gamma linolenic acid can also be further metabolized to arachidonic acid, serving then as a substrate for the formation of eicosanoids. Ultimately, the collective effect of ingesting a diet rich in alpha linolenic acid, EPA, or DHA, is that of an anti-inflammatory environment.

Despite some evidence of their ability to alter the inflammatory response, it is clear that dietary supplementation with omega-3 fatty acids does not provide an immediate benefit, often requiring several weeks of supplementation to evoke changes in the membrane fatty acid profile. To investigate whether changes in lipid composition could be more readily achieved, lipid emulsions enriched with 20% omega-3 or omega-6 fatty acids were infused in healthy horses. Monocyte fatty acid analysis demonstrated incorporation of the parenteral omega-3 and omega-6 fatty acids in monocyte phospholipids immediately after infusion, with changes in the fatty acid composition persisting for up to seven days after infusion. *Ex vivo* production of the inflammatory mediators thromboxane B_2 and tumor necrosis factor by peripheral blood monocytes was diminished by the omega-3 lipid infusion, and was unchanged or increased by omega-6 lipid infusion (McCann, 2000). Thus, use of omega-3 enriched fatty acid emulsions could be beneficial in the treatment of acute inflammatory conditions.

There have been several dietary trials involving omega-3 fatty acids in horses (Henry, 1990; Craig, 1997; Hansen, 2002; Hall, 2004; Khol-Parisini, 2007; O'Connor, 2007; Woodward, 2007; King, 2008; Vineyard, 2010; Hess, 2012). The ability to incorporate dietary omega-3 fatty acids into cell membranes, with subsequent demonstration of modification of the inflammatory response, has been highly variable in horses. These vast differences probably stem from the fact that the source, dose, and duration of use of omega-3 fatty acid supplementation vary considerably from study to study. Flaxseed and linseed oil are affordable and palatable sources of alpha linolenic acid for use in horses, but only small amounts of alpha linolenic acid are metabolized to EPA. In contrast, fish oil is an excellent source of EPA and DHA, but it is more expensive and less palatable to horses, unless the fish oil can be deodorized.

Nonetheless, most studies can demonstrate that omega-3 fatty acid supplementation in horses does, indeed, result in the increased presence of omega-3 fatty acids, or an increase in the omega-3 to omega-6 ratio in plasma or cell membrane fatty acid composition (Henry, 1990; Craig, 1997; Hansen, 2002; Hall, 2004; Khol-Parisini, 2007; Woodward, 2007; King, 2008; Vineyard, 2010; Hess, 2012). Although there have been limited side-by-side comparisons, supplementation with fish oils or sources rich in EPA or DHA may appear to be more successful in significantly altering the omega-3 fatty acid composition of equine cells, compared with other sources of omega-3 fatty acids (O'Connor, 2007; Vineyard, 2010).

The anti-inflammatory effects of omega-3 fatty acid supplementation have also been studied in horses, with demonstration of variable success. This variation is likely associated both with the degree of change in the cell membrane fatty acid profile, and with differences in the models used to test the biological consequences of such alterations. Neither dietary fish oil nor flaxseed supplementation affected *ex vivo* lymphocyte proliferation or endotoxin-induced PGE_2 production in peripheral blood mononuclear cells (Vineyard, 2010). In fact, both omega-3 fatty acid supplements were associated with a more pronounced skin reaction following intradermal injection of phytohemagglutinin, compared with control horses receiving no supplement (Vineyard, 2010).

In another study, flaxseed oil supplementation failed to alter platelet aggregation (Hansen, 2002). In yet another study, involving horses with recurrent airway obstruction, after a ten-week period of dietary supplementation with sunflower oil, rich in linoleic acid or seal blubber oil and source of long chain omega-3 polyunsaturated fatty acids, pulmonary function testing results and clinical signs were not markedly changed (Khol-Parisini, 2007).

Other dietary omega-3 fatty acid trials in horses have shown positive anti-inflammatory effects. After eight weeks, procoagulant activity and thromboxane B_2 production by endotoxin-stimulated monocytes from horses consuming an 8% linseed oil ration decreased by 51% and 71%, respectively, compared with cells obtained from horses consuming the control ration (Henry, 1990). Likewise, endotoxin-induced macrophage production of TNF was significantly less after horses were fed a linseed oil-rich ration (Morris, 1991). In those same horses, anticoagulative properties of the diet were demonstrated by longer mean whole blood recalcification, and activated partial thromboplastin times, before and during endotoxin infusion (Henry, 1991).

In another study involving fish oil supplementation in horses, the leukotrienes B_5 to B_4 ratio from neutrophils stimulated *ex vivo* was four-fold greater (Hall, 2004), and production of the PGE_2 by endotoxin-stimulated bronchoalveolar lavage cells *ex vivo* was significantly reduced, compared with horses receiving the corn oil control diet (Hall, 2004).

Omega-3 fatty acids have been suggested for the management of immune mediated dermatitis with anecdotal reports of success (Scott, 2011). Two clinical studies have evaluated the effect of omega-3 fatty acids in horses with pruritis. Neither study conclusively demonstrated a significant difference in clinical status (Craig, 1997; Friberg, 1999) although, in one of the studies, owners blinded to treatment concluded that horses improved more when supplemented with linseed oil (Friberg, 1999).

Omega-3 fatty acids are also suggested for the management of osteoarthritis, and are often included in joint health supplements, and two clinical studies in horses provide some supportive evidence for use in osteoarthritis. Compared with a corn oil diet, a diet containing stabilized omega-3 fatty acids tended to improve trot stride in horses with lameness (Woodward, 2007). In another study of horses with naturally occurring arthritis, horses treated with EPA at 15 gm/day and DHA at 19.8 gm/day for 90 days had a greater decrease in synovial fluid white blood cell concentration and plasma prostaglandin E_2 concentrations, compared with control horses. There was no difference in lameness when evaluated by force plate method (Manhart, 2009).

23.2.6.6 Lidocaine

Lidocaine is a well-known local anesthetic agent and class IB anti-arrhythmic, which acts by binding to voltage-gated sodium channels, thereby inhibiting the action potential. In the last two decades, popularization of the use of continuous rate infusions of lidocaine for the treatment of postoperative ileus in people and then horses (Malone, 2006) prompted investigations into its prokinetic mechanism of action. Despite these efforts, the prokinetic mechanism of lidocaine remains unclear, and is likely multifaceted. Proposed mechanisms include: decreased sympathetic tone; inhibition of aberrant motility patterns; inhibition of neurohormonal influence; analgesia; and anti-inflammatory effects (Mudge, 2007; Cook, 2008).

Lidocaine is rapidly cleared from the plasma, redistributed, and metabolized in the liver to active metabolites, thus continuous infusion is necessary to maintain therapeutic plasma concentrations between 1–2 mcg/kg body weight (Mudge, 2007). The most commonly reported dose of lidocaine for intravenous use in horses is 1.3 mg/kg body weight IV bolus, given over 5–10 minutes, followed by continuous rate infusion at 0.05 mg/kg/minute (Malone, 2006; Mudge, 2007; Cook, 2009b; Peiró, 2010; Table 23.3). The onset of action is within minutes, although steady state therapeutic levels may not be achieved for approximately an hour after start of the infusion.

Lidocaine and its active metabolites may progressively accumulate in plasma over the course of several days of infusion, and thus infusion doses may need to be adjusted (de Solis, 2007). Signs of lidocaine toxicity include depression, behavioral changes, ataxia, muscular fasciculations, hypotension, bradycardia, seizure, and collapse. Fortunately, these adverse signs typically wane within minutes of discontinuation of the infusion (Mudge, 2007).

The elucidation that lidocaine has anti-inflammatory effects prompted further studies, demonstrating that local or intravenous lidocaine can reduce eicosonaoid and cytokine production and histamine release (Yregard, 2003; Mudge, 2007; Cook, 2008). Furthermore, it has been demonstrated that lidocaine inhibits neutrophil adhesion, migration and accumulation, phagocytic activity, and free radical production. It reduces vascular permeability, lipid peroxidation in membranes, the size of infarcts, and edema (Mudge, 2007; Cook, 2008; Yregard, 2003). By blocking the increase in intracellular sodium that occurs with ischemic inflammation, key pro-inflammatory enzyme activity and apotosis are reduced (Cook, 2008).

To date, four studies have investigated the potential anti-inflammatory actions of lidocaine in equine experimental models, demonstrating mixed degrees of efficacy. When lidocaine was infused intravenously during experimentally induced acute lung inflammation in horses with recurrent airway obstruction, there was no improvement in clinical signs, pulmonary function, or neutrophilic infiltration into bronchioalveolar lavage fluid (Wilson, 2012). Likewise, lidocaine infusion failed to alter cytokine gene expression or neutrophil migration in horses with black walnut-induced laminitis (Williams, 2010). In contrast, in an experimentally induced jejunal ischemia model, intravenous lidocaine reduced plasma PGE_2 concentrations and mucosal COX2 expression (Cook, 2009b).

Further evidence of the anti-inflammatory benefits of lidocaine was demonstrated in an intraperitoneal endotoxin challenge model. Horses treated with intravenous lidocaine had significantly reduced severity of clinical signs and lower serum and peritoneal fluid TNF activity, compared with the control group (Peiró, 2010). Collectively, these later two studies support the clinical use of intravenous lidocaine in patients suffering from endotoxemia and intestinal ischemia.

References

Aleman, M., Nieto, J.E. and Higgins, J.K. (2011). Ulcerative cystitis associated with phenylbutazone administration in two horses. *Journal of the American Veterinary Medical Association* **239**(4), 499–503.

Anderson, F.L., Secombe, C.J. and Lester, G.D. (2013). Clostridial myonecrosis, haemolytic anaemia, hepatopathy, osteitis and transient hypertrophic cardiomyopathy after intramuscular injection in a Thoroughbred gelding. *Australian Veterinary Journal* **91**(5), 204–208.

Andreeta, A., Verde, C., Babusci, M., Muller, R., Simpson, M.I. and Landoni, M.F. (2011). Comparison of diclofenac diethylamine permeation across horse skin from five commercial medical human formulations. *Journal of Equine Veterinary Science* **31**(9), 502–505.

Anfossi, P., Villa, R., Montesissa, C. and Carli, S. (1997). Intramuscular bioavailability of ketoprofen lysine salt in horses. *The Veterinary Quarterly* **19**(2), 65–68.

Arden, W.A., Slocombe, R.F., Stick, J.A. and Parks, A.H. (1990). Morphologic and ultrastructural evaluation of effect of ischemia and dimethyl sulfoxide on equine jejunum. *American Journal of Veterinary Research* **51**(11), 1784–1791.

Armstrong, S. and Lees, P. (1999b). Effects of R and S enantiomers and a racemic mixture of carprofen on the production and release of proteoglycan and prostaglandin E2 from equine chondrocytes and cartilage explants. *American Journal of Veterinary Research* **60**(1), 98–104.

Armstrong, S. and Lees, P. (2002). Effects of carprofen (R and S enantiomers and racemate) on the production of IL-1, IL-6 and TNF-alpha by equine chondrocytes and synoviocytes. *Journal Of Veterinary Pharmacology and Therapeutics* **5**(2), 145–153.

Armstrong, S., Frean, S., Lees, P., Tricklebank, P. and Lake, A. (1999a). Pharmacokinetics of carprofen enantiomers in equine plasma and synovial fluid – a comparison with ketoprofen. *Journal of Veterinary Pharmacology and Therapeutics* **22**(3), 196–201.

Auer, D.E., Ng, J.C. and Seawright, A.A. (1990). Superoxide production by stimulated equine polymorphonuclear leukocytes— inhibition by anti-inflammatory drugs. *Journal of Veterinary Pharmacology and Therapeutics* **13**(1), 59–66.

Aviado, D.M. and Porter, J.M. (1984). Pentoxifylline: a new drug for the treatment of intermittent claudication. *Pharmacotherapy* **4**(6), 297–307.

Azevedo, M.S., de la Côrte, F.D., Brass, K.E., Dalmora, S.L., Machado, F.T., Pompermayer, E., Dau, S.L. and Santa'Ana, L.A. (2013). Bioavailability and tolerability of topical and oral diclofenac sodium administration in healthy ponies. *Journal of Equine Veterinary Science* **33**(1), 22–26.

Back, W., Pollmeier, M., Hanson, P.D., MacAllister, C.G. and van Heel, M.C.V. (2009). The use of force plate measurements to titrate the dosage of a new COX-2 inhibitor in lame horses. *Equine Veterinary Journal* **41**(3), 309–312.

Bailey, C.S., Macpherson, M.L., Graczyk, J., Pozor, M.A., Troedsson, M.H.T., LeBlanc, M.M. and Vickroy, T.W. (2007). Treatment efficacy of trimethoprim sulfamethoxazole, pentoxifylline, and altrenogest in equine placentitis. *Proceedings of the 53rd Annual Convention of the American Association of Equine Practitioners.* Orlando, Florida, USA, 1–5 December, 2007, 339–340.

Baird, J.D., Arroyo, L.G., Vengust, M., McGurrin, M.K.J., Rodriguez-Palacios, A., Kenney, D.G., Aravagiri, M. and Maylin, G.A. (2006). Adverse extrapyramidal effects in four horses given fluphenazine decanoate. *Journal of the American Veterinary Medical Association* **229**(1), 104–110.

Ball, M.A., Rebhun, W., Trepanier, L., Gaarder, J. and Schwark, W.S. (1997). Corneal concentrations and preliminary toxicological evaluation of an itraconazole/dimethyl sulphoxide ophthalmic ointment. *Journal of Veterinary Pharmacology and Therapeutics* **20**(2), 100–104.

Barton, M.H., Ferguson, D., Davis, P.J. and Moore, J.N. (1997). The effects of pentoxifylline infusion on plasma 6-keto-prostaglandin F1α and *ex vivo* endotoxin-induced tumour necrosis factor activity in horses. *Journal of Veterinary Pharmacology and Therapeutics* **20**(6), 487–492.

Barton, M.H. and Moore, J.N. (1994). Pentoxifylline inhibits mediator synthesis in an equine *in vitro* whole blood model of endotoxemia. *Circulatory Shock* **44**(4), 216–220.

Barton, M.H., Moore, J.N. and Norton, N. (1997). Effects of pentoxifylline infusion on response of horses to *in vivo* challenge exposure with endotoxin. *American Journal of Veterinary Research* **58**(11), 1300–1307.

Barton, M.H., Paske, E., Norton, N., King, D., Giguère, S. and Budsberg, S. (2014). Efficacy of cyclooxygenase inhibition by two commercially available firocoxib products in horses. *Equine Veterinary Journal* **46**(1), 72–75.

Beretta, C., Garavaglia, G. and Cavalli, M. (2005). COX-1 and COX-2 inhibition in horse blood by phenylbutazone, flunixin, carprofen and meloxicam: an *in vitro* analysis. *Pharmacological Research: The Official Journal Of The Italian Pharmacological Society* **52**(4), 302–306.

Betley, M., Sutherland, S.F., Gregoricka, M.J. and Pollet, R.A. (1991). The analgesic effect of ketoprofen for use in treating equine colic as compared to flunixin meglumine. *Equine Practice* **13**, 11–16.

Blythe, L. L., Craig, A.M., Christensen, J.M., Appell, L.H. and Slizeski, M.L. (1986). Pharmacokinetic disposition of dimethyl sulfoxide administered intravenously to horses. *American Journal of Veterinary Research* **47**(8), 1739–1743.

Bottoms, G.D., Fessler, J.F., Roesel, O.F., Moore, A.B. and Frauenfelder, H.C. (1981). Endotoxin-induced hemodynamic changes in ponies: effects of flunixin meglumine. *American Journal of Veterinary Research* **42**(9), 1514–1518.

Brainard, B.M., Epstein, K.L., LoBato, D., Kwon, S., Papich, M.G. and Moore, J.N. (2011). Effects of clopidogrel and aspirin on platelet aggregation, thromboxane production, and serotonin secretion in horses. *Journal of Veterinary Internal Medicine* **25**(1), 116–122.

Brayton, C.F. (1986). Dimethyl sulfoxide (DMSO): a review. *The Cornell Veterinarian* **76**(1), 61–90.

Brien, S., Prescott, P., Bashir, N., Lewith, H. and Lewith, G. (2008). Systematic review of the nutritional supplements dimethyl sulfoxide (DMSO) and methylsulfonylmethane (MSM) in the treatment of osteoarthritis. *Osteoarthritis And Cartilage* **16**(11), 1277–1288.

Broome, T.A., Brown, M.P. and Merrit, K.A. (2003). Pharmacokinetics and plasma concentrations of acetylsalicylic acid after intravenous, rectal, and intragastric administration to horses. *Canadian Journal of Veterinary Research* **67**(4), 297–302.

Burns, P.J., Morrow, C., Gilley, R.M. and Papich, M.G. (2010). Evaluation of Pharmacokinetic-Pharmacodynamic Relationships for Bio-Release Meloxicam Formulations in Horses. *Journal of Equine Veterinary Science* **30**(10), 539–544.

Caldwell, F.J., Mueller, P.O.E., Lynn, R.C. and Budsberg, S.C. (2004). Effect of topical application of diclofenac liposomal suspension on experimentally induced subcutaneous inflammation in horses. *American Journal of Veterinary Research* **65**(3), 271–276.

Cambridge, H., Russell, C.S., Hooke, R.E. and Lees, P. (1991). Antithrombotic actions of aspirin in the horse. *Equine Veterinary Journal* **23**(2), 123–127.

Carrick, J.B., Papich, M.G., Middleton, D.M., Naylor, J.M. and Townsend, H.G.G. (1989). Clinical and pathological effects of flunixin meglumine administration to neonatal foals. *Canadian Journal of Veterinary Research* **53**(2), 195–201.

Cazalis, J., Bodet, C., Gagnon, G. and Grenier, D. (2008). Doxycycline reduces lipopolysaccharide-induced inflammatory mediator secretion in macrophage and *ex vivo* human whole blood models. *Journal of Periodontology* **79**(9), 1762–1768.

Chay, S., Woods, W.E., Nugent, T., Blake, J.W. and Tobin, T. (1982). The pharmacology of nonsteroidal anti-inflammatory drugs in the horse: flunixin meglumine (Banamine). *Equine Practice* **4**(10), 16–23.

Coakley, M., Peck, K.E., Taylor, T.S., Matthews, N.S. and Mealey, K.L. (1999). Pharmacokinetics of flunixin meglumine in donkeys, mules, and horses. *American Journal of Veterinary Research* **60**(11), 1441–1444.

Colahan, P.T., Bailey, J.E., Chou, C.C., Johnson, M., Rice, B.L., Jones, G.L. and Cheeks, J.P. (2002). Effect of flunixin meglumine on selected physiologic and performance parameters of athletically conditioned Thoroughbred horses subjected to an incremental exercise stress test. *Veterinary Therapeutics* **3**(1), 37–48.

Cook, V.L. and Blikslager, A.T. (2008). Use of systemically administered lidocaine in horses with gastrointestinal tract disease. *Journal of the American Veterinary Medical Association* **232**(8), 1144–1148.

Cook, V.L., Meyer, C.T., Campbell, N.B. and Blikslager, A.T. (2009a). Effect of firocoxib or flunixin meglumine on recovery of ischemic-injured equine jejunum. *American Journal of Veterinary Research* **70**(8), 992–1000.

Cook, V.L., Davis, J.L., Marshall, J.F., Blikslager, A.T., Jones Shults, J., McDowell, M.R. and Campbell, N.B. (2009b). Anti-inflammatory effects of intravenously administered lidocaine hydrochloride on ischemia-injured jejunum in horses. *American Journal of Veterinary Research* **70**(10), 1259–1268.

Cox, S., Sommardahl, C., Yarbrough, J., Amicucci, A., Reed, K., Breeding, D. and Doherty, T. (2012). Firocoxib loading dose trial in horses. *Journal of Veterinary Internal Medicine* **26**(3), 749.

Craig, J.M., Lloyd, D.H. and Jones, R.D. (1997). A double-blind placebo-controlled trial of an evening primrose and fish oil combination vs. hydrogenated coconut oil in the management of recurrent seasonal pruritus in horses. *Veterinary Dermatology* **8**(3), 177–182.

Cuniberti, B., Odore, R., Barbero, R., Cagnardi, P., Badino, P., Girardi, C. and Re, G. (2012). *In vitro* and *ex vivo* pharmacodynamics of selected non-steroidal anti-inflammatory drugs in equine whole blood. *Veterinary Journal* **191**(3), 327–333.

D'Arcy-Moskwa, E., Noble, G.K., Weston, L.A., Boston, R. and Raidal, S.L. (2012). Effects of meloxicam and phenylbutazone on equine gastric mucosal permeability. *Journal of Veterinary Internal Medicine* **26**(6), 1494–1499.

Dabareiner, R.M., White, N.A., Snyder, J.R., Feldman, B.F. and Donaldson, L.L. (2005). Effects of Carolina rinse solution, dimethyl sulfoxide, and the 21-aminosteroid, U-74389G, on microvascular permeability and morphology of the equine jejunum after low-flow ischemia and reperfusion. *American Journal of Veterinary Research* **66**(3), 525–536.

Davis, J.L., Papich, M.G., Morton, A.J., Gayle, J., Blikslager, A.T. and Campbell, N.B. (2007). Pharmacokinetics of etodolac in the horse following oral and intravenous administration. *Journal of Veterinary Pharmacology and Therapeutics* **30**(1), 43–48.

Davis, J.L., Marshall, J.F., Papich, M.G., Blikslager, A.T. and Campbell, N.B. (2011). The pharmacokinetics and *in vitro* cyclooxygenase selectivity of deracoxib in horses. *Journal of Veterinary Pharmacology and Therapeutics* **34**(1), 12–16.

de Grauw, J.C., van de Lest, C.H.A., Brama, P.A.J., Rambags, B.P.B. and van Weeren, P.R. (2009). *In vivo* effects of meloxicam on inflammatory mediators, MMP activity and cartilage biomarkers in equine joints with acute synovitis. *Equine Veterinary Journal* **41**(7), 693–699.

de Solis, C.N. and McKenzie, H.C. III. (2007). Serum concentrations of lidocaine and its metabolites MEGX and GX during and after prolonged intravenous infusion of lidocaine in horses after colic surgery. *Journal of Equine Veterinary Science* **27**(9), 398–404.

Dirikolu, L., Woods, W.E., Boyles, J., Lehner, A.F., Harkins, J.D., Fisher, M., Schaeffer, D.J. and Tobin, T. (2009a). Nonsteroidal anti-inflammatory agents and musculoskeletal injuries in Thoroughbred racehorses in Kentucky. *Journal of Veterinary Pharmacology and Therapeutics* **32**(3), 271–279.

Dirikolu, L., Lehner, A.F., Harkins, J.D., Woods, W.E., Karpiesiuk, W., Gates, R.S., Fisher, M. and Tobin, T. (2009b). Pyrilamine in the horse: detection and pharmacokinetics of pyrilamine and its major urinary metabolite O-desmethylpyrilamine. *Journal of Veterinary Pharmacology and Therapeutics* **32**(1), 66–78.

Dirikolu, L., Karpiesiuk, W., Lehner, A.F., Hughes, C., Granstrom, D.E. and Tobin, T. (2009c). Synthesis and detection of toltrazuril sulfone and its pharmacokinetics in horses following administration in dimethylsulfoxide. *Journal of Veterinary Pharmacology and Therapeutics* **32**(4), 368–378.

Doucet, M.Y., Bertone, A.L., Hendrickson, D., Hughes, F., MacAllister, C., McClure, S., Reinemeyer, C., Rossier, Y.R., Sifferman, D., Vrins, A.A., White, G., Kunkle, B., Alva, R., Romano, D. and Hanson, P.D. (2008). Comparison of efficacy and safety of paste formulations of firocoxib and phenylbutazone in horses with naturally occurring osteoarthritis. *Journal of the American Veterinary Medical Association* **232**(1), 91–97.

Dyke, T.M., Sams, R.A., Thompson, K.G. and Ashcraft, S.M. (1998). Pharmacokinetics of multiple-dose administration of eltenac in horses. *American Journal of Veterinary Research* **59**(11), 1447–1450.

Erkert, R.S., Clarke, C.R., Payton, M.E. and MacAllister, C.G. (2005). Use of force plate analysis to compare the analgesic effects of intravenous administration of phenylbutazone and flunixin meglumine in horses with navicular syndrome. *American Journal of Veterinary Research* **66**(2), 284–288.

Eyre, P., Hanna, C.J., Wells, P.W. and McBeth, D.G. (1982). Equine immunology 3: Immunopharmacology – Anti-inflammatory and antihypersensitivity drugs. *Equine Veterinary Journal* **14**(4), 277–281.

Farley, J., Sirois, J., MacFarlane, P.H., Kombé, A. and Laverty, S. (2005). Evaluation of coexpression of microsomal prostaglandin E synthase-1 and cyclooxygenase-2 in interleukin-1–stimulated equine articular chondrocytes. *American Journal of Veterinary Research* **66**, 1985–1991.

Frazer, G.S., Rossol, T.J., Threlfall, W.R. and Weisbrode, S.E. (1988). Histopathologic effects of dimethyl sulfoxide on equine endometrium. *American Journal of Veterinary Research* **49**(10), 1774–1781.

Frean, S.P., Lees, P. and Abraham, L.A. (1999). *In vitro* stimulation of equine articular cartilage proteoglycan synthesis by hyaluronan and carprofen. *Research in Veterinary Science* **67**(2), 183–190.

Frellstedt, L. and Slovis, N.M. (2009). Acute renal disease from Leptospira interrogans in three yearlings from the same farm. *Equine Veterinary Education* **21**(9), 478–484.

Friberg, C.A. and Logas, D. (1999). Treatment of Culicoides hypersensitive horses with high-dose n-3 fatty acids: a double-blinded crossover study. *Veterinary Dermatology* **10**(2), 117–122.

Frisbie, D.D., Kawcak, C.E., Werpy, N.M. and McIlwraith, C.W. (2007). Evaluation of topical diclofenac liposomal cream for treatment of equine osteoarthritis using an equine experimental model. *Proceedings* of the 53rd Annual Convention of the American Association of Equine Practitioners. Orlando, Florida, USA, 1–5 December, 2007, 256–257.

Fugler, L.A., Eades, S.C., Moore, R.M., Koch, C.E. and Keowen, M.L. (2013). Plasma matrix metalloproteinase activity in horses after intravenous infusion of lipopolysaccharide and treatment with matrix metalloproteinase inhibitors. *American Journal of Veterinary Research* **74**(3), 473–480.

Geor, R.J., Petrie, L., Papich, M.G. and Rousseaux, C. (1989). The protective effects of sucralfate and ranitidine in foals experimentally intoxicated with phenylbutazone. *Canadian Journal of Veterinary Research* **53**(2), 231–238.

Geor, R.J., Weiss, D.J., Burris, S.M. and Smith, C.M. (1992). Effects of furosemide and pentoxifylline on blood flow properties in horses. *American Journal of Veterinary Research* **53**(11), 2043–2049.

Gerring, E.L., Lees, P. and Taylor, J.B. (1981). Pharmacokinetics of phenylbutazone and its metabolites in the horse. *Equine Veterinary Journal* **13**(3), 152–157.

Gilger, B.C. (2011). *Equine Ophthalmology.* Maryland Heights, MI, Elsevier Saunders.

Goicoechea M., García de Vinuesa, S., Quiroga, B., Verdalles, U., Barraca, D., Yuste, C., Panizo, N., Verde, E., Muñoz, M.A. and Luño, J. (2012). Effects of pentoxifylline on inflammatory parameters in chronic kidney disease patients: a randomized trial. *Journal of Nephrology* **25**(6), 969–975.

Goodrich, L.R. and Nixon, A.J. (2006). Medical treatment of osteoarthritis in the horse – a review. *Veterinary Journal* **171**(1), 51–69.

Goodrich, L.R., Furr, M.O., Robertson, J.L. and Warnick, L.D. (1998). A toxicity study of eltenac, a nonsteroidal anti-inflammatory drug, in horses. *Journal of Veterinary Pharmacology and Therapeutics* **21**(1), 24–33.

Gregoricka, M.J., Busch, K.R., Dedrickson, B.J. and Sutherland, S.F. (1990). Assessment of the intramuscular administration of ketoprofen. *Equine Practice* **12**(7), 15.

Gu, Y., Walker, C., Ryan, M.E., Payne, J.B. and Golub, L.M. (2012). Non-antibacterial tetracycline formulations: clinical applications in dentistry and medicine. *Journal of Oral Microbiology* **4**, 19227–19227.

Gunson, D.E. and Soma, L.R. (1983). Renal papillary necrosis in horses after phenylbutazone and water deprivation. *Veterinary Pathology* **20**(5), 603–610.

Gutierrez-Reyes, G., Lopez-Ortal, P., Sixtos, S., Cruz, S., Ramirez-Iglesias, M.T., Gutierrez-Ruiz, M.C., Sanchez-Avila, F., Roldan, E., Vargas-Vorackova, F. and Kershenobich, D. (2006). Effect of pentoxifylline on levels of pro-inflammatory cytokines during chronic hepatitis C. *Scandinavian Journal of Immunology* **63**(6), 461–467.

Hagedorn, H.W., Meiser, H., Zankl, H. and Schulz, R. (2002). The isomeric metabolites of doxepin in equine serum and urine. *Journal of Pharmaceutical and Biomedical Analysis* **29** (1/2), 317–323.

Hall, J.A., Pearson, E.G., Wander, R.C., Gradin, J.L., Van Saun, R.J. and Tornquist, S.J. (2004). Effect of type of dietary polyunsaturated fatty acid supplement (corn oil or fish oil) on immune responses in healthy horses. *Journal of Veterinary Internal Medicine* **18**(6), 880–886.

Hall, J.A., Wander, R.C. and Van Saun, R.J. (2004). Dietary (n-3) fatty acids from Menhaden fish oil alter plasma fatty acids and leukotriene B synthesis in healthy horses. *Journal of Veterinary Internal Medicine* **18**(6), 871–879.

Hamama, S., Gilbert-Sirieix, M., Vozenin, M-C. and Delanian, S. (2012). Radiation-induced enteropathy: molecular basis of pentoxifylline-vitamin E anti-fibrotic effect involved TGF-β1 cascade inhibition. *Radiotherapy and Oncology: Journal of The European Society For Therapeutic Radiology and Oncology* **105**(3), 305–312.

Hamm, D., Turchi, P., Johnson, J.C., Lockwood, P.W., Thompson, K.C. and Katz, T. (1997). Determination of an effective dose of eltenac and its comparison with that of flunixin meglumine in horses after experimentally induced carpitis. *American Journal of Veterinary Research* **58**(3), 298–302.

Hansen, R.A., Savage, C.J., Reidlinger, K., Traub-Dargatz, J.L., Ogilvie, G.K., Mitchell, D. and Fettman, M.J. (2002). Effects of dietary flaxseed oil supplementation on equine plasma fatty acid concentrations and whole blood platelet aggregation. *Journal of Veterinary Internal Medicine* **16**(4), 457–463.

Henry, M.M., Moore, J.N., Feldman, E.B., Fischer, J.K. and Russell, B. (1990). Effect of dietary alpha-linolenic acid on equine monocyte procoagulant activity and eicosanoid synthesis. *Circulatory Shock* **32**(3), 173–188.

Henry, M.M., Moore, J.N. and Fischer, J.K. (1991). Influence of an omega-3 fatty acid-enriched ration on *in vivo* responses of horses to endotoxin. *American Journal of Veterinary Research* **52**(4), 523–527.

Hess, T.M., Rexford, J.K., Hansen, D.K., Harris, M., Schauermann, N., Ross, T., Engle, T.E., Allen, K.G.D. and Mulligan, C.M. (2012). Effects of two different dietary sources of long chain omega-3, highly unsaturated fatty acids on incorporation into the plasma, red blood cell, and skeletal muscle in horses. *Journal of Animal Science* **90**(9), 3023–3031.

Higgins, A.J., Lees, P., Taylor, J.B.O. and Ewins, C.P. (1986). Flunixin meglumine: quantitative determination in and effects on composition of equine inflammatory exudate. *British Veterinary Journal* **142**(2), 163–169.

Hilton, H.G., Magdesian, K.G., Groth, A.D., Knych, H., Stanley, S.D. and Hollingsworth, S.R. (2011). Distribution of flunixin meglumine and firocoxib into aqueous humor of horses. *Journal of Veterinary Internal Medicine* **25**(5), 1127–1133.

Hinz, B. and Brune, K. (2002). Cyclooxygenase-2-10 years later. *The Journal of Pharmacology and Experimental Therapeutics* **300**(2), 367–375.

Horne, M.M., Pascoe, P.J., Ducharme, N.G., Barker, I.K. and Grovum, W.L. (1994). Attempts to modify reperfusion injury of equine jejunal mucosa using dimethylsulfoxide, allopurinol, and intraluminal oxygen. *Veterinary Surgery* **23**(4), 241–249.

Hough, M.E., Steel, C.M., Bolton, J.R. and Yovich, J.V. (1999). Ulceration and stricture of the right dorsal colon after phenylbutazone administration in four horses. *Australian Veterinary Journal* **77**(12), 785–788.

Hu, H.H., MacAllister, C.G., Payton, M.E. and Erkert, R.S. (2005). Evaluation of the analgesic effects of phenylbutazone administered at a high or low dosage in horses with chronic lameness. *Journal of the American Veterinary Medical Association* **226**(3), 414–417.

Jackman, B.R., Moore, J.N., Barton, M.H. and Morris, D.D. (1994). Comparison of the effects of ketoprofen and flunixin meglumine on the *in vitro* response of equine peripheral blood monocytes to bacterial endotoxin. *Canadian Journal of Veterinary Research* **58**(2), 138–143.

Jarvis, G.E. and Evans, R.J. (1994). Endotoxin-induced platelet aggregation in heparinised equine whole blood *in vitro*. *Research in Veterinary Science* **57**(3), 317–324.

Jarvis, G.E. and Evans, R.J. (1996). Platelet-activating factor and not thromboxane A2 is an important mediator of endotoxin-induced platelet aggregation in equine heparinised whole blood *in vitro*. *Blood Coagulation & Fibrinolysis: An International Journal in Haemostasis and Thrombosis* **7**(2), 194–198.

Jensen, R.C., Fischer, J.H. and Cwik, M.J. (1990). Effect of age and training status on pharmacokinetics of flunixin meglumine in Thoroughbreds. *American Journal of Veterinary Research* **51**(4), 591–594.

Johansson, I.M., Kallings, P. and Hammarlund-Udenaes, M. (1991). Studies of meclofenamic acid and two metabolites in horses-pharmacokinetics and effects on exercise tolerance. *Journal of Veterinary Pharmacology and Therapeutics* **14**(3), 235–242.

Johnson, C.B., Brearley, J.C., Young, S.S. and Taylor, P.M. (1993). Postoperative analgesia using phenylbutazone, flunixin or carprofen in horses. *Veterinary Record* **133**(14), 336–338.

Jones, E.W. and Hamm, D. (1978). Comparative efficacy of PBZ and naproxen in induced equine myositis. *Journal of Equine Medicine and Surgery* **2**, 341–347.

Kabbesh, N., Mallem, M.Y., Desfontis, J.C., Noireaud, J. and Gogny, M. (2010). Vasodilatory effects of pentoxifylline in horses: a study in the veins of fingers 36e Journée de la Recherche Equine, Le Pin au Haras, France, jeudi 4 mars 2010. Le Pin au Haras; France, Les Haras Nationaux, 217–220.

Kelmer, G., Doherty, T.J., Elliott, S., Saxton, A., Fry, M.M. and Andrews, F.M. (2008). Evaluation of dimethyl sulphoxide effects on initial response to endotoxin in the horse. *Equine Veterinary Journal* **40**(4), 358–363.

Khanapure, S.P., Garvey, D.S., Janero, D.R. and Letts, L.G. (2007). Eicosanoids in inflammation: biosynthesis, pharmacology, and therapeutic frontiers. *Current Topics in Medicinal Chemistry* **7**(3), 311–340.

Khol-Parisini, A., Hulan, H.W., Zentek, J., van den Hoven, R. and Leinker, S. (2007). Effects of feeding sunflower oil or seal blubber oil to horses with recurrent airway obstruction. *Canadian Journal of Veterinary Research* **71**(1), 59–65.

King, S.S., AbuGhazaleh, A.A., Webel, S.K. and Jones, K.L. (2008). Circulating fatty acid profiles in response to three levels of dietary omega-3 fatty acid supplementation in horses. *Journal of Animal Science* **86**(5), 1114–1123.

Koblischke, P., Budik, S., Müller, J. and Aurich, C. (2010). Practical experience with the treatment of recipient mares with a non-steroidal anti-inflammatory drug in an equine embryo transfer programme. *Reproduction in Domestic Animals* **45**(6), 1039–1041.

Koene, M., Goupil, X., Kampmann, C., Hanson, P.D., Denton, D. and Pollmeier, M.G. (2010). Field trial validation of the efficacy and acceptability of firocoxib, a highly selective Cox-2 inhibitor, in a group of 96 lame horses. *Journal of Equine Veterinary Science* **30**(5), 237–243.

Kornreich, B., Enyeart, M., Jesty, S.A., Nydam, D.V. and Divers, T. (2010). The effects of pentoxifylline on equine platelet aggregation. *Journal of Veterinary Internal Medicine* **24**(5), 1196–1202.

Kunkle, B.N., Saik, J.E., Attebery, D.K., Targa, N.L., Larsen, D.L. and Hanson, P.D. (2010). Effects of firocoxib and phenylbutazone dosed for 42 days in horses Proceedings of the 56th Annual Convention of the American Association of Equine Practitioners. Baltimore, Maryland, USA, 4–8 December 2010. W. A. Moyer. Lexington; USA, American Association of Equine Practitioners (AAEP).

Kuroda, T., Nagata, S-I., Takizawa, Y., Tamura, N., Kusano, K., Mizobe, F. and Hariu, K. (2013). Pharmacokinetics and pharmacodynamics of d-chlorpheniramine following intravenous and oral administration in healthy Thoroughbred horses. *Veterinary Journal* **197**(2), 433–437.

Kvaternick, V., Pollmeier, M., Fischer, J. and Hanson, P.D. (2007). Pharmacokinetics and metabolism of orally administered firocoxib, a novel second generation coxib, in horses. *Journal of Veterinary Pharmacology and Therapeutics* **30**(3), 208–217.

Landoni, M.F. and Lees, P. (1995). Comparison of the anti-inflammatory actions of flunixin and ketoprofen in horses applying PK/PD modelling. *Equine Veterinary Journal* **27**(4), 247–256.

Landoni, M.F. and Lees, P. (1996). Pharmacokinetics and pharmacodynamics of ketoprofen enantiomers in the horse. *Journal of Veterinary Pharmacology and Therapeutics* **19**(6), 466–474.

Larsen, S.M. and Levine, L.A. (2012). Review of non-surgical treatment options for Peyronie's disease. *International Journal of Impotence Research* **24**(1), 1–10.

Lassaline-Utter, M., Miller, C. and Wotman, K.L. (2014). Eosinophilic keratitis in 46 eyes of 27 horses in the Mid-Atlantic United States (2008–2012). *Veterinary Ophthalmology* **17**(5), 311–320.

Lees, P. and Higgins, A.J. (1985). Clinical pharmacology and therapeutic uses of non-steroidal anti-inflammatory drugs in the horse. *Equine Veterinary Journal* **17**(2), 83–96.

Lees, P. and Landoni, M.F. (2002). Pharmacodynamics and enantioselective pharmacokinetics of racemic carprofen in the horse. *Journal of Veterinary Pharmacology and Therapeutics* **25**(6), 433–448.

Lees, P., Ewins, C.P., Taylor, J.B. and Sedgwick, A.D. (1987). Serum thromboxane in the horse and its inhibition by aspirin, phenylbutazone and flunixin. *The British Veterinary Journal* **143**(5), 462–476.

Lees, P., Sedgwick, A.D., Higgins, A.J., Pugh, K.E. and Busch, U. (1991). Pharmacodynamics and pharmacokinetics of miloxicam in the horse. *The British Veterinary Journal* **147**(2), 97–108.

Lees, P., McKellar, Q., May, S.A. and Ludwig, B. (1994). Pharmacodynamics and pharmacokinetics of carprofen in the horse. *Equine Veterinary Journal* **26**(3), 203–208.

Lees, P., May, S.A., Hoeijmakers, M., Coert, A. and Rens, P.V. (1999). A pharmacodynamic and pharmacokinetic study with vedaprofen in an equine model of acute nonimmune inflammation. *Journal of Veterinary Pharmacology and Therapeutics* **22**(2), 96–106.

Leguillette, R., Desevaux, C. and Lavoie, J.P. (2002). Effects of pentoxifylline on pulmonary function and results of cytologic examination of bronchoalveolar lavage fluid in horses with recurrent airway obstruction. *American Journal of Veterinary Research* **63**(3), 459–463.

Lehnhard, R.A., Adams, A.A., Betancourt, A., Horohov, D.W., Liburt, N.R., Streltsova, J.M., Franke, W.C. and McKeever, K.H. (2010). Phenylbutazone blocks the cytokine response following a high-intensity incremental exercise challenge in horses. *Comparative Exercise Physiology* **7**(3), 103–108.

Letendre, L.T., Tessman, R.K., McClure, S.R., Kvaternick, V.J., Fischer, J.B. and Hanson, P.D. (2008). Pharmacokinetics of firocoxib after administration of multiple consecutive daily doses to horses. *American Journal of Veterinary Research* **69**(11), 1399–1405.

Ley, W.B., Bowen, J.M., Sponenberg, D.P. and Lessard, P.N. (1989). Dimethyl sulfoxide intrauterine therapy in the mare: effects upon endometrial histological features and biopsy classification. *Theriogenology* **32**(2), 263–276.

Lin, H.C., Johnson, C.R., Duran, S.H. and Waldridge, B.M. (2004). Effects of intravenous administration of dimethyl sulfoxide on cardiopulmonary and clinicopathologic variables in awake or halothane-anesthetized horses. *Journal of the American Veterinary Medical Association* **225**(4), 560–566.

Liska, D.A., Akucewich, L.H., Marsella, R., Maxwell, L.K., Barbara, J.E. and Cole, C.A. (2006). Pharmacokinetics of pentoxifylline and its 5-hydroxyhexyl metabolite after oral and intravenous administration of pentoxifylline to healthy adult horses. *American Journal of Veterinary Research* **67**(9), 1621–1627.

Little D., Brown, S.A., Campbell, N.B., Moeser, A.J., Davis, J.L. and Blikslager, A.T. (2007). Effects of the cyclooxygenase inhibitor meloxicam on recovery of ischemia-injured equine jejunum. *American Journal of Veterinary Research* **68**(6), 614–624.

Logas, D., Beale, K.M. and Bauer, J.E. (1991). Potential clinical benefits of dietary supplementation with marine-life oil. *Journal of the American Veterinary Medical Association* **199**(11), 1631–1636.

Lynn, R.C., Hepler, D.I., Kelch, W.J., Bertone, J.J., Smith, B.L. and Vatistas, N.J. (2004). Double-blinded placebo-controlled clinical field trial to evaluate the safety and efficacy of topically applied 1% diclofenac liposomal cream for the relief of lameness in horses. *Veterinary Therapeutics: Research in Applied Veterinary Medicine* **5**(2), 128–138.

MacAllister, C.G., Pollet, R.A., Borne, A.T. and Morgan, S.J. (1993). Comparison of adverse effects of phenylbutazone, flunixin meglumine, and ketoprofen in horses. *Journal of the American Veterinary Medical Association* **202**(1), 71–77.

MacKay, R.J., Daniels, C.A., Bleyaert, H.F., Bailey, J.E., Gillis, K.D., Merritt, A.M., Katz, T.L., Johnson, J.C. and Thompson, K.C. (2000). Effect of eltenac in horses with induced endotoxaemia. *Equine Veterinary Journal Supplement* **32**, 26–31.

Malone, E., Ensink, J., Turner, T., Wilson, J., Andrews, F., Keegan, K. and Lumsden, J. (2006). Intravenous continuous infusion of lidocaine for treatment of equine ileus. *Veterinary Surgery* **35**(1), 60–66.

Manhart, D.R., Scott, B.D., Gibbs, P.G., Coverdale, J.A., Eller, E.M., Honnas, C.M. and Hood, D.M. (2009). Markers of inflammation in arthritic horses fed omega-3 fatty acids. *Professional Animal Scientist* **25**(2), 155–160.

Mathes, R.L., Reber, A.J., Hurley, D.J. and Dietrich, U.M. (2010). Effects of antifungal drugs and delivery vehicles on morphology and proliferation of equine corneal keratocytes *in vitro*. *American Journal of Veterinary Research* **71**(8), 953–959.

Matyjaszek, S.A., Morton, A.J., Freeman, D.E., Grosche, A., Polyak, M.M.R. and Kuck, H. (2009). Effects of flunixin meglumine on recovery of colonic mucosa from ischemia in horses. *American Journal of Veterinary Research* **70**(2), 236–246.

McCann, M.E., Moore, J.N., Carrick, J.B. and Barton, M.H. (2000). Effect of Intravenous Infusion of Omega-3 and Omega-6 Lipid Emulsions on Equine Monocyte Fatty Acid Composition and Inflammatory Mediator Production *in vitro*. *Shock* **14**(2), 222–228.

McCann, M.E., Andersen, D.R., Brideau, C., Black, D.H., Zhang, H. and Hickey, G.J. (2002). *In vitro* activity and *in vivo* efficacy of a novel COX-2 inhibitor in the horse. *Journal of Veterinary Internal Medicine* **16**, 789.

McConnico, R.S., Morgan, T.W., Williams, C.C., Hubert, J.D. and Moore, R.M. (2008). Pathophysiologic effects of phenylbutazone on the right dorsal colon in horses. *American Journal of Veterinary Research* **69**(11), 1496–1505.

McKellar, Q.A., Bogan, J.A., von Fellenberg, R.L., Ludwig, B. and Cawley, G.D. (1991). Pharmacokinetic, biochemical and tolerance studies on carprofen in the horse. *Equine Veterinary Journal* **23**(4), 280–284.

Mealey, K.L., Matthews, N.S., Peck, K.E., Ray, A.C. and Taylor, T.S. (1997). Comparative pharmacokinetics of phenylbutazone and its metabolite oxyphenbutazone in clinically normal horses and donkeys. *American Journal of Veterinary Research* **58**(1), 53–55.

Mealey, K.L., Bennett, B.S., Taylor, T.S., Burchfield, M.L., Matthews, N.S. and Peck, K.E. (2004). Pharmacokinetics of R(−) and S(+) carprofen after administration of racemic carprofen in donkeys and horses. *American Journal of Veterinary Research* **65**(11), 1479–1482.

Milam, S.B., Skelley, L.A. and Mackay, R.J. (1992). Secretion of tumor necrosis factor by endotoxin-treated equine mammary exudate macrophages: effect of dexamethasone and pentoxifylline. *Cornell Veterinarian* **82**(4), 435–446.

Moore, J.N., Hardee, M.M. and Hardee, G.E. (1986). Modulation of arachidonic acid metabolism in endotoxic horses: comparison of flunixin meglumine, phenylbutazone, and a selective thromboxane synthetase inhibitor. *American Journal of Veterinary Research* **47**(1), 110–113.

Moore, R.M., Muir, W.W., Bertone, A.L., Beard, W.L. and Stromberg, P.C. (1995). Effects of dimethyl sulfoxide, allopurinol, 21-aminosteroid U-74839G, and manganese chloride on low-flow ischemia and reperfusion of the large colon in horses. *American Journal of Veterinary Research* **56**(5), 671–687.

Morresey, P.R. (2006). Management of the Acutely Neurologic Patient. *Clinical Techniques in Equine Practice* **5**(2), 104–111.

Morris, D.D., Henry, M.M., Moore, J.N. and Fischer, J.K. (1991). Effect of dietary alpha-linolenic acid on endotoxin-induced production of tumor necrosis factor by peritoneal macrophages in horses. *American Journal of Veterinary Research* **52**(4), 528–532.

Morton, A.J., Campbell, N.B., Gayle, J.M., Redding, W.R. and Blikslager, A.T. (2005). Preferential and non-selective cyclooxygenase inhibitors reduce inflammation during lipopolysaccharide-induced synovitis. *Research in Veterinary Science* **78**(2), 189–192.

Moses, V.S., Hardy, J., Bertone, A.L. and Weisbrode, S.E. (2001). Effects of anti-inflammatory drugs on lipopolysaccharide-challenged and -unchallenged equine synovial explants. *American Journal of Veterinary Research* **62**(1), 54–60.

Mudge, M.C. (2007). Review of the analgesic, prokinetic, and anti-inflammatory uses of IV lidocaine. *Proceedings* of the 53rd Annual Convention of the American Association of Equine Practitioners, Orlando, Florida, USA, 1–5 December, 2007, 245–248.

Nagy, Z., Sipka, R., Ocsovszki, I., Balogh, A. and Mándi, Y. (1999). Suppressive effect of pentoxifylline on natural killer cell activity; experimental and clinical studies. *Naunyn-Schmiedeberg's Archives of Pharmacology* **359**(3), 228–234.

Nakanishi, M., Gokhale, V., Meuillet, E.J. and Rosenberg, D.W. (2010). mPGES-1 as a target for cancer suppression: A comprehensive invited review: Phospholipase A2 and lipid mediators. *Biochimie* **92**(6), 660–664.

Noble, G., Edwards, S., Lievaart, J., Pippia, J., Boston, R. and Raidal, S.L. (2012). Pharmacokinetics and safety of single and multiple oral doses of meloxicam in adult horses. *Journal of Veterinary Internal Medicine* **26**(5), 1192–1201.

O'Connor, C.I., Hayes, S.H. and Lawrence, L.M. (2007). Dietary fish oil supplementation affects serum fatty acid concentrations in horses. *Journal of Animal Science* **85**(9), 2183–2189.

O'Grady, S.E. (2011). How to treat severe laminitis in an ambulatory setting Proceedings of the 57th Annual Convention of the American Association of Equine Practitioners, San Antonio, Texas, USA, 18–22 November 2011. Lexington; USA, American Association of Equine Practitioners (AAEP).

Ollivier, F.J., Brooks, D.E., Kallberg, M.E., Komaromy, A.M., Lassaline, M.E., Andrew, S.E., Gelatt, K.N., Stevens, G.R., Blalock, T.D., van Setten, G-B. and Schultz, G.S. (2003). Evaluation of various compounds to inhibit activity of matrix metalloproteinases in the tear film of horses with ulcerative keratitis. *American Journal of Veterinary Research* **64**(9), 1081–1087.

Olsen, L., Ingvast-Larsson, C., Bondesson, U., Brostrom, H., Tjalve, H. and Larsson, P. (2007). Cetirizine in horses: pharmacokinetics and effect of ivermectin pretreatment [electronic resource]. *Journal Of Veterinary Pharmacology And Therapeutics* **30**(3), 194–200.

Olsen, L., Tjalve, H., Ingvast-Larsson, C., Bondesson, U. and Brostrom, H. (2008). Cetirizine in horses: Pharmacokinetics and pharmacodynamics following repeated oral administration [electronic resource]. *Veterinary Journal* **177**(2), 242–249.

Olsen, L., Bondesson, U., Brostrem, H., Olsson, U., Mazogi, B., Sundqvist, M., Tjälve, H. and Ingvast-Larsson, C. (2011). Pharmacokinetics and effects of cetirizine in horses with insect bite hypersensitivity. *Veterinary Journal* **187**(3), 347–351.

Orsini, J.A., Ryan, W.G., Carithers, D.S. and Boston, R.C. (2012). Evaluation of oral administration of firocoxib for the management of musculoskeletal pain and lameness associated with osteoarthritis in horses. *American Journal of Veterinary Research* **73**(5), 664–671.

Owens, J.G., Kamerling, S.G., Stanton, S.R. and Keowen, M.L. (1995a). Effects of ketoprofen and phenylbutazone on chronic hoof pain and lameness in the horse. *Equine Veterinary Journal* **27**(4), 296–300.

Owens, J.G., Kamerling, S.G. and Barker, S.A. (1995b). Pharmacokinetics of ketoprofen in healthy horses and horses with acute synovitis. *Journal of Veterinary Pharmacology and Therapeutics* **18**(3), 187–195.

Owens, J.G., Kamerling, S.G., Stanton, S.R., Keowen, M.L. and Prescott-Mathews, J.S. (1996). Effects of pretreatment with ketoprofen and phenylbutazone on experimentally induced synovitis in horses. *American Journal of Veterinary Research* **57**(6), 866–874.

Parker, R., Armstrong, M.J., Corbett, C., Rowe, I.A. and Houlihan, D.D. (2013). Systematic review: pentoxifylline for the treatment of severe alcoholic hepatitis. *Alimentary Pharmacology & Therapeutics* **37**(9), 845–854.

Peiró J.R., Barnabé, P.A., Cadioli, F.A., Cunha, F.Q., Lima, V.M., Mendonça, V.H., Santana, A.E., Malheiros, E.B., Perri, S.H. and Valadão, C.A. (2010). Effects of lidocaine infusion during experimental endotoxemia in horses. *Journal of Veterinary Internal Medicine* **24**(4), 940–948.

Pellegrini-Masini, A., Poppenga, R.H. and Sweeney, R.W. (2004). Disposition of flunixin meglumine injectable preparation administered orally to healthy horses. *Journal of Veterinary Pharmacology and Therapeutics* **27**(3), 183–186.

Peters, L.J. and Kovacic, J.P. (2009). Histamine: metabolism, physiology, and pathophysiology with applications in veterinary medicine. *Journal of Veterinary Emergency and Critical Care* **19**(4), 311–328.

Petersen, A. and Schott, H.C., II. (2009). Effects of dexamethasone and hydroxyzine treatment on intradermal testing and allergen-specific IgE serum testing results in horses [electronic resource]. *Veterinary Dermatology* **20** (5–6), 615–622.

Prugner, W., Huber, R. and Luhmann, R. (1991). Eltenac, a new anti-inflammatory and analgesic drug for horses: clinical aspects. *Journal of Veterinary Pharmacology and Therapeutics* **14**(2), 193–199.

Raidal, S.L., Edwards, S., Pippia, J., Boston, R. and Noble, G.K. (2013). Pharmacokinetics and safety of oral administration of meloxicam to foals. *Journal of Veterinary Internal Medicine* **27**(2), 300–307.

Raulo, S.M., Sorsa, T. and Maisi, P. (2006). *In vitro* inhibition of matrix metalloproteinase activity in tracheal epithelial lining fluid from horses with recurrent airway obstruction. *American Journal of Veterinary Research* **67**(7), 1252–1257.

Reed, S.K., Messer, N.T., Tessman, R.K. and Keegan, K.G. (2006). Effects of phenylbutazone alone or in combination with flunixin meglumine on blood protein concentrations in horses. *American Journal of Veterinary Research* **67**(3), 398–402.

Reeves, M.J., Vansteenhouse, J., Stashak, T.S., Yovich, J.V. and Cockerell, G. (1990). Failure to demonstrate reperfusion injury following ischaemia of the equine large colon using dimethyl sulphoxide. *Equine Veterinary Journal* **22**(2), 126–132.

Renault, A., Gerring, E.L., Baker, S., Hoeijmakers, M., Coert, A. and Valks, M. (2003). Comparative study on the use of vedaprofen and flunixin in an endotoxin-induced ileus model in horses. *Bulletin Société Vétérinaire Pratique de France* **87**(3), 138–144.

Rojer, H. and Aurich, C. (2010). Treatment of persistent mating-induced endometritis in mares with the non-steroid anti-inflammatory drug vedaprofen. *Reproduction in Domestic Animals = Zuchthygiene* **45**(6), e458–e460.

Ross, M.W. (2011). Joint therapy: nonsteroidal anti-inflammatory drugs. *Proceedings* of the 57th Annual Convention of the American Association of Equine Practitioners, San Antonio, Texas, USA, 18–22 November 2011. Lexington, USA, American Association of Equine Practitioners (AAEP).

Sagar, J., Sales, K., Seifalian, A. and Winslet, M. (2010). Doxycycline in mitochondrial mediated pathway of apoptosis: a systematic review. *Anti-Cancer Agents in Medicinal Chemistry* **10**(7), 556–563.

Schatzmann, U., Gugelmann, M., Von Cranach, J., Ludwig, B.M. and Rehm, W.F. (1990). Pharmacodynamic evaluation of the peripheral pain inhibition by carprofen and flunixin in the horse. *Schweizer Archiv für Tierheilkunde* **132**(9), 497–504.

Schleining, J.A. and Reinertson, E.L. (2007a). Evidence for dimethyl sulphoxide (DMSO) use in horses. Part 1: DMSO as a topical and intra-articular anti-inflammatory agent. *Equine Veterinary Education* **19**(10), 545–546.

Schleining, J.A. and Reinertson, E.L. (2007b). Evidence for dimethyl sulphoxide (DMSO) use in horses. Part 2: DMSO as a parenteral anti-inflammatory agent and as a pharmacological carrier. *Equine Veterinary Education* **19**(11), 598–599.

Schleining, J.A., McClure, S.R., Evans, R.B., Hyde, W.G., Wulf, L.W. and Kind, A.J. (2008). Liposome-based diclofenac for the treatment of inflammation in an acute synovitis model in horses. *Journal of Veterinary Pharmacology and Therapeutics* **31**(6), 554–561.

Schuh, J.C.L., Ross, C. and Meschter, C. (1988). Concurrent mercuric blister and dimethyl sulphoxide (DMSO) application as a cause of mercury toxicity in two horses. *Equine Veterinary Journal* **20**(1), 68–71.

Scott, D.W. and Miller, W.H. (2011). *Equine Dermatology*. Maryland Heights, MI, Elsevier Saunders.

Semeco, E., Falcon, J., Fernandez, M., Rodriguez, M., Basalo, A., Munoz, T. and Gonzalez, D. (2006). Efficacy of pentoxifylline in the treatment of exercise-induced pulmonary hemorrhage in Thoroughbred racehorses. *Revista Científica Facultad de Ciencias Veterinarias Universidad del Zulia* **16**(5), 481–491.

Semrad, S.D., Hardee, G.E., Hardee, M.M. and Moore, J.N. (1985). Flunixin meglumine given in small doses: pharmacokinetics and prostaglandin inhibition in healthy horses. *American Journal of Veterinary Research* **46**(12), 2474–2479.

Semrad, S.D., Hardee, G.E., Hardee, M.M. and Moore, J.N. (1987). Low dose flunixin meglumine: effects on eicosanoid production and clinical signs induced by experimental endotoxaemia in horses. *Equine Veterinary Journal* **19**(3), 201–206.

Semrad, S.D., Sams, R.A. and Ashcraft, S.M. (1993). Pharmacokinetics of and serum thromboxane suppression by flunixin meglumine in healthy foals during the first month of life. *American Journal of Veterinary Research* **54**(12), 2083–2087.

Sha, M.C. and Callahan, C.M. (2003). The efficacy of pentoxifylline in the treatment of vascular dementia: a systematic review. *Alzheimer Disease And Associated Disorders* **17**(1), 46–54.

Sinclair, M.D., Taylor, T.S., Bennett, B.S., Peck, K.E., Mealey, K.L. and Matthews, N.S. (2006). Comparative pharmacokinetics of meloxicam in clinically normal horses and donkeys. *American Journal of Veterinary Research* **67**(6), 1082–1085.

Smith, C.L., MacDonald, M.H., Tesch, A.M. and Willits, N.H. (2000). *In vitro* evaluation of the effect of dimethyl sulfoxide on equine articular cartilage matrix metabolism. *Veterinary Surgery* **29**(4), 347–357.

Smith, G., Bertone, A.L., Kaeding, C., Simmons, E.J. and Apostoles, S. (1998). Anti-inflammatory effects of topically applied dimethyl sulfoxide gel on endotoxin-induced synovitis in horses. *American Journal of Veterinary Research* **59**(9), 1149–1152.

Snow, D.H., Baxter, P. and Whiting, B. (1981). The pharmacokinetics of meclofenamic acid in the horse. *Journal of Veterinary Pharmacology and Therapeutics* **4**(2), 147–156.

Soma, L.R., Uboh, C.E., Rudy, J.A. and Perkowski, S.Z. (1995). Plasma and synovial fluid kinetics, disposition, and urinary excretion of naproxen in horses. *American Journal of Veterinary Research* **56**(8), 1075–1080.

Soma, L.R., Uboh, C.E. and Maylin, G.M. (2012). The use of phenylbutazone in the horse. *Journal of Veterinary Pharmacology and Therapeutics* **35**(1), 1–12.

Sullins, K.E., White, N.A., Lundin, C.S., Dabareiner, R. and Gaulin, G. (2004). Prevention of ischaemia-induced small intestinal adhesions in foals. *Equine Veterinary Journal* **36**(5), 370–375.

Symonds, K.D., MacAllister, C.G., Erkert, R.S. and Payton, M.E. (2006). Use of force plate analysis to assess the analgesic effects of etodolac in horses with navicular syndrome. *American Journal of Veterinary Research* **67**(4), 557–561.

Taylor, J.B., Walland, A., Lees, P., Gerring, E.L., Maitho, T.E. and Millar, J.D. (1983). Biochemical and haematological effects of a revised dosage schedule of phenylbutazone in horses. *Veterinary Record* **112**(26), 599–602.

Tobin, T. (1979). The nonsteroidal anti-inflammatory drugs: Equiproxen, meclofenamic acid, flunixine meglumine, and others. *Journal of Equine Medicine and Surgery* **3**, 298–302.

Tobin, T., Chay, S., Kamerling, S., Woods, W.E., Weckman, T.J., Blake, J.W. and Lees, P. (1986). Phenylbutazone in the horse: a review. *Journal of Veterinary Pharmacology and Therapeutics* **9**(1), 1–25.

Tomlinson, J.E. and Blikslager, A.T. (2005). Effects of cyclooxygenase inhibitors flunixin and deracoxib on permeability of ischaemic-injured equine jejunum. *Equine Veterinary Journal* **37**(1), 75–80.

Tomlinson, J.E., Wilder, B.O., Young, K.M. and Blikslager, A.T. (2004). Effects of flunixin meglumine or etodolac treatment on mucosal recovery of equine jejunum after ischemia. *American Journal of Veterinary Research* **65**(6), 761–769.

Toutain, P.L. and Cester, C.C. (2004b). Pharmacokinetic-pharmacodynamic relationships and dose response to meloxicam in horses with induced arthritis in the right carpal joint. *American Journal of Veterinary Research* **65**(11), 1533–1541.

Toutain, P.L., Autefage, A., Legrand, C., and Alvinerie, M. (1994). Plasma concentrations and therapeutic efficacy of phenylbutazone and flunixin meglumine in the horse: pharmacokinetic/pharmacodynamic modelling. *Journal of Veterinary Pharmacology and Therapeutics* **17**(6), 459–469.

Toutain, P.L., Bonnaire, Y., Hirsch, A., Narbe, R., Popot, M.A., Reymond, N., Laroute, V. and Garcia, P. (2004a). Pharmacokinetics of meloxicam in plasma and urine of horses. *American Journal of Veterinary Research* **65**(11), 1542–1547.

Traub-Dargatz, J.L., Bertone, J.J., Gould, D.H., Wrigley, R.H., Weiser, M.G. and Forney, S.D. (1988). Chronic flunixin meglumine therapy in foals. *American Journal of Veterinary Research* **49**(1), 7–12.

Turek, J.J., Templeton, C.B., Bottoms, G.D., and Fessler, J.F. (1985). Flunixin meglumine attenuation of endotoxin-induced damage to the cardiopulmonary vascular endothelium of the pony. *American Journal of Veterinary Research* **46**(3), 591–596.

Vander Werf, K.A., Davis, E.G. and Kukanich, B. (2012). Pharmacokinetics and adverse effects of oral meloxicam tablets in healthy adult horses. *Journal of Veterinary Pharmacology and Therapeutics* **36**(4), 376–381.

Verde, C.R., Simpson, M.I., Frigoli, A. and Landoni, M.F. (2001). Enantiospecific pharmacokinetics of ketoprofen in plasma and synovial fluid of horses with acute synovitis. *Journal of Veterinary Pharmacology and Therapeutics* **24**(3), 179–185.

Villarino, N.F., Vispo, T.J., Marcos, F. and Landoni, M.F. (2006). Inefficacy of topical diclofenac in arthritic horses. *American Journal of Animal and Veterinary Sciences* **1**(1), 8–12.

Vineyard, K.R., Warren, L.K. and Kivipelto, J. (2010). Effect of dietary omega-3 fatty acid source on plasma and red blood cell membrane composition and immune function in yearling horses. *Journal of Animal Science* **88**(1), 248–257.

Watts, A.E., Schnabel, L.V., Papich, M. and Fortier, L.A. (2007). Orally administered sub-antimicrobial doxycycline attains synovial fluid levels capable of inhibiting matrix metalloproteinases 3 and 13. *Proceedings* of the 53rd Annual Convention of the American Association of Equine Practitioners, Orlando, Florida, USA, 1–5 December, 2007, 249–250.

Weiss, D.J., Geor, R.J., Burris, S.M. and Smith, C.M. (1992). Effects of pentoxifylline on equine neutrophil function and flow properties. *Canadian Journal of Veterinary Research* **56**(4), 313–317.

Welch, R.D., Watkins, J.P., DeBowes, M. and Leipold, H.W. (1991). Effects of intra-articular administration of dimethylsulfoxide on chemically induced synovitis in immature horses. *American Journal of Veterinary Research* **52**(6), 934–939.

Welsh, J.C.M., Lees, P., Stodulski, G., Cambridge, H. and Foster, A.P. (1992). Influence of feeding schedule on the absorption of orally administered flunixin in the horse. *Equine Veterinary Journal* **24**, 62–65.

White, S.D. (2005). Advances in equine atopic dermatitis, serologic and intradermal allergy testing. *Clinical Techniques in Equine Practice* **4**(4), 311–313.

Wilcke, J.R., Crisman, M.V., Sams, R.A. and Gerken, D.F. (1993). Pharmacokinetics of phenylbutazone in neonatal foals. *American Journal of Veterinary Research* **54**(12), 2064–2067.

Wilcke, J.R., Crisman, M.V., Scarratt, W.K., and Sams, R.A. (1998). Pharmacokinetics of ketoprofen in healthy foals less than twenty-four hours old. *American Journal of Veterinary Research* **59**(3), 290–292.

Williams, J.M., Lin, Y.J., Loftus, J.P., Faleiros, R.R., Peroni, J.F., Hubbell, J.A.E., Ravis, W.R. and Belknap, J.K. (2010). Effect of intravenous lidocaine administration on laminar inflammation in the black walnut extract model of laminitis. *Equine Veterinary Journal* **42**(3), 261–269.

Wilsher, S., Kölling, M. and Allen, W.R. (2006). Meclofenamic acid extends donor-recipient asynchrony in equine embryo transfer. *Equine Veterinary Journal* **38**(5), 428–432.

Wilson, M.E., Berney, C., Behan, A.L. and Robinson, N.E. (2012). The effect of intravenous lidocaine infusion on bronchoalveolar lavage cytology in equine recurrent airway obstruction. *Journal of Veterinary Internal Medicine* **26**(6), 1427–1432.

Woodward, A.D., Nielsen, B.D., O'Connor, C.I., Skelly, C.D., Webel, S.K. and Orth, M.W. (2007). Supplementation of dietary long-chain polyunsaturated omega-3 fatty acids high in docosahexaenoic acid (DHA) increases plasma DHA concentration and may increase trot stride lengths in horses. *Equine and Comparative Exercise Physiology* **4**(2), 71–78.

Yamaga, T., Tsuzuki, N., Seo, J., Oshita, N., Nakao, S., Tanabe, T. and Sasaki, N. (2012). Effects of cyclooxygenase-2 inhibitor on equine gastric mucosa. *Journal of the Japan Veterinary Medical Association* **65**(8), 597–600.

Yregard, L., Cassuto, J., Tarnow, P. and Nilsson, U. (2003). Influence of local anaesthetics on inflammatory activity postburn. *Burns: Journal of The International Society for Burn Injuries* **29**(4), 335–341.

24 Immunosuppressive Therapy

M. Julia B. Felippe

24.1 Definition

Immunosuppressive therapy becomes necessary when immune-mediated tissue damage is life-threatening or causes organ dysfunction. In general, immunosuppressive therapy affects both the humoral and cellular arms of the immune system. However, a combination of drugs that target different sites of cellular metabolism is often used, not only for effectiveness but also to allow use of doses that are tolerated by the patient. Clinical side-effects and systemic susceptibility to infections, particularly to fungal and viral organisms, are risks in patients under immunosuppressive therapy, so appropriate antimicrobial therapy and clinical monitoring are then advised (Sweeney, 1999; Edington, 1985). In addition, understanding of potential drug interactions is recommended in order to prevent patient morbidity and mortality, particularly when using drugs with narrow therapeutic index or unknown safety and pharmacokinetics in horses.

24.2 Types of immunosuppressive drugs

For the horse patient, few immunosuppressive drugs have been studied and are used clinically, including (Suthanthiran, 1996; Gummert, 1999; Allison, 2000; Barshes, 2004):

(a) inhibitors of gene expression or transcription (e.g., corticosteroids);
(b) inhibitors of nucleotide synthesis (e.g., azathioprine, methotrexate);
(c) alkylating agents (cyclophosphamide, chlorambucil, vincristine);
(d) phosphatase and kinase inhibitors (e.g., cyclosporine A, tacrolimus, rapamycin); and
(e) monoclonal antibodies (e.g., against B cell molecules).

24.2.1 Glucocorticoids

Glucocorticoids are potent anti-inflammatory and immunosuppressive drugs, which are frequently used to treat inflammatory, allergic, autoimmune and neoplastic (lymphoma/lymphosarcoma) diseases, and to prevent allograft rejection in transplantation. Commonly used glucocorticoids in horses include hydrocortisone, dexamethasone, prednisolone, methylprednisolone, isoflupredone, triamcinolone, beclomethasone and fluticasone (Rush, 1998; Giguère, 2002; Robinson, 2002; Picandet, 2003; Laan, 2004, 2006; Courouce-Malblanc, 2008; Dauvillier, 2011; Gray, 2012).

In general, therapeutic doses are high and frequent in the initial phase of treatment, and dosage is subsequently tailored to the clinical condition. Undesirable immunosuppressive effects of glucocorticoids are more likely to occur with prolonged treatment of high doses. Nevertheless, glucocorticoids should be used judiciously in the treatment of primary infectious processes (e.g., bacterial, viral, or protozoal) and in neonates, because of their profound immunosuppressive effect.

Glucocorticoids are lipophilic and pass freely through cell membranes (Ashwell, 2000). They bind to a cytosolic glucocorticoid receptor (GR) present in most cells. This interaction allows the GR transcription factor to translocate into the nucleus, and to have two main outcomes (Scheinman, 1995; Auphan, 1995; De Bosscher, 2000; Franchimont, 2004; Wissink, 1998; Smoak, 2004; Clark, 2008):

(a) bind directly to other transcription factors (e.g., nuclear factor kappa B (NF-kappa B), activator protein-1 (AP-1), and cAMP response element-binding protein (CREB)) to suppress their function (*transrepression*) and decrease synthesis of cytokines, chemokines, inflammatory enzymes, and adhesion molecules; or
(b) bind to gene promoters and activate transcription (*transactivation*), with consequent undesirable side-effects of adrenal suppression, hyperglycemia, polyuria/polydipsia, gastrointestinal ulceration, delayed wound healing, growth suppression, osteoporosis, myopathy, hypertension, and hypokalemia (particularly with isoflupredone).

Other mechanisms have also been described, including increase in the synthesis and function of the NF-kappa B inhibitory protein (ikappa B-alpha), which prevents NF-kappa B translocation into the nucleus, and post-translational effects of decreasing stability of messenger RNA (mRNA)-encoding inflammatory cytokines (Scheinman, 1995; Auphan, 1995). Although there are beneficial and detrimental effects caused by both transrepression and transactivation, many current

Equine Clinical Immunology, First Edition. Edited by M. Julia B. Felippe.
© 2016 John Wiley & Sons, Inc. Published 2016 by John Wiley & Sons, Inc.

studies focus on identifying drugs that selectively inhibit adverse effects without removing anti-inflammatory effects.

As anti-inflammatory drugs in the acute phase of disease, glucocorticoids inhibit vasodilation, vascular permeability, chemotaxis, adhesion molecules, and diapedesis, as all these mechanisms require protein synthesis (Perretti, 2000). The effect on neutrophil phagocytosis and bactericidal activity has been variable, depending on the experimental system used (*in vivo* versus *in vitro*), but it seems dose-dependent (Cox, 1995). The more consistent effect on neutrophils is decreased diapedesis and migration to the site of infection (Herzer, 1980).

Glucocorticoids also decrease degranulation of eosinophils and basophils/mast cells (Andrade, 2004). In antigen-presenting cells (macrophages and dendritic cells), glucocorticoids decrease expression of inflammatory cytokines IL-1, IL-6, and TNF-alpha. In addition, lower expression of major histocompatibility (MHC) class II and IL-12 cytokines decreases antigen-presentation capacity to naïve T cells and the differentiation of Th1 lymphocytes (Visser, 1998; Ashwell, 2000; van de Garde, 2014). The expression of IL-10 seems refractory to treatment, which favors a shift to an anti-inflammatory and Th2 response.

As immunosuppressive drugs, glucocorticoids cause profound T cell lymphopenia via inhibition of proliferation (due to decrease IL-2 expression and signaling), sequestration of CD4$^+$ T lymphocytes in the reticuloendothelial system, impaired release from lymphoid tissues, and induction of apoptosis of immature thymocytes (Palliogiani, 1995). Although T cell receptor signaling, expression of cytokines (particularly IFN-gamma), and production of granzymes are all decreased in Th1 lymphocytes, Th17 cells seem resistant to glucocorticoid effects. The effect of low-to-moderate doses of glucocorticoids is milder on the number of circulating B cells and production of antibodies and, depending on the dose and duration of treatment, this may not significantly affect humoral response to vaccines (Kubiet, 1996).

A single intravenous dose (any of 0.05, 0.1 or 0.2 mg/kg body weight) of dexamethasone to a healthy adult horse has shown to induce neutrophilia and lymphopenia, a decrease in the peripheral blood CD4$^+$ T cell population, with a concomitant increase in the CD8$^+$ T cells, and a consequent decrease of CD4:CD8 ratio. These effects are observed at four and 12 hours after the drug administration, and gradually decrease through time in the first 48 hours (Flaminio, 2007; Figures 24.1 and 24.2). The treatment of heaves-affected horses with inhaled fluticasone at therapeutic dosages for 11 months had no statistically significant detectable effect on innate and adaptive (both humoral and cell-mediated) immune parameters, including response to vaccinations (Dauvillier, 2011). Parenteral, oral and aerosolized corticoids reversibly suppress adrenocortical function, while the response to adrenocorticotropic (ACTH) stimulation remains intact (Rush, 1998; Czock, 2005).

24.2.2 Azathioprine

Azathioprine is a prodrug of 6-mercaptopurine, a purine analog that is incorporated into the DNA of lymphocytes and inhibits *de novo* pathway of purine synthesis. Therefore, it inhibits the synthesis of DNA and RNA and, consequently, lymphocyte activation and proliferation. Azathioprine has been used in horse patients for the treatment of immune-mediated anemia, immune-mediated thrombocytopenia, vasculopathy, and pemphigus foliaceus (Humber, 1991; McGurrin, 2004; Winfield, 2013). The use of azathioprine allows reduction in glucocorticoid dose when the two are combined in therapy. Because proliferation of many cell types can also be inhibited, adverse effects associated with azathioprine treatment include leucopenia (with anemia and thrombocytopenia), alopecia or dermatitis, and hepatotoxicity.

A single intravenous dose (1.5 mg/kg) of azathioprine revealed a rapid decrease in plasma drug concentration with a half-life of 1.8 minutes (White, 2005). Oral bioviability at 3 mg/kg was low, and varied from 1–7%. When given daily for 30 days, and subsequently every other day for another 30 days, that oral dose did not cause clinical adverse effects, and abnormal hemogram, leukogram and serum biochemical analysis in most horses. Lymphopenia and immunosuppression was observed in one horse during the experiment. Therefore, periodic complete blood cell counts and blood biochemistry tests are recommended, in order to monitor severe leukopenia and hepatotoxicity, and allow to decrease of dose when necessary.

24.2.3 Cyclophosphamide and vincristine

Cyclophosphamide (phosphoramide and acrolein) and chlorambucil (phenylacetic acid mustard) metabolites alkylate DNA bases, resulting in mutagenic, cytotoxic, antiproliferative, and chemotherapeutic effects. Cyclophosphamide's effect on B cells promotes its application for the treatment of autoantibody-mediated diseases. In horses, these drugs have been used for the treatment of lymphosarcoma (Saulez, 2004). Adverse effects associated with cyclophosphomide and chlorambucil therapies include anemia, leukopenia, alopecia, and secondary malignancies.

Vincristine is a vinca alkaloid that binds to tubulin in the mitotic spindle and prevents purine synthesis. Consequently, it inhibits cell proliferation, resulting in anti-tumor and immunosuppressive effects. In horses, vincristine has been used for the treatment of immune-mediated thrombocytopenia, pemphigus foliaceous, and lymphosarcoma (Vandenabeele, 2004). Mild neurologic adverse effects (proprioceptive deficits) and ileus may occur in the horse.

24.2.4 Cyclosporine, tacrolimus and rapamycin

Cyclosporine is a hydrophobic cyclic peptide isolated from *Tolypocladium inflatum* fungus. It binds to the cytoplasmic receptor cyclophilin and, subsequently, to the catalytic domain of the cytoplasmic phosphatase calcineurin. This binding results in the inhibition of dephosphorylation of transcription factors, importantly the nuclear factor of activated T lymphocyte (NFAT), which prevents its translocation to the nucleus.

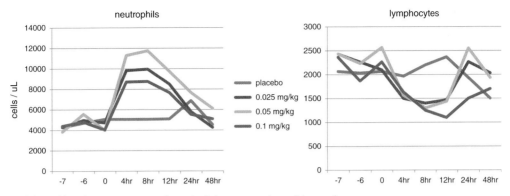

Figure 24.1 Neutrophilia and lymphopenia response after a single intravenous dose of dexamethasone.
Adult healthy horses ($n = 3$ for each treatment) were administered one dose of dexamethasone (0.025, 0.05 or 0.1 mg/kg) or placebo (saline). Complete blood cell counts were obtained on day minus 7 (before moving horses from pasture to a barn for the experiment), on day minus 6 (24 hours after moving the horses), on day 0 (before administration of drug), and at 4, 8, 12, 24 and 48 hours after administration of drug. Note the effect of the dexamethasone for 24 or 48 hours, independent of the dose.

Therefore, the production of key elements of T cell proliferation and activation (IL-2, IL-4, CD40 L, TNF-alpha, IFN-gamma, c-myc) is suppressed. Proto-oncogenes are also inhibited, and cells become arrested in the G0/G1 cell cycle phase (Barshes, 2004).

Cyclosporine has been used in the horse for intravitreal treatment of recurrent uveitis and immune-mediated keratitis (Gilger, 2010). Potential adverse effects of systemic cyclosporine reported in human patients include: vasoconstriction; hypertension; nephrotoxicity (renal failure, hyperkalemia); hepatotoxicity; diarrhea; hyperlipidemia; hyperglycemia (calcineurin inhibitors have toxic effect on the β-cells of the pancreas islets); neurotoxicity (tremors, seizures, coma); hirsutism; and potential susceptibility to infectious organisms that require cell-mediated protection.

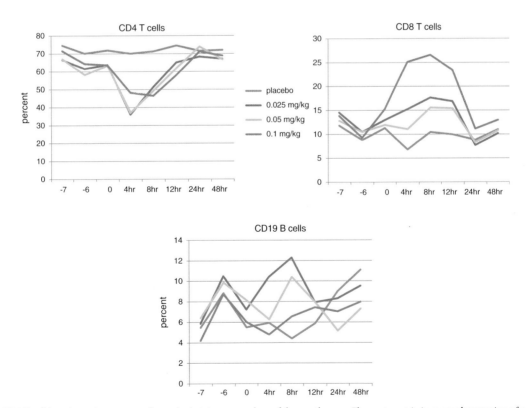

Figure 24.2 CD4 T cell lymphopenia response after a single intravenous dose of dexamethasone. Flow cytometric immunophenotyping of peripheral blood samples from the same horses and at the same time points. Note the marked decrease in CD4 T cell distribution, which lasted 24 hours, independent of the dose. A concomitant increase in the distribution of CD8 T cells and B cells was observed in the same period.

Tacrolimus and rapamycin are macrolide antibiotics that bind to the cytoplasmic FK-binding protein (FK-BP), and the resulting protein complex inhibits calcineurin. The effect includes cell-cycle arrest and decrease in the expression of inflammatory cytokines, similarly to cyclosporine, although tacrolimus is considered to be a more powerful immunosuppressive drug. In the horse, tacrolimus has been used topically for the treatment of hyperkeratosis (Hilton, 2008). Rapamycin ocular toxicity and distribution have been studied for potential clinical use in the horse (Douglas, 2008). Dose-related clinical adverse effects are similar to those promoted by cyclosporine, except hirsutism.

References

Allison, A.C. (2000). Immunosuppressive drugs: the first 50 years and a glance forward. *Immunopharmacology* 47, 63–83.

Andrade, M.V., Hiragun, T. and Beaven, M.A. (2004). Dexamethasone suppresses antigen-induced activation of phosphatidylinositol 3-kinase and downstream responses in mast cells. *Journal of Immunology* 172, 7254.

Ashwell, J.D., Lu, F.W. and Vacchio, M.S. (2000). Glucocorticoids in T cell development and function. *Annual Review of Immunology* 18, 309.

Auphan, N., DiDonato, J.A., Rosette, C., et al. (1995). Immunosuppression by glucocorticoids: inhibition of NF-kappa B activity through induction of I kappa B synthesis. *Science* 270, 286.

Barshes, N.R., Goodpastor, S.E. and Goss, J.A. (2004). Pharmacologic immunosuppression. *Frontiers in Bioscience* 9, 411–20.

Clark, A.R., Martins, J.R. and Tchen, C.R. (2008). Role of dual specificity phosphatases in biological responses to glucocorticoids. *Journal of Biological Chemistry* 283(38), 25765–9.

Couroucé-Malblanc, A., Fortier, G., Pronost, S., Siliart, B. and Brachet, G. (2008). Comparison of prednisolone and dexamethasone effects in the presence of environmental control in heaves-affected horses. *The Veterinary Journal* 175(2), 227–33.

Cox, G. (1995). Glucocorticoid treatment inhibits apoptosis in human neutrophils. Separation of survival and activation outcomes. *Journal of Immunology* 154, 4719.

Czock, D., Keller, F., Rasche, F.M. et al. (2005). Pharmacokinetics and pharmacodynamics of systemically administered glucocorticoids. *Clinical Pharmacokinetics* 44, 61–98.

Dauvillier, J., Felippe, M.J., Lunn, D.P., Lavoie-Lamoureux, A., Leclère, M., Beauchamp, G. and Lavoie, J.P. (2011). Effect of long-term fluticasone treatment on immune function in horses with heaves. *Journal of Veterinary Internal Medicine* 25(3), 549–57.

De Bosscher, K., Vanden Berghe, W. and Haegeman, G. (2000). Mechanisms of anti-inflammatory action and of immunosuppression by glucocorticoids: negative interference of activated glucocorticoid receptor with transcription factors. *Journal of Neuroimmunology* 109, 16–22.

Douglas, L.C., Yi, N.Y. and Davis, J.L. (2008). Ocular toxicity and distribution of subconjunctival and intravitreal rapamycin in horses. *Journal of Veterinary Pharmacology and Therapeutics* 31, 511–6.

Edington, N., Bridges, C.G. and Huckle, A. (1985). Experimental reactivation of equid herpesvirus 1 (EHV 1) following the administration of corticosteroids. *Equine Veterinary Journal* 17, 369–72.

Flaminio, M.J.B.F., Tallmadge, R.L., Secor, E.J., et al. (2007). The effect of glucocorticoid therapy in the immune system of the horse. Proceedings 8th International Veterinary Immunology Symposium (IVIS), August 15–19, 2007, Ouro Preto, Brazil, pp. 144.

Franchimont, D. (2004). Overview of the actions of glucocorticoids on the immune response: a good model to characterize new pathways of immunosuppression for new treatment strategies. *Annals of the New York Academy of Sciences* 1024, 124–37.

Giguère, S., Viel, L., Lee, E., MacKay, R.J., Hernandez, J. and Franchini, M. (2002). Cytokine induction in pulmonary airways of horses with heaves and effect of therapy with inhaled fluticasone propionate. *Veterinary Immunology and Immunopathology* 85(3–4), 147–58.

Gilger, B.C., Wilkie, D.A., Clode, A.B. et al. (2010). Long-term outcome after implantation of a suprachoroidal cyclosporine drug delivery device in horses with recurrent uveitis. *Veterinary Ophthalmology* 13, 294–300.

Gray, B.P., Biddle, S., Pearce, C.M. et al. (2012). Detection of fluticasone propionate in horse plasma and urine following inhaled administration. *Drug Testing and Analysis* [Epub ahead of print].

Gummert, J.F., Ikonen, T. and Morris, R.E. (1999). Newer immunosuppressive drugs: a review. *Journal of the American Society of Nephrology* 10, 1366–80.

Herzer, P. and Lemmel, E.M. (1980). Inhibition of granulocyte function by prednisolone and non-steroid anti-inflammatory drugs. Quantitative evaluation with NBT test and its correlation with phagocytosis. *Immunobiology* 157, 78.

Hilton, H., Affolter, V.K. and White, S.D. (2008). Evaluation of four topical preparations for the treatment of cannon hyperkeratosis in a horse. *Veterinary Dermatology* 19(6), 385–90.

Humber, K.A., Beech, J., Cudd, T.A. et al. (1991). Azathioprine for treatment of immune-mediated thrombocytopenia in two horses. *Journal of the American Veterinary Medical Association* 199, 591–4.

Kubiet, M.A., Gonzalez-Rothi, R.J., Cottey, R. and Bender, B.S. (1996). Serum antibody response to influenza vaccine in pulmonary patients receiving corticosteroids. *Chest* 110, 367.

Laan T.T., Westermann, C.M., Dijkstra, A.V. et al. (2004). Biological availability of inhaled fluticasone propionate in horses. *Veterinary Record* 155, 361–4.

Laan, T.T., Bull, S., van Nieuwstadt, R.A., et al. (2006). The effect of aerosolized and intravenously administered clenbuterol and aerosolized fluticasone propionate on horses challenged with Aspergillus fumigatus antigen. *Veterinary Research Communications* 30, 623–35.

McGurrin, M.K., Arroyo, L.G. and Bienzle, D. (2004). Flow cytometric detection of platelet-bound antibody in three horses with immune-mediated thrombocytopenia. *Journal of the American Veterinary Medical Association* 224(1), 83–7, 53.

Paliogianni, F., Hama, N., Balow, J.E., Valentine, M.A. and Boumpas, D.T. (1995). Glucocorticoid-mediated regulation of protein phosphorylation in primary human T cells. Evidence for induction of phosphatase activity. *Journal of Immunology* 155(4), 1809–17.

Perretti, M. and Ahluwalia, A. (2000). The microcirculation and inflammation: site of action for glucocorticoids. *Microcirculation* 7(3), 147–61.

Picandet, V., Léguillette, R. and Lavoie, J.P. (2003). Comparison of efficacy and tolerability of isoflupredone and dexamethasone in the treatment of horses affected with recurrent airway obstruction ('heaves'). Equine. *The Veterinary Journal* 35(4), 419–24.

Robinson, N.E., Jackson, C., Jefcoat, A. *et al.* (2002). Efficacy of three corticosteroids for the treatment of heaves, Equine. *The Veterinary Journal* 34, 17–22.

Rush, B.R., Worster, A.A., Flaminio, M.J., Matson, C.J. and Hakala, J.E. (1998). Alteration in adrenocortical function in horses with recurrent airway obstruction after aerosol and parenteral administration of beclomethasone dipropionate and dexamethasone, respectively. *American Journal of Veterinary Research* 59(8), 1044–7.

Saulez, M.N., Schlipf, J.W. Jr., Cebra, C.K. *et al.* (2004). Use of chemotherapy for treatment of a mixed-cell thoracic lymphoma in a horse. *Journal of the American Veterinary Medical Association* 224, 733.

Scheinman, R.I., Cogswell, P.C., Lofquist, A.K. and Baldwin, A.S. Jr. (1995). Role of transcriptional activation of I kappa B alpha in mediation of immunosuppression by glucocorticoids. *Science* 270, 283.

Smoak, K.A. and Cidlowski, J.A. (2004). Mechanisms of glucocorticoid receptor signaling during inflammation. *Mechanisms of Ageing and Development* 125(10–11), 697–706.

Suthanthiran, M., Morris, R.E. and Strom, T.B. (1996). Immunosuppressants: cellular and molecular mechanisms of action. *American Journal of Kidney Diseases* 28, 159–72.

Sweeney, C.R. and Habecker, P.L. (1999). Pulmonary aspergillosis in horses: 29 cases (1974–1997). *Journal of the American Veterinary Medical Association* 214, 808–11.

van de Garde, M.D., Martinez, F.O., Melgert, B.N. *et al.* (2014). Chronic exposure to glucocorticoids shapes gene expression and modulates innate and adaptive activation pathways in macrophages with distinct changes in leukocyte attraction. *Journal of Immunology* 192, 1196.

Vandenabeele, S.I., White, S.D., Affolter, V.K. *et al.* (2004). Pemphigus foliaceus in the horse: a retrospective study of 20 cases. *Veterinary Dermatology* 15, 381–8.

van der Burg, B., Liden, J., Okret, S., Delaunay, F., Wissink, S., van der Saag, P.T. and Gustafsson, J.A. (1997). Nuclear factor-kappa B repression in antiinflammation and immunosuppression by glucocorticoids. *Trends in Endocrinology and Metabolism* 8(4), 152–7.

Visser, J., van Boxel-Dezaire, A., Methorst, D. *et al.* (1998). Differential regulation of interleukin-10 (IL-10) and IL-12 by glucocorticoids *in vitro*. *Blood* 91, 4255.

White, S.D., Maxwell, L.K., Szabo, N.J. *et al.* (2005). Pharmacokinetics of azathioprine following single-dose intravenous and oral administration and effects of azathioprine following chronic administration in horses. *American Journal of Veterinary Research* 66, 1578–83.

Winfield, L.D., White, S.D., Affolter, V.K., Renier, A.C., Dawson, D., Olivry, T., Outerbridge, C.A., Wang, Y.H., Iyori, K. and Nishifuji, K. (2013). Pemphigus vulgaris in a Welsh pony stallion: case report and demonstration of antidesmoglein autoantibodies. *Veterinary Dermatology* 24(2), 269–e60.

Wissink, S., van Heerde, E.C., vand der Burg, B. and van der Saag, P.T. (1998). A dual mechanism mediates repression of NF-kappaB activity by glucocorticoids. *Molecular Endocrinology* 12(3), 355–63.

25.1 Definition

Immunostimulant therapy is a common protocol selected for equine patients when the therapeutic goal is non antigen-specific enhancement of endogenous immunity (Figure 25.1). Immune stimulation may be used in a prophylactic manner, prior to pathogen challenge or a stressful situation that may compromise endogenous immunity, such as weaning or long-distance transport. In other settings, immunostimulant therapy is used concurrently with antimicrobial therapy to further enhance endogenous immune clearance mechanisms (i.e., in combination with targeted pathogen treatment to effectively clear pathogens). Immunostimulant preparations should be selected on the basis of demonstrated efficacy and safety in horses (Table 25.1).

25.2 Immunologic mechanisms

Innate immunity allows the host to destroy invading pathogens rapidly. This activity does not depend on memory, nor does it provide antigenic specificity, yet it distinguishes *self* from *nonself* antigens, based on host detection of classes of pathogens. Innate immunity typically not only provides immediate immune activation, but also serves as a bridge to activation of adaptive responses via antigen presenting cells (APCs). Immediate innate responses rely on germline-encoded pattern recognition receptors (PRR) expressed by a variety of cells that render immune protection to the host, both vertebrate and invertebrate.

Evolutionary conservation has ensured that similar innate components are expressed in some plant, invertebrate and mammalian species. Studies performed in the fruit fly *Drosophila* spp. illustrate the importance of the Toll receptor, a conserved surface-expressed PRR. Following exposure of *Drosophila* to bacteria or purified LPS, cell signaling is induced, yielding nuclear translocation of the nuclear factor NF-kappa B. Activation of this signaling pathway enhances gene transcription for inflammatory mediators and antimicrobial factors. In contrast, Toll receptor-deficient flies lack the ability to kill fungi, leading to the insect's demise. Subsequent reports involving the

elucidation of NF-kappa B signaling have described similar patterns of activation in mammalian hosts, and the discovery of Toll-like receptors (TLRs).

A list of pattern recognition receptors includes mannose receptor, CD14, peptidoglycan recognition protein (PGRP), scavenger receptors (SR), TLRs, and nucleotide oligomerization domain/caspase recruitment domain (NOD/CARD). Certain inflammatory responses are triggered when pathogen-associated molecular patterns (PAMPs) bind to host cell receptors. Pattern recognition receptors that recognize PAMPs are expressed by various leukocyte and epithelial subsets on the cell membrane, or intracellularly, to maintain effective barriers of protection against different types of invading microorganisms.

TLRs are involved in innate immunity and recognize microbial, viral, and fungal conserved structures. While many TLRs are type 1 transmembrane receptors, and recognize extracellular organisms, many are strategically placed intracellularly. For example, Toll-like recptor-9 (TLR-9) recognizes unmethylated CpG-containing DNA motifs, frequently found in the genome of intracellular bacteria and viruses but not vertebrates. Toll-like receptor-7 (TLR-7), also intracellular, recognizes small synthetic immune modifiers, including imiquimod, R-848, loxoribine, and bropirimine, all of which are already applied or promising for clinical use against viral infections and cancers. Plasmacytoid dendritic cells express TLR-7 and TLR-9, and respond to TLR-7 and TLR-9 ligands by producing a large amount of interferon (IFN)-alpha.

Stimulation of TLRs by pathogen-derived compounds leads to activation of APCs, which facilitate the induction of protective acquired immunity. This phenomenon is the basis of most adjuvant formulations currently in development (Figure 25.2). The ability of TLR-3, TLR-5, TLR-7 and TLR-9 signaling to enhance cytotoxic T cell (CTL) responses has been well established. For example, upon vaccination with virus-like particles, it has been shown that stimulation of TLR-2 and TLR-4 failed to increase CTL response, whereas ligands for TLR-3, TLR-5, TLR-7 or TLR-9 exhibited significant adjuvant function. Consequently, each type of immunostimulant has an immune outcome depending on its structure (PAMPs) and the receptors (PRR) that they bind to for cell signaling activation.

Equine Clinical Immunology, First Edition. Edited by M. Julia B. Felippe.
© 2016 John Wiley & Sons, Inc. Published 2016 by John Wiley & Sons, Inc.

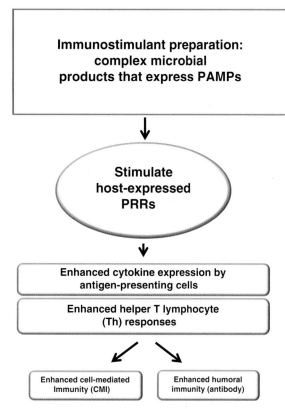

Immunostimulant preparation: complex microbial products that express PAMPs

↓

Stimulate host-expressed PRRs

↓

Enhanced cytokine expression by antigen-presenting cells

Enhanced helper T lymphocyte (Th) responses

Enhanced cell-mediated Immunity (CMI) **Enhanced humoral immunity (antibody)**

Figure 25.1 General mechanism of action of immunostimulants. Activation of the immune system of the equine host starts with detection of pathogen-associated molecular pattern (PAMP) in immunostimulant preparations.

25.3 Commercially available immunostimulants for use in horses

25.3.1 Inactivated Parapoxvirus ovis

Parapoxvirus ovis (Orf virus) is a double-stranded DNA virus member of the *Poxviridie* family. This zoonotic virus is associated with the induction of skin lesions in small ruminants. *Parapoxvirus ovis* was selected as an immunomodulator, based on the fact that this poxvirus induced immunomodulatory proteins that support viral replication in the presence of a marked host immune response (Figure 25.3). Immunomodulator proteins expressed by PPVO include granulocyte-monocyte colony stimulating factor (GM-CSF) inhibitor factor (GIF), interleukin IL-2, and a viral homologue of IL-10. Interleukin-10 is a cytokine recognized with immunesuppressive activates, particularly with regard to the down-regulation of Th1 immune responses. The collective effect from this response is immune activation via IL-2, while tissue destruction is minimized via IL-10 and GIF.

Additional immunologic evidence to support the favorable immune benefits induced by PPVO include the activation of APCs with up-regulation of inflammatory cytokines IL-6, IL-8, TNF-alpha, and Th1 response-inducing cytokines IL-12 and IL-18. In addition, it activates T lymphocyte expression of IL-2, IFN-alpha/beta and IFN-gamma (Fachinger, 2000). Immunomodulatory activity of PPVO has been demonstrated to be maintained following viral inactivation, making this an appropriate agent to induce host-protective mechanisms. Original experimental evidence to support the efficacy of inactivated-PPVO (iPPVO) as an immunostimulant agent *in vivo* came from murine experimental models, in which *P. ovis* resulted in

Table 25.1 Immunostimulant preparations used in equine medicine.

Immunostimulant		Trade name	Label	Indications for use	Treatment protocol
Parapoxvirus ovis	Inactivated Pox virus family APC activation	Zylexis® (Zoetis)	Equine	Upper respiratory disease EHV-1/4	2 mL IM Days 0, 2 and 9
Propionibacterium acnes	Inactivated bacteria TLR9 agonist APC activation	EqStim® (Neogen)	Equine	Respiratory disease complex	1 mL/250 lbs IV Days 0, 3 and 5
Mycobacterial cell wall extract	Mycobacterial cell wall extract APC activation	Settle® (Bioniche) Equimune IV® (Bioniche)	Equine ⫼Equine	Post breeding endometritis Respiratory disease complex	1.5 mL IV once ⫼1.5 mL IV once
Granulocyte-colony stimulating factor	Bone marrow stimulation	Neupogen	Human	Neonatal sepsis, alloimmune neutropenia, neutropenia	6 mcg/kg SC once consider co-administration NSAID for bone pain
Interferon alpha	IFN-alpha2b	Intron A	Human	Non-mast cell or eosinophil lower airway inflammation	0.22–2.0 IU/kg sublingual SID 5–10 days
Imiquimod	TLR-7 agonist	Aldera	Human	Aural plaques, sarcoid, papilloma	Topical administration

APC – antigen presenting cells; TLR – toll-like receptor; IFN – interferon; IU – international units; IV – intravenous; IM – intramuscular; SC – subcutaneous; lbs – pounds body weight; SID – *semel in die* or once a day.

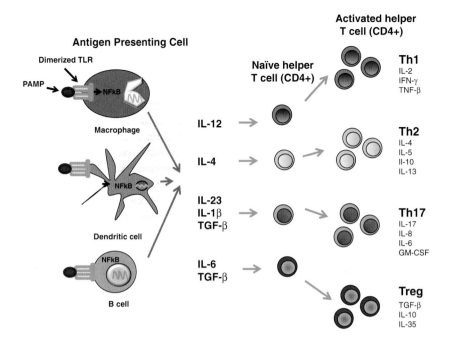

Figure 25.2 Antigen presenting cells detect the presence of immunostimulants and initiate immune response. Pattern-recognition receptor (PRR) interaction with pathogen-associated molecular patterns (PAMPs) induces activation of antigen-presenting cells with cytokine expression. Depending on the type of PRR involved and, consequently, cytokine expressed, T cells may differentiate into a variety of subsets. Therefore, both innate, humoral and cell-mediated immunity outcomes are associated with the type of PAMP involved.

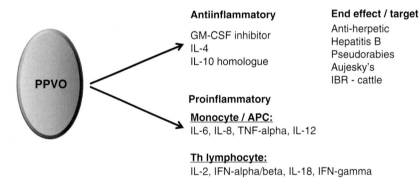

Figure 25.3 Example of an immunostimulant preparation. Inactivated Parapoxvirus ovis (iPPVO) is a commercially available immunostimulant for use in equine patients. iPPVO induces expression of inflammatory (e.g., IL-12, TNF-alpha), as well as immunosuppressive (e.g., IL-10) cytokines that induce immunomodulatory outcomes.

herpes-viral clearance, in a severe infection challenge (Weber, 2003).

Inactivated PPVO is marketed for horses as Zylexis (Zoetis Animal Health, Inc.), and indicated for enhanced immunity before an stressful event or during disease, aimed at the resolution of respiratory disorders caused by viral respiratory pathogens, particularly equine herpes virus-1 (EHV-1) and EHV-4. Treatment recommendations include a 2 mL intramuscular injection on days 0 (before the stressful event), 2 and 9, or similar three-dose series treatment during a disease episode.

Immunologic evidence to support the use of iPPVO in horses includes an investigation that demonstrated enhanced peripheral blood mononuclear cell (PBMC) cytokine expression in healthy yearlings treated with iPPVO compared with saline-treated horses (Horohov, 2008). Enhanced phagocytosis and oxidative burst activity of foal neutrophils has also been demonstrated following systemic administration of a three-dose series iPPVO. Moreover, iPPVO has been tested as an immunostimulant in young foals for the prevention of *Rhodococcus equi* pyogranulomatous pneumona and enteritis. Although the exact etiopathogenesis continues to be investigated, a key immunologic risk factor for disease development is the fact that foals are IFN-gamma deficient early in life (Breathnach, 2006). Therapeutic strategies aimed at enhancing expression of this key cytokine may provide an immunologic advantage, perhaps similar to a protective Th1/IFN-gamma expression profile developed for adult horses.

Administration of a three-dose series of PPVO resulted in monocyte-derived dendritic cells to express IL-12p40 and TNF-alpha when cultured *ex vivo* (Ryan, 2010). The efficacy of iPPVO immunostimulant therapy was tested in a separate randomized trial that evaluated 28 foals treated with iPPVO, and 31 control foals administered with placebo (Sturgill, 2011). Immunostimulant therapy was initiated on the first day of life, followed by a second dose at 24 hours, and a final dose at nine days following the initial dose. When the foals were evaluated at one and two weeks old, treatment foals PBMC had a higher level of IFN-gamma expression, compared with control foals. However, when foals were prospectively evaluated twice weekly for three months for the development of pneumonia, disease manifestation was similar among the two groups. These findings were consistent with a separate study that failed to demonstrate an increase of IFN-gamma expression in foals that received iPPVO in the immediate post-natal period (Ryan, 2010).

These data suggest that, although IFN-gamma may be upregulated following immunostimulant therapy, there is not a universal response in all foals. In addition, even if IFN-gamma is upregulated in some foals, these foals may remain susceptible to infection, supporting the fact that disease manifestation is truly multifactorial, and not simply a result of IFN-gamma deficiency.

Overall, the use of iPPVO in horses appears to be safe, and may provide some benefit with regard to improved recovery from respiratory disease. It is likely that the predominant cytokine response that provides host-protective mechanisms is IFN-gamma expression. Although this preparation is not protective in neonatal foals exposed to R. equi challenge, there is an apparent shift in cytokine expression following immunostimulant administration. This cytokine shift is believed to provide an immunologic advantage through the combination of anti-viral and cytokine inducing mechanisms.

25.3.2 Propionibacterium acnes extract

Propionibacterium acnes is a commensal bacterium among skin microbiota in healthy individuals. Previous nomenclature for this organism was Corynebacterium parvum. Propionibacterium acnes provides pronounced immunomodulatory activity that has been recognized for more than three decades. The DNA sequence of P. acnes contains repetitive unmethylated CpG motifs that are, in part, responsible for its immunostimulatory activity through TLR9 binding (Figure 25.2). Immune activation induced by P. acnes involves both TLR9-dependent and -independent mechanisms, which result in global systemic immune activation (Tchaptchet, 2012).

When administered systemically, P. acnes is taken up by splenic macrophages, Kupffer cells and pulmonary intravascular macrophages. The organism is retained in the cytoplasmic space with a delay in degradation, providing prolonged immune system exposure. In laboratory animals, administration of P. acnes stimulates macrophage function, natural killer cytotoxicity, cytokine production (IL-1, IFN-gamma), and prophylactic protection against lethal bacterial challenge. Stimulation of systemic immunity has been observed in laboratory animals for up to five days after intravenous or intraperitoneal

administration, although prolonged immunostimulant activity has not been demonstrated.

In equine medicine, inactivated Propionibacterium acnes, marketed as EqStim® (Neogen, Inc.), is recommended for treatment of chronic, exudative respiratory disease that is unresponsive to conventional antibiotic treatment. In addition, it is recommended for prophylactic administration prior to stressful events that may impair pulmonary defense mechanisms, including weaning and long-distance transport. EqStim® is prepared as suspension in 12.5% ethanol in saline, and the product requires shaking to ensure that a uniform suspension is collected. EqStim® is administered as an intravenous dose of 1 mL/113 kg (or 250 lbs), with administration on days 1, 3 (or 4) and 7.

Evidence to support the use of P. acnes in equine patients comes from increased distribution of T helper and cytotoxic lymphocyte populations, function via IL-2-induced cellular cytotoxicity, and non-opsonized phagocytic activity when P. acnes was administered to healthy, yearling horses using the three-dose protocol. Although other hematologic changes were not observed in horses following P. acnes administration, cellularity of bronchoalveolar lavage fluid (BALF) was reduced, and was characterized by a reduction in BALF lymphocytes. Reduced lymphocyte counts were attributed to result from margination of pulmonary lymphocytes into regional lymphoid tissues, or resolution of sub-clinical pulmonary infection (Flaminio, 1998). Subsequent work to support the immune-stimulating capability of P. acnes administration demonstrated enhanced PBMC IFN-gamma and host defense peptide expression (Davis, 2003).

An independent investigation aimed at determining the benefits of inactivated P. acnes in the treatment of adult horses with naturally occurring equine respiratory disease. Inactivated P. acnes was administered, as an adjunct to conventional therapy, for the treatment of equine infectious respiratory disease complex. Horses were enrolled based on clinical evidence of infectious respiratory disease, randomized with treatment to include three doses of P. acnes, administered intravenously on days 1, 3 (or 4), and 7, based on enrollment into the investigation (Evans, 1988). Control horses were similarly enrolled, and received conventional standard of care therapy and placebo (drug carrier 12.5% ethanol in saline solution). At 14 days post-enrollment, there was a clinical improvement or complete recovery from clinical disease in 100% (28/28) of the cases that received P. acnes, whereas 67% (10/15) of the control group demonstrated improvement or complete recovery ($p = 0.006$).

In a later, but similarly designed investigation, 45 horses were randomly assigned to treatment for respiratory disease that included conventional therapy with or without the administration of three doses of P. acnes, using the recommended protocol (Vail, 1990). In this randomized, controlled, blinded investigation, 96% (24/25) of the horses that received conventional therapy with P. acnes demonstrated clinical recovery or improvement of clinical signs whereas, among the control group, 35% (7/20) of the horses demonstrated an improvement or recovery from respiratory disease.

When combined, data from these two investigations provide evidence that 98% (52/53) of the horses that received *P. acnes* with conventional therapy improved or recovered from clinical respiratory disease, while 49% (17/35) of the horses that received control treatment with conventional therapy for respiratory disease recovered or improved over 14 days of evaluation.

Additional evidence to support the use of *P. acnes* as an immunostimulant in horses prior to long-distance transport is brought by an investigation that evaluated 450 horses transported distances ranging from 390 miles to 2300 miles (Nestved, 1996). However, one difference in this investigation was that horses received one or two doses of *P. acnes*, rather than the three-dose series. Among the transported horses, 217 received *P. acnes* prior to transport, while control horses did not receive any pre-treatment. Overall, among the horses that received pre-treatment with *P. acnes*, 81.5% (177/217) of the horses did not have clinical evidence of respiratory disease seven days following transportation, while the control group included only 39% (91/233) that were free from clinical evidence of respiratory disease seven days following long-distance transport (Nestved, 1996). Collectively, the experimental evidence supports the use of inactivated *P. acnes* as an immunostimulant, and as an adjunct in the treatment of adult horses with respiratory disease, or as an immunostimulant in adult horses prior to long-distance transport.

The potential for *P. acnes* effectiveness in young foals that were at risk for the development of *R. equi* pneumonia and enteritis was also investigated. Foals were treated after birth and at 30 days old with a three-dose series of intravenous *P. acnes*, and PBMCs were examined for IFN-gamma expression (Sturgill, 2011). Although there was not a significant increase in IFN-gamma expression after the initial series at birth, there was an apparent increase in cytokine expression following a second series initiated at 28 days old. Induction of IFN-gamma expression at 1 month old unlikely provides timely protection in all foals that encounter virulent *R. equi* earlier than this period. Nevertheless, these results suggest plasticity of the foal immune response by 30 days of life that may allow for immunomodulatory therapy.

An additional study compared the efficacy of two commercially available immunostimulant preparations in young foals. Inactivated *P. acnes*, inactivated *Parapoxvirus ovis* or placebo were administered at one week old, according to label recommendations, and subsequently compared for their ability to induce bactericidal activity in foal leukocytes *ex vivo*. There was a reduced *R. equi* proliferation within monocyte-derived macrophages collected on study day 12, when compared with control foals, but there was no difference when compared with iPPVO treated foals (Ryan, 2010).

Neutrophil phagocytosis and oxidative burst activity were increased in the iPPVO treated foals on study days 12 and 24, compared with baseline values, and foals treated with iPPVO had increased phagocytosis and oxidative burst activity on day 24 when compared with *P. acnes* treated foals. Foals treated with iPPVO also demonstrated increased TNF-alpha expression in monocyte-derived macrophages, and increased BALF IL-12 p40 expression when compared with control foals. Treatment with *P. acnes* resulted in an increase in leukocyte IL-10 expression on day 24, when compared with control foals or those that received iPPVO. Despite the valuable understanding of immunomodulatory effects of these commercially available products, there is no evidence to date of effectiveness of a product that significantly alters the frequency of *R. equi* pneumonia in foals.

There are numerous anatomic and physiologic factors that lead to persistent uterine inflammation and fluid retention in mares. In addition, impaired neutrophil function has been suggested as a contributing condition for disease susceptibility (Troedsson, 1993), and the efficacy of *P. acnes* administration in mares with endometritis was evaluated. When *P. acnes* was administered on days 1, 3 and 7, following the cytologic confirmation of uterine inflammation, there was a significant improvement of uterine inflammation in treated mares (Zingher, 1996).

In a separate double-blinded investigation that involved the administration of *P. acnes* in combination with standard of care therapy, an increased pregnancy rate was observed. In the mares that conceived and maintained pregnancy, the optimal effect was detected when mares were bred within eight days after the first *P. acnes* treatment (Rohrbach, 2007).

25.3.3 Mycobacterial cell wall extract

Mycobacterial products are potent stimulators of nonspecific immunity. The bacillus Calmette-Guerin (BCG) vaccine was developed from a strain of *Mycobacterium bovis* attenuated through serial passage in culture. Live BCG, whole-inactivated BCG, and mycobacterial cell wall fractions, have been used as non-specific immunostimulant agents, and all three preparations demonstrate adjuvant activity when administered with antigen. Currently marketed preparations include *Mycobacterium phlei* cell wall extract (MCWE). Whole, inactivated BCG preparations induce tuberculin sensitivity, so deproteinized mycobacterial cell wall products (muramyl dipeptide and lipoarabinomannan) have been developed to prevent induction of tuberculin positivity in treated animals.

Purified muramyl dipeptides are the smallest subunit of the mycobacterial cell wall that retains immunostimulant activity. In equine medicine, mycobacterial cell wall products are used to treat infectious respiratory disease (Equimune IV®, Bioniche Animal Health Inc.), and post-breeding endometritis (Settle® Bioniche Animal Health Inc.). Dosing recommendations are for a single intravenous injection (1.5 mL) at the time of desired immune stimulation.

In a recent investigation, MCWE was tested for the ability to reduce post-breeding inflammation in mares (Fumuso, 2003). Mares were classified as resistant or susceptible to post-breeding endometritis. Susceptible mares demonstrated an increased inflammatory cytokine profile, represented by increased IL-1beta, IL-6 and TNF-alpha in endometrial tissues that were collected during estrus. When susceptible mares received MCWE at the time of breeding, there was a significant reduction in IL-1beta expression, with a trend for reduced IL-6 expression. Collectively, the data generated in this study suggest that, when susceptible mares are treated with MCWE at the time of breeding, reduced inflammation may allow these mares to have reproductive capacity that is more similar to resistant mares.

In human patients, an effective therapeutic strategy for the management of certain forms of bladder cancer is the intravesical instillation of BCG. Instillation of live or attenuated BCG organisms into the bladder prevents recurrence or progression of non-muscle-invasive bladder tumors. Attenuation through heat inactivation appears to reduce the anti-tumor activity of this therapy. Depending on the stage of disease, BCG therapy is sometimes used independently, or in combination with chemotherapeutic agents. Stimulation of both local and systemic immune function has been documented after intravesical BCG therapy in patients with urinary bladder carcinoma.

Suspected adverse pulmonary reactions to intravenous purified mycobacterial cell wall extract have been reported in humans and horses. In horses, adverse reactions have occurred after multiple intravenous administrations of the product. Pulmonary lesions include multifocal granulomatous pneumonitis, bronchiolitis, and progressive pulmonary fibrosis, with clinical signs of cough, fever, tachypnea, lethargy, and leukocytosis. A similar adverse pulmonary reaction (interstitial pneumonitis with disseminated pulmonary granulomas) occurs in approximately 1% of human patients after intravesical BCG therapy. Pulmonary lesions are suspected to result from either a pulmonary hypersensitivity reaction against the BCG protein component, or BCG mycobacteremia resulting in pulmonary infection. Mycobacterial organisms are rarely recovered from the pulmonary lesions. Therefore, hypersensitivity reaction is considered to be the origin of these pulmonary lesions.

25.3.4 Interferon-alpha

Interferon-alpha (IFN-alpha) is an naturally occurring cytokine protein that demonstrates antiviral, immunomodulatory, and antiproliferative properties (Moore, 1997, 2004). In a murine model, exogenously administered IFN-alpha stimulates subsequent additional lymphocyte IFN-alpha expression, as well as Th1 cellular activation that enhances natural killer cell cytotoxicity, macrophage activation, and cytokine production. Interferon-alpha suppresses B cell proliferation, differentiation, and immunoglobulin production, and inhibits delayed-type hypersensitivity reactions.

Oral administration of IFN-alpha reduces inflammation in the lower respiratory tract of racehorses with inflammatory airway disease (IAD), characterized by a high BALF total cell count and neutrophilia (approximately 15%). Low-dose (50–150 IU), natural, human IFN-alpha reduces exudate in the respiratory tract, lowers total cell counts in BALF, and converts the differential cell count to a non-inflammatory cytologic profile (Moore, 1993). Interferon-alpha administration is not indicated, or effective, in horses with mast cell-rich or eosinophilic BALF. In addition, IFN-alpha is not beneficial in the treatment of acute, fulminant viral respiratory infection in horses. Oral administration of low-dose (0.2–2.2 IU/kg) recombinant IFN-alpha-2a does not diminish the severity of clinical disease or duration of viral shedding in horses with experimental equine herpes virus-1 infection.

The pathway for dissemination of the biologic effects of IFN-alpha, following oral administration, does not occur via small intestinal absorption and peripheral circulation of the cytokine, since this protein is degraded by digestive enzymes and cannot be detected in peripheral blood after enteral administration. It is hypothesized that oropharyngeal-associated lymphoid tissue is recruited to antiviral activity by orally administered IFN-alpha. Local lymphocytes exposed to IFN-alpha secrete more IFN-alpha, and transfer antiviral activity to naive lymphocytes. Recruited lymphocytes then enter systemic circulation and confer antiviral capability to cells at distant sites (e.g., the surface of the respiratory tract, gastrointestinal tract, and eye), representing a major mechanism for amplification and dissemination of endogenous IFN-alpha activity.

Patients can become unresponsive to IFN-alpha therapy after prolonged administration due to production of anti-IFN-alpha antibody, or down-regulation of receptors. The conformational structure of recombinant IFN-alpha is more likely to induce neutralizing antibody production than natural IFNs. Production of neutralizing antibodies to recombinant IFN-alpha correlates with treatment failure in human cancer patients, and anti-IFN-alpha antibody has been identified in calves, following treatment with the recombinant product.

25.3.5 Imiquimod

Imiquimod is a synthetic imidazoquinoline amine-based immune response modifier, with potent antiviral and antitumor activities in humans and horses. Imiquimod serves as a TLR-7 ligand that stimulates dendritic cells to secrete proinflammatory cytokines for T cell activation. It has recognized antiviral effects, demonstrated efficacy in humans for the treatment of with virus-associated skin lesions, including external genital and perianal warts. In horses, imiquimod treatment has shown favorable results in patients with aural plaques, sarcoid skin tumors, or sweat gland ductal carcinoma.

A clinical trial assessed the efficacy of imiquimod (Aldara™) for the treatment of aural plaques in sixteen horses (Torres, 2010). The treatment protocol involved application of a thin layer of imiquimod 5% cream to the lesions on three (nonconsecutive) days a week, every other week, to complete six treatments per month. Complete resolution of aural plaques were observed in 16 horses with a treatment protocol that ranged from 1.5 to 8 months. Owner perception of treatment efficacy for the majority of cases was considered excellent. Although most horses required sedation or restraint for treatment, ten out of 12 horse owners involved in the study reported that they would repeat the same therapeutic protocol in the future if needed, based on the favorable outcome. When considering the lack of efficacy of other therapeutic protocols that have been utilized for the treatment of aural plaques in horses, this immunomodulator therapy appears to be an appropriate treatment protocol for this equine condition.

Additional investigations have included sarcoid skin tumors (Nogueira, 2006) and sweat gland ductal carcinoma (Cihocki, 2007). An individual case report provides support for the use of imiquimod as an adjunct to standard of care surgical resection for sweat gland ductal carcinoma lesions. In this report, treatment provided partial resolution for skin lesions that could not be resected. Eight of 12 (67%) lesions resolved or were smaller, while the remaining four out of 12 (33%) were unchanged following imiquimod therapy. Five months following therapy, the lesions remained static, and no further therapy was implemented. Imiquimod alone was noted to induce a mild cellulitis, and topical application of bandage material following topical administration worsened the local inflammatory response. Therefore, bandage is not recommended after treatment (Cihocki, 2007).

Equine patients with sarcoid tumors have also been tested in a pilot study that suggests partial response to topical imiquimod administration, but further studies are required to more fully elucidate the efficacy of this therapy for this condition (Nogueira, 2006). The treatment protocol for this investigation involved topical administration three times weekly, on non-consecutive days, for a minimum of 16 weeks, although some horses were treated for up to 32 weeks. Treatment duration was extended to 32 weeks if improvement was noted by 16 weeks but lesion resolution was incomplete. Sixteen weeks was selected as a minimum treatment protocol, based on human protocols for dermal skin lesions.

Nineteen lesions on 15 horses were tested, and treatment was completed for 15 lesions. Twelve of 15 sarcoids (80%) demonstrated a greater than 75% reduction in tumor size. Among the 12 lesions that improved, nine of these (60%) completely resolved. Treatment protocols for those lesions that responded to therapy ranged from 8–32 weeks. Four lesions were withdrawn from the study due to difficulty with treatments, inability to maintain follow-up appointment, and two that failed to respond to therapy. In total, when all 19 lesions were included in the analysis, there was a 68% success rate. This pilot study demonstrated that the topical application of 5% imiquimod cream SID three times weekly resulted in greater than 75% reduction in 80% of the lesions present on horses that completed the investigation. It was also noted by the investigators that, if no improvement is noted by 16 weeks, it is unlikely that this therapy will be effective.

25.3.6 Granulocyte-colony stimulating factor

Granulocyte-colony stimulating factor (G-CSF) is an endogenous immunomodulator that induces proliferation and differentiation of g progenitor cells. Granulocyte-colony stimulating increases the number of precursor cells into the myeloblast compartment, increases the rate of neutrophil production (9.4 fold), and shortens the time required for neutrophils to mature (from five days to one day). The half-life of circulating neutrophils remains normal (eight hours).

In horses, G-CSF has been used for treatment and prophylaxis of neutropenia resulting from sepsis, endotoxemia, and drug-induced myeloid hypoplasia (Sullivan, 1993). Canine, recombinant G-CSF administered to healthy neonatal foals (20 mcg/kg IM SID) increases neutrophil counts by approximately three-fold after a single dose, and approximately seven-fold after 14 days of administration. Granulocyte-colony stimulating factor may be an efficacious prophylactic measure for neonatal infection, and may aid in the treatment of endotoxin-induced neutropenia in septic foals.

Administration of canine, recombinant G-CSF (10 mcg/kg IM SID) improves recovery of adult horses after experimentally-induced ischemia and resection of the ascending colon (Sullivan, 1993). Administration of G-CSF may enhance immunity in post-operative patients by promoting the number and function of circulating neutrophils; therapeutic recommendations include G-CSF 6 mcg/kg SQ single dose (Davis, 2003; Wong, 2012).

25.3.7 Levamisole phosphate

Levamisole phosphate is a synthetic anthelmintic labeled for treatment of nematode infection in cattle. It has been suggested to have immune-stimulating capabilities applicable to stress, aging or immaturity of the immune system. Controlled investigation of the immunostimulatory effects of levamisole in healthy or immunocompromised horses has not been reported. Levamisole has been anecdotally recommended as an adjunct treatment of equine protozoal myelitis (EPM) at 1 mg/kg PO SID (Furr, 2010). A recent *in vitro* investigation, aimed at determining the potential synergistic effects of levamisole with decoquinate against *Sarcocystis neurona*, demonstrated that levamisole has a direct toxic effect on pathogen survival (Lindsay, 2013).

In humans, levamisole has been shown to enhance lympho-proliferative responses in post-operative patients, and reduce viremia in patients with chronic hepatitis B infection. Levamisole improves cell-mediated immune responses and lymphocyte cytotoxicity in children with severe protein-calorie malnutrition and chronic respiratory infection. It is reported to be an effective adjunct treatment for rheumatoid arthritis and chronic bronchitis (Miescher, 1984).

References

Breathnach, C.C., Sturgill-Wright, T., Stiltner, J.L., Adams, A.A. and Horohov, D.W. (2006). Foals are interferon gamma deficient at birth. *Veterinary Immunology Immunopathology* 112(3–4), 199–209.

Cihocki, L.M., Divers, T.J., Johnson, A.L., Warren, A.L., Schramme, M., Rassnick, K.M. and Scott, D.W. (2007). A case of multiple epitrichial sweat gland ductal carcinomas in a horse. *Veterinary Dermatology* **18**, 134–137.

Davis, E.G., Rush, B.R. and Blecha, F. (2003). Increased in cytokine and antimicrobial peptide gene expression in horses by immunomodulation with *Propionibacterium acnes*. *Veterinary Therapeutics* **4**(1), 5–11.

Evans, D., Brent Rollins, J., Huff, G.K., Hartgrove, T.B. and Kampen, K.R. (1988). Inactivated *Priopionibacterium acnes* as an adjunct to conventional therapy in the treatment of equine respiratory disease. *Equine Practice* **10**(6), 17–21.

Flaminio, M.J.B.F., Rush, B.R. and Shuman, W. (1998). Immunologic Function in horses after non-specific immunostimulant administration. *Veterinary Immunology Immunopathology* **63**(4), 303–315.

Fumuso, E., Giguère, J., Wade, J., Rogan, D., Videla-Dorna, I. and Bowden, R.A. (2003). Endometrial IL-1β, IL-6 and THNF-α, mRNA expression in mares resistant or suceptible to post breeding endometritis Effects of estrous cycle, artificial insemination and immunomodulation. *Veterinary Immunology Immunopathology* **96**(1–2), 31–41.

Furr, M. (2010). Equine Protozoal Myelitis. In: Reed, S.M., Bayly, W.M. and Sellon, D.C. (eds). *Equine Internal Medicine*, second edition, p 614. Saunders, St. Louis, MO.

Horohov, D.W., Breatnach, C.C., Sturgill, T.R., Stiltner, J.L., Strong, D., Nieman, N. and Holland, R.E. (2008). *In vitro* and *in vivo* modulation of the equine immune response by parapoxvirus ovis. *Equine Veterinary Journal* **40**(5), 468–472.

Lindsay, D.S., Nazir, M.M., Maqbool, A., Ellison, S.P. and Strobl, J.S. (2013). Efficacy of decoquinate against *Sarcocystis neurona* in cell cultures. *Veterinary Parasitology* **19**, 21–23.

Miescher, P.A. and Beris, P. (1984). Immunosuppressive therapy in the treatment of autoimmune diseases. *Springer Seminars in Immunopathology* **7**(1), 69–90.

Moore, B.R., Krakowka, S., Cummins, J.M. and Robertson, J.T. (1996). Changes in airway inflammatory cell populations in standardbred racehorses after interferon-alpha administration. *Veterinary Immunology and Immunopathology* **49**, 347–358.

Moore, B.R., Krakowka, S., McVey, D.S., Cummings, J.M. and Robertson, J.T. (1997). Inflammatory markers in bronchoalveolar lavage fluid of standardbred racehorses with inflammatory airway disease: response to interferon-alpha. *Equine Veterinary Journal* **29**(2), 142–147.

Moore, I., Horney, B., Lofstedt, J. and Cribb, A.E. (2004). Treatment of inflammatory airway disease in young standardbreds with interferon alpha. *Canadian Veterinary Journal* **45**(7), 594–601.

Nestved, A. (1996). Evaluation of an immunostimulant in preventing shipping stress related respiratory disease. *Journal of Equine Veterinary Science* **16**(2), 78–82.

Nogueira, S.A., Torres, S.M.F., Malone, E.D., Diaz, S.F., Jensen, C. and Gilbert, S. (2006). Efficacy of imiquimod 5% cream in the treatment of equine sarcoids: a pilot study. *Veterinary Dermatology* **17**(4), 259–265.

Rohrbach, B.W., Sheerin, P.C., Cantrell, C.K., Matthews, P.M., Steiner, J.V. and Dodds, L.E. (2007). Effect of adjunctive treatment with intravenously administered *Propionibacterium acnes* on reproductive performance in mares with persistent endometritis. *Journal of American Veterinary Medical Association* **231**, 107–113.

Ryan, C., Giguère, S., Fultz, L., Long, M.T. and Crawford, P.C. (2010). Effects of two commercially available immunostimulants on leukocyte function of foals following *ex vivo* exposure to *Rhodococcus equi*. *Veterinary Immunology Immunopathology* **138**(3), 198–205.

Sturgill, T.L., Strong, D., Rashid, C., Betancourt, A. and Horohov, D.W. (2011). Effect of Proionibacterium acnes-containing immunostimulant on interferon-gamma production in the neonatal foal. *Veterinary Immunology Immunopathology* **141**(1–2), 124–127.

Sullivan, K.E., Snyder, J.R., Madigan, J.E., Pascoe, J.R., Farver, T.B., Thurmond, M.C. and Andresen, J.W. (1993). Effects of perioperative granulocyte colony-stimulating factor on horses with ascending colonic ischemia. *Veterinary Surgery* **22**, 343–350.

Tchaptchet, S., Gumenscheimer, M., Kalis, C., Freudenberg, N., Hölscher, C. and Kirschning, C.J. (2012). TLR-9 dependent and independent pathways drive activation of the immune system by Propionibacterium acnes. *PLoS One* **7**(6), e39155.

Terlou, A., van Seters, M., Kleinjan, A., Heijmans-Antonissen, C., Santegoets, L.A., Beckmann, I., van Beurden, M., Helmerhorst, T.J. and Blok, L.J. (2010). Imiquimod-induced clearance of HPV is associated with normalization of immune cell counts in usual type vulvar intraepithelial neoplasia. *International Journal of Cancer* **127**(12), 2831–2840.

Torres, S.M., Malone, E.D., White, S.D., Koch, S.N. and Watson, J.L. (2010). The efficacy of imiquimod 5% cream (Aldara®) in the treatment of aural plaques in horses: a pilot open-label clinical trial. *Veterinary Dermatology* **21**(5), 503–509.

Troedsson, M.H., Liu, I.K. and Thurmond, M. (1993). Function of uterine and blood-derived polymorphonuclear neutrophils in mares susceptible and resistant to chronic uterine infection: phagocytosis and chemotaxis. *Biology of Reproduction* **49**, 507–514.

Vail, C.D., Nestved, A.J., Clapper, J.J., Van Kampen, K.R., Peters, B.A. and Hay, C.A. (1990). Adjunct treatment of equine respiratory disease complex (ERDC) with the Propionibacterium immunostimulant, EqStim®. *Equine Veterinary Science* **10**(6), 399–403.

Weber, O., Siegling, A., Friebe, A., Limmer, A., Schlapp, T., Knolle, P., Mercer, A., Schaller, H. and Volk, H.D. (2003). Inactivated parapoxvirus ovis (Orf virus) has antiviral activity against hepatitis B virus and herpes simplex virus. *Journal of General Virology* **84**(7), 1843–1852.

Wong, D.M., Alcott, C.J., Clark, S.K., Jones, D.E., Fisher, P.G. and Sponseller, B.A. (2012). Alloimmune neonatal neutropenia and neonatal isoerythrolysis in a Thoroughbred colt. *Journal of Veterinary Diagnostic Investigation* **24**(1), 219–226.

Zingher, A.C. (1996). Effects of immunostimulation with Propionibacterium acnes (EqStim) in mares cytologically positive for endometritis. *Journal of Equine Veterinary Science* **16**(3), 100–103.

26 Immunoglobulin Therapy

Elizabeth G. Davis

26.1 Definition

Immunoglobulin administration is a blood product therapy that is utilized in equine practice for a variety of clinical conditions. Formulations for administration include plasma, serum or concentrated immunoglobulin proteins. Therapeutic indications for immunoglobulin therapy vary, and include: provision of passive immunity to neonatal foals with failure of passive transfer; prophylaxis from infectious disease such as *Rhodococcus equi*; clinical management of infectious gastrointestinal disease, such as enteric pathogens *Salmonella* spp. and *Clostridium* spp; conditions of hypoproteinemia; neutralization of endotoxin; and immunomodulation for immune-mediated thrombocytopenia.

The decision-making process for the equine practitioner, regarding immunoglobulin therapy and determination of the ideal product to administer, can be challenging when one considers all of the available commercial products. In 2009, the AAEP Biologics and Therapeutic Agents Committee posted a White Paper to aid the equine clinician with the selection process, entitled *Information on Equine Plasma and Serum Products for the Equine Practitioner*. The entire document can be downloaded from http://www.aaep.org/info/white-papers.

An important focus of this manuscript is to inform equine veterinarians that there are *licensed* and *non-licensed* products on the market. Through information provided in this document, such as the requirements needed to produce a licensed plasma or serum product, practitioners can establish therapeutic decisions consistent with the current standard of care. When possible, the use of a licensed product is preferred over a non-licensed product. If uncertainty regarding the licensing process exists, one can contact the USDA Center for Veterinary Biologics at: CVB@APHIS.USDA.gov, visit the website http://www.aphis.usda.gov/wps/portal/aphis/ourfocus/animalhealth/sa_vet_biologics, or call (800) 752-6255.

Some non-licensed products or licensed products that make unapproved claims may provide therapeutic benefit. However, without appropriate regulatory oversight, equine practitioners are unable to determine the efficacy, safety and potency of commercial products. Therefore, it is recommended by the AAEP that, in the best interest of equine patients and, when possible, the use of plasma and serum products should be limited to licensed products, and administered according to their approved label indications.

Licensed products are prepared from healthy horses that are routinely tested for infectious diseases, at manufacturing facilities frequently audited, following standard operating procedure (SOP) for all production methods, to ensure safety and efficacy of all product(s). At the time of writing, there are eight plasma products licensed for treatment of failure of passive transfer, three for *Rhodococcus equi* prevention; and others for the management of Gram-negative sepsis in foals, general treatment of sepsis, and a conditionally licensed product for the treatment of *Streptococcus equi* in horses (Table 26.1). When administering any serum or plasma product, close patient monitoring is imperative, due to the potential for immediate or delayed adverse hypersensitivity reaction which may develop, particularly during repeat administration.

26.2 Immunologic mechanisms

26.2.1 Failure of passive transfer

Fresh-frozen plasma administration is a standard of care therapeutic strategy for the management of neonatal foals with failure of passive transfer (FPT) of immunoglobulins through colostrum. The goal of such therapy is to increase the circulating IgG concentration to an acceptable level of > 800 mg/dL (Tizard, 2013) or, ideally, above 1000 mg/dL. Enhanced bactericidal activity results from the opsonizing and neutralizing activities of antibodies, primarily IgG. Immunoglobulin and other opsonins are essential for efficient phagocytosis and pathogen killing. In addition, immunoglobulins have neutralization properties that are particularly valuable against endotoxins released from Gram-negative bacteria, the most prevalent isolate from septic equine neonates (Wilson, 1989; Marsh, 2001). As a bonus, plasma also provides the foal with a colloidal fluid, which enhances oncotic pressure and improves cardiovascular stability often needed in sepsis.

Semi-quantitative ELISA (SNAP, Idexx) and quantitative radioimmunodiffusion assay (RID) are the standard methods

Equine Clinical Immunology, First Edition. Edited by M. Julia B. Felippe.
© 2016 John Wiley & Sons, Inc. Published 2016 by John Wiley & Sons, Inc.

Table 26.1 USDA licensed antibody products for use in equine patients.

Manufacturer	Product	Indication for administration	Dose
Plasvacc	**Equiplas** IgG	Failure of passive transfer	Foal 1 unit/50 kg
Plasvacc	**Equiplas Plus** IgG	Failure of passive transfer	Foal 1 unit/50 kg
Lake Immunogenics	**Plasmune (Foalimmune)** IgG	Failure of passive transfer	Foal 20 ml/kg
Lake Immunogenics	**Higamm-Equi** IgG	Failure of passive transfer	Foal 20 ml/kg
Sera	**Seramune IV** IgG	Failure of passive transfer	Foal 250 mL
Sera	**Seramune Oral** IgG	Failure of passive transfer	Foal 250 mL
MG Biologics	**High-Glo Equine** IgG	Failure of passive transfer	Foal 1 unit/50 kg
American Veterinary Reference Labs	**Equine IgG** IgG	Failure of passive transfer	Foal 1 unit/5 kg
Colorado Serum	**Normal Equine Serum** serum	Treatment of non-specific infections and disease conditions	50–250 mL up to the discretion of the DVM
Professional Biologic	**Normal Serum Equine** serum	Treatment of non-specific infections and disease conditions	50–250 mL up to the discretion of the DVM
Plasvacc	**Equiplas R** *Rhodococcus equi* antibody	Treatment of FPT and prophylaxis for *R. equi*	Foal 1 unit/50 kg
Plasvacc	**Equiplas REA** *Rhodococcus equi* antibody	Prophylaxis for *R. equi* pneumonia	Foal 1 unit/50 kg
Lake Immunogenics	**Pneumomune-Re** *Rhodococcus equi* antibody	Prophylaxis for *R. equi* pneumonia in foals < 5 days old	Foal 1 L
MG Biologics	***Streptococcus equi*** antibody	Treatment of *S. equi* Conditionally licensed by USDA	200 mL/100 pounds
Plasvacc	**Equiplas J** *Escherichia coli* antibody	Treatment of endotoxemia	Adult horse 2–4 L Foal 1–2 L
Plasvacc	**Equiplas B** *Clostridium botulinum* Type B antibody	Treatment of botulism	Adult horse 200 mL Foal 5 mL
Immvac	**Endoserum** *Salmonella typhimurium* antiserum	Attenuation of symptoms associated with *S. typhimerium* and *E. coli* when administered prior to challenge	Adult horse 500 mL to 1 L Foal 100 mL
Novartis	**Equine Coli Endotox** *Escherichia coli* antibody	Use in neonatal foals less than 12 hours old for prevention of colibacillosis and septicemia from K99 piliated *E. coli*	Foal 10 mL

used to establish the diagnosis of FPT. It is the goal of the practitioner to raise the IgG value to > 800 mg/dL, in order to provide an adequate level of serum IgG so that the foal is protected from locally encountered pathogens, which may pose a risk to health and well-being during the perinatal period. The standard dose of fresh frozen plasma is 20 mL/kg, approximately 1 L of plasma per 50 kg foal, particularly if the foal has partial failure of passive transfer. In the event that the foal absorbed a negligible quantity of colostrum, this volume may need to be increased to a total dose of 2 L, in order to raise the IgG to adequate levels.

Specific treatment protocols for plasma administration include an aseptically placed indwelling intravenous catheter. Typically, a 16-gauge polypropylene or Teflon catheter is selected for use in neonatal foals. After proper thawing of fresh frozen plasma, plasma administration is performed through an inline filter with a pore diameter of 210 μm. Administration should be initiated slowly, with frequent monitoring of vital parameters to detect symptoms associated with a hypersensitivity reaction.

Although uncommon, adverse reactions occasionally develop in neonatal foals receiving plasma transfusion. Similar to adult horses, if an adverse reaction is observed, represented by elevated respiratory rate or effort, tachycardia, or pyrexia, administration should be discontinued, vitals monitored and, if needed, treatment for anaphylaxis initiated.

Approximately 2–4 hours following plasma transfusion, circulating IgG concentration should be re-evaluated, in order to establish that an adequate level of passive immunity has been achieved. In addition, in the foal that encounters significant pathogen challenge, or that has ongoing evidence of septicemia, IgG levels should be monitored through the course of illness, due to the potential that a repeat plasma transfusion may be required. Ongoing sepsis and pathogen challenge will result in enhanced catabolism of circulating antibody proteins, which may result in an abbreviated half-life of circulating antibody proteins received from an initial plasma transfusion.

Passive administration of immunoglobulins is an important strategy to provide the neonatal foal with antibody proteins in the first several weeks of life. After this time, the foal will initiate endogenous adaptive immune responsiveness, which will include humoral immunity, with the production of antigen-specific antibody proteins.

26.2.2   Management of sepsis

Horses with serious gastrointestinal disease, such as enterocolitis or strangulating intestinal lesions, commonly endure marked Gram-negative bacterial challenge and subsequent endotoxemia. Clinical evidence of endotoxemia includes: altered core body temperature (pyrexia or hypothermia); tachycardia; injected mucous membranes; prolonged capillary refill time; dark *toxic* line along the incisors; and intestinal hypomotility.

Subsequent to the development of endotoxin challenge, affected patients are at increased risk for the development of clinically relevant consequences, such as disseminated intravascular coagulation, vascular thrombosis, and/or laminitis. Therefore, therapeutic management of the endotoxemic equine patient is aimed at attenuation or neutralization of circulating endotoxin.

More specifically endotoxin is defined as a biologically active, outer cell membrane component of Gram-negative bacteria termed lipopolysaccharide (LPS). Among licensed products, selection of a product originating from horses hyperimmunized against *Salmonella* and *E. coli* is preferred for endotoxemic patients. In such settings, the therapeutic goal is to neutralize Gram-negative cell wall products, and reduce expression and signaling through host inflammatory mediator pathways (Morris, 1986). Although data is limited, there is support that such a therapeutic strategy may attenuate the biologically active form of TNF-alpha. Additional investigation is required to determine the merit of this therapy in a variety of clinical patients. Among the licensed products, serum and plasma products targeted against LPS are available (see Table 26.1).

Fresh frozen plasma contains proteins that include not only immunoglobulin, but also albumin, which is important for the management of conditions where oncotic pressure is reduced and protein loss may be ongoing, such as severe enterocolitis secondary to sepsis with enteric pathogens. Additional proteins that are likely to provide benefit to the septic equine patient also include protein C, fibronectin and antithrombin. Evidence to support the administration of fresh frozen plasma to septic equine patients comes from the fact that activated protein C has demonstrated an improved survival rate when administered to septic human patients (Kager, 2013). Although published evidence does not

provide an equine clinical trial, in addition to the supportive evidence from endotoxemic human patients, there is strong anecdote to support the fact that plasma therapy is commonplace, and has provided an observed benefit in endotoxemic equine patients with severe gastrointestinal diseases.

Fibronectin is a large plasma glycoprotein produced by hepatocytes and fibroblasts that, among other functions, such as facilitating wound healing and stabilizing blood clot organization, can serve as an opsonin that aids with the clearance of immune complexes, damaged platelets, and associated particulate matter secondary to systemic pathogen challenge. Circulating fibronectin levels are markedly reduced in response to acute inflammation, particularly in septic patients (Mamani, 2012). Therefore, fibronectin, as a component of fresh frozen plasma, is expected to provide a therapeutic benefit to equine patients with sepsis and/or endotoxemia that receive plasma transfusion.

Septic equine patients may present disseminated intravascular coagulation which is associated with reduced antithrombin levels (formerly antithrombin III, AT III) (Dolente, 2002). Reduced antithrombin levels correlate with mortality in human patients, and restoration is therefore an important therapeutic goal when managing septic horses. In addition to anticoagulant effects, antithrombin also provides notable anti-inflammatory properties, such as the attenuation of factor X and thrombin (factor II), which facilitate inflammatory mediator expression (Wiedermann, 2002, 2006). Antithrombin has been shown to demonstrate a marked anti-inflammatory effect through the inhibition of apoptosis which attenuated inflammation in a reperfusion injury model (Isik, 2012). Therefore, restoration of depleted antithrombin stores can be expected to provide septic patients with anti-inflammatory effects that can aid in resolution of systemic inflammatory response.

It has been suggested that the anti-inflammatory effects of antithrombin may be attenuated in the presence of heparin, suggesting that, although heparin has previously been considered beneficial for patient outcome, it may prove detrimental. It is, therefore, not recommended as a combination therapy when performing plasma transfusion. Septic patients may present hemostatic disorders, and those with coagulopathies associated with prolongation of clotting times, represented by delayed prothrombin time and/or partial thromboplastin time concurrent with spontaneous hemorrhage, or are in need of immediate surgical procedures, will also benefit from immunoglobulin therapy. In addition to conditions that are associated with gastrointestinal disorders, two equine serum products have been licensed for the treatment of non-specific infections and disease conditions (see Table 26.1).

Administration of immunoglobulin therapy to septic equine patients is aimed at regulating altered coagulation profiles and balancing inflammatory pathways to improve overall patient stability. Although it is anticipated that allogeneic plasma will provide therapeutic benefit to the septic patient, there are risks associated with the administration of any foreign protein-containing product to any patient.

In general, it is assumed that, when using a licensed product, harvesting was performed from a healthy donor that that is free from infectious disease. The potential for adverse events following administration are uncommon, but may manifest as immediate or delayed hypersensitivity reactions, hypocalcemia secondary to reduced availability of ionized calcium and/or, intravascular volume over expansion, particularly if renal compromise exists. Uncommon, but also possible is the development of hepatic necrosis (Theiler's) following administration of plasma products, consistent with risks following administration of any equine biologic agent (Aleman, 2005). This apparent adverse reaction is uncommon, and does not provide evidence to withhold any form of plasma therapy, but is a consideration for the clinician, who may observe a change in clinical condition, concurrent with elevation of hepatic enzymes, days to weeks following plasma or serum administration.

Human albumin has been reported to be safe and efficacious as a colloidal therapy in equine patients, although no large-scale (equine subject) clinical trials have been performed at the time of writing. Extrapolation from use in other species, combined with an equine abstract, provides evidence that this is a therapeutic option for the hypoalbuminemic/hypoproteinemic equine patient (DeWitt, 2004). Dosing recommendations are somewhat empiric, but in the reported study the dose range was 2–5 mL 25% human albumin/kg, diluted and subsequently administered as a 10% solution. Adverse events have been reported in small animal patients, and these may include facial swelling that may have resulted as a hypersensitivity reaction (Mathews, 2008). Delayed-type hypersensitivity reactions may also occur, but are reportedly infrequent.

26.2.3 Prophylaxis for *Rhodococcus equi* infection in foals

Administration of a commercially available and licensed plasma-containing antibody against *Rhodococcus equi* is recommended as an aid for the prevention of *R. equi*-associated pneumonia on endemic farms (Giguere, 2011). Although transfusion with hyperimmune *R. equi* plasma does not confer immunity in all patients, it is recommended as a preventative strategy aimed at reducing risk of disease on endemic farms. Other important factors for controlling disease include monitoring and formal screening of at-risk foals. Overall, intravenous administration of hyperimmune plasma harvested from hyperimmunized donors has evidence to demonstrate efficacy, as reducing the severity of *R. equi* pneumonia in foals, following an *R. equi* experimental challenge (Caston, 2006).

Other studies have shown equivocal results, which result in conflicting data. Specifically, immunoglobulins targeted against VapA and VapC are responsible for the protection provided by hyperimmune plasma, so administration of plasma harvested from horses that have not been hyperimmunized against *R. equi* is not recommended. In addition, administration of hyperimmune plasma licensed as an aid in the control of *R. equi* pneumonia is recommended but, in contrast to plasma obtained from horses hyperimmunized against *R. equi*, is not licensed. Licensure of the plasma product ensures potency, purity and safety.

Dosing recommendations for the administration of *R. equi* hyperimmune plasma to foals should be aimed at providing protection prior to challenge, as evidenced by a failure for foals to be protected from disease when plasma administration occurred following aerosol infection with *R. equi*. Therefore the 2011 ACVIM *R. equi* consensus statement recommendations suggest that at least 1 L of licensed hyperimmune plasma is administered no later than the second day of life. When the potential for ongoing challenge is high, it is recommended that an additional liter of plasma be administered while the foal remains susceptible to challenge, at approximately 14–32 days of age.

26.2.4 Intravenous immunoglobulin therapy for thrombocytopenia

Human patients with primary immune thrombocytopenia that is non-responsive to conventional immunosuppressive therapy typically undergo intravenous immunoglobulin (IVIg) therapy. Although the mechanism is not completely understood, it is believed that dilution (and removal) of antibodies targeted against platelet surface proteins provides a therapeutic benefit. A recent report in the human literature describes a surgical patient with immune-mediated thrombocytopenic purpura. Immunoglobulin therapy was administered post-operatively and was reported to provide safe, effective therapy for the management of IMT (Toyomasu, 2013).

Similar to human patients, concentrated immunoglobulin therapy has also been utilized for equine patients with profound thrombocytopenia. The recommended dose is 20 ml/kg/day for 2–5 days (9 L plasma/450 kg horse; IgG 1.5–2.0 g/dl). In addition to the previously mentioned dilutional effects, the mechanism of treatment success when using high-dose plasma transfusion for the treatment of IMT is multifaceted, through blocked Fc receptor binding, steric hindrance of immune complex adherence, enhanced T-lymphocyte suppressor activity, and reduced B-lymphocyte function.

References

Aleman, M., Nieto, J.E., Carr, E.A. and Carlson, G.P. (2005). Serum hepatitis associated with commercial plasma transfusion in horses. *Journal of Veterinary Internal Medicine* **19**(1), 120–122.

Caston, S., McClure, S.R., Martens, R.J., Chaffin, M.K., Miles, K.G., Griffith, R.W. and Cohen, N.D. (2006). Effect of hyperimmune plasma on the severity of pneumonia caused by *Rhodococcus equi* in experimentally infected horses. *Veterinary Therapeutics* **7**(4), 361–375.

DeWitt, S.F. and Paradis, M.R. (2004). *Use of human albumin as a colloidal therapy in the hypoproteinemic equine.* In: Proceedings of the 22nd Annual ACVIM Forum, p. 394.

Dolente, B., Wilkins, P.A. and Boston, R.C. (2002). Clinicopathologic evidence of disseminated intravascular coagulation in horses with acute colitis. *Journal of the American Veterinary Medical Association* **220**(7), 1034–1038.

Giguere, S., Cohen, N.D., Chaffin, M.K., Slovis, N.M., Hondalus, M.K., Hines, S.A. and Prescott, J.F. (2011). Diagnosis, treatment, control, and prevention of infections caused by *Rhodococcus equi* in foals. *Journal of Veterinary Internal Medicine* **25**(6), 1209–1220.

Isik S., Tuncyurek, P., Zengin, N.I., Demirbag, A.E., Atalay, F., Yilmaz, S. and Orug, T. (2012). Antithrombin prevents apoptosis by regulating inflammation in the liver in a model of cold ischemia/warm perfusion injury. *Hepatogastroenterology* **59**(114), 453–457.

Kager L.M., Wiersinga, W.J., Roelofs, J.J., Meijers, J.C., Zeerleder, S.S., Esmon, C.T., van't Veer, C. and van der Poll, T. (2013). Endogenous protein C has a protective role during Gram-negative pneumosepsis (melioidosis). *Journal of Thrombosis and Haemostasis* **11**(2), 282–292.

Mamani, M., Hashemi, S.H., Hajilooi, M., Saedi, F., Niayesh, A. and Fallah, M. (2012). Evaluation of fibronectin and C-reactive protein levels in patients with sepsis: a case-control study. *Acta Medica Iranica* **50**, 404–410.

Marsh P. and Palmer, J.E. (2001). Bacterial isolates and their susceptibility patterns in critically ill foals: 543 cases (1991–1998). *Journal of American Veterinary Medical Association* **218**(10), 1608–1610.

Mathews, K. (2008). The therapeutic use of 25% human serum albumin in critically ill dogs and cats. *Veterinary Clinics of North America Small Animal Practice* **38**(3), 595–605.

Morris, D.D., Whitlock, R.H. and Corbeil, L.B. (1986). Endotoxemia in horses: protection provided by antiserum to core lipopolysaccharide. *American Journal of Veterinary Research* **47**(3), 544–550.

Tizard, I. (2013). *Veterinary Immunology*, ninth edition. St. Louis, Elsevier. 231–236.

Toyomasu, Y., Shimabukuro, R., Moriyama, H., Eguchi, D., Ishikawa, K., Kishihara, F., Fukuyama, Y., Matsumata, T., Mochiki, E. and Kuwano, H. (2013). Successful perioperative management of a patient with idiopathic thrombocytopenic purpura undergoing emergent appendectomy: Report of a case. *International Journal of Surgery Case Reports* **4**(10), 898–900.

Wiedermann, Ch.J. and Römisch, J. (2002). The anti-inflammatory actions of antithrombin – a review. *Acta Medica Austriaca* **29**, 89–92.

Wiedermann, C.J. (2006). Clinical review: molecular mechanisms underlying the role of antithrombin in sepsis. *Critical Care* **10**, 209.

Wilson, W.D. and Madigan, J.E. (1989). Comparison of bacteriologic culture of blood and necropsy specimens for determining the cause of foal septicemia: 47 cases (1978–1987). *Journal of American Veterinary Medical Association* **195**, 1759–1763.

27 Plasmapheresis

Nathan M. Slovis

27.1 Definition

Plasmapheresis is a procedure in which extracorporeal separation of blood components results in a filtered plasma product. The plasma product can be returned to the patient or administered to another patient. The basis for therapeutic plasmapheresis (TP) is the removal of proteins, protein-bound or high molecular weight solutes, including: autoantibodies; circulating immune (antibody-antigen) complexes; excess lipids or hormones; aromatic amino acids; ammonia; bilirubin; endotoxin; lipids and phenols; and exogenous toxins from circulation. A current literature search revealed no published manuscripts describing TP in the equine patient, although this author has used this form of treatment in a few equine clinical cases reported below.

27.2 Methods for preparing plasma products

27.2.1 Manual blood centrifugation and gravity sedimentation

Blood bag centrifugation and gravity sedimentation are two common methods used in ambulatory equine medicine to produce a plasma product. Blood centrifugation can be used because of the different specific gravities inherent to red cells, white cells, platelets and plasma. *Gravity sedimentation* relies on the rapid erythrocyte sedimentation rate of equine blood that separates from plasma (Feige, 2003). *Membrane plasma separation* uses differences in particle size to filter plasma from the cellular components of blood (Siami, 2001). Plasma obtained from both centrifugation and gravity sedimentation preparations have significantly more erythrocytes and leukocytes, compared with automated methods (Feige, 2003).

For whole-blood collection, a 12 or 10 gauge (13 cm) indwelling catheter is placed aseptically into a jugular vein. A volume of 15 ml/kg body weight of blood can be collected into evacuated 500 ml glass bottles containing 50 ml of anticoagulant citrate dextrose (ACD) solution. Blood is then allowed to sediment for 24 hours at 4°C, after which plasma is carefully decanted into 500 ml glass bottles.

27.2.2 Automated plasmapheresis

The introduction of automated in-line blood cell separators in the early 1980s revolutionized plasmapheresis procedures. These instruments attach sterile disposable collection sets to intravenous catheters inserted into donors. The instrument removes whole blood from the donors and infuses anticoagulant (ACD) into the extracted blood at a controlled rate. The blood with anticoagulant is then introduced into a disposable separation chamber for automated centrifugation and separation of the blood components. After centrifugation, the plasma is diverted to attached bags while, simultaneously, concentrated cells are returned to the donor.

The automated plasmapheresis is considered a closed system for harvesting of plasma, in contrast to the plasma harvesting techniques above, which increase the possibility of bacterial contamination. Although designed for use in humans, this equipment has been modified for use in automated procedures of equine blood donors. The automated procedure is more efficient for harvesting plasma (20 minutes to harvest one liter of plasma), compared with the other techniques (Feige, 2003).

Feige and colleagues demonstrated that the number of erythrocytes during automated plasmapheresis was reduced by a factor of more than 100, and there was a 100–1000-fold lower leukocyte count compared to the other methods. The use of an automated plasmapheresis (Autopheresis-C A-200 unit, Fenwal, Inc.) procedure for the harvest of equine plasma has been described (Ziska, 2012). The thorough removal of erythrocytes minimizes the risk of immunological and non-immunological adverse reactions in the recipient (Vengelen-Tyler, 1999a, 1999b). A low cell count is also important for reducing the activation of coagulation proteins and, therefore, decreasing the normal coagulation activity of plasma. Leukocyte removal from plasma is beneficial because leukocytes may degranulate and fragment during storage, releasing substances that may promote febrile or allergic reactions in the recipient (Feige, 2003). The main criteria for assessment of plasma quality are, therefore, low blood cell counts and normal coagulation activity of the plasma (Vengelen-Tyler, 1999a, 1999b).

Coagulation factors in harvested plasma obtained by either plasmapheresis or blood centrifugation were not altered from normal when compared, and both methods are suitable for the

Equine Clinical Immunology, First Edition. Edited by M. Julia B. Felippe.
© 2016 John Wiley & Sons, Inc. Published 2016 by John Wiley & Sons, Inc.

production of plasma for coagulation factor substitution (Schneider, 1995; Feige, 2003). A glass bottle cannot be used to harvest plasma for this purpose because it reduces platelets and coagulation factors VII, VIII and XII (Vengelen-Tyler, 1999a, 1999b).

Equine plasma transfusion has been recognized as a valuable resource for the treatment of various medical conditions. Plasma harvested from equine donors has been used for the treatment of coagulopathies, protein-losing enteropathies, endotoxemia, failure of passive transfer, and protection against naturally acquired infections (e.g., *Rhodococcus equi, Salmonella, Clostridium difficile and Clostridium perferingens*). Plasma is also the most common biologic colloid utilized for supportive therapy in horses, and offers the advantage of providing a broad range of proteins in addition to its principle colloid, albumin. These additional proteins include coagulation factors, antithrombin, and immunoglobulin (Magdesian, 2003).

In the author's experience of increasing the plasma albumin levels in a 500 kg horse, it has been noted that, for every 1 L of plasma administered, the clinician could expect a 0.1–0.2 g/dl increase in plasma albumin levels. In a study consisting of septic and critically ill foals, it was noted, for the entire study population, a higher survival rate to discharge for those foals receiving hyperimmune plasma rich in antiendotoxin antibodies. Administration of plasma rich in antiendotoxin antibodies also was associated with greater survival in septic foals (Peek, 2006).

27.3 Apheresis

Apheresis is a procedure in which blood of the patient or donor is passed through a medical device that separates out one or more components of blood, and returns the remaining blood products to the patient or donor with, or without, extracorporeal treatment or replacement of the separated component. In the field of human medicine, the Apheresis Applications Committee of the American Society of Apheresis has categorized the use of apheresis (Category I to IV), and periodically evaluates the literature for its indications (Szczepiorkowski, 2010):

- *Category I* – Disorders for which apheresis is accepted as a first-line therapy, either as a primary standalone treatment or in conjunction with other modes of treatment (e.g., Guillain-Barre Syndrome and myasthenia gravis).
- *Category II* – Disorders for which apheresis is accepted as a second-line therapy, either as a standalone treatment or in conjunction with other modes of treatment (e.g., multiple sclerosis, mushroom poisoning, and hemolytic uremic syndrome).
- *Category III* – Disorders for which the optimum role of apheresis therapy has not been established, and decision-making is individualized (e.g., immune-mediated hemolytic anemia).
- *Category IV* – Disorders in which published evidence demonstrates or suggests apheresis to be ineffective or harmful (e.g., Stiff Person Syndrome and immune-mediated thrombocytopenia).

27.4 Therapeutic plasmapheresis

Therapeutic plasmapheresis (TP) has been used in small animal and human medicine for many years, but is underutilized in the equine patient (Szczepiorkowski, 2010). TP is the process by which plasma-containing components causing, or thought to cause, disease are removed from the circulation, and harmless plasma returned to the patient.

TP primarily removes protein-bound solutes or high molecular weight solutes, such as circulating protein-bound toxins, autoantibodies, immune complexes, or other abnormally occurring molecules. Plasmapheresis has been used in the treatment of more than 100 diseases in human medicine, including immune-mediated diseases, neoplasia, infectious diseases, sepsis, hyperlipidemia, thyrotoxicosis, and removal of toxins. In immune-mediated disease, it is most useful to rapidly decrease plasma concentrations of antibodies or immune complexes, while other immunosuppressive measures are used to prolong the effect (Bartges, 1990, 1997; Szczepiorkowski, 2010; Kim, 2013).

In the following section, the rationale for the use of TP will be presented. Where applicable, the author will share some of his experiences utilizing this type of treatment in equine medicine.

Take home message

Apheresis is a procedure in which blood of the patient or donor is passed through a medical device that separates out one or more components of blood, and returns the remaining blood products to the patient or donor, with or without extracorporeal treatment or replacement of the separated component.

Therapeutic plasmapheresis is the process by which plasma-containing components causing or thought to cause disease are removed from the circulation, and harmless plasma returned to the patient.

Plasmapheresis has been used in the treatment of immune-mediated diseases, neoplasia, infectious diseases, sepsis, hyperlipidemia, and removal of toxins.

Adverse effects of therapeutic plasmapheresis include return of concentrated blood cells into the subcutaneous tissue, neurological abnormalities, citrate toxicity, hypercoagulability, hypogammaglobulinemia, hypotension (foals), and non-specific inflammatory response to the extracorporeal circulation devices.

27.4.1 Immune-mediated hemolytic anemia

Immune-mediated hemolytic anemia is caused by autoantibodies that induce intravascular or extravascular red cell destruction. TP removes circulating autoantibodies, immunocomplexes, and activated complement components, and it is used in patients with poor response to blood transfusions and life-threatening hemolysis (Szczepiorkowski, 2010). TP treatment helps until immunosuppressive therapy takes effect, or when other treatments have failed.

In human patients, most auto-immune IgG is found extravascularly and bound to the red cells, and is not always efficiently removed when plasma is filtered, so TP does not always show clinical improvement. The duration of treatment is based on the control of hemolysis, the effect of immunosuppressive therapy, and the need of blood transfusions. Frequency of the procedure in humans is typically every other day.

In human medicine, approximately 1–1.5 L of total plasma volume can be removed and replaced with albumin. While this volume may not be realistic in the equine patient, the removal of 7–8 L of plasma in a 500 kg patient may be adequate without the need of plasma replacement from a donor.

27.4.2 Immune-mediated dermatoses

Pemphigus foliaceus is the most common autoimmune skin disease of the horse (Zabel, 2005). The disease may take weeks to months to control with the use of glucocorticoids and/or azathioprine. In a retrospective study, only four out of 11 (36%) equine patients remained in remission for more than a year after immunosuppressive therapy (Vandenabelle, 2004).

The author has applied TP in four adult equine patients diagnosed with pemphigus foliaceus that did not respond to high doses of glucocorticoids (dexamethasone). TP consisted of the removal of 22 ml of plasma/kg body weight at monthly intervals, without exchange transfusion of equivalent donor plasma volume. However, crystalloid therapy of 20 ml/kg body weight was used during the TP. The clinical condition in these patients was responsive to lower doses of dexamethasone.

27.4.3 Purpura hemorrhagica

Purpura hemorrhagica is an immune-mediated severe necrotizing vasculitis that causes lesions of the skin and mucous membranes, with larger hemorrhagic and edematous damage in the muscles and subcutaneous tissues (Pusterla, 2003). The author used TP in two cases of severe purpura hemorrhagica that were not responsive to glucocorticoids. TP consisted of a one-time removal of 22 ml of plasma/kg body weight, in order to aid removal of the antibody-antigen complexes until the immunosuppressive therapy became effective.

27.4.4 Hypertriglyceridemia

Hypertriglyceridemia can be secondary to diabetes mellitus, hypothyroidism, pregnancy, and the use of certain medications in human patients. In equid cases, this disorder is more frequently observed in miniature horses and miniature donkeys, secondary to a primary systemic disease, including septicemia, colitis, esophageal obstruction, gastric impaction or rupture, fecalith, excessive parasitism, and pituitary adenoma (Rush, 1994). Even though therapy in equid patients usually consists of specific treatment for the primary disease, supportive care, and nutritional support, TP may be a viable option for animals that do not respond to conventional treatment.

Human reports and a single non-randomized controlled trial have examined the use of TP to treat acute pancreatitis due to hypertriglyceridemia (Szczepiorkowski, 2010). Reductions in human triglyceride levels of 46–80% have been reported, with improvements of symptoms following one to three TP procedures (Swoboda, 1993; Bolan, 2002). In equid patients, TP may be a viable option for animals that do not respond to conventional treatment. The volume of plasma removal needed to reduce triglyceride level in an equid is unknown, but a volume of plasma no larger than 15–20 ml/kg body weight could be considered. If TP needs to be repeated more than twice, transfusion with an equivalent amount of donor plasma would be necessary.

27.4.5 Liver failure and kernicterus

The liver has more than 500 different functions that are impossible to be replaced by one or a few substitute methods; therefore, liver transplantation is the principle method for treatment of hepatic failure in humans (Naruse, 2005). Despite the advances in transplantation medicine, many patients still die waiting for a transplant, because of the severe shortage of donors. The use of TP in human patients with hepatic failure in exchange with an equivalent volume of donor plasma has been shown to reverse hepatic coma and to improve coagulation in human patients (Yamazaki, 1992; Szczepiorkowski, 2010). The major difficulty with this method of treatment is the need for a large volume of normal plasma as a substitute.

This author has attempted using TP in foals with kernicterus and neurological signs (e.g., seizures). The procedure involves the removal of 15–20 ml of plasma/kg body weight, and the concurrent administration of an equivalent volume of donor plasma. To date, TP has not been successful in preventing the death of these equine patients. However, further therapeutic trials are warranted, because it is possible that TP would have a more successful outcome if treatment were initiated before the presence of neurological signs.

27.4.6 Sepsis and multiple organ dysfunction syndrome

Sepsis induces a systemic inflammatory response that affects the health and function of organs, and can cause death. Cytokines and other mediators of sepsis include tumor necrosis factor alpha (TNF-alpha), interleukin (IL)-1, IL-2, IL-6, IL-8, leukotrienes, prostaglandins, endotoxin, and tumor necrosis factor beta (TGF-beta) (Buscund, 2002; McMaster, 2003). Clinical management of sepsis includes antimicrobial agents to control the source of infection, hemodynamic support with fluids and vasopressors, and therapies to interrupt the cascade of inflammation. Attempts to block or remove single mediators of sepsis have been somewhat successful in human medicine (Buscund, 2002; McMaster, 2003).

TP has the potential to remove multiple toxic mediators of sepsis and can, therefore, be more effective than blocking single components. Randomized clinical trials in human patients with sepsis resulted in significantly reduced mortality rates in the TP group (33%), compared with the control group (54%), with one or two therapies (Buscund, 2002). Other case series have treated patients daily until improvements were noted, and replacement fluids during the TP consisted of albumin or plasma but not crystalloid. The use of TP may have a benefit in the treatment of sepsis in the equine patient, but there has been no report to date.

27.5 Complications of therapeutic plasmapheresis

In one study evaluating a protocol for automated plasmapheresis, several adverse events were observed in horses, including the inadvertent return of concentrated blood cells into the subcutaneous tissue, ataxia and inability to stand, unilateral or bilateral blindness, and death (Feige, 2003). The described neurological abnormalities were temporary, and resolved within hours to days after the procedure, except for one horse that had bilateral blindness. Other possible complications of plasmapheresis reported in human patients include transient hypercoagulable state during the procedure due to the loss of antithrombin, hypogammaglobulinemia, and non-specific inflammatory response to the extracorporeal circulation filter and/or drains (Seczynska, 2013).

This author believes that therapeutic plasmapheresis is a safe method when planned for the removal of 22 ml of plasma/kg body weight from an equine patient as frequently as every 14 days without exchange plasma transfusions (Feige, 2003; Ziska, 2012). If an exchange transfusion with donor plasma is performed, TP can even be performed daily. Nevertheless, hypovolemia can be observed in foals that undergo TP, and monitoring of vital signs and urine production is essential to adjust colloid or crystalloid therapy accordingly.

References

Bartges, J.W. (1997). Therapeutic plasmapheresis, *Seminars in Veterinary Medicine and Surgery (Small Animal)* **12**(3), 170–177.

Bartges, J.W., Klausner, J.S., Bostwick, E.F., Hakala, J.E. and Lennon, V.A. (1990). Clinical remission following plasmapheresis and corticosteroid treatment in a dog with acquired myasthenia gravis. *Journal of the American Veterinary Medical Association* **196**(8), 1276–8.

Bolan, C., Oral, E.A., Gorden, P., Taylor, S. and Leitman, S.F. (2002). Intensive, long-term plasma exchange therapy for severe hypertriglyceridemia in acquired generalized lipoatrophy. *The Journal of Clinical Endocrinology and Metabolism* **87**(1), 380–384.

Buscund, R., Koukline, V., Utrobin, U. and Nedashkovsky, E. (2002). Plasmapheresis in severe sepsis and septic shock: a prospective, randomized, controlled trial. *Intensive Care Medicine* **28**(10), 1434–1439.

Feige, K., Ehrat, F., Kastner, S. and Schwarzwald, C.C. (2003). Automated plasmapheresis compared with other plasma collection methods in a horse. *Journal of Veterinary Medicine, A, Physiology, Pathology, Clinical Medicine* **50**(4), 185–189.

Kim, Y.A. and Sloan, S.R. (2013). Pediatric Therapeutic Apheresis: Rationale and Indications for Plasmapheresis, Cytapheresis, Extracorporeal Photopheresis, and LDL Apheresis. *Pediatric Clinics of North America* **60**(6), 1569–1580.

Magdesian, G.K. (2003). Colloid Replacement in the ICU. *Clinical Techniques in Equine Practice* **2**, 130–137.

McMaster, P. and Shann, F. (2003). The use of extracorporeal techniques to remove humoral factors in sepsis. *Pediatric Critical Care Medicine* **4**(1), 2–7.

Naruse, K., Nagashima, H., Sakai, Y., Kokudo, N. and Makuuchi, M. (2005). Development and perspectives of perfusion treatment for liver failure. *Surgery Today* **35**(7), 507–517.

Peek, S.F., Semrad, S., McGuirk, S.M., Riseberg, A., Slack, J.A., Marques, F., Coombs, D., Lien, L., Keuler, N. and Darien, B.J. (2006). Prognostic value of clinicopathologic variables obtained at admission and effect of antiendotoxin plasma on survival in septic and critically ill foals. *Journal of Veterinary Internal Medicine* **20**(3), 569–574.

Pusterla, N., Watson, J.L., Affolter, V.K., Magdesian, K.G., Wilson, W.D. and Carlson, G.P. (2003). Purpura haemorrhagica in 53 horses. *The Veterinary Record* **153**(4), 118–121.

Rush, B.M., Abood, S.K. and Hinchcliff, K.W. (1994). Hyperlipemia in 9 Miniature Horses and Miniature Donkeys. *Journal of Veterinary Internal Medicine* **8**(5), 376–381.

Schneider, A. (1995). Blood components: collection, processing and storage. *The Veterinary Clinics of North America. Small Animal Practice* **25**(6), 1245–1261.

Seczynska, B., Nowak, I., Sega, A., Kozka, M., Wodkowski, M., Krolikowski, W. and Szczeklik, W. (2013). Supportive Therapy for a Patient with Toxic Epidermal Necrolysis Undergoing Plasmapheresis. *Critical Care Nurse* **33**(4), 26–39.

Siami, G.A. and Siami, F.S. (2001). Membrane plasmapheresis in the United States: a review over the last 20 years. *Therapeutic Apheresis and Dialysis* **5**(4), 315–320.

Swoboda, K., Derfler, K., Koppensteiner, R., Langer, M., Pamberger, P., Brehm, R., Ehringer, H., Druml, W. and Widhalm, K. (1993). Extracorporeal lipid elimination for treatment of gestational hyperlipidemic pancreatitis. *Gastroentrology* **104**(5), 1527–1531.

Szczepiorkowski, Z.M., Winters, J.L., Bandarenko, N., Kim, H.C., Linenberger, M.L., Marques, M.B., Sarode, R., Schwartz, J., Weinstein, R., Shaz, B.H. and Apheresis Applications Committee of the American Society for Apheresis. (2010). Guidelines on the Use of Therapeutic Apheresis in Clinical Practice – Evidence Based Approach from the Apheresis Applications Committee of the American Society for Apheresis. *Journal of Clinical Apheresis* **25**(3), 83–177.

Vandenabelle, S.I., White, S.D. and Affolter, V.K. (2004). Pemphigus foliaceus in the horse: a retrospective study of 20 cases. *Veterinary Dermatology* **15**(6), 381–388.

Vengelen-Tyler, V. (1999a). Blood component preparation, storage, shipping, and transportation. In: Vengelen-Tyler, V. (ed). *Technical Manual*, pp. 162–192. Bethesda, American Association of Blood Banks.

Vengelen-Tyler, V. (1999b). Platelet and granulocyte antigens and antibodies. In: Vengelen-Tyler, V. (ed). *Technical Manual*, pp. 339–356. Betheseda, American Association of Blood Banks.

Yamazaki, Z., Kamai, F., Ideduki, Y. and Inoue, N. (1992). Extracorporeal methods of liver failure treatment. *Biomaterials, Artificial Cells, and Artificial Organs* **15**(4), 296–299.

Zabel, S., Mueller, R.D., Fieseler, K.V., Bettenay, S.V., Littlewood, J.D. and Wagner, R. (2005). Review of 15 cases of pemphigus foliaceus in horses and a survey of the literature. *The Veterinary Record* **157**(17), 505–509.

Ziska, S.M., Schumaker, J., Duran, S.H. and Brock, K.V. (2012). Development of an automated plasmapheresis procedure for the harvest of equine plasma in accordance with current good manufacturing practice. *American Journal of Veterinary Research* **73**(6), 762–769.

28 Principles of Vaccination

Noah D. Cohen and Angela I. Bordin

28.1 Definition

Although a call for cure is generally more compelling to veterinarians and clients than that for prevention, control of infectious diseases is more effectively accomplished through preventative practices, and vaccination is an important method for disease control and prevention. Protocols for vaccinating horses have been published elsewhere, and guidelines for vaccinating horses in North America are provided by the American Association of Equine Practitioners (AAEP) at http://www.aaep. org/info/vaccination-guidelines-265. In addition, summary tables of the AAEP guidelines for foals and broodmares are provided below (Tables 28.1 to 28.5).

28.2 Efficacy and effectiveness of vaccines

Vaccinologists and epidemiologists distinguish between vaccine efficacy and vaccine effectiveness (Fedson, 1998; Weinberg, 2010). *Vaccine efficacy* refers to the proportional reduction in disease incidence in a vaccinated group, compared with an unvaccinated group under optimal conditions (i.e., a randomized controlled trial, RCT). In equine medicine, experimental infections of research horses (controlled experiments) are generally used to evaluate vaccine efficacy rather than RCTs. The strength of these laboratory or epidemiological experimental study designs are that they permit detailed, accurate measurement of a variety of primary and secondary clinical, clinicopathological, and microbiological outcomes. They also help control for biases through randomization of assignment, and systematic sampling for evaluation of vaccine immunogenicity. A limitation of vaccine efficacy studies is that their results may not accurately reflect the performance of the vaccine under field conditions, because the effects of drugs among patients selected for study in RCTs may not accurately reflect their performance in the more general population.

The term vaccine *effectiveness* is used to refer to the performance of vaccines in the *real world* or primary care setting, where there is less stringency for inclusion criteria for receipt of vaccines, and where assessment of outcomes (including disease and adverse reactions) is less rigorous, but more reflective of actual performance of the vaccine for reducing disease in the population. Vaccine effectiveness studies generally permit larger sample sizes, in which both effectiveness and safety can be more comprehensively assessed.

Vaccine effectiveness is influenced by how well the vaccine is administered, including such factors as storage and proper dilution.

The principal limitation of vaccine effectiveness studies is the same as their principal advantage: the data are conducted in the real-world setting, which provide many biases that can influence the results of vaccine studies. Examples of possible biases from field evaluation of vaccines include: differential case identification between vaccinates and non-vaccinates (i.e., perhaps a diagnosis is less likely to be considered if the horse has been vaccinated against the disease); differences in reference population of vaccinates relative to non-vaccinates (e.g., a situation in which non-vaccinated horses might be less likely to have flying insect control than vaccinated horses); or differences in access to health care (e.g., horses that are vaccinated may be more likely to be examined by a veterinarian and diagnosed with a disease than are horses that are not vaccinated).

In general, vaccine efficacy is expected to be greater than effectiveness because of the strict, controlled conditions and circumstances under which efficacy studies are conducted. Although this is not always the case, it is likely that efficacy is higher than effectiveness for equine vaccines, because equine vaccines are evaluated using experimental study populations, rather than general populations.

28.2.1 Calculating vaccine efficacy and vaccine effectiveness

Vaccine efficacy can be calculated by knowing the incidence (or cumulative incidence) of *disease* in the vaccinated group and in the unvaccinated group, using the following formula:

$$\text{Efficacy} = \frac{\text{incidence unvaccinated} - \text{incidence vaccinated}}{\text{incidence unvaccinated}} \times 100.$$

Equine Clinical Immunology, First Edition. Edited by M. Julia B. Felippe.
© 2016 John Wiley & Sons, Inc. Published 2016 by John Wiley & Sons, Inc.

Table 28.1 Vaccination recommendations for foals from vaccinated dams.

VACCINE (Foals and weanlings of mares vaccinated in prepartum against the disease indicated)	DOSE (D)	Schedule	COMMENTS
Botulism	1	① D1 (Month 2)	Foals at high risk may be vaccinated as early as two weeks old.
	2	② 4 weeks after D1	
	3	③ 4 weeks after D2	
Eastern/Western Equine Encephalomyelitis	1	① Initial Dose, D1	Foals at high risk may be given an initial dose at three months old.
	2	② 4–6 weeks after D1	
	3	③ 10–12 months old	
West Nile Virus	1	① Initial Dose, D1	Suggested dosage for inactivated whole virus vaccine and inactivated flavivirus chimera
	2	② 4–6 weeks after D1	
	3	③ 10–12 months old	
Tetanus	1	① D1	
	2	② 4–6 weeks after D1	
	3	③ 10–12 months old	
Equine Herpesvirus	1	① D1	Revaccinate at six-month intervals.
	2	② 4–6 weeks after D1	
	3		
Strangles – Streptococcus equi	1	① D1	Recommended dosage is for killed vaccine only.
	2	② 4–6 weeks after D1	
	3	③ 4–6 weeks after D2	
Potomac Horse Fever	1	① D1	Subsequent doses to be administered at four-week intervals until six months old.
	2	② 3–4 weeks after D1	
Rabies	1	① D1	
	2	② 4–6 weeks after D1	
Equine Viral Arteritis	1	① COLTS ONLY: Single dose at 6–12 months old	Prior to initial vaccination, colts should undergo serologic testing and be confirmed negative.
Equine Influenza	1	① D1	Suggested dosage for inactivated vaccine only.
	2	② 3–4 weeks after D1	
	3	③ 10–12 months old	
Anthrax	N/A – See comments		Not applicable because mares are not vaccinated during pregnancy.
Rotavirus	N/A – See comments		Not recommended in foals.

Timeline header: MONTH 1 (WEEKS 1 2 3 4), MONTH 2 (5 6 7 8), MONTH 3 (9 10 11 12), MONTH 4 (13 14 15 16), MONTH 5 (17 18 19 20), MONTH 6 (21 22 23 24), MONTH 7 (25 26 27 28), MONTH 8 (29 30 31 32), MONTH 9 (33 34 35 36), MONTH 10 (37 38 39 40), MONTH 11 (41 42 43 44), MONTH 12 (45 46 47 48)

Legend: ■ Core Vaccine ■ Non-core Vaccine

Table 28.2 Vaccination recommendations for foals from unvaccinated dams.

FOALS AND WEANLINGS of unvaccinated mares or mares with unknown vaccination history

Vaccine	Dose (D)	Schedule	Comments
Tetanus	1	D1 (Month 1)	
	2	4 weeks after D1	
	3	60 days after D2	
Botulism	1	D1 (Month 1)	Foals at high risk may be vaccinated as early as two weeks old.
	2	4 weeks after D1	
	3	4 weeks after D2	
Eastern/Western Equine Encephalomyelitis	1	D1 (Month 3)	Foals at high risk may be given initial dose at three months old.
	2	4 weeks after D1	
	3	60 days after D2	
Rabies	1	D1 (Month 3)	
	2	4–6 weeks after D1	
West Nile Virus	1	D1 (Month 3)	Suggested dosage for inactivated whole and flavivirus chimera vaccine, as well recombinant canary pox vaccine.
	2	30 days after D1	
	3	60 days after D2	
Equine Herpesvirus	1	D1 (Month 4)	Revaccinate at six-month intervals.
	2	4–6 weeks after D1	
	3	10–12 months old	
Strangles – Streptococcus equi	1	D1 (Month 4)	Recommended dosage is for killed vaccine only.
	2	4–6 weeks after D1	
	3	4–6 weeks after D2	
Potomac Horse Fever	1	D1 (Month 5)	Subsequent doses to be administered at four-week intervals until six months old.
	2	3–4 weeks after D1	
Equine Viral Arteritis	1	COLTS ONLY: Single dose at 6–12 months old	Prior to initial vaccination, colts should undergo serologic testing and be confirmed negative.
Equine Influenza	1	D1 (Month 5)	Suggested dosage for inactivated vaccine only.
	2	3–4 weeks after D1	
	3	10–12 months old	
Anthrax	N/A – See comments		No age-specific guidelines. Give primary series of two doses administered subcutaneously at a 2–3 week interval.
Rotavirus	N/A – See comments		Not recommended in foals.

■ Core Vaccine   ■ Non-core Vaccine

Table 28.3 Vaccination recommendations for vaccinated broodmares.

Vaccine	Dose (D)	Timing	Comments
Equine Herpesvirus	1	① 5 months GEST*	Give with product labeled for protection against EHV abortion.
	2	② 7 months GEST*	
	3	③ 9 months GEST*	
Rotavirus	1	① 8 months GEST*	
	2	② 4 weeks after D1	
	3	③ 4 weeks after D2	
Tetanus	1	① 4–6 weeks PP†	Revaccinate annually. Booster at time of penetrating injury or prior to surgery if last dose was administered over six months previously.
Eastern/Western Equine Encephalomyelitis	1	① 4–6 weeks PP†	Revaccinate annually.
West Nile Virus	1	① 4–6 weeks PP†	Revaccinate annually.
Rabies	1	① 4–6 weeks PP†	Can be given prior to breeding due to relatively long duration of immunity. Revaccinate annually.
Botulism	1	① 4–6 weeks PP†	Revaccinate annually.
Equine Influenza	1	① 4–6 weeks PP†	Suggested dosage for either inactivated vaccine or canary pox vector vaccine. Revaccinate semi-annually.
Potomac Horse Fever	1	① 4–6 weeks PP†	Semi-annual or annual booster. A revaccination interval of 3–4 months may be considered for high-risk areas.
Strangles – Streptococcus equi	1	① 4–6 weeks PP†	Suggested dosage for killed vaccine containing M-protein. Revaccinate semi-annually.
Anthrax	N/A – See comments		Not recommended during gestation.
Equine Viral Arteritis	N/A – See comments		Not recommended unless high-risk.

ADULT HORSES: BROODMARES previously vaccinated against the disease indicated

Timeline columns: MONTH 1 (Week 1 2 3 4) · MONTH 2 (5 6 7 8) · MONTH 3 (9 10 11 12) · MONTH 4 (13 14 15 16) · MONTH 5 (17 18 19 20) · MONTH 6 (21 22 23 24) · MONTH 7 (25 26 27 28) · MONTH 8 (29 30 31 32) · MONTH 9 (33 34 35 36) · MONTH 10 (37 38 39 40) · MONTH 11 (41 42 43 44) · PARTURITION · COMMENTS

GEST* Gestation
PP† Pre-partum

Legend: ▮ Core Vaccine   ▮ Gestation   ▮ Non-core Vaccine   Pre-partum

Table 28.4 Vaccination recommendations for unvaccinated broodmares.

VACCINE (ADULT HORSES: BROODMARES previously unvaccinated against the disease indicated)	DOSE (D)	Schedule	COMMENTS
Tetanus	1	① D1	Booster at time of penetrating injury or prior to surgery if last dose was administered over 6 months previously.
	2	② 4–6 weeks after D1	
	3	③ 4–6 weeks PP†	
Eastern/Western Equine Encephalomyelitis	1	① D1	Consider six-month revaccination interval for immunocompromised horses or horses in endemic areas.
	2	② 4 weeks after D1	
	3	③ 4–6 weeks PP†	
Equine Influenza	1	① D1	Suggested dosage for inactivated vaccine only.
	2	② 4–6 weeks after D1	
	3	③ 4–6 weeks PP†	
Strangles – Streptococcus equi	1	① D1	Suggested dosage for killed vaccine containing M-protein.
	2	② 2–4 weeks after D1	
	3	③ 4–6 weeks PP†	
Equine Herpesvirus	1	① 5 mo GEST*	Give with product labeled for protection against EHV abortion.
	2	② 7 mo GEST*	
	3	③ 9 mo GEST*	
Botulism	1	① D1	
	2	② 4 weeks after D1	
	3	③ 4 weeks after D2	
Rotavirus	1	① D1	
	2	② 4 weeks after D1	
	3	③ 4 weeks after D2	
Potomac Horse Fever	1	① 7–9 weeks PP†	Semi-annual or annual booster. A revaccination interval of 3–4 months may be considered for high-risk areas.
	2	② 4–6 weeks PP†	
Rabies	1	① 4–6 weeks PP†	Can be given prior to breeding due to relatively long duration of immunity.
West Nile Virus	N/A – See comments		Preferable to vaccinate when open or according to unvaccinated adult horse guidelines if high risk.
Anthrax	N/A – See comments		Not recommended during gestation.
Equine Viral Arteritis	N/A – See comments		Not recommended unless high-risk.

Legend: ■ Core Vaccine ■ Non-core Vaccine — GEST* Gestation — PP† Pre-partum

Table 28.5 Vaccination recommendations for unvaccinated adult horses.

ADULT HORSES unvaccinated or lacking vaccination history — VACCINE	DOSE	Schedule	COMMENTS
Tetanus (Tet)	1	① Tet	Booster at time of penetrating injury or prior to surgery if last dose was administered over six months ago.
	2	② Tet: 4–6 wks after Dose 1	
Eastern/Western Equine Encephalomyelitis (EEE/WEE)	1	① EEE/WEE	Consider six-month revaccination interval for immunocompromised horses or horses in endemic areas.
	2	② EEE/WEE: 4–6 wks after Dose 1	
West Nile Virus (WNV)	1	① WNV	Suggested dosage for inactivated whole virus and inactivated flavivirus chimera vaccines.
	2	② WNV: 4–6 wks after Dose 1	
Rabies (Rab)	1	① Rab	Revaccinate annually.
Anthrax (Anthr)	1	① Anthr	Revaccinate annually.
	2	② Anthr: 4 wks after Dose 1	
	3	③ Anthr: 4 wks after Dose 2	
Botulism (Botu)	1	① Botu	Revaccinate annually.
	2	② Botu: 4 wks after Dose 1	
	3	③ Botu: 4 wks after Dose 2	
Equine Herpesvirus (EHV)	1	① EHV	Consider six-month revaccination interval for horses < 5 years old, horses on breeding farms, or high risk horses.
	2	② EHV: 4–6 wks after Dose 1	
	3	③ EHV: 4–6 wks after Dose 2	
Equine Viral Arteritis (EVA)	1	① EVA	Prior to initial vaccination, horses should be serologically tested and confirmed negative.
Equine Influenza (EI)	1	① EI	Suggested dosage for inactivated vaccine only. Revaccinate semi-annually to annually.
	2	② EI: 4–6 wks after Dose 1	
	3	③ EI: 3–6 months after Dose 2	
Potomac Horse Fever (PHF)	1	① PHF	Semi-annual or annual booster. A revaccination interval of 3–4 months may be considered for high-risk areas.
	2	② PHF: 3–4 wks after Dose 1	
Strangles Streptococcus equi (Strang)	1	① Strang	Suggested dosage for killed vaccine containing M-protein. Give third dose where recommended by manufacturer.
	2	② Strang: 2–4 wks after Dose 1	
	3	③ Strang: 2–4 wks after Dose 2 (see comments)	
Rotavirus (Rota)	N/A – See comments		Not applicable for adult horses – disease mainly affects foals.

Timeline columns: MONTH 1 (WK 1 2 3 4), MONTH 2 (5 6 7 8), MONTH 3 (9 10 11 12), MONTH 4 (13 14 15 16), MONTH 5 (17 18 19 20 21 22 23 24), MONTH 6 (24), MONTH 7 (25 26 27 28), MONTH 8 (29 30 31 32), MONTH 9 (33 34 35 36), MONTH 10 (37 38 39 40), MONTH 11 (41 42 43 44), MONTH 12 (45 46 47 48).

Legend: ■ Core Vaccine　■ Noncore Vaccine

Alternatively, if the vaccine efficacy is measured using a risk ratio (RR), it may be calculated as:

$$\text{Efficacy} = (1 - \text{RR}) \times 100.$$

The RR of disease among vaccinated relative to unvaccinated requires a cohort (prospective design), so that incidence data (attack rates) may be calculated for the vaccinated and unvaccinated groups.

It is also possible to use a case-control study design to evaluate vaccine effectiveness. If the disease is rare, and cases and controls are representative of the reference population, then effectiveness can be calculated using the odds ratio (OR) estimated from a case-control study:

$$\text{Effectiveness} = (1 - \text{OR}) \times 100.$$

Vaccine effectiveness may be evaluated using either cohort or case-control study designs (Comstock, 1990, 1994; Halloran, 1999; Orenstein, 1988; Rodrigues, 1999). In a cohort study, vaccinates (exposed cohort) and non-vaccinates (unexposed cohorts) would be followed forward in time after vaccination, and evaluated for development of disease and other outcomes of interest. If the vaccine is effective against the disease of interest, the incidence of disease will be lower among vaccinates than among unvaccinated horses. The case-control study design also is used commonly in human medicine to assess vaccine effectiveness. The odds of vaccination in cases of a disease of interest are compared to the odds of vaccination in healthy controls and, if the odds of vaccination among cases are significantly less than the odds among controls, then the vaccine is considered to be effective.

28.2.2   Rationale

The rationale for evaluating vaccine efficacy and effectiveness is manifold. Evidence of *efficacy* is required for licensure in the United States (http://www.aphis.usda.gov/wps/portal/aphis/ourfocus/animalhealth/sa_vet_biologics; accessed 7/31/2013). Once a vaccine is licensed, however, there are no governmental requirements in the United States for evaluating effectiveness of veterinary vaccines, and there is little incentive for manufacturers to evaluate *effectiveness*.

Effectiveness can be less than efficacy, irrespective of any changes in the antigenic biotype of circulating organism. With organisms like equine influenza virus, with potential for antigenic drift and antigenic shift, effectiveness of licensed vaccines may differ substantially from the efficacy studies used for licensure when the biotype of the vaccine differs sufficiently from circulating biotypes. Indeed, pivotal studies of effectiveness led to updated equine influenza vaccines in horses (Morley, 1999; Yates, 2000). Thus, evaluating vaccine effectiveness is important for development of better vaccines. Demonstration of vaccine efficacy/effectiveness is critical for stimulating and sustaining use of vaccines. For example, evidence of effectiveness of West Nile virus (WNV) vaccine (Epp, 2007) has been important in sustaining vaccination following the initial trans-continental spread of WNV westward across North America.

Vaccine effectiveness is also important for informing *cost-effectiveness*. The balance between cost of disease and cost of vaccination depends on the proportion of the disease that is preventable by vaccination (i.e., vaccine effectiveness). The most cost-effective vaccines are the ones for which both the burden of disease is large and the proportion of disease that is vaccine-preventable is large. An example of such a situation would be WNV vaccination of horses (Table 28.6).

Vaccination against even uncommon diseases may be deemed cost-effective when vaccine effectiveness is high, such as tetanus. Indeed, the disease is likely rare, because vaccination is highly effective and commonly administered. Anecdotally, there has been some debate in Australia regarding the cost-effectiveness of the Hendra virus vaccine. The cost of the vaccine is quite high, and there are regions of Australia where the disease is exceedingly rare. Therefore, veterinarians and horse-owners question the cost-effectiveness of Hendra virus vaccination in regions of very low risk. Cost-effectiveness is by no means the sole consideration of the value of a vaccine: vaccinating horses and other animals against rabies has an impact on human health, irrespective of the fact that rabies is a rare disease in horses.

The expectation that an effective vaccine will reduce the incidence of disease among vaccinates relative to unvaccinates, or that the odds of disease will be lower among vaccinates than among unvaccinated individuals, can lead to the misunderstanding that disease should always be less common among vaccinates than non-vaccinates when the vaccine is effective (Chen, 1996). In fact, when the vaccine is highly effective (but less than 100% effective), and vaccine coverage (i.e., the proportion of the population that is vaccinated) is high, most cases of a disease will occur among horses that have been vaccinated (see Table 28.7, adapted from Chen, 1996). This paradoxical result can lead to the misperception that a vaccine is not helping when it is, in fact, highly effective. For example, if vaccine coverage is very high, then it is likely that most cases will be found among *vaccinated*, rather than unvaccinated, horses. It also is worth noting that the proportion of diseased cases does not account for the severity of disease, which might be less severe among vaccinates than non-vaccinates.

The clinical outcome to demonstrate efficacy required for licensure is not always prevention of the disease of interest. For example, initial licensure of WNV vaccines for horses was based on reduction of the proportion of viremic horses. This outcome was selected, in part, due to the ability to induce viremia with WNV in horses experimentally, the absence of an equine model of WNV encephalomyelitis at the time of licensure, and the need to act swiftly to provide protection for horses during the WNV epidemic. This approach was ultimately successful, given the apparent effectiveness of licensed vaccines (Epp, 2007; Seino, 2007).

Table 28.6 Summary of West Nile virus efficacy and effectiveness studies: experimental and field studies.

Source	Design	Population	N	Vaccine type	Clinical outcome evaluated	Efficacy/effectiveness*
Chiang, 2005	Experimental	Foals	30	DNA	Viremia	83% (49–98%)
Epp, 2007	Field	Horses	300	Killed	Neurological disease	96% (67–99%)
Gardner, 2007	Field	Horses	192	**1** Inactivated virus **2** Canarypox recombinant	Neurological disease	100% (93–100%)
Long, 2007	Experimental	Horses	30	*Flavivirus* chimera	Neurological disease	95% (85–100%)
Ng, 2003	Experimental	Horses	30	Canarypox recombinant	Viremia	94% (69–100%)
Schuler, 2004	Field	Horses	569	Not reported	Death from WNV infection	94% (42–99%) when vaccinated according to manufacturers' recommendations 68% (32–85%) when receiving one or two doses not given per manufacturers' recommendation
Seino, 2007	Experimental	Horses	24	Inactivated Canarypox recombinant *Flavivirus* chimera	Neurological disease	71% (49% to 92%) for all three vaccines
Siger, 2004	Experimental	Horses	19	Canarypox recombinant	Viremia	86% (54–100%)
Siger, 2006	Experimental	Horses	20	Canarypox recombinant	Neurological disease	88% (58–100%)

* Numbers in parentheses are 95% confidence intervals.

28.2.3 Evidence of efficacy and effectiveness

In North America, the USDA and the Canadian Food Inspection Agency have placed greater emphasis on documenting purity, stability, and safety rather than efficacy. As mentioned previously, efficacy of equine vaccines is on data from small, experimental challenge studies. Because there is no requirement for manufacturers to publish their results, the design and results of efficacy studies are generally not presented in peer-reviewed publications (Townsend, 2000; Wilson, 2007). Therefore, our knowledge about the effectiveness of vaccines is relatively impoverished.

The perception of many people, including veterinarians, is that the effectiveness of commercially available vaccines is very high, if not 100%. In some instances, evidence indicates that this perception is justified. For example, experimental and field data indicate that the effectiveness of vaccines against WNV encephalomyelitis is high (Table 28.6). Although only two post-licensure field studies of effectiveness have been reported, both

Table 28.7 Hypothetical data demonstrating that if the effectiveness of vaccine is high and vaccine coverage is high, most cases will occur among vaccinates.*

Population of horses	100	100	100	100	100
Vaccine effectiveness	90%	90%	90%	90%	90%
Number vaccinated	60	80	90	95	100
Number protected by vaccine	54	72	81	86	90
Number vaccinated but susceptible	6	8	9	9	10
Number unvaccinated (all susceptible)	40	20	10	5	0
Total susceptible	46 (6 + 40)	28 (8 + 20)	19 (9 + 10)	14 (9 + 5)	10 (10 + 0)
Proportion susceptible that were vaccinated	13% (6/46)	29% (8/28)	47% (9/19)	64% (9/14)	100% (10/10)

* after Chen, 1996.

document very high effectiveness (Epp, 2007; Gardner, 2007). A third field trial documented high *apparent* effectiveness for preventing WNV clinical disease that resulted in death or euthanasia of the horse (Schuler, 2004). It is worth noting that reports of effectiveness are as high as, or higher than, efficacy studies using experimental intrathecal infection with WNV. The reasons for this phenomenon may reflect the small sample sizes, differences in outcomes evaluated (viremia, neurological disease, and mortality from neurologic disease), and the severity of the intrathecal challenge model relative to the spectrum of naturally-occurring disease.

For other diseases, vaccine effectiveness is lower than that reported for WNV vaccines. Several experimental and field studies have been published since documented low vaccine effectiveness for equine influenza vaccine among horses at a racetrack in western Canada, but none specifically quantified vaccine effectiveness (Morley, 1999; Newton, 2000, 2006; Cullinane, 2001; Townsend, 2001, 2003; Toulemonde, 2005; Paillot, 2008, 2010, 2013; Heldens, 2010). Nevertheless, these reports suggest that vaccine effectiveness for influenza vaccines is considerably lower than that for WNV encephalomyelitis.

In humans, reports indicate that vaccine effectiveness against influenza is approximately 50–60% (Osterholm, 2012; Centers for Disease Control, 2013), with markedly lower vaccine effectiveness reported for persons over 65 years old. Although vaccine effectiveness for vaccination against influenza is lower than widely regarded, influenza vaccine is helpful for protecting against disease. The success of influenza vaccination in people and horses, despite vaccine effectiveness being lower than is generally perceived, is most likely attributable to the impact of herd immunity.

Herd immunity refers to the phenomenon whereby vaccination or protection of a significant proportion of the population (herd) provides protection to the whole herd, including individuals that have not developed immunity (Fine, 1993). This protection to those that lack specific immunity often occurs by interrupting transmission of infection and, thus, decreasing the chances of susceptible individuals contacting infectious individuals. Herd immunity is a principle that applies to infections that are spread from animal to animal by direct contact. Aerosolized respiratory tract infections are particularly efficient at such transmission, and very effective at causing disease outbreaks. In contrast, for a disease like WNV encephalomyelitis, which is not transmitted from horse to horse, herd immunity is unlikely to be an applicable concept, since infection is vector-borne, with horses being dead-end hosts. Thus, the relatively high vaccine effectiveness for WNV is clinically crucial.

28.3 Safety of vaccines

Vaccination is one of the most effective tools for controlling and preventing disease. However, just as no vaccine is completely effective, no vaccine is completely safe, and all vaccines carry the risk of adverse reactions. The safety of vaccines may be perceived differently than other medical interventions (e.g., medications or surgery), because vaccines are administered primarily to healthy individuals, whereas other medical interventions are administered generally to individuals with disease. This may partially explain the aforementioned prioritization of demonstration of safety for licensure by regulatory agencies in North America.

28.3.1 Classifying adverse events

Adverse events following vaccination can be classified in a number of ways, including their cause, frequency, and severity. From the standpoint of cause, the United States Centers for Disease Control and Prevention (CDC) defines four types of vaccine-associated adverse events (Centers for Disease Control, 2012):

1 vaccine-induced events;
2 vaccine-potentiated events;
3 programmatic error; and
4 coincidental.

Vaccine-induced adverse events are those that would not have occurred in the absence of vaccination. Vaccine-induced events are attributable to properties of the vaccine and characteristics of the response of the individual vaccine (e.g., vaccine-associated strangles, after administration of modified live *Streptococcus equi* subspecies *equi* (SE) vaccine).

Vaccine-potentiated reactions are those that would have or might have occurred anyway but have been precipitated by vaccination (e.g., first febrile seizure in a predisposed individual, or purpura hemorrhagica following SE vaccination in a predisposed individual).

Programmatic error is an adverse event that occurs due to technical errors in vaccine storage, preparation, handling, or administration (e.g., abscesses of SE caused by contamination of other vaccines with modified-live SE vaccine).

Coincidental events are those that are reported as associated with vaccination, but that happened by chance or due to an underlying illness (e.g., mild colic following vaccination with live, intranasal SE vaccine).

Vaccine-induced and vaccine-potentiated events are those that should be considered to be vaccine-associated adverse effects. Adverse events that result from errors in vaccine delivery are a form of adverse reaction that is iatrogenic and preventable. Coincidental events are not causally associated with vaccination. Because adverse reactions to vaccines that are in the advanced stages of development or licensed are generally quite rare, epidemiological studies are usually required in order to identify and clarify associations. For example, anecdotal reports indicating that WNV vaccination of pregnant mares was associated with abortions and deformity of foals. Subsequent systematic epidemiological evaluation, however, indicated that vaccination of pregnant mares was not associated with abortion (Vest, 2004).

The vast majority of vaccines are recommended to be stored at temperatures between 35°–45°F (2–7°C) (Wilson, 2005).

(i.e., mare-foal pairs). Thus, when vaccination is delayed until six months, an ill-defined sub-population of foals remains vulnerable during a window of time when maternally-derived antibody has waned, but specific humoral and cell-mediated immune responses have not yet developed. For some infections (e.g., *Rhodococcus equi* or equine herpersvirus-1), cell-mediated immunity is more critical for protection than humoral immunity and, in these cases, humoral immune responses may be poor markers of protective immunity. For vaccines given by the mucosal route or for live-organism vaccines, interference from circulating maternal antibody may play little or no role in modulating immune responses to vaccination of foals.

There is considerable need to further evaluate the current blanket recommendation that foal vaccination be delayed until six months of age, and the development of vaccines that overcome maternal antibody interference. Although evidence exists that three-day-old foals produce less strong humoral and cell-mediated immune responses to vaccination than do foals three months of age, responses were stronger among adult horses than three-month-old foals (Ryan, 2010).

28.4.3 Number of vaccines or antigens

Horses, including pregnant mares during late gestation, are often vaccinated simultaneously with multiple vaccines, and many vaccines are manufactured to include multiple antigens. Simultaneous vaccination with multiple antigens offers advantages. First, it promotes higher vaccine coverage and compliance, by reducing confusion about scheduling multiple vaccinations administered at varying times. Second, it reduces the number of times the horse has to be subjected to the stress and discomfort of vaccination. Third, combination products reduce the costs of shipping, stocking, and (often) purchasing. Fourth, it reduces costs of veterinary visits for the owner. Finally, new antigens may be incorporated into existing vaccines (e.g., inclusion of WNV antigens in products for other core vaccines, such as Eastern and Western encephalitis vaccines).

Nevertheless, potential disadvantages to combination vaccines exist. Adverse events may occur more often with combination products than when individual components are administered separately (Thompson, 2006; Centers for Disease Control, 2010). There may be confusion about the need or impact for extra antigens (e.g., an additional dose of tetanus toxoid in a combination vaccine given more than once annually to protect against Eastern and Western encephalitis viruses). Perhaps most importantly, the impact of immunogenicity on one or more components of the vaccine might be reduced (Insel, 1995; Dagan, 1998; Denoël, 2007). To the authors' knowledge, systematic evaluation of this question has not been addressed for equine vaccines, and may be difficult to assess for at least two reasons.

1 The principal outcome measured in such studies is often serological (titers against the antigen), but serological titers may not represent the principal correlate of protective immunity (Plotkin, 2010, 2012).

2 The outcome of primary interest is protection against disease, rather than immunogenicity. However, given the rarity of most vaccine-preventable diseases, cohort studies would need to follow extremely large numbers of horses, and case-control studies would require exceptional historical recording of vaccination, along with accumulation of sufficient cases and controls.

Thus, it is unlikely that a reliable answer to the question of the impact of vaccinating with multiple antigens at once will be addressed among horses in the foreseeable future.

Clinical experience with equine and human medicine indicates that multiple antigens can be delivered efficaciously, but the extent to which this is true across all products and preparations is ill defined. In human medicine, with considerably greater resources and number of studies, questions remain about the immunogenicity of protocols and products when multiple antigens are delivered simultaneously (Bar-On, 2012).

28.4.4 Anti-inflammatory administration for horses with reactions to vaccines

As mentioned previously, some horses may experience localized swelling or low-grade fever in response to vaccination. In some of those horses, reactions may be avoided or reduced by switching vaccines. Some other horses, however, experience adverse effects irrespective of the type of vaccine or needle used. In such cases, veterinarians elect to concurrently administer either a non-steroidal anti-inflammatory drug (e.g., flunixin meglumine) or a glucocorticoid (e.g., dexamethasone) to counteract the inflammatory response to the vaccine.

Whether this process negatively impacts the immune response in horses is not clear. To the authors' knowledge, this question has not been systematically evaluated in horses. In people, there is some evidence that non-steroidal anti-inflammatory drugs can reduce immune responses to experimental rhinovirus infection (Graham, 1990). Current recommendations from the CDC indicate that evidence is lacking to support the use of antipyretics before or at the time of vaccination, to avoid adverse effects (Centers for Disease Control, 2010). Antipyretics do not prevent febrile seizures in children with previous febrile seizures (American Academy of Pediatrics, 2008).

Corticosteroids are known to suppress immune responses, including antibody production (Butler, 1975; Baxter, 1975). Nevertheless the Committee on Infectious Diseases of the American Academy of Pediatrics states that corticosteroids administered for brief periods appear to have only a minimal effect on antibody response to influenza vaccine (American Academy of Pediatrics, 2000). Although asthmatic people taking high-dose inhaled corticosteroids or oral corticosteroids had diminished immune responses to the B, but not the A, antigen of influenza vaccine, they were otherwise similar in immune response to influenza vaccination to individuals who were taking low-dose corticosteroids or no corticosteroids (Hanania, 2004).

Steroids did not alter the immune response to influenza vaccination among elderly patients with chronic obstructive pulmonary disease (de Roux, 2006). On the other hand, varicella vaccine failure was associated with administration of oral (but not inhaled) corticosteroids in children (Verstraeten, 2003). In horses, one dose of dexamethasone (0.05 mg/kg, 0.1 mg/kg, or 0.2 mg/kg IV) administered four hours before vaccination did not prevent horses from producing antibodies against tetanus toxoid; all these horses were healthy adult horses that had been vaccinated with tetanus toxoid at least yearly (Flaminio, 2009).

It remains unclear whether pre-treatment or concurrent treatment with anti-inflammatory drugs is effective at preventing or mitigating adverse events, or whether the drugs have a deleterious effect on immune responses. Current opinion and evidence in human medicine suggests that short-term use of low to moderate doses of anti-inflammatory drugs should not impact vaccinal responses.

28.5 Protocols for vaccination

Blanket recommendations for vaccination cannot be made reasonably because risk differs amongst groups of horses based on geographical, environmental, and individual characteristics (e.g., activity, age). Vaccination protocols might vary even for horses residing within the same barn. For example, a middle-aged gelding retired from competition that has limited exposure to other horses has a different level of risk than a young filly actively engaged in showing. Of course, one needs to be aware that the hypothetical gelding is at risk of being exposed to agents carried back by the hypothetical filly from her exposures at shows.

As stated and summarized in this chapter's tables, guidelines exist for vaccinating horses. The American Veterinary Medical Association (AVMA, 2011) defines core vaccines as those that protect from:

1 diseases that are endemic to a region;
2 diseases that have potential public health significance, so that vaccination is required by law;
3 virulent/highly infectious organisms and/or those posing a risk of severe disease.

In addition, core vaccines are those that *have clearly demonstrated efficacy and safety, and thus exhibit a high enough level of patient benefit and low enough level of risk to justify their use in the majority of patients.* On the basis of these definitions, the AAEP considers vaccines against the following agents to be core vaccines in the United States: tetanus toxoid; Eastern and Western equine encephalitis virus; rabies virus; and WNV.

Even for these core vaccines, however, risk-based decisions may define differences in schedule. For example, annual revaccination against Eastern and Western equine encephalitis is recommended in the United States, yet many veterinarians in areas where mosquitoes are active for most of the year (e.g., much of Florida and Texas) elect to vaccinate horses more frequently than once annually (American Association of Equine Practitioners, 2011). The rationale for this practice is that, if horses are vaccinated early in the spring, antibodies may be waning later in the fall, when disease risk may still be high in warm areas (Davidson, 2005; Wilson, 2005).

Interestingly, evidence exists that vaccinated horses were protected against experimental challenge with Eastern equine encephalitis virus even when antibody levels were not detectable (Barber, 1978). It is possible, if not likely, that the correlates of protective immunity extend beyond humoral responses for many vaccines, and that variation in serological responses among individuals, or measurement error in laboratory testing, render titers effective but weak tools for studying immune responses to vaccination.

In addition to core vaccines, licensed vaccines exist for other agents that may be considered risk-based. These include SE, equine influenza, equine herpesviruses-1 and -4, Venezuelan equine encephalomyelitis (VEE), equine viral arteritis (EVA), rotavirus, anthrax, botulism, *Neorickettsia risticii*, and endotoxin derived from *Salmonella enterica*. Specific recommendations for these vaccines are beyond the scope of this chapter, but recommendations relevant to North America are available from the AAEP guidelines at http://www.aaep.org/info/riskbased-vaccination-guidelines (and are summarized for foals and broodmares in Tables 28.1 and 28.2).

The onus is thus on the veterinarian to assess the risk of exposure to individual horses or individual facilities, farms or barns, in designing vaccine protocols. The risk of infectious disease may vary by region. For example, a mare from Texas being shipped to Kentucky to foal-out and be bred back may be vaccinated against botulism to protect her foal, that will be at greater risk of botulism in Kentucky than in Texas. Risk of infectious disease may also vary by activity. For instance, a yearling being shown frequently in futurity classes will have greater need for vaccination against influenza than a horse in a closed herd, where influenza exposure is unlikely.

Risk of infectious disease may vary by season. In many regions, the risk of mosquito-borne diseases (e.g., WNV encephalomyelitis) begins in the spring, and vaccinations against these vector-borne diseases should be timed accordingly in order to provide adequate protection prior to the beginning of vector activity. Although evidence is scant, age probably contributes to the risk of infection. Neonatal foals and geriatric horses appear to be at increased risk of infectious disease, and there is some evidence they may be less responsive to vaccines (Horohov, 1999; Muirhead, 2008; Ryan, 2010). Thus, neonatal foals and geriatric horses will require special consideration for vaccination protocols.

Risk-based vaccination continues to evolve, as new information about efficacy and safety of vaccines is provided, new vaccine technologies are licensed, and new and old infectious diseases emerge. Current recommendations for vaccination protocols may become out of date, and following the current literature and AAEP guidelines is recommended.

References

American Academy of Pediatrics (2000). Report of the Committee of Infectious Diseases: Influenza. In: Pickering, L.K. (ed). *2000 Red Book*, pp. 354–355. Grove Village, Ill, American Academy of Pediatrics.

American Academy of Pediatrics: Steering Committee on Quality Improvement and Management, Subcommittee on Febrile Seizures. (2008). Febrile seizures: clinical practice guideline for the long-term management of the child with simple febrile seizures. *Pediatrics* **121**(6), 1281–1286.

American Association of Equine Practitioners (2011). Vaccination guidelines. Accessed on August 2, 2013 at http://www.aaep.org/info/vaccination-guidelines-265 and http://www.aaep.org/info/riskbased-vaccination-guidelines

American Veterinary Medical Association. (2011). Veterinary biologics, p.6. Accessed on August 2, 2013 at https://ebusiness.avma.org/ProductCatalog/ProductCatalog.aspx under veterinary biologics.

Balasuriya, U., Go, Y.Y. and MacLachlan, N.J. (2013). Equine arteritis virus. *Veterinary Microbiology* **167**(1–2), 93–122.

Ball, B.A. (1988). Embryonic loss in mares: incidence, possible causes, and diagnostic considerations. *Veterinary Clinics of North America [Equine Practice]* **4**(2), 263–290.

Barber, T.L., Walton, T.E. and Lewis, K.J. (1978). Efficacy of trivalent inactivated encephalomyelitis virus vaccine in horses. *American Journal of Veterinary Research* **39**(4), 621–625.

Bar-On, E.S., Goldberg, E., Hellman, S. and Leibovici, L. (2012). Combined DTP-HBV-HIB vaccine versus separately administered DTP-HBV and HIB vaccines for primary prevention of diptheria, tetanus, pertussis, hepatitis B and Haemophilus influenzae B (HIB) (Review). *Cochrane Database of Systematic Reviews* 2012, Issue 4. rt. No.: CD005530.

Baxter, J.D. and Harris, A.W. (1975). Mechanism of glucocorticoid action: general features, with reference to steroid-mediated immunosuppression. *Transplantation Proceedings* **7**, 55–65.

Bofetta, P., Merler, E. and Vaino, H. (1993). Carcinogenicity of mercury and mercury compounds. *Scandinavian Journal of Work, Environment & Health* **19**(1), 1–7.

Brown, C., Kaneene, J.B. and Walker, R.D. (1988). Intramuscular injection techniques and the development of clostridial myositis or cellulitis in horses. *Journal of the American Veterinary Medical Association* **193**(6), 668–670.

Butler, W.T. (1975). Corticosteroids and immunoglobulin synthesis. *Transplantation Proceedings* **7**, 49–53.

Centers for Disease Control and Prevention. (2010). Recommendations from the Advisory Committee on Immunization Practices (ACIP) regarding administration of combination MMRV vaccine. *Morbidity and Mortality Weekly Reports* **59**(RR-3), 1–16.

Centers for Disease Control and Prevention. (2012). Vaccine safety. In: Atkinson, W., Wolfe, S. and Hamborsky, J. (eds). *Epidemiology and Prevention of Vaccine-Preventable Diseases*, 12th edition, pp. 45–60. Washington DC, Public Health Foundation.

Centers for Disease Control and Prevention. (2013). Interim adjusted estimates of seasonal influenza vaccine effectiveness – United States, February 2013. *Morbidity and Mortality Weekly Reports* **62**(07), 119–123.

Chen, R.T. and Orenstein, W.A. (1996). Epidemiologic methods in immunization programs. *Epidemiologic Reviews* **18**(2), 99–117.

Chiang, Y-W., Jennen, C.M., Holt, T.M., Waldbillig, C.P., Hathaway, D.K., Jennings, N.J., Ng, T. and Chu, H-J. (2005). Demonstration of efficacy of a West Nile virus DNA vaccine in foals. *Proceedings of the 51st Annual Convention of the American Association of Equine Practitioners* **51**, 183–190.

Comstock, G.W. (1990). Vaccine evaluation by case-control or prospective studies. *American Journal of Epidemiology* **131**, 205–207.

Comstock, G.W. (1994). Evaluating vaccination effectiveness and vaccine efficacy by means of case-control studies. *Epidemiologic Reviews* **16**(1), 77–89.

Conboy, H.S., Berry, D.B., Fallon, E.H., Holland, R.E., Powell, D.G. and Chambers, T.M. (1997). Failure of foal seroconversion following equine influenza vaccination. *Proceedings of the 43rd Annual Convention of the American Association of Equine Practitioners* **43**, 22–23.

Cullinane, A., Weld, J., Osborne, M., Nelly, M., McBride, C. and Walsh, C. (2001). Field studies of equine influenza vaccination regimes in Thoroughbred foals and yearlings. *The Veterinary Journal* **161**(2), 174–185.

Dagan, R., Eskola, J., Juhani, L., Leclerc, C. and Leroy, O. (1998). Reduced response to multiple vaccines sharing common protein epitopes that are administered simultaneously to infants. *Infection and Immunity* **66**(5), 2093–2098.

Davidson, A.H., Traub-Dargatz, J.L., Rodeheaver, R.M., Ostlund, E.N., Pederson, D.D., Moorhead, R.G., Stricklin, J.B., Dewell, R.D., Roach, S.D., Long, R.E., Albers, S.J., Callan, R.J. and Salman, M.D. (2005). Immunologic responses to West Nile virus in vaccinated and clinically affected horses. *Journal of the American Veterinary Medical Association* **226**(2), 240–245.

Denoël, P.A., Goldblatt, D., de Vleeschauver, I., Jacquet, J-M., Pichichero, M.E. and Poolman, J.T. (2007). Quality of the *Haemophilus influenzae* type b (Hib) antibody response induced by diphtheria-tetanus-acellular pertussis/Hib combination vaccines. *Clinical and Vaccine Immunology* **14**(10), 1362–1369.

de Roux, A., Marx, A., Burkhardt, O., Schweiger, B., Borkowski, A., Banzhoff, A., Pletz, M.W.R. and Lode, H. (2006). Impact of corticosteroids on the immune response to a MF59-adjuvanted influenza vaccine in elderly COPD-patients. *Vaccine* **24**(10), 1537–1542.

Domingo, J.L. (1994). Metal-induced developmental toxicity in mammals: a review. *Journal of Toxicology and Environmental Health* **42**(2), 123–141.

Epp, T., Waldner, C., and Townsend, H.H.G. (2007). A case-control study of factors associated with development of clinical disease due to West Nile virus, Saskatchewan 2003. *Equine Veterinary Journal* **39**(6), 498–503.

Fedson, D.S. (1998). Measuring protection: efficacy versus effectiveness. *Developments in Biological Standardization* **95**, 195–201.

Fine, P. (1993). Herd immunity: history, theory, practice. *Epidemiologic Reviews* **15**(2), 265–302.

Flaminio, M.J.B. (2009). Proceedings and abstracts of the 8th International Veterinary Immunology Symposium, August 15–19, 2007, Ouro Preto, Brazil. *Veterinary Immunology Immunopathology* **128**(1–3), 1–347.

Gardner, I.A., Wong, S.J., Ferraro, G.L., Balasuriya, U.B., Hullinger, P.J., Wilson, W.D., Shi, P-Y. and MacLachlan, N.J. (2007). Incidence and effects of West Nile virus infection in vaccinated and unvaccinated horses in California. *Veterinary Research* **38**, 109–116.

Graham, N.M.H., Burrell, C.J., Douglas, R.M., Debelle, P. and Davies, L. (1990). Adverse effects of aspirin, acetaminophen, and ibuprofen on immune function, viral shedding, and clinical status *in rhinovirus-infected volunteers. Journal of Infectious Diseases* **162**, 1277–1282.

Halloran, M.E., Longini, I.M., Jr. and Struchiner, C.J. (1999). Design and interpretation of vaccine field studies. *Epidemiologic Reviews* **21**(1), 73–88.

Hanania, N.A., Sockrider, M., Castro, M., Holbrook, J.T., Tonascia, J., Wise, R. and Atmar, R.L. (2004). Immune response to influenza vaccination in children and adults with asthma: effect of corticosteroid therapy. *Journal of Allergy and Clinical Immunology* **113**(4), 717–724.

Heldens, J.G.M., Pouwelsa, H.G.W., Derska, C.G.G., Van de Zandea, S.M.A. and Hoeijmakers, M.J.H. (2010). Duration of immunity induced by an equine influenza and tetanus combination vaccine formulation adjuvanted with ISCOM-Matrix. *Vaccine* **28**, 6989–6996.

Horohov, D.W., Dimock, A., Guirnalda, P., Folsom, R.W., McKeever, K.H. and Malinowski, K. (1999). Effect of exercise on the immune response of young and old horses. *American Journal of Veterinary Research* **60**, 643–647.

Insel, R.A. (1995). Potential alterations in immunogenicity by combining or simultaneously administering vaccine components. *Annals of the New York Academy of Sciences* **754**, 35–47.

Kaese, H.J., Valberg, S.J., Hayden, D.W., Wilson, J.H., Charlton, P., Ames, T.T. and Al-Ghamdi, G.H. (2005). Infarctive purpura hemorrhagica in five horses. *Journal of the American Veterinary Medical Association* **226**(11), 1893–1898.

Long, M.T., Gibbs, E.P.J., Mellencamp, W., Bowen, R.A., Seino, K.K., Zhang, S., Beachboard, S.E. and Humphrey, P.P. (2007). Efficacy, duration, and onset of immunogenicity of a West Nile virus vaccine, live *Flavirus* chimera, in horses with a clinical disease challenge model. *Equine Veterinary Journal* **39**(6), 491–497.

Morley, P.S., Townsend, H.H.G., Bogdan, J.R. and Haines, D.M. (1999). Efficacy of a commercial vaccine for preventing disease caused by influenza virus infection in horses. *Journal of the American Veterinary Medical Association* **215**(1), 61–66.

Muirhead, T.L., McClure, J.T., Wichtel, J.J., Stryhn, H., Frederick Markham, R.J., McFarlane, D. and Lunn, D.P. (2008). The effect of age on serum antibody titers after rabies and influenza vaccination in healthy horses. *Journal of Veterinary Internal Medicine* **22**, 654–661.

Newton, J.R., Townsend, H.H.G., Wood, J.L.N., Sinclair, R., Hannant, D. and Mumford, J.A. (2000). Immunity to equine influenza: relationship of vaccine-induced antibody in young Thoroughbred racehorses to protection against field infection with influenza A/equine-2 viruses (H3N8). *Equine Veterinary Journal* **32**(1), 65–74.

Newton, J.R., Daly, J.M., Spencer, L. and Mumford, J.A. (2006). Description of the outbreak of equine influenza (H3N8) in the United Kingdom in 2003, during which recently vaccinated horses in Newmarket developed respiratory disease. *The Veterinary Record* **158**(6), 185–192.

Ng, T., Hathaway, D., Jennings, N., Champ, D., Chiang, Y-W. and Chu, H-J. (2003). Equine vaccine for West Nile virus. *Developments in Biologicals* **114**, 221–227.

Orenstein, W.A., Bernier, R.A. and Hinman, A.R. (1988). Assessing vaccine efficacy in the field: further observations. *Epidemiologic Reviews* **10**(1), 212–241.

Osterholm, M.T., Kelly, N.S., Sommer, A. and Belongia, E.A. (2012). Efficacy and effectiveness of influenza vaccines: a systematic review and meta-analysis. *The Lancet* **12**(1), 36–44.

Paillot, R., Grimmett, H., Elton, D. and Daly, J.M. (2008). Protection, systemic IFN-gamma, and antibody responses induced by an ISCOM-based vaccine against a recent equine influenza virus in its natural host. *Veterinary Research* **39**, 21.

Paillot, R., Prowse, L., Donald, C., Medcalf, E., Montessoa, F., Bryant, N., Watson, J., Jeggob, M., Eltona, D., Newton, R., Trail, P. and Barneset, H. (2010). Efficacy of a whole inactivated EI vaccine against a recent EIV outbreak isolate and comparative detection of virus shedding. *Veterinary Immunology and Immunopathology* **136**, 272–283.

Paillot, R., Prowse, L., Montesso, F., Huang, C.M., Barnes, H. and Escala, J. (2013). Whole inactivated equine influenza vaccine: Efficacy against a representative clade 2 equine influenza virus, IFN-gamma synthesis and duration of humoral immunity. *Veterinary Microbiology* **162**, 396–407.

Peek, S.F., Semrad, S.D. and Perkins, G.A. (2003). Clostridial myonecrosis in horses (37 cases 1985–2000). *Equine Veterinary Journal* **35**(1), 86–92.

Plotkin, S.A. (2010). Correlates of protection induced by vaccination. *Clinical and Vaccine Immunology* **17**(7), 1055–1065.

Plotkin, S.A. and Gilbert, P.B. (2012). Nomenclature for immune correlates of protection after vaccination. *Clinical Infectious Diseases* **54**(11), 1615–1617.

Pusterla, N., Watson, J.L., Affolter, V.K., Magdesian, K.G., Wilson, W.D. and Carlson, G.P. (2003). Purpura haemorrhagica in 53 horses. *Veterinary Record* **153**(4), 118–121.

Rodrigues, L.C. and Smith, P.G. (1999). Use of the case-control approach in vaccine evaluation: efficacy and adverse effects. *Epidemiologic Reviews* **21**(1), 56–72.

Ryan, C. and Giguère, S. (2010). Equine neonates have attenuated humoral and cell-mediated immune responses to a killed adjuvanted vaccine compared to adult horses. *Clinical and Vaccine Immunology* **17**(12), 1896–1902.

Schuler, L.A., Khaitsa, M.L., Dwyer, N.W. and Stoltenow, C.L. (2004). Evaluation of an outbreak of West Nile virus infection in horses: 569 cases (2002). *Journal of the American Veterinary Medical Association* **225**(7), 1084–1089.

Seino, K.K., Long, M.T., Gibbs, E.P.J., Bowen, R.A., Beachboard, S.E., Humphrey, P.P., Dixon, M.A. and Bourgeois, M.A. (2007). Comparative efficacies of three commercially available vaccines against West Nile virus (WNV) in a short-duration challenge trial involving an equine WNV encephalitis model. *Clinical and Vaccine Immunology* **14**(11), 1465–1471.

Siger, L., Bowen, R.A., Karaca, K., Murray, M.J., Gordy, P.W., Loosemore, S.M., Audonnet, J-C., Nordgren, R.M. and Minke, J.M. (2004). Assessment of the efficacy of a single dose of a recombinant vaccine against West Nile virus in response to natural challenge with West Nile virus-infected mosquitoes in horses. *American Journal of Veterinary Research* **65**(11), 1459–1462.

Siger, L., Bowen, R.A., Karaca, K., Murray, M.J., Jagannantha, S., Echols, S., Nordgren, R. and Minke, J.M. (2006). Evaluation of the efficacy provided by a recombinant canarypox-vectored equine West Nile virus vaccine against an experimental West Nile virus intrathecal challenge in horses. *Veterinary Therapeutics* **7**(3), 249–256.

Slovis, N.M., Watson, J.L., Affolter, V.K. and Stannard, A.A. (1999). Injecton site eosinophilic granulomas and collagenolysis in 3 horses. *Journal of Veterinary Internal Medicine* **13**(6), 606–612.

Steven, D.H. (1982). Placentation in the mare. *Journal of Reproduction and Fertility Suppl*, **31**, 41–55.

Thompson, L.A., Irigoyen, M., Matiz, L.A., LaRussa, P.S., Chen, S. and Chimkin, F. (2006). The impact of DTaP-IPV-HB vaccine on use of health services for young infants. *Pediatric Infectious Diseases Journal* **25**(9), 826–31.

Timoney, P.J. and McCollum, W.H. (1993). Equine viral arteritis. *Veterinary Clinics of North America [Equine Practice]* **9**(2), 295–309.

Toulemonde, C.E., Daly, J., Sindle, T., Guigal, P.M., Audonnet, J.C. and Minke, J.M. (2005). Efficacy of a recombinant equine influenza vaccine against challenge with an American lineage H3N8 influenza virus responsible for the 2003 outbreak in the United Kingdom. *The Veterinary Record* **156**, 367–371.

Townsend, H.H.G. (2000). The role of vaccines and their efficacy in the control of infectious respiratory disease of the horse. *Proceedings of the 46th Annual Convention of the American Association of Equine Practitioners* **46**, 21–26.

Townsend, H.H.G., Penner, S.J., Watts, T.C., Cook, A., Bogdan, J., Haines, D.M., Griffin, S., Chambers, T., Holland, R.E., Whitaker-Dowling, P., Youngner, J.S. and Sebring, R.W. (2001). Efficacy of a cold-adapted, intranasal, equine influenza vaccine: challenge trials. *Equine Veterinary Journal* **33**(7), 637–643.

Townsend, H.G.G., Lunn, D.P., Bogdan, J., Griffin, S., Holland, R. and Barnett, C. (2003). Comparative efficacy of commercial vaccines in naïve horses: serologic responses and protection after influenza challenge. *Proceedings of the 49th Annual Convention of the American Association of Equine Practitioners* **49**, 227–229.

van Maanen, C., Bruin, G., deBoer-Luijtze, E., Smolders, G. and de Boer, G.F. (1992). Interference of maternal antibodies with immune response of the foals after vaccination against equine influenza. *Veterinary Quarterly* **14**(1), 13–17.

Verstraeten, T., Jumaan, A.O., Mullooly, J.P., Seward, J.F., Izurieta, H.S., DeStefano, F., Black, S.B. and Chen, R.T. (2003). A retrospective cohort study of the association of varicella vaccine failure with asthma, steroid use, age at vaccination, and measles-mumps-rubella vaccination. *Pediatrics* **112**(2), e98–e103.

Vest, D.J., Cohen, N.D., Berezowski, C.J., Morehead, J.P., Blodgett, G.P. and Blanchard, T.L. (2004). Evaluation of administration of West Nile virus vaccine to pregnant broodmares. *Journal of the American Veterinary Medical Association* **225**(12), 1894–1897.

Weinberg, G.A. and Szilagyi, P.G. (2010). Vaccine epidemiology: efficacy, effectiveness, and the translational research roadmap. *Journal of Infectious Diseases* **201**(11), 1607–1610.

Wilson, J.H., Gibbs, P.J., Calisher, C.H., Buergelt, C.D. and Schneider, C. (1995). Investigation of vaccine-induced tolerance to Eastern equine encephalitis virus in foals. *Proceedings of the 41st Annual Convention of the American Association of Equine Practitioners* **41**, 178–180.

Wilson, J.H. (2005). Vaccine efficacy and controversies. *Proceedings of the 51st Annual Convention of the American Association of Equine Practitioners* **51**, 409–420.

Wilson, W.D., Mihalyi, J.E., Hussey, S. and Lunn, D.P. (2001). Passive transfer of maternal immunoglobulin isotype antibodies against tetanus and influenza and their effect on the response of foals to vaccination. *Equine Veterinary Journal* **33**(7), 644–650.

Wilson, W.D. and Pusterla, N. (2007). Immunoprophylaxis. In: Sellon, D.C. and Long, M.T. (eds). *Equine Infectious Diseases*, pp. 556–570. St. Louis, Saunders Elsevier.

Yates, P. and Mumford, J.A. (2000). Equine influenza vaccine efficacy: the significance of antigenic variation. *Veterinary Microbiology* **74**(1–2), 173–177.

29 Types of Vaccines

Angela I. Bordin and Noah D. Cohen

29.1 Definition

Active immunization, or the use of antigens (formulated as a vaccine) to stimulate an immune response, is one of the best strategies to control and prevent infectious diseases in horses and other domestic animals. Re-immunization, or natural exposure to the pathogen in the vaccinated animal, results in a secondary immune response and enhanced immunity (Tizard, 2009). Immunization of horses is common. According to the United States Department of Agriculture's (USDA) National Animal Health Monitoring System (NAHMS) report in 2005, approximately 75% of equids in the USA received some type of vaccine during their initial 12 months of life (http://www.aphis. usda.gov/animal_health/nahms/equine/downloads/equine05/ Equine05_is_PartII_Highlights.pdf).

An ideal vaccine should be safe and should induce a potent and long-lasting immune response (Bachmann, 2010), mimicking as much as possible the immune response elicited by the infection. A vaccine should not, however, induce clinical signs associated with the disease, and should cause either minimal or no adverse side-effects. Ideally, a vaccine should, in the face of an outbreak, enable discrimination of naturally-infected animals from those vaccinated. In addition, the protective immune responses induced by vaccination should ideally include both humoral and cellular components, such as high-affinity antibodies and cell-mediated immune (CMI) responses.

29.2 Immunologic mechanisms

29.2.1 Types of licensed equine vaccines

The types of vaccines licensed for use in horses are: attenuated or modified live vaccines (MLV); killed or inactivated vaccines; subunit vaccines; nucleic acid-based vaccines; and chimera vaccines (see Table 29.1 for examples of licensed monovalent vaccines for use in horses in the USA).

29.2.1.1 Attenuated or modified live vaccines (MLV)

Live vaccines are composed of viable attenuated organisms that have limited replication in host cells, while they stimulate an immune response comparable to that elicited by natural infection (Ellis, 2008), but without causing disease in the recipient of the vaccine. Such microorganisms are attenuated by methods that will reduce their virulence or render a vaccine strain avirulent, while conserving immunogenicity (Shams, 2005). Several methods of attenuation are available, including cell culture attenuation, use of variants from other pathogen species, temperature-sensitive mutants (Ellis, 2008), and the use of internal ribosome entry site (IRES) (Volkova, 2008; Rossi, 2013).

The principal advantage of MLVs is that they are usually more effective than killed or inactivated vaccines (Abbas, 2007a), because they replicate and send danger signals to the host, stimulating both innate and adaptive immune responses (Siegrist, 2008). They elicit a greater number of effector mechanisms, such as activation of CD4$^+$ T cells and cytotoxic CD8$^+$ T cells (CTLs) (Murphy, 2012). Usually, MLVs are administered at a mucosal site of infection. This has many advantages, as discussed later (see mucosal vaccines section).

Nevertheless, MLVs have disadvantages. Virulence reversion or virulent opportunistic infections in immunodeficient patients can potentially occur with MLVs (Murphy, 2012). The manufacturing process, storage, and handling of live vaccines is more challenging and laborious than for other types of vaccines (Shams, 2005). Safety and phenotypic stability are also critical issues regarding MLVs (Youngner, 2001), as well as a risk for environmental contamination (Meeusen, 2007).

There are a few MLVs commercially available for equine diseases in the USA (Table 29.1). An intranasal MLV attenuated by cold adaptation in embryonated eggs (Flu Avert®, Heska Corporation) is available against equine influenza virus (EIV). A single dose in naïve horses protects against challenge from the homologous wild type (Townsend, 1999; Chambers, 2001; Youngner, 2001). Another example of an intranasal MLV is against *Streptococcus equi* subspecies *equi* (hereafter termed *Strep. equi*) infection (Pinnacle® I.N., Pfizer/Zoetis), which stimulates both innate and mucosal immune responses. This is particularly important, because protection against *Strep. equi* depends on both nasopharynx mucosal IgG and IgA antibodies against M (seM) protein, as well as opsonic IgG antibodies in the serum (Timoney, 1993). In horses resistant to reinfection with

Equine Clinical Immunology, First Edition. Edited by M. Julia B. Felippe.
© 2016 John Wiley & Sons, Inc. Published 2016 by John Wiley & Sons, Inc.

Table 29.1 Examples of monovalent equine vaccines licensed in the United States.

Agent	Commercial name	Type	Route	Manufacturer
Equine arteritis virus	Arvac®	MLV	IM	Pfizer/Zoetis
Eastern and Western	Equiloid Innovator®***	Killed	IM	Pfizer/Zoetis
equine	Encevac®-T with Havlogen***	Killed	IM	Merck/Intervet
encephalomyelitis virus	Encephalomyelitis Vaccine Eastern & Western	Killed	IM	Colorado Serum Co.
Equine herpesvirus-1	Calvenza™ EHV	Killed	IM or IN*	Boehringer Ingelheim
and -4	Rhinomune®	MLV	IM	Boehringer Ingelheim
	EquiVac® Innovator	Killed	IM	Pfizer/Zoetis
	Prestige® with Havlogen®	Killed	IM	Merck/Intervet
	Prodigy (EHV-1) with Havlogen®	Killed	IM	Merck/Intervet
Equine influenza virus	Fluvac Innovator®	Killed	IM	Pfizer/Zoetis
	FluAvert® I.N.	MLV	IN	Merck/Intervet
	Calvenza™ EIV	Killed	IM	Boehringer Ingelheim
	Recombitek® rFLU	Recombinant – live canary pox vector	IM	Merial
Rabies virus	IMRAB®	Killed	IM	Merial
Rotavirus A	Equine Rotavirus Vaccine**	Killed vaccine	IM	Pfizer/Zoetis
	Vetera® West Nile	Killed	IM	Boehringer Ingelheim
	Recombitek® rWNV	Recombinant – live canary pox vector	IM	Merial
West Nile virus	West Nile Innovator®	Killed	IM	Pfizer/Zoetis
	West Nile Innovator® – DNA	Plasmid-DNA based	IM	Pfizer/Zoetis
	Equi-Nile™ WNV with Havlogen®	Killed flavivirus chimera	IM	Merck/Intervet
Clostridium botulinum	Botvax® B	Killed	IM	Neogen
Type B	Tetanus Toxoid	Toxoid	IM	Pfizer/Zoetis
Clostridium tetani	Tetanus Toxoid Concentrate	Toxoid	IM	Colorado Serum Co.
	Tetanus Toxoid Unconcentrated	Toxoid	IM	Colorado Serum Co.
Neorickettsia risticii	Potomavac®	Bacterin	IM	Merial
	Strepvax® II	Bacterin	IM	Boehringer Ingelheim
Streptococcus equi	Pinnacle® IN	MLV	IN	Pfizer/Zoetis

MLV: Modified Live vaccine, IN: intranasal, IM: intramuscular.
* Initial dose intramuscular, revaccination IN or IM;.
** Conditional licensed;.
*** Contains Tetanus Toxoid.

Strep. equi, mucosal immunity functions to block entry of *Strep. equi* (Sweeney, 2005).

The only MLV against equine herpesvirus-1 (EHV-1) is Rhinomune® (Boehringer Ingelheim Vetmedica, Inc), which stimulates a strong EHV-1-specific $IgG_{4/7}$ antibody response, an important isotype for protection, as well as more interferon (IFN)-gamma-producing lymphocytes after restimulation of PBMCs with EHV-1 (Goodman, 2012). Other commercially available MLVs for horses include products against anthrax (Anthrax spore vaccine, Colorado Serum) and equine arteritis virus (EAV) (Arvac®, Zoetis).

29.2.1.2 Killed or inactivated vaccines

Inactivated or killed vaccines are prepared with killed microorganisms that are rendered unable to replicate in the host. Methods of inactivation include chemical agents that inactivate bacteria and viruses and detoxify bacterial toxins while preserving their antigenicity, such as formaldehyde, glutaraldehyde, and hydrogen peroxidase (Finn, 2008). Other methods include heat-killing (Srivastava, 1985) and irradiation (Fine, 2010).

Killed or inactivated vaccines are easier to manufacture than live vaccines (Ellis, 2008), are more stable than live vaccines, and cannot revert to the virulent form (Meeusen, 2007), making them safer for immunosuppressed animals. Inactivated vaccines usually require multiple injections to elicit an immune response (Minke, 2004; Tizard, 2009), but induce less adverse reactions. In general, they induce humoral immune responses (Meeusen, 2007) but, when combined with an adjuvant or a delivery system, they may stimulate CTLs (Ellis, 2008).

Immunization with an inactivated vaccine against West Nile virus has been shown to provide protection against severe disease (Davidson, 2005; Gardner, 2007; Salazar, 2004; Seino, 2007). Several inactivated vaccines are commercially available for use in horses in the US, in both monovalent and multivalent formats. Examples of such vaccines are those against EHV-1, EHV-4, EIV, equine encephalitis viruses (Eastern, Western, and Venezuelan), West Nile virus, rotavirus, *Strep. equi*, *Neoreckettsia risticii*, and rabies virus (Table 29.1).

29.2.1.3 Protein or subunit vaccines

Subunit vaccines are those that combine a portion (subunit) of the pathogen that causes a disease (Roth, 2001), composed of antigens purified from microbes or inactivated toxins, usually combined with an adjuvant (Abbas, 2007a). Evidence exists that toxins can be rendered harmless without loss of immunogenicity, and these toxins can induce strong antibody responses (Abbas, 2007a). For example, bacterial-extract vaccines against *Strep. equi*, when administered intramuscularly or subcutaneously, elicit serum antibody responses 7–10 days later (Sweeney, 2005).

Advantages of subunit vaccines include increased safety without the risk of reverting back to virulence, when compared with live vaccines, reduced antigenic competition relative to whole organisms, and the possibility to differentiate vaccinated animals from infected animals (marker vaccines). Another advantage of subunit vaccines is the potential for reducing the antigen load in the final product. Reducing the antigen load may reduce the immune response to irrelevant antigens, down-regulate immunosuppressive or pro-inflammatory responses, and enhance efficiency of vaccine production (Roth, 2001).

Subunit vaccines, nevertheless, have disadvantages. They can require strong adjuvants to stimulate effective immune responses with, consequently, more tissue adverse reactions (Roth, 2001). The duration of immunity is generally shorter for subunit vaccines than for live vaccines (Ellis, 2008). Subunit vaccines do not colonize mucosal surfaces, and do not generate mucosal antibodies. Last, subunit vaccines generally do not replicate intracellularly and, therefore, do not generate cell-mediated immune responses (Roth, 2001).

A subunit vaccine against *Strep. equi* (Strepvax® II, Boehringer Ingelheim), made with a purified M-protein, is available in the US. Other examples of subunit vaccines commonly used in horses are the toxoids that protect against tetanus and botulism (Table 29.1). In Europe, a sub-unit vaccine against EAV has been evaluated (Castillo-Olivares, 2001). It is a recombinant glycoprotein G_L (the immunodominant viral antigen), with varying degrees of protection observed in experimental challenges.

29.2.1.4 Recombinant vectored vaccines

Recombinant vectored vaccines use a virus or bacterium vector to express selected genes from the target pathogen coding for protective antigens. The vector can be either live or killed. Live recombinant vector vaccines are built by inserting the aforementioned selected genes into live, infectious, non-disease-causing viruses (Paillot, 2006a).

The great advantage of a viral vector is the induction of a full range of immune responses, including CTLs (Abbas, 2007a).

With virus-based live vector vaccines, viral antigens are expressed and synthesized *de novo* within the infected cells, presented via major histocompatibility complex (MHC) class-I and class-II antigen-processing routes, and stimulating both humoral and CMI responses (Paillot, 2006a).

One concern of vectored vaccines is the pre-existence of immunity against the vector (Paillot, 2006a), or the potential to initiate an immune response against the vector as a result of repeated vaccinations, limiting the immune response against the target pathogen.

Recombinant vaccines using a canary pox-vectored platform are available for use in horses against EIV (Recombitek® rFLU, Merial Limited) and West Nile virus (Recombitek® rWNV, Merial Limited). The recombinant vaccine against EIV contains two canary pox viruses expressing genes encoding for the hemagglutinin of two lineages of influenza virus (Adams, 2010). The use of live, non-replicating canary pox-vectored EIV vaccine resulted in specific antibody and CMI immune responses, as well as protection from clinical disease in naïve horses (Paillot, 2006b, 2007; Adams, 2010). In aged horses, even though the response to canary pox vectored EIV vaccine was limited, the animals were protected from disease (Adams, 2010).

29.2.1.5 Deoxyribonucleic acid (DNA)-based vaccines

DNA vaccines are produced by manufacturing and inserting genes coding for protective antigens into bacterial plasmids that enter the host cells and direct their own synthesis of the vaccine protein (Rogan, 2005). Therefore, the plasmid DNA encodes the antigen of interest and, with its expression controlled by a mammalian promoter, the host is responsible for expressing the antigen, to which its own immune system will be exposed (Coban, 2011). DNA uptake can be facilitated by chemical formulation or delivery through a non-replicating virus or bacterium (Ellis, 2008). Inoculation of a plasmid containing complementary DNA encoding an immunogenic protein leads to strong and long-lived humoral and CMI responses to the protein's antigen(s) (Coban, 2011; Ghanem, 2013).

DNA vaccines have a number of important advantages. They are considered safe, because they lack the ability to replicate, infect, or induce disease in the host (Rogan, 2005). They provide the only approach, other than live viruses, for eliciting strong CTL responses, because the DNA-encoded proteins are synthesized in the cytosol of transfected cells (Abbas, 2007a), in addition to humoral response (Ellis, 2008). They are also stable, which facilitates shipping and storage, and they are easy and inexpensive to manufacture, compared with isolated proteins or whole organisms (Ghanem, 2011). Plasmid DNA also has intrinsic adjuvant-like activities detected by immune cells, and it is possible to incorporate co-stimulators or cytokines into plasmid DNA vaccines (Abbas, 2007a).

Plasmid-based DNA vaccines have a few disadvantages. The DNA uptake by cells apparently decreases with increased body size, a finding that does not bode well for most breeds of horses. DNA vaccines can result in extended immunostimulation, which might result in either chronic inflammation or auto-antibody production. The immune response of DNA vaccines is limited to protein immunogens. DNA vaccines have the potential to affect genes responsible for cell growth (Ghanem, 2013), which might lead to tumor development.

The first USDA-approved DNA vaccine was an equine West Nile virus vaccine (West Nile-Innovator® DNA, Fort Dodge Animal Health). This was the only plasmid-DNA licensed for use in horses, but this vaccine was discontinued (De Filette, 2012). More DNA vaccines are being studied in horses, but none has yet been licensed or commercialized in the USA. Examples are recombinant vaccines for EAV (Zhang, 2012), EIV (Soboll, 2003; Ault, 2012), and equine infectious anemia virus (EIAV; Meng, 2012), with variable efficacy and protection.

29.2.1.6 Chimera vaccines

The USDA classifies chimeras as hybrid organisms created by the combination of nucleic acid fragments from two or more different organisms, with at least two of the fragments containing essential genes necessary for replication (http://www.aphis .usda.gov/animal_health/vet_biologics/publications/notice_05_ 23.pdf). The chimera vaccines available commercially use the Chimerivax technology, in which a live, attenuated recombinant virus is engineered from yellow fever virus strain 17D (YF-17D) by replacing the envelope protein genes of YF-17D with the corresponding genes of another flavivurus (Monath, 2002).

In horses, the West Nile (WN)-YF chimera vaccine is safe (Long, 2007a) and stimulates protective immune responses by ten days after a single vaccination, with a duration of immunity of 12 months against encephalitis and viremia (Long, 2007b). It also significantly reduces the frequency and severity of clinical signs among vaccinated horses, relative to unvaccinated control horses following severe intrathecal challenge (Seino, 2007). One of the limitations of the chimera vaccine is that the immunogenic protein(s) of the pathogenic virus must be known in order to produce the chimera. Also, chimeras are made from two viruses from the same family, making it challenging to find viruses from all families that are harmless and, thus, suitable to be used as backbone for the vaccine.

Examples of chimera vaccines licensed in US are the live West Nile virus flavivirus chimera (PreveNile™ with Havlogen®, Merck/Intervet), and West Nile virus killed flavivirus chimera (EquiNile™ with Havlogen®, Merck/Intervet). The live chimera vaccine PreveNile™ was removed from the market because of adverse effects, such as acute anaphylaxis, colic, respiratory distress and death (De Filette, 2012).

29.2.1.7 Marker vaccines (DIVA)

Marker or so-called DIVA (differentiating infected from vaccinated animals) vaccines lack one or more proteins (or part of a protein) of the virulent organism, enabling the differentiation of a vaccinated animal from those that are infected naturally. Currently, there is no licensed marker vaccine in the USA for use in horses, although a few attempts to produce a marker vaccine against EAV have been made, with promising results (Castillo-Olivares, 2003; Zhang, 2012).

In one study, the gene segment specifying residues 66 to 112 of the GL protein was deleted to create a mutant EAV (Castillo-Olivares, 2003). This mutant vaccine protected ponies against challenge with virulent EAV, even though *in vitro* experiments demonstrated poor neutralization of wild-type EAV strain. A limitation of this study was that only a small number of animals were challenged. Also, the mutant vaccine was not tested in pregnant mares, and no information on duration of immunity was presented.

Another study used a recombinant EAV as a MLV, with a single silent nucleotide substitution in the nucleocapsid gene (Zhang, 2012). This recombinant virus was similar to a parental MLV vaccine, but allowed differentiation of the vaccine from other field and laboratory strains of EAV by allelic discrimination, using a real-time reverse transcription polymerase chain reaction (RT-PCR) assay. In this study, the recombinant virus was shown to be immunogenic, but vaccinated horses were not fully protected.

29.3 Immune responses to vaccination

Vaccination induces protection against infections by stimulating the development of antibodies, long-lived effector cells, and memory cells (Abbas, 2007a). The type of vaccine influences which type of immune effectors are predominantly elicited, and is also related to protective efficacy (Siegrist, 2008). In addition to the vaccine's intrinsic characteristics (type of vaccine, antigen load, adjuvant or delivery system), the immune response can be influenced by host factors, such as genetics, degree of existing immunity to the antigen (i.e., first time versus subsequent exposure) (Fine, 2007; Vidor, 2007a), age (Boyd, 2003; Siegrist, 2001, 2009; Morein, 2007), the immune status of the vaccinated animal (Flaminio, 2002), presence of maternal antibodies (Jonsdottir, 2007; Vidor, 2007b), and pregnancy status (Matthiesen, 1996). Below is a brief summary of the types of immune responses induced by vaccines (see Figure 29.1).

29.3.1 Innate immunity

A vaccine will initially induce an immune response by sending danger signals to the host through stimulation of pathogen recognition receptors (PRR) of the innate immune cells. During a natural infection, this stimulation is achieved by signature microbial molecules known as pathogen-associated molecular patterns (PAMPs) (Abbas, 2007b). Toll-like receptors (TLRs) and NOD-like receptors (NLRs) are two examples of PRRs, and these families include cell-surface and cytoplasmic specific receptors that are each stimulated by different ligands expressed on extracellular or intracellular organisms, respectively.

Live vaccines are able to stimulate the innate immune system because they still contain PAMPs, regardless of the attenuation.

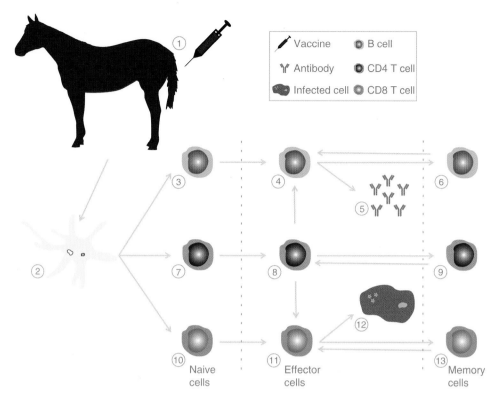

Figure 29.1 Intramuscular or subcutaneous vaccine in the horse.

1) Intramuscular or subcutaneous administration of vaccine in the horse.

2) Antigen (Ag) travels to lymphoid organs via lymph or captured by dendritic cells (DC) in the periphery.

3) Naïve B cells encounter and internalize the Ag in its native form, interact with T cells, become activated and differentiate into plasma cells.

4) Antibody-secreting plasma cells (effector B cells).

5) High-affinity antibodies against the vaccine Ag specific to a pathogen.

6) Some B cells become memory cells, which might differentiate into plasma cells whenever activated by antigen.

7) Naïve CD4$^+$ T cells encounter processed antigen-loaded DCs in lymphoid organs and become activated into T helper cells.

8) T helper cells proliferate and produce cytokines and modulate the immune response of both B cells and cytotoxic T cells (CTLs).

9) Some T helper cells become memory T cells, that might become effector cells when processed antigen is presented by DCs or other antigen presenting cells.

10) Naïve CD8$^+$ T cells encounter processed antigen-loaded DCs in lymphoid organs, and become activated into CTLs.

11) CTLs proliferate and perform surveillance of infected cells with related antigen.

12) CTLs identify and kill infected cells expressing related antigen.

13) Some CTLs become memory CD8$^+$ T cells, that might become activated in case of infection with specific intracellular pathogen.

In the case of inactivated, subunit, or DNA vaccines, stimulation of innate immunity usually results primarily from the adjuvants added to the vaccine (types of adjuvants are discussed later in this chapter). Adjuvants promote inflammation at the site of the vaccination, attracting antigen-presenting cells (APCs) that become activated by the vaccine PAMPs. The APCs subsequently migrate to the regional lymph nodes, and initiate T and B cell activation (Siegrist, 2008).

B cell receptors can recognize a wide range of molecules, such as proteins, lipids, carbohydrates, and nucleic acids. Therefore, non-replicating vaccines (including whole inactivated organism, subunit, and DNA vaccines) generally induce a strong antibody response (Abbas, 2007a). T cells, however, can only recognize peptides that have been displayed on MHC molecules, which confines their activation to vaccines containing protein antigens

that can be processed by APCs and presented via MHCs. Accordingly, inactivated viruses do not produce proteins in the cytosol and, consequently, their peptides are not presented via MHC class I molecules. Therefore, they do not induce a CTL response (Murphy, 2012).

On the other hand, plasmid-DNA vaccines that replicate in the host cell are potentially capable of activating both arms of the adaptive immune system. Nevertheless, certain adjuvants added to vaccines can initially activate APCs to secrete cytokines (e.g., interleukin IL-12) that can activate T cells (Abbas, 2007c).

29.3.2 Humoral immunity

Humoral immunity, along with complement activation, is quite efficient in controlling extracellular infections (Shams, 2005).

Following injection of a vaccine, the relevant antigens reach the regional lymph nodes through lymph, or the spleen through blood, and are stored on the surface of follicular cells of lymphoid tissues. Naïve B cells may recognize specific vaccine antigens via their B cell receptor (BCR), which consists of membrane-bound IgM and adjacent signaling molecules. For T-cell-dependent antigens, their binding to the BCR provides signal 1 for B cell activation, and subsequent interaction with CD4+ T helper cells provides signal 2 for clonal proliferation.

Some of the activated B cells immediately become plasma cells and secrete IgM for an early-phase humoral immune. Other cells develop a germinal center with highly-proliferative cells that undergo somatic hypermutation, affinity maturation and isotype switching, with further differentiation into plasma cells and memory cells. This process takes days, but results in the production of antibodies with high affinity and avidity for the antigens, and of different isotypes than IgM (e.g., IgG, IgA and IgE). There are also T cell-independent antigens, exemplified by polysaccharides, membrane glycolipids, and nucleic acids vaccines. These antigens are polyvalent and, therefore, induce strong B cell activation without the need of T cell interaction (Abbas, 2007c).

29.3.3 Cell-mediated immunity

Immunity against intracellular pathogens requires CMI responses. The ability to generate CMI responses is an important feature in a vaccine, and not all vaccines have this quality. Modified-live vaccines are particularly effective at inducing CMI responses.

When APCs migrate to lymphoid tissues from the site of injection in the periphery (i.e., intramuscular or subcutaneous injections, or mucosally administrated vaccines) after phagocytizing extracellular antigen, they become activated and process the vaccine antigen for presentation to CD4+ T cells via the MHC class II molecules. The MHC class II molecule, loaded with the antigen, binds to the T cell receptor (TCR), establishing the first signal for T cell activation. The interaction of additional costimulatory molecules expressed on T cells (CD40 L and CD28) and APCs (CD40 and CD86/CD80), respectively, is needed for complete activation of T cells. Antigens can also be presented by APCs (cross-presentation) through MHC class I molecules, and are recognized by CD8+ T cells (CTLs). Subsequent recognition of antigens by CTLs happens when infected cells express the antigen via MHC class I.

After activation, T cells undergo clonal expansion and differentiation into effector cells. CD4+ T helper effector cells produce cytokines that activate not only B cells but, importantly, CD8+ T cells and macrophages, leading to the production of antibodies, destruction of infected cells, and removal of pathogens, respectively (Siegrist, 2008). Indeed, cytotoxic T lymphocytes are responsible for T cell-mediated cytotoxicity of host cells containing intracellular pathogens. Activated CD4+ and CD8+ T cells can generate long-lived memory cells.

29.4 Routes of vaccination

The route of administration is an important consideration for vaccine development and delivery (Siegrist, 2008), as they aim to reach local APCs and induce immunity as similar as possible to a natural challenge. Several vaccines, however, are designed for administration via a parenteral route (intramuscular or subcutaneous), and these vaccines may not mimic the usual route of entry of targeted pathogens (Murphy, 2012). Inactivated vaccines administered parentally induce immune responses in the regional lymph nodes close to the site of injection, and the produced antibodies circulate through blood and lymph to all sites and tissues.

An ideal vaccine would use the same route as the targeted infecting agent (Murphy, 2012). Generation of mucosal immunity is the main goal of vaccination against those diseases caused by organisms that enter through mucosal surfaces. Examples of pathogens with mucosal entry include EIV, EHV-1, *Strep. equi, Rhodococcus equi, Salmonella enterica*, and *Escherichia coli*. When using mucosal MLVs, limited replication of the organism occurs at the site of administration, mimicking natural infection and, therefore, inducing an immune response tailored to the pathogen. Several routes can be used for mucosal vaccination, including intranasal, oral, sublingual, vaginal, ocular, and aerosol (Pavot, 2012).

The mucosal immune system has both inductive and effector sites (Smith, 2013). An inductive site is where the immune response will be induced, including the mucosa-associated lymphoid tissue (MALT) structures and lymph nodes. The MALT and lymph nodes are concentrated in areas where pathogens invade the body (Neutra, 2006). Effector sites are the mucosal epithelia and lamina propria, and stromal cells and connective tissue stroma (Smith, 2013). These sites are, essentially, where the B and T cells generated during the immune response at the inductive site will be directed.

One interesting feature of the mucosal immune system is that immunization at one mucosal site can induce specific responses at distant sites (De Magistris, 2006). As an example, the inductive sites for generation of immune responses to EIV with administration of an intra-nasal vaccine are in the upper respiratory tract (Smith, 2013). However, the effector sites are both in the upper and lower respiratory tract (Paillot, 2006a). Both B and T cells primed in the mucosa acquire specific migration patterns, migrating to the effector sites or back to the mucosal priming site via blood circulation (Pasetti, 2011).

Oral vaccines can activate all arms of the immune system, from secretory IgA (sIgA), systemic IgG, CMI responses, and antibody-dependent cellular cytotoxicity (Holmgren, 2005; De Magistris, 2006; Pasetti, 2011). This may explain why the only method demonstrated to date to protect foals against experimental intrabronchial infection with *R. equi* has been the oral/enteral administration of live, virulent organisms, while a number of other strategies have failed. Humoral mucosal immune responses develop earlier than systemic immune responses (Holmgren, 2005), which is an especially important consideration when vaccinating newborns, for example.

A needle-free vaccine delivery is being studied in horses as an alternative method for administration. This approach has been demonstrated to be as efficient and effective as parenteral administration with a syringe and needle (Ault, 2012).

29.5 Adjuvants and vaccine delivery systems

Adjuvants are substances added to a vaccine product to enhance and modulate protective immunity (Awate, 2013). Proposed mechanisms of action of adjuvants include: formation of depot; induction of inflammatory cytokines and chemokines; recruitment of immune cells; enhancement of antigen uptake and presentation; and, increased expression of costimulatory molecules and cytokines that stimulate T and B cell proliferation and differentiation (Abbas, 2007a; Ellis, 2008; Awate, 2013).

The addition of adjuvants to vaccines not only enhances the immunogenicity of antigens, but also reduces the number of immunizations required and improves the efficacy of vaccines in immunocompromised individuals, including newborns and the elderly (Montomoli, 2011). Modified-live vaccines usually do not need an adjuvant because they send danger signals when the organism replicates *in vivo*. Inactivated-organism, subunit, and DNA-based vaccines, however, may require an adjuvant or delivery system in order to enhance their immunogenicity (Ellis, 2008).

Adjuvants are used in equine vaccines. Most licensed vaccines contain a proprietary adjuvant and, therefore, both their composition and mechanism of action remain unclear. Below, we describe a few examples of substances that have been the focus of research on adjuvants in horses.

Toll-like receptors (TLRs) are structures in innate immune cells that recognize danger signals sent by pathogens. Activation of TLRs initiates a cascade of events that enhance the environment for activation of cells of the adaptive immune system. Examples of TLRs studied in horses that are potential sources of stimulation are TLR2, 3, 4, 6, 8, and 9 (Flaminio, 2007; Astakhova, 2009; Figueiredo, 2009; Liu, 2009; Sturgill, 2009; Gornik, 2011; Kwon, 2011; Bordin, 2012; Harrington, 2012). Because TLR8 is expressed in foal phagocytes, it could potentially be stimulated by its ligands, such as R848 (Harrington, 2012). Bacterial DNA is rich in cytosine-phosphate guanine (CpG) dinucleotides, and synthetic oligodeoxynucleotides containing bacterial CpG motifs (CpG-ODNs) are known to activate TLR9 in horses, with stimulation of protective immune responses against intracellular pathogens (Liu, 2009; Bordin, 2012).

Cholera toxin (CT) or CT subunit B (CTB), alone or coupled with protein antigens, are potent adjuvants for use in oral vaccines, and stimulate mucosal immune responses and production of sIgA (Kim, 1998). Cholera toxin can also be administered parentally (Lavelle, 2004). Genetically coupling CT to an epitope of a seM-protein was used in studying an intranasal vaccine against *Strep. equi* in ponies (Sheoran, 2002). Despite the production of specific antibodies, however, the vaccine did not protect the animals from challenge. Intragastric administration of an inactivated *R. equi* vaccine adjuvanted with CTB did not cause changes in the fecal microbiome of foals (Bordin, 2013).

Nanoparticles and microparticles are antigen delivery systems with dimensions similar to pathogens (Bachmann, 2010). Recently, it has been described that polymeric particles also have adjuvant properties, such as complementing the activity of TLR ligands and engaging NALP3 inflammasome (Rice-Ficht, 2010). In Europe, surface modified poly-lactic acid (PLA) nanoparticles, containing a *Strep. equi* enzymatic extract adsorbed onto the surface, were immunogenic in mice (Florindo, 2009, 2010).

Immune-stimulating complex (ISCOM) is a nanoparticle used as delivery system for vaccine antigens for both mucosal and parenteral administration (Morein, 2004). The ISCOM are 40-nm, partially purified fractions of saponin that induce cytokines such as IL-12 and IFN-gamma, enhancing APC function and inducing T-cell responses (Montomoli, 2011). Microparticles have been used with success against *Brucella abortus* in deer by using alginate-vitelline protein B microencapsulation (Arenas-Gamboa, 2009).

29.6 Important diseases with unavailable effective vaccines

There are several vaccines commercially available for equine diseases, with impact on both animal health and productivity. Several important diseases of horses, however, still remain without licensed vaccines, including vaccines against *R. equi*, *Burkholderia mallei* (glanders), *Leptospira interrogans*, *Sarcocystis neurona*, equine infectious anemia virus, *Lawsonia intracellularis*, and *Taylorella equigenitalis*, among others.

Most of the commercially available vaccines for use in horses are discussed in this chapter, such as modified live and inactivated whole organisms, protein and subunits, recombinant proteins, chimeras, and marker vaccines. Nevertheless, there are other types of vaccines still being studied (both against microorganisms that have effective vaccines and those pathogens for which an effective vaccine is lacking), as well as new adjuvants and delivery systems. Increasing knowledge of genetics is permitting the generation of several different approaches to vaccine development. Most of the attempts at novel vaccine strategies are to ensure a safe and reliable approach of protecting horses against infectious diseases, in which adequately protective immune responses are generated without severe side-effects.

References

Abbas, A.K., Lichtman, A.H., and Pillai, S. (2007a). Immunity to microbes. In: Abbas, A.K., Lichtman, A.H., and Pillai, S. (eds). *Cellular and Molecular Immunology*, pp. 351–373. Philadelphia, Saunders.

Abbas, A.K., Lichtman, A.H., and Pillai, S. (2007b). Innate immunity. In: Abbas, A.K., Lichtman, A.H., and Pillai, S. (eds). *Cellular and Molecular Immunology*, pp. 19–46. Philadelphia, Saunders.

Abbas, A.K., Lichtman, A.H., and Pillai, S. (2007c). *Cellular and Molecular Immunology*, First Edition. Elsevier Saunders.

Adams, A.A., Sturgill, T.L., Breathnach, C.C., Chambers, T.M., Siger, L., Minke, J.M. and Horohov, D.W. (2010). Humoral and cell-mediated immune responses of old horses following recombinant canarypox virus vaccination and subsequent challenge infection. *Veterinary Immunology and Immunopathology* 139(2–4), 128–140.

Arenas-Gamboa, A.M., Ficht, T.A., Davis, D.S., Elzer, P.H., Kahl-McDonagh, M., Wong-Gonzalez, A. and Rice-Ficht, A.C. (2009). Oral vaccination with microencapsuled strain 19 vaccine confers enhanced protection against *Brucella abortus* strain 2308 challenge in red deer (*Cervus elaphus elaphus*). *Journal Wildlife Diseases* 45(4), 1021–1029.

Astakhova, N.M., Perelygin, A.A., Zharkikh, A.A., Lear, T.L., Coleman, S.J., MacLeod, J.N. and Brinton, M.A. (2009). Characterization of equine and other vertebrate TLR3, TLR7, and TLR8 genes. *Immunogenetics* 61(7), 529–539.

Ault, A., Zajac, A.M., Kong, W., Gorres, J., Royals, M., Wei, C., Bao, S., Yang, Z., Reedy, S., Sturgill, T., Page, A., Donofrio-Newman, J., Adams, A., Balasuriya, U., Horohov, D., Chambers, T., Nabel, G. and Rao, S. (2012). Immunogenicity and clinical protection against equine influenza by gene-based DNA vaccination of ponies. *Vaccine* 30(26), 3965–3974.

Awate S., Babiuk, L.A. and Mutwiri, G. (2013). Mechanisms of action of adjuvants. *Frontiers in Immunology* 4, 114.

Babiuk, L.A. (2013). Modern vaccines. In *Sustainable animal production. Workshop discussion online resources*. http://www.agriculture.de/acms1/conf6/ws5bvacc.htm. Accessed on July 1 2013.

Bachmann, M.F. and Jennings, G.T. (2010). Vaccine delivery: a matter of size, geometry, kinetics and molecular patterns. *Nature Review Immunology* 10(11), 787–796.

Bordin, A., Liu, M., Nerren, J., Buntain, S., Brake, C., Kogut, M. and Cohen, N. (2012). Neutrophil function of neonatal foals is enhanced *in vitro* by CpG oligodeoxynucleotide stimulation. *Veterinary Immunology and Immunopathology* 145(1–2), 290–297.

Bordin, A.I., Suchodolski, J.S., Markel, M.E., Weaver, K.B., Steiner, J.M., Dowd, S.E., Pillai, S. and Cohen, N.D. (2013). Effects of administration of live or inactivated virulent *Rhodococccus equi* and age on the fecal microbiome of neonatal foals. *PLoS One* 8(6), e66640.

Boyd, N.K., Cohen, N.D., Lim, W.S., Martens, R.J., Chaffin, K.M. and Ball, J.M. (2003). Temporal changes in cytokine expression of foals during the first month of life. *Veterinary Immunology and Immunopathology* 92(1–2), 75–85.

Castillo-Olivares, J., de Vries, A. and Raamsman, M.J. (2001). Evaluation of a prototype sub-unit vaccine against equine arteritis virus comprising the entire ectodomain of the virus large envelope glycoprotein (GL): induction of virus-neutralizing antibody and assessment of protection in ponies. *Journal of General Virology* 82(10), 2425–2435.

Castillo-Olivares, J., Wieringa, R., Tamás, B., de Vries, A.A.F., Davis-Poynter, N.J. and Rottier, P.J.M. (2003). Generation of a candidate live marker vaccine for Equine Arteritis virus by deletion of the major virus neutralization domain. *Journal of Virology* 77(15), 8470–8480.

Center for Veterinary Biologics, NOTICE NO. 05–23. (2005). United States Department of Agriculture, Animal and Plant Health Inspection Service. http://www.aphis.usda.gov/animal_health/vet_biologics/publications/notice_05_23.pdf. Accessed on July 1 2013.

Chambers, T.M., Holland, R.E., Tudor, L.R., Townsend, H.G., Cook, A., Bogdan, J., Lunn, D.P., Hussey, S., Whitaker-Dowling, P., Youngner, J.S., Sebring, R.W., Penner, S.J. and Stiegler, G.L. (2001). A new modified live equine influenza virus vaccine: phenotypic stability, restricted spread and efficacy against heterologous virus challenge. *Equine Veterinary Journal* 33(7), 630–636.

Coban, C., Kobiyama, K., Aoshi, T., Takeshita, F., Horii, T., Akira, S. and Ishii, K. (2011). Novel strategies to improve DNA vaccine immunogenicity. *Current Gene Therapy* 11(6), 479–484.

Davidson, A.H., Traub-Dargatz, J.L., Rodeheaver, R.M., Ostlund, E.N., Pedersen, D.D., Moorhead, R.G., Stricklin, J.B., Dewell, R.D., Roach, S.D., Long, R.E., Albers, S.J., Callan, R.J. and Salman, M.D. (2005). Immunologic responses to West Nile virus in vaccinated and clinically affected horses. *Journal of the American Veterinary Medical Association* 226(2), 240–245.

De Filette, M., Ulbert, S., Diamond, M.S. and Sanders, N.N. (2012). Recent progress in West Nile virus diagnosis and vaccination. *Veterinary Research* 43(1), 16.

De Magistris, M.T. (2006). Mucosal delivery of vaccine antigens and its advantages in pediatrics. *Advanced Drug Delivery Reviews* 58(1), 52–67.

Ellis, R.W. (2008). Technologies for making new vaccines. In: Plotkin, S., Orenstein, W. and Offit, P. (eds). *Vaccines*, pp. 1335–1355. Philadelphia, Saunders.

Figueiredo, M.D., Vandenplas, M.L., Hurley, D.J. and Moore, J.N. (2009). Differential induction of MyD88- and TRIF- dependent pathways in equine monocytes by Toll-like receptor agonists. *Veterinary Immunology and Immunopathology* 127(1–2), 125–134.

Fine, D.L., Roberts, B.A., Teehee, M.L., Terpening, S.J., Kelly, C.L., Raetz, J.L., Baker, D.C., Powers, A.M. and Bowen, R.A. (2007). Venezuelan equine encephalitis virus vaccine candidate (V3526) safety, immunogenicity and efficacy in horses. *Vaccine* 25, 1868–1876.

Fine, D.L., Jenkins, E., Martin, S.S., Glass, P., Parker, M.D. and Grimm, B. (2010). A multisystem approach for development and evaluation of inactivated vaccines for Venezuelan Equine Encephalitis virus (VEEV). *Journal of Virology Methods* 163(2), 424.

Finn, T.M. and Egan, W. (2008). Vaccine additives and manufacturing residuals in United States-licensed vaccines. In: Plotkin, S., Orenstein, W. and Offit, P. (eds). *Vaccines*, pp. 73–81. Philadelphia, Saunders.

Flaminio, M.J., LaCombe, V., Kohn, C.W. and Antczak, D. (2002). Common variable immunodeficiency in a horse. *Journal of the American Veterinary Medical Association* 221(9), 1296–1302.

Flaminio, M.J., Borges, A.S., Nydam, D.V., Horohov, D.W., Hecker, R. and Matychak, M.B. (2007). The effect of CpG-ODN on antigen presenting cells of the foal. *Journal of Immune Based Therapies and Vaccines* 25(5), 1–17.

Florindo, H.F., Pandit, S., Gonçalves, L.M.D., Alpar, H.O. and Almeida, A.J. (2009). New approach on the development of a mucosal vaccine against strangles: Systemic and mucosal immune responses in a mouse model. *Vaccine* **27**(8), 1230–1241.

Florindo, H.F., Pandit, S., Gonçalves, L.M.D., Alpar, H.O. and Almeida, A.J. (2010). Surface modified polymeric nanoparticles for immunization against equine strangles. *International Journal of Pharmaceutics* **390**(1), 25–31.

Gardner, I.A., Wong, S.J., Ferraro, G.L., Balasuriya, U.B., Hullinger, P.J., Wilson, W.D., Shi, P.Y. and MacLachlan, N.J. (2007). Incidence and effects of west Nile virus infection in vaccinated and unvaccinated horses in California. *Veterinary Research* **38**(1), 109–116.

Ghanem, A., Healey, R. and Adly, F. (2013). Current trends in separation of plasmid DNA vaccines: a review. *Analytica Chimica Acta* **760**, 1–15.

Goodman, L., Wimer, C., Dubovi, E., Gold, C. and Wagner, B. (2012). Immunological correlates of vaccination and infection for equine herpesvirus 1. *Clinical and Vaccine Immunology* **19**(2), 235–241.

Gornik, K., Moore, P., Figueiredo, M. and Vandenplas, M. (2011). Expression of Toll-like receptors 2, 3, 4, 6, 9, and MD-2 in the normal equine cornea, limbus, and conjunctiva. *Veterinary Ophthalmology* **14**(2), 80–85.

Harrington, J.R., Wilkerson, C.P., Brake, C.B. and Cohen, N.D. (2012). Effects of age and R848 stimulation on expression of Toll-like receptor 8 mRNA by foal neutrophils. *Veterinary Immunology and Immunopathology* **150**(1–2), 10–18.

Holmgren, J. and Czerkinsky, C. (2005). Mucosal immunity and vaccines. *Nature Medicine*, **11**(4), S45–S53.

Jonsdottir, I. (2007). Maturation of mucosal immune responses and influence of maternal antibodies. *Journal of Comparative Pathology* **137**(Suppl. 1), S20–S26.

Kim, P.-H., Eckmann, L., Lee, W.J., Han, W. and Kagnoff, M. (1998). Cholera toxin and cholera toxin B subunit induce IgA switching through the action of TGF- β1. *The Journal of Immunology* **160**(3), 1198–1203.

Kwon, S., Vandenplas, M.L., Figueiredo, M.D., Salter, C.E., Andrietti, A.L., Robertson, T.P., Moore, J.N. and Hurley, D.J. (2011). Differential induction of Toll-like receptor gene expression in equine monocytes activated by Toll-like receptor ligands or TNF- alpha. *Veterinary Immunology and Immunopathology* **138**(3), 213–217.

Lavelle, E.C., Jarnicki, A., McNeela, E., Armstrong, M.E., Higgins, S.C., Leavy, O. and Mills, K.H.G. (2004). Effects of cholera toxin on innate and adaptive immunity and its application as an immunomodulatory agent. *Journal of Leukocyte Biology* **75**(5), 756–763.

Liu, M., Liu, T., Bordin, A., Nerren, J. and Cohen, N. (2009). Activation of foal neutrophils at different ages by CpG oligodeoxynucleotides and Rhodococcus equi. *Cytokine* **48**(3), 280–289.

Long, M.T., Gibbs, E.P.J., Mellencamp, M.W., Zhang, S., Barnett, D.C., Seino, K.K., Beachboard, S.E. and Humphrey, P.P. (2007a). Safety of an attenuated West Nile virus vaccine, live Flavivirus chimera in horses. *Equine Veterinary Journal* **39**(6), 486–490.

Long, M.T., Gibbs, E.P.J., Mellencamp, M.W., Bowen, R.A., Seino, K.K., Zhang, S., Beachboard, S.E. and Humphrey, P.P. (2007b). Efficacy, duration, and onset of immunogenicity of a West Nile virus vaccine, live Flavivirus chimera, in horses with a clinical disease challenge model. *Equine Veterinary Journal* **39**(6), 491–497.

Lunn, P.D., Davis-Poynter, N., Flaminio, M.J.B.F., Horohov, D.W., Osterrieder, K., Pusterla, N. and Townsend, H.G.G. (2009). Equine herpesvirus-1 consensus statement. *Journal of Veterinary Internal Medicine* **23**, 450–461.

Matthiesen, L., Berg, G., Ernerudh, J. and Hakansson, L. (1996). Lymphocyte subsets and mitogen stimulation of blood lymphocytes in normal pregnancy. *American Journal Reproductive Immunology* **35**(2), 70–79.

Meeusen, E.N., Walker, J., Petters, A., Pastoret, P.-P. and Jungersen, G. (2007). Current status of veterinary vaccines. *Clinical Microbiology Reviews* **20**(3), 489–510.

Meng, Q., Lin, Y., Ma, J., Ma, Y., Zhao, L., Li, S., Yang, K., Zhou, J., Shen, R., Zhang, X. and Shao, Y. (2012). A pilot study comparing the development of EIAV Env-specific antibodies induced by DNA/recombinant vaccinia-vectored vaccines and an attenuated Chinese EIAV vaccine. *Viral Immunology* **25**(6), 477–484.

Minke, J.M., Audonnet, J.-C. and Fischer, L. (2004). Equine viral vaccines: the past, present and future. *Veterinary Research* **35**(4), 425–443.

Monath, T.P., McCarthy, K., Bedford, P., Johnson, C.T., Nichols, R., Yoksan, S., Marchesani, R., Knauber, M., Well, K.H., Arroyoa, J. and Guirakhoo, F. (2002). Clinical proof of principle for ChimeriVax^{TM}: recombinant live, attenuated vaccines against flavivirus infections. *Vaccine* **20**(7–8), 1004–1018.

Montomoli, E., Piccirella, S., Khadang, B., Mennitto, E., Camerini, R. and de Rosa, A. (2011). Current adjuvants and new perspectives in vaccine formulation. *Expert Review of Vaccines* **10**(7), 1053–1061.

Morein, B., Hu, K-F. and Abusugra, I. (2004). Current status and potential application of ISCOMs in veterinary medicine. *Advanced Drug Delivery Reviews* **56**(10), 1367–1382.

Morein, B., Blomqvist, G. and Hu, K. (2007). Immune responsiveness in the neonatal period. *Journal of Comparative Pathology* **137**(Suppl. 1), S27–S31.

Murphy, K. (2012). *Janeway's Immunobiology*, eighth edition. New York, Garland Science.

Neutra, M. and Kozlowski, P. (2006). Mucosal vaccines: the promise and the challenge. *Nature Review Immunology* **6**(2), 148–158.

Paillot, R., Hannant, D., Kydd, J.H. and Daly, J.M. (2006a). Vaccination against equine influenza: Quid novi? *Vaccine* **24**(19), 4047–4061.

Paillot, R., Kydd, J.H., Sindle, T., Hannant, D., Edlund Toulemonde, C., Audonnet, J.C., Minke, J.M. and Daly, J.M. (2006b). Antibody and IFN-gamma responses induced by a recombinant canarypox vaccine and challenge infection with equine influenza virus. *Veterinary Immunology and Immunopathology* **112**(3–4), 225–233.

Paillot, R., Kydd, J.H., MacRae, S., Minke, J.M., Hannant, D. and Daly, J.M. (2007). New assays to measure equine influenza virus-specific Type 1 immunity in horses. *Vaccine* **25**(42), 7385–7398.

Pasetti, M., Simon, J.K., Sztein, M.B. and Levine, M.M. (2011). Immunology of gut mucosal vaccines. *Immunological Reviews* **239**(1), 125–148.

Pavot, V., Rochereau, N., Genin, C., Verrier, B. and Paul, S. (2012). New insights in mucosal vaccine development. *Vaccine* **30**(2), 142, 154.

Rice-Ficht, A.C., Arenas-Gamboa, A.M., Kahl-McDonagh, M.M. and Ficht, T.A. (2010). Polymeric particles in vaccine delivery. *Current Opinion in Microbiology* **13**(1), 106–112.

Rogan, D. and Babiuk, L.A. (2005). Novel vaccines from biotechnology. *Revue scientifique et technique* **24**, 159–74.

Rossi, S.L., Guerbois, M., Gorchakov, R., Plante, K.S., Forrester, N.L. and Weaver, S.C. (2013). IRES-based Venezuelan equine encephalitis vaccine candidate elicits protective immunity in mice. *Virology* **437**(2), 81–88.

Roth, J.A. and Henderson, L.M. (2001). New technology for improved vaccine safety and efficacy. *Veterinary Clinics of North America: food animal practice* **17**(3), 585–597.

Salazar, P., Traub-Dargatz, J.L., Morley, P.S., Wilmot, D.D., Steffen, D.J., Cunningham, W.E. and Salman, M.D. (2004). Outcome of equids with clinical signs of West Nile virus infection and factors associated with death. *Journal of the American Veterinary Medical Association* **225**(2), 267–274.

Seino, K.K., Long, M.T., Gibbs, E.P.J., Bowen, R.A., Beachboard, S.E., Humphrey, P.P., Dixon, M.A. and Bourgeois, M.A. (2007). Comparative efficacies of three commercially available vaccines against West Nile Virus (WNV) in a short-duration challenge trial involving an equine WNV encephalitis model. *Clinical and Vaccine Immunology* **14**(11), 1465–1471.

Shams, H. (2005). Recent developments in veterinary vaccinology. *The Veterinary Journal* **170**(3), 289–299.

Sheoran, A.S., Artiushin, S. and Timoney, J.F. (2002). Nasal mucosal immunogenicity for the horse of a SeM peptide of *Streptococcus equi* genetically coupled to cholera toxin. *Vaccine* **20**(11), 1653–1659.

Siegrist, C-A. (2001). Neonatal and early life vaccinology. *Vaccine* **19**(25–26), 3331–3346.

Siegrist, C.-A. (2008). Vaccine Immunology. In: Plotkin, S., Orenstein, W. and Offit, P. (eds). *Vaccines*, pp. 17–35. Philadelphia, Saunders.

Siegrist, C.-A., and Aspinall, R. (2009). B-cell reponses to vaccination at the extremes of age. *Nature Review Immunology* **9**(3), 185–194.

Smith, P.D., MacDonald, T.T. and Blumberg, R.S. (2013). Immunological and functional differences between individual compartments of the mucosal immune system. In: Smith, P.D., MacDonald, T.T. and Blumberg, R.S. (eds). *Principles of Mucosal Immunology*, pp. 27–36. New York, Garland Science.

Soboll, G., Horohov, D.W., Aldridge, B.M., Olsen, C.W., McGregor, M.W., Drape, R.J., Macklin, M.D., Swain, W.F. and Lunn, D.P. (2003). Regional antibody and cellular immune responses to equine influenza virus infection, and particle mediated DNA vaccination. *Veterinary Immunology and Immunopathology* **94**(1–2), 47–62.

Srivastava S.K. and Barnum, D.A. (1985). Studies on the immunogenicity of Streptococcus equi vaccines in foals. *Canadian Journal Comparative Medicine* **49**(4), 351–356.

Sturgill, T.L., Strong, D., Rashid, C., Betancourt, A. and Horohov, D.W. (2009). Effect of Propionibacterium acnes-containing immunostimulant on interferon-gamma (IFN-γ) production in the neonatal foal. *Veterinary Immunology and Immunopathology* **141**(1–2), 124–127.

Sweeney C.R., Timoney, J.F., Newton, J.R. and Hines, M. (2005). Streptococcus equi infection in horses: guidelines for treatment, control, and prevention of strangles. *Journal of Veterinary Internal Medicine* **19**, 123–134. ACVIM Consensus Statement.

Timoney, J. (1993). Strangles. *Veterinary Clinics of North America: Equine Practice* **9**(2), 365–374.

Tizard, I.R. (2009). *The use of vaccines. In: Veterinary Immunology: An introduction*, eighth edition. Philadelphia, Saunders.

Townsend, H.G.G., Cook, A., Watts, T.C., Bogdan, J., Haines, D.M., Grifffin, S., Chambers, T.M., Holland, R.E., Whitaker-Dowling, P., Youngner, J., Penner, S.J. and Sebring, R.W. (1999). Efficacy of a cold-adapted, modified-live virus influenza vaccine: a double-blinded challenge trial. *Proceedings of the 45th Annual Convention of the American Association of Equine Practitioners* **45**, 41–42.

Veterinary Services Centers for Epidemiology and Animal Health. (2006). *Vaccination Practices on U.S. Equine Operations*. United States Department of Agriculture, Animal and Plant Health Inspection Service. Accessed on: July 1 2013. http://www.aphis.usda.gov/animal_health/nahms/equine/downloads/equine05/Equine05_is_Vaccination.pdf. Accessed on: July 1 2013.

Veterinary Services Centers for Epidemiology and Animal Health. (2007). *Highlights of Equine 2005 Part II: Changes in the U.S Equine Industry, 1998–2005*. United States Department of Agriculture, Animal and Plant Health Inspection Service. Accessed on: July 1 2013. http://www.aphis.usda.gov/animal_health/nahms/equine/downloads/equine05/Equine05_is_PartII_Highlights.pdf.

Vidor, E. (2007a). The nature and consequences of intra-and inter-vaccine interference. *Journal of Comparative Pathology* **137**(Suppl. 1), S62–S66.

Vidor, E. (2007b). Vaccination of newborns against Hepatitis A in the presence of maternally derived antibodies. *Journal of Comparative Pathology* **137**(Suppl. 1), S42–S45.

Volkova, E., Frolova, E., Darwin, J.R., Forrester, N.L., Weaver, S.C. and Frolov, I. (2008). IRES-dependent replication of Venezuelan equine encephalitis virus makes it highly attenuated and incapable of replicating in mosquito cells. *Virology* **377**, 160–169.

Youngner, J.S., Whitaker-Dowling, P., Chambers, T.M., Rushlow, K.E. and Sebring, R. (2001). Derivation and characterization of a live attenuated equine influenza vaccine virus. *American Journal Veterinary Research* **62**(8), 1290–4.

Zhang, J., Go, Y.Y., Huang, C., Meade, B., Lu, Z., Snijder, E., Timoney, P. and Balasuriya, U. (2012). Development and characterization of an infectious cDNA clone of the modified live virus vaccine strain of equine arteritis virus. *Clinical and Vaccine Immunology* **19**(8), 1312–1321.

30 Transplantation Immunology

Rebecca L. Tallmadge

30.1 Definition

Histocompatibility refers to whether a foreign donor cell is likely to be accepted and engraft in a recipient, most often when sharing identical genes. The *Major Histocompatibility Complex (MHC)* encompasses the main set of genes that rule transplantation acceptance or rejection, and the two classes of MHC molecules are referred to as MHC class I and MHC class II. Many variants of these genes are found within a population, and the constellation of alleles, or types, at each of these genes within an individual, determines their *haplotype*.

> **Take home message: Definitions**
>
> **Allograft–**Cells or tissue harvested from one individual and transplanted to another individual with a different haplotype.
>
> **Haplotype–**an individual's set of alleles of histocompatibility loci.
>
> **ELA – Equine Leukocyte Antigen–**haplotype of a horse's MHC class I and MHC class II antigens, often determined by serology.
>
> **Major Histocompatibility Complex (MHC)–**encompasses the main set of genes that rule transplantation acceptance or rejection, referred to as MHC class I and MHC class II molecules.
>
> **Microsatellites–**short repeating sequences of DNA that are used as molecular markers in small groups or large population studies and fingerprinting.
>
> **Autograft–**Cells or tissue harvested and transplanted within an individual.

Other genes that may cause a graft to be rejected more slowly encode *minor* histocompatibility (H) antigens, and these are not linked to the MHC genomic region. Minor histocompatibility antigens are peptides from other cellular proteins that differ between individuals; for example, H-Y proteins, encoded on the Y chromosome and, hence, foreign to female recipients (Billingham, 1960; Dierselhuis, 2009). Proteins expressed on red blood cells (RBCs) may also differ between individuals and define blood groups on a population level. In contrast to the relatively simple human ABO blood groups, seven blood groups have been identified in the horse (A, C, D, K, P, Q, and U), and 34 unique blood group factors are derived from these (Sandberg, 1996). Proteins (antigens) not shared between individuals induce an immune response, including at least antibody production.

MHC class I molecules play a key role in immune surveillance, because they present peptide segments from intracellular proteins to the T cell receptor on CD8[+] T cells. MHC class I molecules are expressed on most nucleated cells. Prior to cell surface expression, MHC class I molecules must form stable trimers with a peptide and beta-2-microglobulin; the peptide may derive from intracellular self or non-self proteins. If a nucleated cell lacks MHC class I expression – a possibility with certain viral infections or types of tumors, in an attempt to escape immunity – it will be destroyed. In the absence of MHC class I molecules to bind killer inhibitory receptors (KIRs) expressed on natural killer (NK) cells, killing mechanisms are activated when NK cells interact with the bare nucleated cell. Therefore, MHC class I molecules also participate in immune surveillance. Classical MHC class I molecules are traditionally defined as highly polymorphic (many allelic variants exist in the population), and non-classical MHC class I molecules generally have one, or few, alleles in a population.

The function of *MHC class II* molecules is to present peptides derived from exogenous proteins to CD4[+] T cells. The peptides are processed and complexed with MHC class II alpha and beta heterodimers, encoded by DRA, DRB, DQA or DQB loci. MHC class II molecules are expressed on antigen-presenting cells (APCs, dendritic cells, macrophages, and B lymphocytes), and T lymphocytes in horses (Crepaldi, 1986).

30.2 Equine MHC genes: genomic organization and variation

To understand the genomic organization of the equine MHC class I and class II genes, a contig of large insert (bacterial artificial chromosome or BAC) clones spanning the equine leukocyte antigen ELA-A3 MHC was created (Gustafson, 2003). Because of the similarity within MHC class I and class II genes, other non-immune genes present in the MHC genomic region were used to anchor the contig. This led to the sequencing and localization of 15 distinct MHC class I genes and

Equine Clinical Immunology, First Edition. Edited by M. Julia B. Felippe.

pseudogenes in the ELA-A3 haplotype: seven are expressed in a variety of tissues, while the other eight genes harbor protein-coding defects, so are designated as pseudogenes (Tallmadge, 2005).

Recovery of the full genomic sequence for each locus (including coding sequence, introns, and flanking untranslated regions) was instructive for defining individual genes, as opposed to alleles of the same gene. This work was then extended across ELA haplotypes to define allelic groups of expressed MHC class I genes. The use of ELA-A2, ELA-A3, ELA-A5, ELA-A9, and ELA-A10 MHC homozygous horses from Dr. D.F. Antczak's Equine Genetics Center at Cornell University was essential for this phase. Five to eight MHC class I sequences were obtained from each individual horse, comprised of 3–5 classical and 2–3 non-classical sequences (Tallmadge, 2010). Comparison of sequences across serologically-defined haplotypes revealed that several genes are expressed by many haplotypes (locus 1, 2, 5, 6, 7, and 16), but many haplotypes also express a relatively unique MHC class I gene (locus 3, 4). For this MHC discussion, the terms *gene* and *locus* are equivalent.

Genomic analysis of the horse MHC class II region revealed one DRA gene, three DQA genes, three DQB genes, and three DRB genes in the ELA-A3 haplotype (D.C. Miller and D.F. Antczak, personal communication). Comparison of the ELA-A3 expressed DR and DQ sequences with those expressed by other common haplotypes (ELA-A2, ELA-A5, ELA-A9, and ELA-A10) revealed little variation in the DRA gene, whereas high levels of variation were encoded by DRB, DQA, and DQB genes (D.C. Miller and D.F. Antczak, personal communication, sequences available on the Immuno Polymorphism database, http://www.ebi.ac.uk/ipd/mhc/ela/index.html). MHC class II DRA, DRB, DQA and DQB sequence variations have been investigated by several groups: 17 DRA alleles (Albright-Fraser, 1996; Brown, 2004; Díaz, 2008; Janova, 2009); 14 DRB alleles (Gustafsson, 1994; Fraser, 1996; Díaz, 2001); 27 DQA alleles (Fraser, 1998; Janova, 2009); and more than 17 DQB alleles (Szalai, 1994; Horín, 2002; Villegas-Castagnasso, 2003).

30.3 Determining equine MHC haplotypes

Variation of horse MHC class I proteins has been traditionally assessed *serologically* by the lymphocyte microcytotoxicity assay, which is able to discern 19 distinct specificities or haplotypes. International workshops have developed panels of antisera for this purpose, and established the Equine Leukocyte Antigen (ELA) nomenclature, where haplotypes are designated by ELA-A1, ELA-A2, and so forth (Lazary, 1988). Application of this method across 12 common breeds revealed that each breed differs in ELA gene frequency, but that nearly all American Standardbreds, French Standardbreds, and American Saddlebreds could be typed with antisera against ELA-A1 through ELA-11, as could greater than 73% of Thoroughbreds, Quarter Horses, Morgan Horses, Peruvian Paso Finos, and Draft Horses

(Antczak, 1986). Although the serological assay provides a cell-based read-out, limited specificities and amount of typing sera, and the possibility of polyclonal alloantisera are considerable drawbacks.

With the advent of genome sequence information and tools, molecular alternatives to the lymphocyte microcytotoxicity assay have been explored. Given the collection of *MHC class I sequences linked to common ELA haplotypes* (ELA-A2, -A3, -A5, -A9, -A10) and sequences defined in ELA-A1, -A4, -A6, -A7, and -W11 haplotypes, it is possible to perform limited ELA typing via polymerase chain reaction (PCR) and sequencing (Chung, 2003; Ramsay, 2010; Tallmadge, 2010). A major limitation of this approach is that not all ELA haplotypes are recognized by the established serological panels. Consequently, MHC sequences associated with these unknown haplotypes have not been characterized.

Table 30.1 illustrates the different complements of MHC class I sequences expressed by common ELA haplotypes. Each column displays the group of sequences identified in the respective haplotype, and the rows display the prevalence of a locus across haplotypes. For example, locus 1 alleles have been detected in seven of the 10 haplotypes investigated (not found in ELA-A1, -A2, or –A5 to date), but each allele is distinct; hence, the designation Eqca-1*00101 through -1*00701 (1 denotes the locus; *00X01 denotes the allele).

In contrast, locus 3 and 4 appear to be unique to the ELA-A3 haplotype. The UN sequences are also unique to a haplotype (for example, sequence Eqca-N*00101 has only been detected in the ELA-A2 haplotype), but their position in the genome is undefined. The non-classical loci are frequently shared across haplotypes and exhibit low polymorphism (e.g., only one allele of locus 5 has been defined to date – Eqca-5*00101, in 5 of 6 ELA haplotypes).

The use of polymorphic *microsatellite* markers located within the MHC genomic region as proxies for serologically-defined markers is attractive, because microsatellite typing is rapid, inexpensive, and accurate. Strong correlations were found between this method and serology (r values ranged from 0.75 to 0.95) (Tseng, 2010). However, microsatellites reveal more genetic diversity than serological methods, as five ELA serotypes were associated with multiple microsatellite haplotypes. This increase in MHC diversity hinders their use in horses that have not been serotyped or are not related. Furthermore, while these microsatellites were very useful in identifying haplotypes in greater than or equal to 90% of the Thoroughbreds and Standardbreds tested, they were less successful in Arabian horses (63%). Overall, this approach has great potential, but practical application is limited at present, due to the small number of horses that have been typed, and the limited number of ELA-linked microsatellite haplotypes.

The utility of a custom DNA *microarray* has also been assessed for equine MHC class I typing (Ramsay, 2010). Expressed MHC class I sequences were determined from a population of interest and corresponding allele-specific probes

Table 30.1 MHC class I sequences linked to ELA haplotypes.

		ELA haplotype									
		A1	A2	A3	A4	A5	A6	A7	A9	A10	W11
	Classical loci										
	1	-	-	1*00101	1*00401	-	1*00501	1*00601	1*00201	1*00301	1*00701
	2	2*00202	2*00201	2*00101	2*00301	2*00302	-	2*00401	2*00102	2*00303	2*00304
	3	-	-	3*00101	-	-	-	-	-	-	-
	4	-	-	4*00101	-	-	-	-	-	-	-
	16	-	16*00101	-	-	16*00201	16*00401	16*00501	16*00301	-	16*00601
	17	N*00302	-	-	-	N*00201	-	-	N*00301	N*00401	N*00201
	18	N*00601	-	-	-	-	-	-	-	N*00501	-
MHC class I locu	19	N*01301	-	-	-	-	-	-	-	-	-
	UN	-	N*00101	-	-	-	-	-	-	-	-
	UN	-	-	-	N*00801	-	-	-	-	-	-
	UN	-	-	-	-	-	N*00901	-	-	-	-
	UN	-	-	-	-	-	-	N*01001	-	-	-
	UN	-	-	-	-	-	-	-	N*00701	-	-
	Non-classical loci										
	5	NT	5*00101	5*00101	NT	-	5*00101	NT	5*00101	5*00101	NT
	6	NT	6*00101	6*00101	NT	6*00101	NT	NT	6*00201	6*00201	NT
	7	NT	7*00101	7*00201	NT	7*00101	NT	NT	7*00101	7*00101	NT

Published allele suffix provided, all have *Eqca*-prefix. Dash (−) indicates that an allele has not been identified for that haplotype and **NT** indicates that the haplotype has not been tested for presence of allele. **UN** loci are unlinked to a genomic location and are not assigned to an allelic series. Data from Ramsay, 2010 and Tallmadge, 2010.

were designed. MHC class I reverse transcriptase PCR (RT-PCR) products were then labeled and hybridized to the array. In this closed population, the microarray was specific, consistent, and efficient. Provided a great deal of MHC class I haplotype sequence information and probe optimization, this method could be implemented on a larger scale.

30.4 Immunosuppression and engraftment

To promote graft acceptance, immunosuppressive drugs may be administered to the recipient before and transiently after transplantation. Many immunosuppressive drugs have been used in human transplantation, but few have been rigorously studied in the horse. In addition, many of these drugs can become cost-prohibitive when doses are scaled up to a horse's body weight. Drugs that induce death of particular T cells, such as cyclophosphamide, are often used in human medicine. Cyclophosphamide has been used in the horse as a chemotherapeutic agent (Saulez, 2004).

Allograft acceptance may occur if immunological *tolerance* is induced. Immunotolerance is present when the recipient is unresponsive to foreign donor antigens. Tolerance normally takes place to avoid inflammatory responses to self-antigens and innocuous antigens common in food and the environment. Transplantation studies in miniature swine with selective MHC matching indicate that cyclosporine A can prevent early

rejection of incompatible renal allografts, and tolerance could be induced after cyclosporine A treatment ended, if at least one MHC locus matched (Gianello, 1996).

Induction of tolerance can be achieved by lymphocyte receptor activation without co-stimulation. However, it can be affected by the differentiation stage of the responding lymphocytes when first encountering the antigen, the number of responding lymphocytes, the antigen presenting cells, and the site of antigen encounter. Human and animal clinical studies have demonstrated that anti-lymphocyte antibodies against T cell receptor or T cell co-receptor CD8 and CD4 antigens can induce tolerance of allografts (Siemionow, 2003; Graca, 2006).

Chimerism is the mosaic status of a recipient harboring engrafted donor cells. Depending on the impetus for transplantation, clinical parameters may be sufficient to determine successful engraftment, such as replacement of a depleted cell population. One alternative and sensitive measurement of graft acceptance is to quantify genetic determinants unique to the donor cells. For example, quantification of the SRY gene inherent to male cells transplanted into female recipients revealed that approximately 1% donor cells persisted at eight months post-transplant (Hidaka, 2003).

Recently, our laboratory performed bone marrow transplantation between a full-sister pair. An MHC-matched donor was identified by typing the affected horse and family members with polymorphic microsatellites in the MHC region (Figure 30.1). Only the full-sister carried the same MHC haplotype as the affected horse. To quantify donor cells present in the recipient,

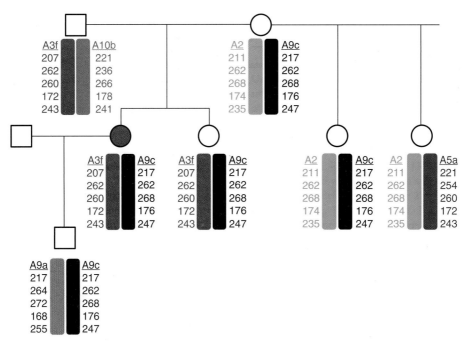

Figure 30.1 Major histocompatibility class (MHC) microsatellite typing of a horse family identified a full sibling MHC-matched donor for the patient. MHC microsatellite typing results of a horse family are shown for parents, siblings, and offspring of a patient with common variable immunodeficiency. Females are indicated by circles, males are indicated by squares, and the patient is indicated by a filled circle. The typing results are presented by haplotype (chromosome), and microsatellite alleles are listed below in the following order: COR110, COR112, COR113, UM011, COR114. Haplotype A2 is presented in green, A3f is in red, A5a is in purple, A9a is in gray, A9c is in black, and A10b is in blue.

we employed discordant microsatellite markers (i.e., sites where donor and recipient genome harbor different alleles) to quantify chimerism post-transplantation, but the sensitivity of the microsatellite assay was not sufficient to detect donor cells (lower limit of 10% donor DNA, unpublished data by C.T. Tseng, R.L. Tallmadge, and M.J. Felippe).

We then took advantage of the availability of genome-wide single nucleotide polymorphism (SNP) typing to identify places in the genome where the full-siblings differed (that is, donor genome carried *GG* genotype and recipient genome carried *AA* genotype), and developed a quantitative PCR assay specific for the *GG* genotype. Standard curves in which the donor genomic DNA was diluted in the recipient genomic DNA revealed that levels of 0.1% donor DNA could be detected with this assay. Although small and transient, donor DNA was detected in the recipient's circulating peripheral blood cells.

30.5 Graft rejection

Graft rejection will occur if the recipient recognizes the transplanted tissue as foreign. Immune responses against the graft are generally mounted by the adaptive immune system, mediated by either T cells or antibodies. The non-self MHC molecules expressed on allogeneic grafts are usually targeted by the recipient's immune system. Attempts are therefore made to match MHC haplotypes between donor and recipient.

Hyperacute graft rejection occurs within minutes to hours if the recipient harbors pre-existing antibodies against antigens expressed on donor cells. These may have formed in response to previous blood or tissue transfusions, or pregnancy. During pregnancy, paternal MHC class I molecules are transiently expressed by trophoblast and, if they are incompatible with the mare, strong maternal humoral and cytotoxic responses are induced (Crump, 1987; Baker, 2000). Antibody binding to the foreign graft antigens induces activation of the complement cascade and mediates tissue destruction and rejection.

Acute graft rejection generally occurs within days of transplantation or the cessation of immunosuppressive drugs. In acute rejection, the recipient is naïve to the donor tissue (i.e., the recipient does not have pre-existing donor-specific antibodies or T cells), but the foreign graft antigens are recognized either by direct or indirect allorecognition. Direct allorecognition occurs when antigen-presenting cells (APCs) from the transplanted tissue travel to the recipient's lymph nodes and present peptides to the recipient's lymphocytes. The peptide and accompanying co-stimulatory molecules expressed by the donor's APCs then stimulate an immune response – often a CD8[+] T cell-mediated graft rejection. Indirect allorecognition is the immune response generated by the recipient's own APCs presenting donor-derived peptides and, frequently, rejection is mediated by a CD4[+] T cell response, with accompanying antibody production. These antigenic peptides may be generated from mismatched donor MHC molecules or other minor histocompatibility antigens.

Chronic graft rejection develops months or years after transplantation. The pathogenesis of chronic graft rejection is similar to that of acute graft rejection, in which graft-specific T cells or antibodies are generated.

Graft-versus-host disease ensues when the donor's mature T cells initiate an immune response against recipient antigens. This is often seen in bone marrow transplant recipients, when the donor cells replace the recipient's ablated cells. Host APCs are able to present peptides to the mature donor T cells, resulting in activation of an anti-host immune response. Graft-versus-host immune responses have been documented in transplantation of severe combined immunodeficiency (SCID, lack B and T lymphocytes) foals with immune competent incompatible donor tissues (Perryman, 1987).

Take home message

Transplantation of cells or tissues between individuals that differ genetically (allografts), and correspondingly in expression of cell antigens, may result in immunological rejection of the graft.

MHC class I and MHC class II are the main set of genes that govern transplantation acceptance or rejection.

Minor histocompatibility antigens, like blood group antigens or sex-specific antigens, may also cause a graft to be rejected.

Better understanding of equine MHC class I and MHC class II gene variability has been attained, and will facilitate better matching between donor and recipient cells.

Immunosuppressive treatment regimens may delay rejection, induce graft tolerance and decrease graft-versus-host disease.

Chimerism (engrafted donor cells) can be precisely quantified.

Transplantation is an active area of basic and clinical research in the horse.

30.6 Current transplantation applications

Ongoing basic and clinical research has unveiled a great deal about successful transplantation in the horse, on both immunogenetic and regenerative fronts. However, significant barriers remain in developing rapid and inexpensive MHC typing assays, equine-specific reagents for donor cell/tissue isolation and phenotyping, immunosuppressive regimes, and optimal graft administration parameters of cell numbers, timing, frequency, and route.

Blood transfusions may be warranted, pursuant to severe blood loss, decreased erythrocyte production or non-regenerative conditions, immune-mediated hemolytic anemia, or neonatal isoerythrolysis. Prior to blood transfusion, it is important to identify compatible blood donors and recipients, because blood group frequencies are known to vary between breeds (Trommershausen Bowling, 1985), and incompatible transfusions may result in hemolysis of donor cells.

Blood compatibility is determined serologically by cross-matching, or typing of an individual may be performed with monoclonal or polyclonal antisera of defined specificity. In the major cross-match, recipient serum is incubated with donor erythrocytes to assess pre-existing antibodies in the recipient; agglutination indicates a positive test and incompatibility. In the minor cross-match, donor serum is incubated with recipient erythrocytes to determine whether pre-existing antibodies in the donor serum could hemolyze recipient red cells in the presence of complement. Blood typing or cross-match services are offered by the Animal Health Diagnostic Center at Cornell University, the Animal Genetic Testing & Research Laboratory at the University of Kentucky, and the University of California at Davis Veterinary Medical Teaching Hospital.

Neonatal isoerythrolysis is the most common cause of hemolytic anemia in neonatal foals and it results from fetal-maternal blood group incompatibility – maternal alloantibodies absorbed from colostrum mediate lysis of neonatal RBCs. Anti-red blood cell antibodies can be produced by sensitized mares from previous blood transfusions or pregnancies with incompatible blood groups. Indeed, anti-RBC antibodies were detected in serum from 10% of Thoroughbred and 20% of Standardbred mares tested (Bailey, 1982). The diagnosis may be confirmed by mare/foal RBC compatibility tests that are similar to the major cross-match. Severely affected foals may require RBC transfusion, and the mare is the ideal donor, provided only her RBCs are transfused (washed RBCs), because the serum contains alloantibody specific for the foal's RBCs. Alternatively, blood from a gelding can be used, although cross-matching is recommended.

Skin grafts are performed in horses most often to promote healing of large wounds, and vary in success from 50–100% within the same surgical technique (modified Meek technique, Wilmink, 2006; pinch grafts, Schumacher, 1989; mesh grafts, Booth, 1982). Autografts are used in most of these studies, because immune-mediated rejected of skin allografts can occur within 14 days of grafting (Adams, 2001).

Corneal transplants have an 88% success rate in overall vision retention in horses, when performed with penetrating keratoplasty, posterior lamellar keratoplasty, or deep lamellar endothelial keratoplasty surgical procedures (Brooks, 2008). However, despite the immunologic privilege of the cornea, the most common postoperative surgical complication is graft rejection, primarily mediated by CD4[+] T lymphocytes (Panda, 2007). The immune privilege normally present appears to be breached by keratitis and neovascularization (Panda, 2007).

The use of transplantation to repair joint, cartilage, and bone defects has been an active area of research. Autologous *chondrocyte and osteochondral grafting* has been successful, albeit requiring matching physical properties of donor and recipient sites (Hurtig, 2001; Bodo, 2004; Nixon, 2011). Allogeneic osteochondral grafts, without any typing efforts, may result in synovitis and leukocyte infiltration of the synovial membrane (Hurtig, 1988), although osteochondral and chondrocyte allografts have been reported successful in more recent studies (Hidaka, 2003; Pearce, 2003). By transplanting male cells into female recipients and measuring the male SRY gene, Hidaka and co-workers (2003) demonstrated that few ($\approx$ 1%) donor chondrocytes persisted in the repair tissue at eight months post-transplant. Based on these successful allografts, it has been posited that cartilage is an immune-privileged site (Sams, 1995; Hidaka, 2003).

Stem cell transplantation is an attractive regenerative treatment for a variety of conditions, due to intrinsic abilities of self-renewing and differentiation into a variety of cell types. In the horse, most research has been published on the use of bone marrow-derived mesenchymal stem cells (MSCs), which are able to differentiate into osteoblasts, adipocytes, and chondroblasts. MSCs derived from adipose, umbilical, and placental tissues have been described (Schnabel, 2013).

MSCs differ from hematopoietic stem cells (HSCs), which are able to repopulate erythroid, myeloid, and lymphoid blood lineages. Although MSC phenotyping is inconsistent between reports and is hampered by lack of reagents, conventionally MSCs express MHC class I molecules on the cell surface but lack immune co-stimulatory molecules (Burk, 2013). In the horse, MHC class II expression on MSCs may vary between individuals and between passages (Schnabel, 2014). It has been suggested that MSCs exert immunomodulatory and anti-inflammatory effects via soluble factors and direct interactions with immune cells, which may facilitate engraftment (Peroni, 2011). Notably, intradermal injections of allogeneic MSCs repeated after 3–4 weeks did not induce donor-specific cellular immune responses (Carrade, 2011).

Autologous MSC transplants have been performed to repair cases of soft palate defect and induced tendon lesion (Carstanjen, 2006; Pacini, 2007; Schnabel, 2009). Transplantation of autologous bone-marrow derived MSCs expanded *in vitro* yielded significantly better healing of articular defects than controls over 30 days, although this difference was not appreciated at eight months (Wilke, 2007). Similarly, injection of fetal-derived embryonic-like stem cells from an allogeneic commercial cell line promoted healing of induced tendon injury, and donor cells were identified eight weeks post-injection. These cells did not express MHC class I or MHC class II on their cell surface (Watts, 2011).

References

Adams, A.P. and Antczak, D.F. (2001). Ectopic transplantation of equine invasive trophoblast. *Biology of Reproduction* **64**(3), 753–763.

Albright-Fraser, D.G., Reid, R., Gerber, V. and Bailey, E. (1996). Polymorphism of DRA among equids. *Immunogenetics* **43**, 315–317.

Antczak, D.F., Bailey, E., Barger, B., Guerin, G., Lazary, S., McClure, J., Mottironi, V.D., Symons, R., Templeton, J. and Varewyck, H. (1986). Joint report of the Third International Workshop on Lymphocyte Alloantigens of the Horse, Kennett Square, Pennsylvania, 25–27 April 1984. *Animal Genetics* **17**, 363–373.

Bailey, E. (1982). Prevalence of anti-red blood cel antibodies in the serum and colostrum of mares and its relationship to neonatal isoerythrolysis. *American Journal of Veterinary Research* **43**, 1917–1921.

Baker, J.M., Bamford, A.I., Carlson, M.L., Mcculloch, C.E. and Antczak, D.F. (2000). Equine trophoblast as an immunological target. *Journal of Reproduction and Fertility Supplement* (**56**), 635–644.

Billingham, R.E. and Silvers, W.K. (1960). Studies on tolerance of the Y chromosome antigen in mice. *Journal of Immunology* **85**, 14–26.

Bodo, G., Hangody, L., Modis, L. and Hurtig, M. (2004). Autologous osteochondral grafting (mosaic arthroplasty) for treatment of subchondral cystic lesions in the equine stifle and fetlock joints. *Veterinary Surgery* **33**, 588–596.

Booth, L.C. (1982). Split-thickness autogenous skin transplantation in the horse. *Journal of the American Veterinary Medical Association* **180**, 754–757.

Brooks, D.E., Plummer, C.E., Kallberg, M.E., Barrie, K.P., Ollivier, F.J., Hendrix, D.V., Baker, A., Scotty, N.C., Utter, M.E., Blackwood, S.E., Nunnery, C.M., Ben-Shlomo, G. and Gelatt, K.N. (2008). Corneal transplantation for inflammatory keratopathies in the horse: visual outcome in 206 cases (1993–2007). *Veterinary Ophthalmology* **11**, 123–133.

Brown, J.J., Thomson, W., Clegg, P., Eyre, S., Kennedy, L.J., Matthews, J., Carter, S. and Ollier, W.E. (2004). Polymorphisms of the equine major histocompatibility complex class II DRA locus. *Tissue Antigens* **64**, 173–179.

Burk, J., Badylak, S.F., Kelly, J. and Brehm, W. (2013). Equine cellular therapy – from stall to bench to bedside? *Cytometry A* **83**, 103–113.

Carrade, D.D., Affolter, V.K., Outerbridge, C.A., Watson, J.L., Galuppo, L.D., Buerchler, S., Kumar, V., Walker, N.J. and Borjesson, D.L. (2011). Intradermal injections of equine allogeneic umbilical cord-derived mesenchymal stem cells are well tolerated and do not elicit immediate or delayed hypersensitivity reactions. *Cytotherapy* **13**, 1180–1192.

Carstanjen, B., Desbois, C., Hekmati, M. and Behr, L. (2006). Successful engraftment of cultured autologous mesenchymal stem cells in a surgically repaired soft palate defect in an adult horse. *Canadian Journal of Veterinary Research* **70**, 143–147.

Chung, C., Leib, S.R., Fraser, D.G., Ellis, S.A. and McGuire, T.C. (2003). Novel classical MHC class I alleles identified in horses by sequencing clones of reverse transcription-PCR products. *European Journal of Immunogenetics* **30**, 387–396.

Crepaldi, T., Crump, A., Newman, M., Ferrone, S. and Antczak, D.F. (1986). Equine T lymphocytes express class II MHC antigens. *Journal of Immunogenetics* **13**, 349–360.

Crump, A., Donaldson, W.L., Miller, J., Kydd, J.H., Allen, W.R. and Antczak, D.F. (1987). Expression of major histocompatibility complex (MHC) antigens on horse trophoblast. *Journal of Reproduction and Fertility Supplement* **35**, 379–388.

Díaz, S., Giovambattista, G., Dulout, F.N. and Peral-García, P. (2001). Genetic variation of the second exon of ELA-DRB genes in Argentine Creole horses. *Animal Genetics* **32**, 257–263.

Díaz, S., Echeverría, M.G., It, V., Posik, D.M., Rogberg-Muñoz, A., Pena, N.L., Peral-García, P., Vega-Pla, J.L. and Giovambattista, G. (2008). Development of an ELA-DRA gene typing method based on pyrosequencing technology. *Tissue Antigens* **72**, 464–468.

Dierselhuis, M. and Goulmy, E. (2009). The relevance of minor histocompatibility antigens in solid organ transplantation. *Current Opinion in Organ Transplantation* **14**(4), 419–425.

Fraser, D.G. and Bailey, E. (1996). Demonstration of three DRB loci in a domestic horse family. *Immunogenetics* **44**, 441–445.

Fraser, D.G. and Bailey, E. (1998). Polymorphism and multiple loci for the horse DQA gene. *Immunogenetics* **47**, 487–490.

Gianello, P.R. and Sachs, D.H. (1996). Effect of major histocompatibility complex matching on the development of tolerance to primarily vascularized renal allografts: a study in miniature swine. *Human Immunology* **50**, 1–10.

Graca, L., Daley, S., Fairchild, P.J., Cobbold, S.P. and Waldmann, H. (2006). Co-receptor and co-stimulation blockade for mixed chimerism and tolerance without myelosuppressive conditioning. *BMC Immunology* **7**, 9.

Gustafson, A.L., Tallmadge, R.L., Ramlachan, N., Miller, D., Bird, H., Antczak, D.F., Raudsepp, T., Chowdhary, B.P. and Skow, L.C. (2003). An ordered BAC contig map of the equine major histocompatibility complex. *Cytogenetic and Genome Research* **102**, 189–195.

Gustafsson, K. and Andersson, L. (1994). Structure and polymorphism of horse MHC class II DRB genes: convergent evolution in the antigen binding site. *Immunogenetics* **39**, 355–358.

Hidaka, C., Goodrich, L.R., Chen, C.T., Warren, R.F., Crystal, R.G. and Nixon, A.J. (2003). Acceleration of cartilage repair by genetically modified chondrocytes over expressing bone morphogenetic protein-7. *Journal of Orthopaedic Research* **21**, 573–583.

Horín, P. and Matiasovic, J. (2002). A second locus and new alleles in the major histocompatibility complex class II (ELA-DQB) region in the horse. *Animal Genetics* **33**, 196–200.

Hurtig, M.B. (1988). Experimental use of small osteochondral grafts for resurfacing the equine third carpal bone. *Equine Veterinary Journal Supplement* **(6)**, 23–27.

Hurtig, M., Pearce, S., Warren, S., Kalra, M. and Miniaci, A. (2001). Arthroscopic mosaic arthroplasty in the equine third carpal bone. *Veterinary Surgery* **30**, 228–239.

Janova, E., Matiasovic, J., Vahala, J., Vodicka, R., Van Dyk, E. and Horin, P. (2009). Polymorphism and selection in the major histocompatibility complex DRA and DQA genes in the family Equidae. *Immunogenetics* **61**, 513–527.

Lazary, S., Antczak, D.F., Bailey, E., Bell, T.K., Bernoco, D., Byrns, G. and McClure, J.J. (1988). Joint Report of the Fifth International Workshop on Lymphocyte Alloantigens of the Horse, Baton Rouge, Louisiana, 31 October – 1 November 1987. *Animal Genetics* **19**, 447–456.

Nixon, A.J., Begum, L., Mohammed, H.O., Huibregtse, B., O'Callaghan, M.M. and Matthews, G.L. (2011). Autologous chondrocyte implantation drives early chondrogenesis and organized repair in extensive full- and partial-thickness cartilage defects in an equine model. *Journal of Orthopaedic Research* **29**, 1121–1130.

Pacini, S., Spinabella, S., Trombi, L., Fazzi, R., Galimberti, S., Dini, F., Carlucci, F. and Petrini, M. (2007). Suspension of bone marrow-derived undifferentiated mesenchymal stromal cells for repair of superficial digital flexor tendon in race horses. *Tissue Engineering* **13**, 2949–2955.

Panda, A., Vanathi, M., Kumar, A., Dash, Y. and Priya, S. (2007). Corneal graft rejection. *Survey of Ophthalmology* **52**, 375–396.

Pearce, S.G., Hurtig, M.B., Boure, L.P., Radcliffe, R.M. and Richardson, D.W. (2003). Cylindrical press-fit osteochondral allografts for resurfacing the equine metatarsophalangeal joint. *Veterinary Surgery* **32**, 220–230.

Peroni, J.F. and Borjesson, D.L. (2011). Anti-inflammatory and immunomodulatory activities of stem cells. *Veterinary Clinics of North America: Equine Practice* **27**, 351–362.

Perryman, L.E., Bue, C.M., Magnuson, N.A., Mottironi, V.D., Ochs, H.S. and Wyatt, C.R. (1987). Immunologic reconstitution of foals with combined immunodeficiency. *Veterinary Immunology and Immunopathology* **17**, 495–508.

Ramsay, J.D., Leib, S.R., Orfe, L., Call, D.R., Tallmadge, R.L., Fraser, D.G. and Mealey, R.H. (2010). Development of a DNA microarray for detection of expressed equine classical MHC class I sequences in a defined population. *Immunogenetics* **62**(9), 633–639.

Sams, A.E. and Nixon, A.J. (1995). Chondrocyte-laden collagen scaffolds for resurfacing extensive articular cartilage defects. *Osteoarthritis Cartilage* **3**, 47–59.

Sandberg, K. (1996). *Guidelines for the interpretation of blood typing tests in horses.* International Society for Animal Genetics 1–9.

Saulez, M.N., Schlipf, J.W., Jr, Cebra, C.K., McDonough, S.P. and Bird, K.E. (2004). Use of chemotherapy for treatment of a mixed-cell thoracic lymphoma in a horse. *Journal of the American Veterinary Medical Association* **224**, 733–738.

Schnabel, L.V., Lynch, M.E., van der Meulen, M.C., Yeager, A.E., Kornatowski, M.A. and Nixon, A.J. (2009). Mesenchymal stem cells and insulin-like growth factor-I gene-enhanced mesenchymal stem cells improve structural aspects of healing in equine flexor digitorum superficialis tendons. *Journal of Orthopaedic Research* **27**, 1392–1398.

Schnabel, L.V., Fortier, L.A., Wayne McIlwraith, C. and Nobert, K.M. (2013). Therapeutic use of stem cells in horses: Which type, how, and when? *The Veterinary Journal* **197**(3), 570–577.

Schnabel, L.V., Pezzanite, L.M., Antczak, D.F., Felippe, M.J. and Fortier, L.A. (2014). Equine bone marrow-derived mesenchymal stromal cells are heterogeneous in MHC class II expression and capable of inciting an immune response in vitro. *Stem Cell Research and Therapy* **5**(1), 1–13.

Schumacher, J. and Hanselka, D.V. (1989). Skin grafting of the horse. *Veterinary Clinics of North America: Equine Practice* **5**, 591–614.

Siemionow, M.Z., Izycki, D.M. and Zielinski, M. (2003). Donor-specific tolerance in fully major histocompatibility major histocompatibility complex-mismatched limb allograft transplants under an anti-alpha-beta T-cell receptor monoclonal antibody and cyclosporine A protocol. *Transplantation* **76**, 1662–1668.

Szalai, G., Antczak, D.F., Gerber, H. and Lazary, S. (1994). Molecular cloning and characterization of horse DQB cDNA. *Immunogenetics* **40**, 458.

Tallmadge, R.L., Lear, T.L. and Antczak, D.F. (2005). Genomic characterization of MHC class I genes of the horse. *Immunogenetics* **57**, 763–774.

Tallmadge, R.L., Campbell, J.A., Miller, D.C. and Antczak, D.F. (2010). Analysis of MHC class I genes across horse MHC haplotypes. *Immunogenetics* **62**, 159–172.

Trommershausen Bowling, A. and Clark, R.S. (1985). Blood group and protein polymorphism gene frequencies for seven breeds of horses in the United States. *Animal Blood Groups and Biochemical Genetics* **16**, 93–108.

Tseng, C.T., Miller, D., Cassano, J., Bailey, E. and Antczak, D.F. (2010). Identification of equine major histocompatibility complex haplotypes using polymorphic microsatellites. *Animal Genetics* **41**(suppl 2), 150–153.

Villegas-Castagnasso, E.E., Díaz, S., Giovambattista, G., Dulout, F.N. and Peral-García, P. (2003). Analysis of ELA-DQB exon 2 polymorphism in Argentine Creole horses by PCR-RFLP and PCR-SSCP. *Journal of Veterinary Medicine Series A, Physiology, Pathology, Clinical Medicine* **50**, 280–285.

Watts, A.E., Yeager, A.E., Kopyov, O.V. and Nixon, A.J. (2011). Fetal derived embryonic-like stem cells improve healing in a large animal flexor tendonitis model. *Stem Cell Research & Therapy* **2**, 4.

Wilke, M.M., Nydam, D.V. and Nixon, A.J. (2007). Enhanced early chondrogenesis in articular defects following arthroscopic mesenchymal stem cell implantation in an equine model. *Journal of Orthopaedic Research* **25**, 913–925.

Wilmink, J.M., van den Boom, R., van Weeren, P.R. and Barneveld, A. (2006). The modified Meek technique as a novel method for skin grafting in horses: evaluation of acceptance, wound contraction and closure in chronic wounds. *Equine Veterinary Journal* **38**, 324–329.

31 Mesenchymal Stem Cell Therapy

Gerlinde R. Van de Walle, Catharina De Schauwer and Lisa A. Fortier

31.1 Definition

Stem cells can be broadly classified as either embryonic (ESC) or adult stem cells (ASC), depending on the developmental stage of the donor from which they are obtained (Fortier, 2005). A schematic overview of the classification of stem cells is depicted in Figure 31.1.

Embryonic stem cells can be either totipotent or pluripotent. The zygote, up to the 8-cell stage of the morula, is capable of forming the germ cells and cells of the endo-, meso-, and ectoderm layers, as well as the supporting trophoblast, that are required for the survival of the developing embryo. These cells are, therefore, termed totipotent (Lakshmipathy, 2005). Pluripotent stem cells are isolated from the inner cell mass of the blastocyst and give rise to endo-, meso- and ectoderm, but not to extra-embryonic tissues.

Adult stem cells have traditionally been viewed as a resident population of cells within each tissue that are necessary to maintain organ mass during normal cellular turnover (Fortier, 2005). Examples include: the hematopoietic stem cells that differentiate to all hematopoietic cells; neural stem cells that give rise to neurons, astrocytes, and oligodendrocytes; and mesenchymal stem cells (MSC) that differentiate into fibroblasts, osteoblasts, chondroblasts, adipocytes, and skeletal muscle (Verfaillie, 2002). In addition, ASC have the potential to differentiate into cell types of tissue lineages different from their tissue of origin – a concept called stem cell plasticity (Fortier, 2005; Koch, 2008; Baer, 2012).

The use of MSC for the treatment of equine injuries and diseases holds immense potential, and is expanding from its original application in orthopedics into the treatment of ischemic, inflammatory, and neurologic disorders (De Schauwer, 2013b). Nevertheless, sustained in-depth characterization of the MSC, and investigations using well-designed prospective clinical trials, remain indispensable for optimal clinical application and patient benefit. It should be a collective goal of the equine veterinary community to use clinical trials that include sufficient similar cases and a consistent and standardized panel of objective outcome measures.

31.2 Regenerative functions of mesenchymal stem cells

The use of MSC for primary tissue regeneration was initially advocated on the basis of their ability to differentiate into various tissue types. For example, a MSC would differentiate into a hepatocyte and secrete liver enzymes. As such, the regeneration of damaged tissues would be directly stimulated, since injected MSC colonize the injury site, differentiate into the appropriate mesenchymal tissue type, and affect repair (Stewart, 2011b). However, it is becoming increasingly clear that MSC also stimulate tissue regeneration indirectly, by secreting immunomodulatory and bioactive trophic factors (Borjesson, 2011; Fortier, 2011).

In general, tissue injury is associated with the activation of immune and/or inflammatory cells. Phagocytes, such as macrophages and neutrophils, secrete inflammatory molecules in response to factors (e.g., histamine, bradykinin, and prostaglandins) released by damaged cells. In addition, these factors will attract and activate B and T lymphocytes. These changes in the local microenvironment will result in mobilization and differentiation of MSCs, either tissue-resident or recruited from the bone-marrow, into damaged tissue. Under the influence of these inflammatory molecules (e.g., IFN-gamma, IL-1 or TNF-alpha), MSC will produce a variety of growth factors such as epidermal growth factor (EGF), fibroblast growth factor (FGF), vascular endothelial growth factor (VEGF), keratinocyte growth factor (KGF) and/or others. These growth factors, in turn, activate endothelial cells, fibroblasts and tissue-intrinsic stem cells, to promote tissue repair through enhanced angiogenesis, inhibition of leukocyte transmigration, and stimulation of stem cell differentiation (Ma, 2014).

Taken together, complex interactions exist between MSC and the cells present in injured tissue. Moreover, the secretion of growth factors by MSC might explain the remarkable regenerative effects, even if the locally injected MSC themselves do not engraft and/or differentiate.

Equine Clinical Immunology, First Edition. Edited by M. Julia B. Felippe.
© 2016 John Wiley & Sons, Inc. Published 2016 by John Wiley & Sons, Inc.

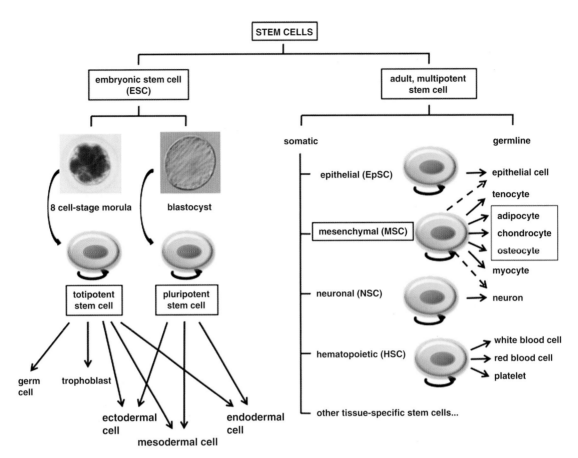

Figure 31.1 Classification of embryonic and adult stem cells.

31.3 Immunologic mechanisms and associations

Mesenchymal stem cells have potent immunomodulatory activities, affecting both innate and adaptive immunity. These immunomodulatory effects are mediated either through direct cell-cell contact with cells of the immune system or indirectly, via the production of multiple soluble factors (Kode, 2009; Peroni, 2011). The underlying mechanisms for these activities are not fully understood, and available data are sometimes controversial. This uncertainty can, in part, be explained by the fact that not all immunomodulatory functions of MSC are constitutively expressed, but some are induced by pro-inflammatory cytokines secreted by activated leukocytes. These cytokines, in turn, will stimulate MSC to secrete various soluble factors mediating immunosuppression.

In addition, the majority of information regarding the immunomodulatory activities of MSC comes from rodent and human studies, and there are important species differences. For example, the immunosuppressive effects of murine MSC are mediated by the production of the (inducible) nitric oxide synthase (iNOS), while human MSC utilize indolamine 2,3-dioxygenase (IDO) (Ling, 2014). However, several studies have shown that

equine MSC appear to possess similar immunomodulatory profiles (Peroni, 2011; Carrade, 2012; De Schauwer, 2014).

While the immunosuppressive activities of MSC support the concept of using stem cells in immune-mediated diseases, MSC have other immunomodulatory properties. Depending on the level of inflammation, MSC will either be immunosuppressive, or will enhance immune responses. Indeed, when inflammation levels are low, or MSC factors that mediate immunosuppression are inhibited, MSCs can promote immune responses instead of suppressing them (Ma, 2014). This concept of MSC plasticity, depending on the level of inflammation in the micro-environment, has important implications for the need to accurately determine the route of injection, the timing of the injection, and the cell number administered in order to obtain a successful clinical outcome of MSC treatments.

31.3.1 Immunosuppressive properties

Damaged tissues are normally accompanied by inflammation, with increased IFN-gamma expression in combination with pro-inflammatory cytokines TNF-alpha and IL-1. This inflammatory environment triggers MSC to synthesize and secrete a variety of potent immunosuppressive factors, as well as promoting expression of chemokines and adhesion molecules,

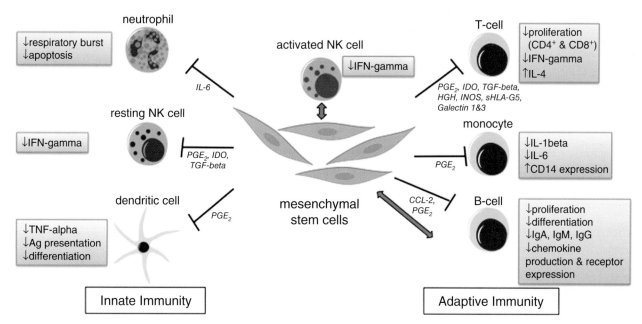

Figure 31.2 A schematic overview of the immunosuppressive properties of mesenchymal stem cells (MSC).

including intercellular adhesion molecule 1 (ICAM-1), vascular cell adhesion molecule 1 (VCAM-1), and ligands of chemokine receptors CXCR3 and CCR5 (Figure 31.2). The latter factors induce accumulation of immune cells to the site of injury, resulting in a microenvironment, where MSC can closely interact with the attracted immune cells. Locally produced MSC and direct cell-to-cell contact will, therefore, result in potent immunosuppression (Ma, 2014).

The cytokine IL-6 produced by MSCs not only decreases respiratory burst and protects neutrophils from apoptosis, but is also involved in inhibition of monocyte differentiation into dendritic cells (DC). Moreover, MSC, via the secretion of prostaglandin 2 (PGE$_2$), retain DC in their immature state, by inhibiting expression of antigen-presenting molecule major histocompatibility (MHC) class II and the co-stimulatory molecules CD40, CD80 and CD86 involved in the activation of T cells, and also by suppressing production of pro-inflammatory cytokines such as TNF-alpha. MSC have been shown to induce IL-10 producing macrophages, and IL-10 is an anti-inflammatory cytokine that is produced by a variety of immune cells as well as MSC. MSC also suppress natural killer (NK) cells, via soluble factors PGE$_2$, TGF-beta and IDO, and through direct cell-cell contact.

Aside from the immunosuppressive effects on cells from the innate immune system, MSC also influence adaptive immune responses. MSC inhibit T cell proliferation via many different stimuli, including PGE$_2$, IDO, TGF-beta, hepatocyte growth factor (HGF), iNOS, soluble HLA-5 and galectins 1 and 3. TGF-beta and HGF function synergistically to suppress T cell proliferation (Di Nicola, 2002; Klyushnenkova, 2005), and are expressed in equine MSC (De Schauwer, 2014). IDO most likely

does not play an important role in the immunosuppressive activities of equine MSC, since equine MSC, even in the presence of activated T cells, do not express IDO (Carrade, 2012; De Schauwer, 2014). In addition, MSC decrease B cell proliferation, differentiation, antibody and chemokine production, and reduce the expression of chemokine receptors on B cells via direct cell-cell contact, as well as via MSC-secreted soluble factors (Bunnell, 2010; Hoogduijn, 2010; Ben-Ami, 2011; Deuse, 2011; Ma, 2014).

31.3.2 Immunostimulant properties

Besides having immunosuppressive properties, MSC can also upregulate immune responses. Indeed, low level IFN-gamma stimulation of human or murine MSC can induce MHC class II-mediated antigen presentation to CD4$^+$ T cells and cross-presentation (a process by which extracellular antigens are presented via MHC class I) to CD8$^+$ T cells (Francois, 2009). Stimulation of equine MSC with equine IFN-gamma can induce MHC class II expression with stimulation of an *in vitro* immune response (Schnabel, 2014). The capacity of MSC to behave as antigen-presenting cells (APC) makes them attractive candidates for therapeutic cell-based treatments against cancer and/or infectious diseases.

31.4 Sources of equine mesenchymal stem cells

Bone marrow (BM) and adipose tissue (AdT) are the most commonly used sources of MSCs in equine regenerative medicine, although less invasive alternative sources, such as blood samples, including umbilical cord blood (UCB), and peripheral

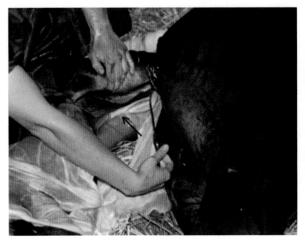
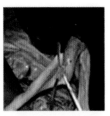
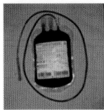

Figure 31.3 Collection of umbilical cord blood (UCB). Immediately after parturition, the umbilical cord is clamped as closely as possible by the vulva of the mare, and disinfected with 70% alcohol. The natural stricture where the umbilical cord usually ruptures is indicated by the arrow. After puncturing the umbilical vessel, as shown in the upper right panel, the UCB is drained by gravity into a sterile blood donor bag (lower right panel).

blood (PB), are gaining more interest. In addition, MSC have also been identified in other equine non-invasive tissues including, but not limited to, umbilical cord matrix, amnion, tendon, muscle and periosteal tissue.

Recent comparative studies evaluating the properties of equine MSC from different sources demonstrate both overlapping, as well as unique, mechanisms of these cells (Burk, 2013; Radtke, 2013; Carrade Holt, 2014; De Schauwer, 2014). Better understanding of the unique characteristics of equine MSC from a specific source will have practical implications for their selection in MSC therapy, with best application to the condition or injury to be treated.

31.4.1 Bone marrow

Since equine MSC were originally isolated from BM, this source is the most studied and best characterized for equine MSC to date (Fortier, 2011). The sternum is most commonly used to aspirate BM, although alternative sites, such as tuber coxae, tibia and humerus, have been used (Taylor, 2011). Harvesting BM has potential drawbacks, such as low cell yield, pain associated with the collection, and potential pericardial laceration during collection (Nixon, 2008). Safety concerns for the clinician must also be considered when harvesting BM from adult horses (Berg, 2009). Furthermore, 2–6 weeks of culture after the isolation of BM-derived MSC are required to allow cellular expansion, in order to obtain a sufficient number of MSC for treatment (Berg, 2009; Fortier, 2011).

31.4.2 Adipose tissue

Fat can be collected from the tail head of horses, the dorsal gluteal muscles, and the inguinal and sternal fat depots (Nixon, 2008; Taylor, 2011). In highly trained athletic horses, the collection can be difficult because of the small amount of accessible fat (Carrade, 2011a). In general, AdT yields higher numbers of MSC per unit volume than BM (Toupadakis, 2010). A mixture of cells, called the stromal vascular fraction (SVF), isolated from the AdT are injected into the patient without a cell culture step, giving the advantage of supplying cells within 48

hours (Fortier, 2011). However, SVF will contain adipocytes and leukocytes, and characteristics of adipose stem cells may or may not be applicable to SVF.

31.4.3 Umbilical cord blood

Umbilical cord blood (UCB) is a non-invasive source for MSC that can be easily collected at parturition before the umbilical cord ruptures (Carrade, 2011b; Taylor, 2011; De Schauwer, 2011a, 2013a). In earlier times, there was a widespread belief that the mare was still passing blood towards the foal through the umbilical cord immediately after parturition (Bartholomew, 2009). However, using Doppler ultrasound, no blood flow has been detected through the cord, indicating that UCB can be collected without harming the foal (Doarn, 1987). An illustration on how to collect UCB is shown in Figure 31.3. High numbers of MSC can be expanded from UCB (Carrade, 2011b).

31.4.4 Peripheral blood

Another non-invasive source for equine MSC is peripheral blood (PB). The collection of a sterile blood sample can be performed easily in the field by an equine practitioner, and is practically always available. This makes PB-derived MSC a readily accessible source of MSC when injuries occur (Spaas, 2013). A disadvantage is the varying success rate of MSC isolation from equine PB, which ranges from 40–66% (Koerner, 2006; Giovannini, 2008; Martinello, 2010).

31.5 Characterization of equine mesenchymal stem cells

In contrast to human MSC, no uniform characterization criteria are available to date for MSC from animal origin, including of equine origin (Jiang, 2002; Dominici, 2006). As a result, different research groups and/or companies use different methods to isolate and characterize equine MSC, which makes it difficult not only to compare research findings, but also to compare clinical outcomes of equine MSC therapies.

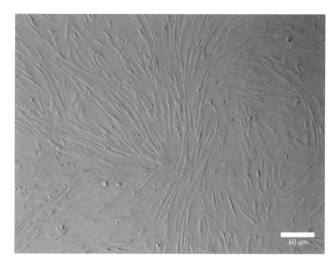

Figure 31.4 Equine mesenchymal stem cells (MSC). Light microscopic image of a monolayer of undifferentiated, plastic-adherent and spindle-shaped equine MSC in culture (40×).

While MSC from multiple species can easily be identified by their ability of plastic-adherence and tri-lineage differentiation, their surface antigen expression is not well characterized universally (Dominici, 2006). A limited availability of species-specific or cross-reacting antibodies in veterinary medicine in general, and in equine medicine, hampers the possibilities for the proper immunophenotyping of MSC (Ibrahim, 2007; Rozemuller, 2010).

31.5.1 Morphological characterization

The ability of MSC to adhere to tissue culture plastic was originally described for the isolation of murine MSC (Frieden-stein, 1976), but plastic-adherence is a common characteristic for all MSC populations (Taylor, 2007). Moreover, MSC, including equine MSC, are morphologically identified as spindle-shaped cells that grow in a monolayer, and they show a varying cellular morphology, ranging from very slender and elongated, towards more cuboidal, with shorter cytoplasmatic extensions (Figure 31.4).

31.5.2 Immunophenotyping

The International Society for Cellular Therapy (ISCT) has proposed strict guidelines for characterization of human MSC, based on the presence and absence of certain cell markers. It is defined that MSCs must express CD73, CD90, and CD105, while they must lack the expression of CD14, CD34, CD45, CD79α and MHC II (Dominici, 2006). The lack of a single marker specific for MSC, and the currently limited availability of antibodies recognizing equine molecules, are major complicating factors for the immunophenotypical characterization of equine MSC. Moreover, contradicting results on the cross-reactivity of antibodies with equine epitopes are reported. This can be explained in part by the lack of proper control groups, or the use of different available antibodies, since it has

been shown that different clones of antibodies against the same antigen can result in different outcomes in expression (Zuk, 2009).

Testing antibodies for human molecules for cross-reactivity in other species should always be performed with great care in order to avoid incorrect conclusions. Firstly, cross-reactive antibodies must be thoroughly characterized, since some reagents have been reported to identify alternative epitopes on different proteins (Ibrahim, 2007). Secondly, some surface molecules are only expressed transiently, and their expression might be missed (Mitchell, 2006; Radcliffe, 2010). Lastly, the use of isotype controls and appropriate positive and negative controls while testing antibody cross-reactivity is crucial, especially when looking for negative expression of markers (De Schauwer, 2011, 2012).

In general, immunophenotyping of MSC is mostly performed by flow cytometry, as this technique allows for a rapid identification of cells. Ideally, a multicolor flow cytometric assay should be used to simultaneously identify the presence and absence of markers on individual cells (Dominici, 2006). Flow cytometry is a highly sensitive and specific method for the qualitative and quantitative assessment of multiple parameters of individual cells in suspension (Reggeti, 2011), although the technique is susceptible to false-positive signals (Radcliffe, 2010; Reggeti, 2011). Therefore, it is important to ensure the quality of instrument performance and the use of appropriate and sufficient controls, and to verify that the detected signals indeed correspond to a specific antigen-antibody interaction. Therefore, examining cytospin slides by fluorescence microscopy is a commonly used confirmatory method (Reggeti, 2011). Table 31.1 provides an overview of the expression of cellular protein markers on human and equine MSC.

31.5.3 Differentiation

Under specific culture conditions, MSC have a multi-lineage differentiation potential, with mainly osteogenic, chondrogenic, and adipogenic differentiation capacities. In addition, myogenic, tenogenic, neuronal and hepatogenic differentiation potential of equine MSC have been reported (De Schauwer, 2011b). Table 31.2 is an overview of the methods used to characterize differentiated equine MSC.

31.5.4 Autologous versus allogeneic

MSC are considered minimally or non-immunogenic, since they express low levels of MHC class I antigens, and do not express MHC class II and co-stimulatory molecules such as CD40, CD80, and CD86 (Sensebé, 2009). However, there are differences in the expression of these molecules among species, as well as differences between different sources of MSC within one species. For example, equine bone marrow-derived MSC can express MHC class II antigens, depending on the donor horse (Schnabel, 2014), whereas umbilical cord blood-derived MSC appear always to be MHC class II negative (De Schauwer, 2012, 2013a, 2014).

Table 31.1 Expression of cell surface protein markers on equine and human mesenchymal stem cells.

Cellular protein marker	Synonyms	Expression in:		Positive control
		Human MSC	Equine MSC	
CD29	β1-integrin	+	+	T and B cells, Mo
CD44		+	+	Mo, granulocytes, lymphocytes
CD73	Ecto 5'nucleotidase, SH3, SH4	+	?	T and B cells
CD90	Thy-1	+	+	T cells, thymocytes, neurons, EC and fibroblasts
CD105	Endoglin, SH2	+	+	EC
CD106	VCAM-1	+	?	EC after stimulation with cytokines
CD166	SB-10, ALCAM	+	?	Thymic EpC, activated T cells, B cells, Mo
MHC I	HLA-I	+	+	Leukocytes
CD11b	ITGAM, CR3A	–	?	Mo, Mφ
CD14		–	–	Mo, Mφ
CD19		–	?	B cells
CD34		–	–	Primitive HP and EC
CD45	LCA, B220, T200	–	–	All leukocytes
CD79α		–	–	B cells
MHC II	HLA-DR, HLA-II	–	–	Lymphocytes

+ present; – absent; ?: unknown; Mo: Monocytes; Mφ: Macrophages; EC: Endothelial cells; EpC: Epithelial cells; HP: Hematopoietic progenitors. Cells from the positive control group can be used to validate cross-reactivity when no anti-horse antibodies are available.

Table 31.2 Overview of the methods used to characterize differentiated equine MSCs.

Differentiation lineage	Histological staining	Gene expression	Protein expression
Osteogenic	Alkaline phosphatase activity Alizarine Red S Von Kossa	Runx2 Osteonectin SPP1	Runx2 Collagen I Osteocalcin β₁ integrin Osteonectin
Chondrogenic	Toluidine Blue Alcian Blue Saffranin O Masson trichrom	Sox-9 Collagen II Collagen II/ collagen I Aggrecan/ Versican	Collagen II β₁ integrin
Adipogenic	Oil Red O	PPAR-γ	Adiponectin β₁ integrin
Myogenic	HE Masson	Desmin	Desmin Phalloidin Myf5 MyoD Smooth muscle Actin
Tenogenic	HE	Tenomodulin Decorin	ND

HE: Hematoxylin and eosin staining; ND: not done.

Because of this low immunogenicity, allogeneic (different donor horse and recipient horse) MSC is being considered a safe alternative to autologous MSC treatments, where MSC from the patient itself are used. Indeed, several clinical studies suggest that allogeneic MSC can be used without eliciting an apparent cell-mediated immune response in horses (Guest, 2008,

Carrade, 2011a, 2011b), although it should be emphasized that the available studies included only a limited number of horses and a very short-term monitoring period. Therefore, larger controlled clinical studies, with longer follow-up periods, are needed in order to ensure the safety and efficacy of equine allogeneic MSC use (Koch, 2009).

At present, most cell-based therapies in horses are using autologous MSC, primarily due to the regulatory uncertainty that exist in the commercial market of veterinary stem cell therapy (Schnabel, 2013). Nevertheless, an allogeneic source would provide an off-the-shelf, more standardized and readily available product, without the inherent lag period associated with isolation and expansion of autologous MSC (Alves, 2011). On the other hand, it is questionable if the use of allogeneic MSC would be more cost-effective, since there are additional storage expenses and extra tests needed to ensure that no infectious diseases are transmitted (Fortier, 2011).

31.6 Applications of equine mesenchymal stem cells in equine regenerative medicine

The therapeutic use of equine MSC for orthopedic injuries was described for the first time in 2003, with less than five peer-reviewed fundamental research articles published at that time. Since then, the clinical use of MSC has exploded, with thousands of horses now being treated worldwide. Although the fundamental research has also expanded, it lags substantially behind when considering the rapid product development and clinical experimentation using equine MSC (Borjesson, 2011). Many of the disorders that seem ideally suited for MSC treatment have a long history of potential revolutionary therapies that have subsequently been shown either to be not efficacious or deleterious for the patient's recovery (Clegg, 2011).

The efficacy of equine MSC therapy is difficult to evaluate, because appropriate control groups are not always included, and MSC treatment is often combined with other biological factors, including BM supernatants, autologous serum, or platelet-rich plasma (Koch, 2009). Nevertheless, demonstrating true efficacy should be a collective goal of the equine veterinary community, by performing clinical trials that include a sufficient amount of similar cases, and a consistent and standardized panel of objective outcome measures (Stewart, 2011a). For example, magnetic resonance imaging, radiology and ultrasonography are possible tools to evaluate reparative responses in tendon, ligament, bone, and articular lesions, while force plate and gait analysis measurements can provide quantitative data of functional recovery to confirm the clinicians' diagnostic findings and return-to-competition results (Stewart, 2011a).

The current clinical literature frequently relies on study designs that often do not respond to the gold standard of evidence-based medicine (i.e., blinded randomized control trials). Indeed, the latter set-up is difficult to undertake in equine veterinary science, because of the logistical and economical hurdles of such a study (Clegg, 2011). Although several studies are controlled, the experimental power is often lacking, because of the limited sample size in horse-based studies and the inter-animal variability of the pathological conditions (Clegg, 2011).

Most equine clinical studies report on the use of BM-derived MSC that have been expanded *in vitro* prior to *in vivo* use, thereby providing a certain degree of quality control and the expectation that the obtained effect of the treatment is actually caused by the MSC (Koch, 2009). On the other hand, cell suspensions containing a mixture of cells can also be administered immediately without an *in vitro* expansion step, which reduces the *in vitro* selection pressure on the pertinent cells.

It is apparent that many fundamental questions remain to be answered regarding the clinical use of MSC in equine medicine, such as the efficacy of treatment, the MSC dose, the tissue source, the route of administration, adjuvant products, whether scaffolds are necessary or not, the timing of administration, and the use of autologous or allogeneic MSC (Borjesson, 2011; Fortier, 2011).

31.6.1 Orthopedic injuries

The ability of MSC to differentiate into various tissues of mesodermal origin holds great potential for the repair and regeneration of tendon, cartilage and bone (Taylor, 2007). An overview of clinical studies using equine MSC to treat musculoskeletal diseases in the horse is given in Table 31.3.

31.6.1.1 Tendon

Injuries to superficial digital flexor tendon, deep digital flexor tendon, and the suspensory ligament, are very common in competition horses subjected to high-intensity exercise. These tissues accumulate degenerative damage as they operate close to their functional limits (Richardson, 2007; Spaas, 2012). In response to acute injury, there is an initial temporary inflammatory reaction, characterized by edema and pain. During the healing process, the newly formed collagen of the scar tissue is less highly cross-linked and functionally more deficient, when compared with a normal tendon. Consequently, there is a substantial risk of reduced performance and/or re-injury. Standard conservative treatment includes prolonged confinement and controlled exercise for up to 12 months after injury (Guest, 2008; Spaas, 2012).

The poor success with conventional therapy further supports the need to search for novel treatments that aim at restoring functionality and regenerating with a tissue as close to the tendon as possible. Frequently, the typical *core lesion* in the superficial digital flexor tendon occurs centrally within the tendon, extended in length, and surrounded by intact tendon tissue (Brehm, 2012). Therefore, the equine MSC suspension can be administered into the lesion without the need for artificial scaffold material. Intralesional administration of MSC in horses with tendinitis may stimulate the intrinsic healing, decrease the initial inflammatory reaction and scar tissue formation, and reduce the re-injury rate (Gutierrez-Nibeyro, 2011). Overall, a positive therapeutic effect of MSC for the treatment of tendon lesions has been suggested in several studies using either experimentally-induced tendinitis or naturally occurring lesions (see Table 31.3).

Since the presence of mature fibrous tissue within the tendon would make MSC implantation more difficult, and its persistence would reduce the benefits of the MSC therapy, chronic recurrent injuries are not considered ideal cases for stem cell therapy (Richardson, 2007). Some studies recommend to apply stem cell therapy within one month of injury (i.e., after the initial inflammatory phase but before fibrous scar tissue is formed) (Richardson, 2007; Godwin, 2012).

31.6.1.2 Cartilage

The possibility of obtaining effective repair of injured articular cartilage is limited, due to its hypocellular and avascular nature (Frisbie, 2011). Full thickness cartilage defects in horses heal with fibrocartilage that has inferior biomechanical properties, compared with articular hyaline cartilage (Taylor, 2007). Given the ability of MSC to undergo chondrogenic differentiation, much of the recent research on cartilage resurfacing in the horse has focused on the use of these cells (Frisbie, 2011). Although chondrogenic differentiation of equine MSC is known to occur *in vitro*, the *in vivo* use of MSC-based therapy might be hampered by the compressive load exerted on the injected cells and scaffolds (Koch, 2009).

The surgical technique *microfracture* provides access for chondrogenic progenitor cells and growth factors of the subchondral BM compartment into the base of the cartilage defect, and stimulates cartilage repair (Taylor, 2007; Frisbie, 2011). The outcome of this technique could be substantially improved when

Q1 **Table 31.3** An overview of clinical studies using equine MSC to treat musculoskeletal diseases in the horse.

Study	N horses	Control group	Nature of the lesion	Diagnosis	Follow-up period	Efficacy MSC treatment vs control
Tendon						
Smith, 2003	1	NI	Natural	CE + U	6 weeks	NA
Pacini, 2007	11	Conservative treatment	Natural	CE + U	2 years	18.2% vs 100%
Del Bue, 2008	16	NI	Natural	CE + U	240 days	12.5% vs NI
Guest, 2008	2	NI	Induced	IHC	10 and 34 days	No significant effect
Nixon, 2008	8	PBS	Induced	U + H + IHC + PCR + BA	6 weeks	Positive effect
Smith, 2008	500	NI	Natural	CE + U	> 1 year	13–36%* vs NI
Ferris, 2009	97	NI	Natural	CE	7–39 months	15–27%
Leppänen, 2009	58	NI	Natural	PI	18–24 months	26.4% vs NI
Schnabel, 2009	12	Control limb: PBS	Induced	U + MT + H + PCR + BA	8 weeks	Positive effect
Crovace, 2010	6	Saline	Induced	CE + U + H + IHC	21 weeks	Positive effect
De Mattos Carvalho, 2011	8	Control limb: no MSC	Induced	CE + U + H + IHC	8–21 weeks	Positive effect
Godwin, 2012	141	NI	Natural	CE + U + S + H	3 years	27.4% vs NI
Marfe, 2012a	3	Conservative treatment	Natural	U	3 years	0% vs 100%
Cartilage						
Wilke, 2007	6	Control limb: PBS	Induced	A + H + (I)HC + ISH	8 months	No significant effect
Ferris, 2009, 2014	40	NI	Natural	PI	21 months	28% vs NI
Frisbie, 2009	24	Placebo	Induced	CE + RX + H + punction	70 days	No significant effect
McIlwraith, 2011	10	Control limb: hyaluron alone	Induced	CE + RX + A + MRI + H + HM + IHC + BA	12 months	No significant effect

Where applicable, the efficacy of the MSC treatment (i.e. effect as assessed by diagnostic tools or percentage (%) of horses re-injured after MSC treatment versus the control group) is indicated

NI not included; CE clinical examination; U ultrasonography; NA not applicable; IHC immunohistochemistry; RX radiography; H histopathology; PCR polymerase chain reaction; BA biochemical analysis; PI phone interview; MT mechanical testing; S scintigraphy; A arthroscopy; ISH *in situ* hybridization; HM histomorphometry; MRI magnetic resonance imaging; *depending on discipline.

MSC are co-administered into the joint space. However, this synergism needs to be further studied, since one study did not reveal significant clinical improvements or histological differences between microfracture alone, and microfracture in combination with the intra-articular administration of BM-derived MSC (McIlwraith, 2011).

The treatment of osteoarthritis, also known as degenerative joint disease, using conventional therapy or cell-based therapy, is more challenging than the repair of focal cartilage defects. The articular cartilage damage in osteoarthritis is often more diffuse, and periarticular tissues, such as the synovial membrane, the joint capsule, ligaments, menisci, and subchondral bone, can be impaired (Frisbie, 2011). A beneficial effect of MSC on cartilage morphology and histology has been demonstrated in various osteoarthritis animal models, and can be explained both by MSC differentiation and by the effect of the soluble factors secreted by these cells (Matsumoto, 2009; van Buul, 2012).

In human patients, clinical studies have been conducted using BM-derived MSC to treat osteoarthritis, and several finished trials have shown positive outcomes (Gupta, 2012). In a controlled experimental study of equine osteoarthritis, induced by bone and cartilage debris with a negligible destabilization of the joint, BM- or AdT-derived MSC in the carpal osteochondral fragment reported a slight improvement in clinical signs, and found an up-regulation of pro-inflammatory cytokines in the synovial fluid concentrations (Frisbie, 2009). In another clinical trial of moderate to severe osteoarthritis, about one-third of the horses treated intra-articularly with autologous BM-derived MSC returned to their prior or superior level of performance (Ferris, 2009). The use of MSC to treat equine osteoarthritis is indicated in cases of impairment of soft tissue structures leading to joint instability, for instance when meniscal damage is present (Frisbie, 2010).

31.6.1.3 Bone

In contrast to tendon and cartilage repair, bone fractures usually regenerate with similar biochemical and biomechanical properties to those of the original tissue (Taylor, 2007). However, when large quantities of bone need to be regenerated, stimulation of the natural processes of bone repair may be necessary (Kraus,

2006), including: substantial loss of host bone from trauma or tumor resection; arthrodesis; spinal fusion; non- or delayed unions; osseous cyst-like lesions; metabolic disease; arthroplasty or insufficient healing potential of the host because of local or systemic disease, old age or drug treatment (Kraus, 2006; Taylor, 2007).

In veterinary orthopedics, many of the current techniques to aid fracture healing and stimulate bone formation involve the use of autologous bone grafts that provide both osteogenic cells and osseous matrix (Milner, 2011). However, such an autologous graft must be harvested from another site of the patient's body, which can result in donor-site morbidity (Vertenten, 2009). Furthermore, the number of osteoprogenitor cells has been reported to vary between donor sites, and might be less potent, due either to an age-related decline in MSC number or to a reduced metabolic function with increasing age (Koch, 2009). Allogeneic grafts, on the other hand, have a lower osteogenic capacity, a higher resorption rate, a larger immunogenic response, and less extensive revascularization, besides the risk of a possible viral contamination of the graft material (Vertenten, 2009). Therefore, combining grafts with equine MSC might stimulate bone regeneration.

To date, a few preliminary experiments have been performed, in which a pastern joint arthrodesis was supported by a combined therapy of stem cells and a bone replacement material, resulting in a good development of bone fusion (Brehm, 2012). However, no controlled clinical studies on the application of MSC in bone regeneration in horses have been reported.

31.6.2 Non-orthopedic injuries

31.6.2.1 Immune-mediated and inflammatory disease

Mesenchymal stromal cells are known to modulate local inflammatory responses, and recruit autologous stem cells inside injured tissues to stimulate cell survival and tissue repair (Stewart, 2011b). MSC are considered useful resources in cases of organ transplantation, inflammatory and auto-immune diseases (Sensebe, 2009). There is no evidence of systemic immunosuppression or increased risk of infections as possible side-effects when MSC are administered to immune-competent patients, suggesting that the immunomodulatory effects of MSC are restricted to inflamed tissues (Sensebe, 2009). A number of studies with animal models have demonstrated the efficacy of human MSC as a tool for immunomodulation in the protection against allograft rejection, autoimmune encephalomyelitis, collagen-induced arthritis, sepsis, systemic lupus erythematosus, and autoimmune myocarditis (De Schauwer, 2013b).

Examples of equine autoimmune diseases for which MSC therapy can be of relevance are equine recurrent uveitis (Deeg, 2008) and pemphigus foliaceus (Vandenabeele, 2004). Although not evaluated in clinical studies thus far, equine MSC treatment could be of relevance for these diseases with autoimmune and inflammatory pathophysiological components.

31.6.2.2 Ischemic diseases

Stem cell therapy has been investigated in ischemic diseases that cause cell injury and related organ dysfunction. Although ischemic injuries are usually local in nature, they are often a part of disorders with a highly complex pathophysiology that involve biochemical changes in different cell types (Lange, 2005; Chen, 2006). The multi-differentiation and immunomodulatory properties of MSC provide the opportunity for using these cells in the treatment of a variety of diseases such as stroke, ischemic retinopathy, myocardial infarction, ischemic diseases of the liver, ischemic renal failure, and ischemic limb dysfunction. The functional recovery of the damaged tissue is supported by circulating endogenous stem cells that migrate specifically to ischemic regions (Chen, 2006).

It has been proposed that MSC therapy can improve the current treatment options for laminitis in horses (Koch, 2009). Laminitis is a multifactorial disease of the equine foot, with various initiating causes, including local ischemia (Engiles, 2010). Although many practitioners are currently administering stem cells from different sources to laminitic horses, it is important to acknowledge that no controlled studies have been performed to evaluate the safety or efficacy of equine MSC for the treatment of this devastating condition. In general, most horses are treated with stem cells twice – once as early as possible during an acute episode, and again at 14 days after the first injection (Schnabel, 2013).

31.6.2.3 Wound repair

Horses are predisposed to traumatic wounds that can be labor-intensive and expensive to manage, and equine MSC can play an important role in wound repair, considering their potential to improve the healing of skin defects (Sensebe, 2009; Theoret, 2009). The historical gold standard treatment to replace lost skin is an autologous skin graft but, unfortunately, graft failure is relatively common in equine patients, due to infection, inflammation, fluid accumulation beneath the graft, and motion. Also, full-thickness autografting is limited to relatively small wounds, since the horse lacks redundant donor skin (Theoret, 2009).

So far, only one study describes the use of equine MSC at the site of a surgically repaired soft palate defect (Carstanjen, 2006). Labeled autologous BM-derived MSC were implanted into the repaired defect at surgery, and the horse was submitted to euthanasia 14 days later. Microscopic examination revealed that the MSC were oriented and integrated along the axis of the skeletal myocytes under the epithelium, which is indicative for a successful engraftment.

31.6.2.4 Ophthalmology

In veterinary ophthalmology, there is only one recent study describing the use of equine MSC, in four chronic cases of corneal ulcer and one case of retinal detachment in horses. These patients were non-responsive to conventional treatment, and all four patients showed significant improvement within three months after MSC treatment (Marfe, 2012b).

31.6.2.5 Neurological disorders

Based on the capacity of MSC to differentiate *in vitro* into neurogenic progenitors expressing specific neuronal markers, the potential efficacy of MSC for functional repair of nervous tissues has been studied in several animal models, including a dog model of spinal cord injury (Jung, 2009; Jamnig, 2012). In this model, exogenous transplanted canine MSC migrated towards the injured spinal cord lesion and provided a suitable environment for neuronal repair, due the immunosuppressive, anti-inflammatory and trophic effects of these MSC (Jung, 2009).

Since neurodegenerative diseases in horses display common pathological processes, a specific therapeutic agent, such as equine MSC, could improve the clinical signs of several neurodegenerative disorders, based on their ability to replace damaged cells or secrete trophic factors and immunomodulating cytokines (Sadan, 2009). Equine myeloencephalopathy, equine motor neuron disease, and laryngeal hemiplegia are examples of neurodegenerative disorders for which MSC therapy might be of interest. However, it remains to be demonstrated whether equine MSC display sufficient neurogenic differentiation capacity and survival *in vivo* to support the treatment of neurodegenerative disorders.

References

Alves, A.G., Stewart, A.A., Dudhia, J., Kasashima, Y., Goodship, A.E. and Smith, R.K.W. (2011). Cell-based therapies for tendon and ligament injuries. *The Veterinary Clinics of North America: Equine Practice* 27(2), 315–333.

Baer, P.C. and Geiger, H. (2012). Adipose-derived mesenchymal stromal/stem cells: tissue localization, characterization, and heterogeneity. *Stem Cells International* 2012, 812693.

Bartholomew, S., Owens, S.D., Ferraro, G.L., Carrade, D.D., Lara, D.J., Librach, F.A., Borjesson, D.L. and Galuppo, L.D. (2009). Collection of equine cord blood and placental tissues in 40 Thoroughbred mares. *Equine Veterinary Journal* 41(8), 724–728.

Ben-Ami, E., Berrih-Aknin, S. and Miller, A. (2011). Mesenchymal stem cells as an immunomodulatory therapeutic strategy for autoimmune diseases. *Autoimmunity Reviews* 10(7), 410–415.

Berg, L.C., Koch, T., Heerkens, T., Bessonov, K., Thomsen, P. and Betts, D.H. (2009). Chondrogenic potential of mesenchymal stromal cells derived from equine bone marrow and umbilical cord blood. *Veterinary and Comparative Orthopaedics and Traumatology* 22(5), 363–370.

Borjesson, D.L. and Peroni, J.F. (2011). The regenerative medicine laboratory: facilitating stem cell therapy for equine disease. *Clinics in Laboratory Medicine* 31(1), 109–123.

Brehm, W., Burk, J., Delling, U., Gittel, C. and Ribitsch, I. (2012). Stem cell-based tissue engineering in veterinary orthopaedics. *Cell and Tissue Research* 347, 677–688.

Broeckx, S., Zimmerman, M., Crocetti, S., Suls, M., Mariën, T., Ferguson, S.J., Chiers, K., Duchateau, L., Franco-Obregon, A., Wuertz, K. and Spaas, J.H. (2014). Regenerative therapies for equine degenerative joint disease: a preliminary study. *Plos One* 9(1), e85917.

Bunnell, B.A., Betancourt, A.M. and Sullivan, D.E. (2010). New concepts on the immune modulation mediated by mesenchymal stem cells. *Stem Cell Research and Therapy* 11(5), 34.

Burk, J., Badylak, S.F., Kelly, J. and Brehm, W. (2013). Equine cellular therapy – from stall to bench to bedside? *Cytometry* 83A, 103–113.

Carrade, D.D., Affolter, V.K., Outerbridge, C.A., Watson, J.L., Galuppo, L.D., Buerchler, S., Kumar, V., Walker, N.J. and Borjesson, D.L. (2011a). Intradermal injections of equine allogeneic umbilical cord-derived mesenchymal stem cells are well tolerated and do not elicit immediate or delayed hypersensitivity reactions. *Cytotherapy* 13(10), 1180–1192.

Carrade, D.D., Owens, S.D., Galuppo, L.D., Vidal, M.A., Ferraro, G.L., Librach, F.A., Buerchler, S., Friedman, M.S., Walker, N.J. and Borjesson, D.L. (2011b). Clinicopathologic findings following intra-articular injection of autologous and allogeneic placentally derived equine mesenchymal stem cells in horses. *Cytotherapy* 13(4), 419–430.

Carrade, D.L., Lame, M.W., Kent, M.S., Clark, K.C., Walker, N.J. and Borjesson, D.L. (2012). Comparative analysis of the immunomodulatory properties of equine adult-derived mesenchymal stem cells. *Cell Medicine* 4(1), 1–11.

Carrade, D.L. and Borjesson, D.L. (2013). Immunomodulation by mesenchymal stem cells in veterinary species. *Comparative Medicine* 63(3), 207–217.

Carrade Holt, D.D., Wood, J.A., Granick, J.L., Walker, N.J., Clark, K.C. and Borjesson, D.L. (2014). Equine mesenchymal stem cells inhibit T cell proliferation through different mechanisms depending on tissue source. *Stem Cells and Development* 23(11), 1258–1265.

Carstanjen, B., Desbois, C., Hekmati, M. and Behr, L. (2006). Successful engraftment of cultured autologous mesenchymal stem cells in a surgically repaired soft palate defect in an adult horse. *Canadian Journal of Veterinary Research* 70(2), 143–147.

Chen, C.P., Lee, Y.J., Chiu, S.T., Shyu, W.C., Lee, M.Y., Huang, S.P. and Li, H. (2006). The application of stem cells in the treatment of ischemic diseases. *Histology and Histopathology* 21, 1209–1216.

Clegg, P.D. and Pinchbeck, G.L. (2011). Evidence-based medicine and stem cell therapy: how do we know such technologies are safe and efficacious? *The Veterinary Clinics of North America: Equine Practice* 27(2), 373–382.

Crovace, A., Lacitignola, L., Rossi, G. and Francioso, E. (2010). Histological and immunohistochemical evaluation of autologous cultured bone marrow mesenchymal stem cells and bone marrow mononucleated cells in collagenase-induced tendinitis of equine superficial digital flexor tendon. *Veterinary Medicine International* 2010, 250978.

Deeg, C.A., Hauck, S.M., amann, B., Pompetzki, D., Altmann, F., Raith, A., Schmalzl, T., Stangassinger, M. and Ueffing, M. (2008). Equine recurrent uveïtis – a spontaneous horse model of uveitis. *Opthalmic Research* 40(3–4), 151–153.

Del Bue, M., Ricco, S., Ramoni, R., Conti, V., Gnudi, G. and Grolli, S. (2008). Equine adipose-tissue derived mesenchymal stem cells and platelet concentrates: their association *in vitro* and *in vivo*. *Veterinary Research Communications* 32, S51–S55.

de Mattos Carvalho, A., Garcia Alves, A.L., Galvao Gomes de Oliveira, P., Cisneros Alvarez, L.E., amorin, R.L., Hussni, C.A. and Deffune, E. (2011). Use of adipose-derived mesenchymal stem cells for experimental tendinitis therapy in equines. *Journal of Equine Veterinary Science* 31, 26–34.

de Mattos Carvalho, A., Ramos Badial, P., Cisneros Alvarez, L.E., Miluzzi Yamada, A.L., Borges, A.S., Deffune, E., Hussni, C.A. and Alves, A.L.G. (2013). Equine tendonitis therapy using mesenchymal stem cells and platelet concentrates: a randomized controlled trial. *Stem Cell Research and Therapy* **4**, 85.

De Schauwer, C., Meyer, E., Cornillie, P., De Vliegher, S., Van de Walle, G.R., Hoogewijs, M., Declercq, H., Govaere, J., Demeyere, K., Cornelissen, M. and Van Soom, A. (2011a). Optimization of the isolation, culture and characterization of equine umbilical cord blood mesenchymal stromal cells. *Tissue Engineering Part C* **17**(11), 1061–1070.

De Schauwer, C., Meyer, E., Van de Walle, G.R. and Van Soom, A. (2011b). Markers of stemness in equine mesenchymal stem cells: a plea for uniformity. *Theriogenology* **75**, 1431–1443.

De Schauwer, C., Piepers, S., Van de Walle, G.R., Demeyere, K., Hoogewijs, M.K., Govaere, J.L.J., Braeckmans, K., Van Soom, A. and Meyer, E. (2012). In search for cross-reactivity to immunophenotype equine mesenchymal stromal cells by multicolor flow cytometry. *Cytometry part A* **81**, 312–323.

De Schauwer, C., Van de Walle, G.R., Piepers, S., Hoogewijs, M.K., Govaere, J.L.J., Meyer, E. and Van Soom, A. (2013a). Successful isolation of equine mesenchymal stromal cells from cryopreserved umbilical cord blood-derived mononuclear cell fractions. *Equine Veterinary Journal* **45**(4), 518–522.

De Schauwer, C., Van de Walle, G.R., Van Soom, A. and Meyer, E. (2013b). Mesenchymal stem cell therapy in horses: useful beyond orthopedic injuries? *The Veterinary Quarterly* **33**(4), 234–241.

De Schauwer, C., Goossens, K., Piepers, S., Hoogewijs, M.K., Govaere, J.L.J., Smits, K., Meyer, E., Van Soom, A. and Van de Walle, G.R. (2014). Characterization and profiling of immunomodulatory genes of equine mesenchymal stromal cells from non-invasive sources. *Stem Cell Research and Therapy* **5**(1), 6.

Deuse, T., Stubbendorff, M., Tang-Quan, K., Philips, N., Kay, M.A., Eiermann, T., Phan, T.T., Volk, H.D., Reichenspurner, H., Robbins, R.C. and Schrepfer, S. (2011). Immunogenicity and immunomodulatory properties of umbilical cord lining mesenchymal stem cells. *Cell Transplantation* **20**(5), 655–667.

Di Nicola, M., Carlo-Stella, C., Magni, M., Milanesi, M., Longoni, P.D., Matteucci, P., Grisanti, S. and Gianni, A. (2002). Human bone marrow stromal cells suppress T-lymphocyte proliferation induced by cellular or nonspecific mitogenic stimuli. *Blood* **99**(10), 3838–3843.

Doarn, R.T., Threlfall, W.R. and Kline, R. (1987). Umbilical blood flow and the effects of premature severance in the neonatal horse. *Theriogenology* **78**, 789–790.

Dominici, M., Le Blanc, K., Mueller, I., Slaper-Cortenbach, I., Marini, F.C., Krause, D.S., Deans, R.J., Keating, A., Prockop, D.J. and Horwitz, E. (2006). Minimal criteria for defining multipotent mesenchymal stromal cells. The International Society for Cellular Therapy position statement. *Cytotherapy* **8**, 315.

Engiles, J.B. (2010). Pathology of the distal phalanx in equine laminitis: more than just a skin deep. *The Veterinary Clinics of North America: Equine Practice* **26**(1), 155–165.

Ferris, D.J., Frisbie, D.D., Kisiday, J.D., McIlwraith, C.W., Hague, B.A., Major, M.D., Schneider, R.K., Zubrod, C.J., Watkins, J.J., Kawcak, C.E. and Goodrich, L.R. (2009). Clinical follow-up of horses treated with bone marrow-derived mesenchymal stem cells for musculoskeletal lesions. *AAEP Proceedings* **55**, 59–60.

Ferris, D.J., Frisbie, D.D., Kisiday, J.D., McIlwraith, C.W., Hague, B.A., Major, M.D., Schneider, R.K., Zubrod, C.J., Kawcak, C.E. and Goodrich, L.R. (2014). Clinical outcome after intra-articular administration of bone marrow derived mesenchymal stem cells in 33 horses with stifle injury. *Veterinary Surgery* **43**(3), 255–265.

Fortier, L.A. (2005). Stem cells: classifications, controversies, and clinical applications. *Veterinary Surgery* **34**(5), 415–423.

Fortier, L.A. and Travis, A.J. (2011). Stem cells in veterinary medicine. *Stem Cell Research & Therapy* **2**, 9.

François, M., Romieu-Mourez, R., Stock-Martineau, S., Boivin, M.N., Bramson, J.L. and Galipeau, J. (2009). Mesenchymal stromal cells cross-present soluble exogenous antigens as part of their antigen-presenting cell properties. *Blood* **114**, 2632–2638.

Friedenstein, A.J., Gorskaja, U.F. and Kulagina, N.N. (1976). Fibroblast precursors in normal and irradiated mouse hematopoietic organs. *Experimental Hematology* **4**, 267–274.

Frisbie, D.D., Kisiday, J.D., Kawcak, C.E., Werpy, N.M. and McIlwraith, C.W. (2009). Evaluation of adipose-derived stromal vascular fraction or bone marrow-derived mesenchymal stem cells for treatment of osteoarthritis. *Journal of Orthopaedic Research* **27**(12), 1675–1680.

Frisbie, D.D. and Smith, R.K.W. (2010). Clinical update on the use of mesenchymal stem cells in equine orthopaedics. *Equine Veterinary Journal* **42**(1), 86–89.

Frisbie, D.D. and Stewart, M.C. (2011). Cell-based therapies for equine joint disease. *The Veterinary Clinics of North America: Equine Practice* **27**(2), 335–349.

Giovannini, S., Brehm, W., Mainil-Varlet, P. and Nesic, D. (2008). Multilineage differentiation potential of equine blood-derived fibroblast-like cells. *Differentiation* **76**, 118–129.

Godwin, E.E., Young, N.J., Dudhia, J., Beamish, I.C. and Smith, R.K.W. (2012). Implantation of bone marrow-derived mesenchymal stem cells demonstrates improved outcome in horses with overstrain injury of the superficial digital flexor tendon. *Equine Veterinary Journal* **44**(1), 25–32.

Guest, D.J., Smith, M.R. and Allen, W.R. (2008). Monitoring the fate of autologous and allogeneic mesenchymal progenitor cells injected into the superficial digital flexor tendon of horses: preliminary study. *Equine Veterinary Journal* **40**(2), 178–181.

Gupta, P.K., Das, A.K., Chullikana, A. and Majumdar, A.S. (2012). Mesenchymal stem cells for cartilage repair in osteoarthritis. *Stem Cell Research and Therapy* **3**, 25.

Gutierrez-Nibeyro, S.D. (2011). Commercial cell-based therapies for musculoskeletal injuries in horses. *The Veterinary Clinics of North America: Equine Practice* **27**(2), 363–371.

Hoogduijn, M.J., Popp, F., Verbeek, R., Masoodi, M., Nicolaou, A., Baan, C. and Dahlke, M.H. (2010). The immunomodulatory properties of mesenchymal stem cells and their use for immunotherapy. *International Immunopharmacology* **10**(12), 1496–1500.

Ibrahim, S., Saunders, K., Kydd, J.H., Lunn, D.P. and Steinbach, F. (2007). Screening of anti-human leukocyte monoclonal antibodies for reactivity with equine leukocytes. *Veterinary Immunology and Immunopathology* **119**, 63–80.

Jamnig, A. and Lepperdinger, G. (2012). From tendon to nerve: an MSC for all seasons. *Canadian Journal of Physiology and Pharmacology* **90**(3), 295–306.

Jiang, Y., Jahagirdar, B.N., Reinhardt, R.L., Schwartz, R.E., Keene, C.D., Ortiz-Gonzalez, X.R., Reyes, M., Lenvik, T., Lund, T., Blackstad, M., Du, J., aldrich, S., Lisberg, A., Low, W.C., Largaespada, D.A. and Verfaillie, C.M. (2002). Pluripotency of mesenchymal stem cells derived from adult marrow. *Nature* **418**, 41–49.

Jung, D.I., Ha, J., Kang, B.T., Kim, J.W., Quan, F.S., Lee, J.H., Woo, E.J. and Park, H.M. (2009). A comparison of autologous and allogenic bone marrow-derived mesenchymal stem cell transplantation in canine spinal cord injury. *Journal of Neurological Sciences* **285**, 67–77.

Klyushnenkova, E., Mosca, J.D., Zernetkina, V., Majumdar, M.K., Beggs, K.J., Simonetti, D.W., Deans, R.J. and McIntosh, K.R. (2005). T cell responses to allogeneic human mesenchymal stem cells: immunogenicity, tolerance, and suppression. *Journal of Biomedical Science* **12**(1), 47–57.

Koch, T.G., Berg, L.C. and Betts, D.H. (2008). Concepts for the clinical use of stem cells in equine medicine. *Canadian Veterinary Journal* **49**, 1009–1017.

Koch, T.G., Berg, L.C. and Betts, D.H. (2009). Current and future regenerative medicine – principles, concepts, and therapeutic use of stem cell therapy and tissue engineering in equine medicine. *Canadian Veterinary Journal* **50**, 155–165.

Kode, J.A., Mukherjee, S., Joglekar, M.V. and Hardikar, A.A. (2009). Mesenchymal stem cells: immunobiology and role in immunomodulation and tissue regeneration. *Cytotherapy* **11**(4), 377–391.

Koerner, J., Nesic, D., Romero, J.D., Brehm, W., Mainil-Varlet, P. and Grogan, S.P. (2006). Equine peripheral blood-derived progenitors in comparison to bone marrow-derived mesenchymal stem cells. *Stem Cells* **24**, 1613–1619.

Kraus, K.H. and Kirker-Head, C. (2006). Mesenchymal stem cells and bone regeneration. *Veterinary Surgery* **35**(3), 232–242.

Lakshmipathy, U. and Verfaillie, C. (2005). Stem cell plasticity. *Blood Reviews* **19**, 29–38.

Lange, C., Tögel, F., Ittrich, H., Clayton, F., Nolte-Ernsting, C., Zander, A.R. and Westenfelder, C. (2005). Administered mesenchymal stem cells enhance recovery from ischemia/reperfusion-induced acute renal failure in rats. *Kidney International* **68**, 1613–1617.

Lange-Consiglio, A., Tassan, S., Corradetti, B., Meucci, A., Perego, R., Bizzaro, D. and Cremonesi, F. (2013). Investigating the efficacy of amnion-derived compared with bone marrow-derived mesenchymal stromal cells in equine tendon and ligament injuries. *Cytotherapy* **15**, 1011–1020.

Leppänen, M., Tulamo, R., Heikkilä, P. and Katiskalahti, T. (2009). Follow-up of equine tendon and ligament injuries 18-24 months after treatment with enriched autologous adipose-derived mesenchymal stem cells – a clinical study. *Regenerative Medicine* **4**(6), S21–22.

Ling, W., Zhang, J., Yuan, Z., Ren, G., Zhang, L., Chen, X., Rabson, A.B., Roberts, A.I., Wang, Y. and Shi, Y. (2014). Mesenchymal stem cells use IDO to regulate immunity in tumor microenvironment. *Cancer Research* **74**(5), 1576–1587.

Ma S., Xie, N., Li, W., Yuan, B., Shi, Y. and Wang, Y. (2014). Immunobiology of mesenchymal stem cells. *Cell Death and Differentiation* **21**, 216–225.

Marfe, G., Rotta, G., De Martino, L., Tafani, M., Fiorito, F., Di Stefano, C., Polettini, M., Ranalli, M., Russo, M.A. and Gambacurta, A. (2012a). A new clinical approach: use of blood-derived stem cells (BDSCs) for superficial digital flexor tendon injuries in horses. *Life Sciences* **90**, 825–830.

Marfe, G., Massaro-Giordano, M., Ranalli, M., Cozzoli, E., Di Stefano, C., Malafoglia, V., Polettini, M. and Gambacurta, A. (2012b). Blood derived stem cells: an ameliorative therapy in veterinary ophthalmology. *Journal of Cellular Physiology* **227**(3), 1250–1256.

Martinello, T., Bronzini, I., Maccatrozzo, L., Iacopetti, I., Sampaolesi, M., Mascarello, F. and Patruno, M. (2010). Cryopreservation does *not affect the stem characteristics of multipotent cells isolated from equine peripheral blood. Tissue Engineering Part C* **16**(4), 771–781.

Matsumoto, T., Cooper, G.M., Gharaibeh, B., Meszaros, L.B., Li, G., Usas, A., Fu, F.H. and Huard, J. (2009). Cartilage repair in a rat model of osteoarthritis through intraarticular transplantation of muscle-derived stem cells expressing bone morphogenetic protein 4 and soluble Flt-1. *Arthritis and Rheumatism* **60**, 1390–1405.

McIlwraith, C.W., Frisbie, D.D., Rodkey, W.G., Kisiday, J.D., Werpy, N.M., Kawcak, C.E. and Steadman, J.R. (2011). Evaluation of intra-articular mesenchymal stem cells to augment healing of microfractured chondral defects. *Arthroscopy* **27**(11), 1552–1561.

Milner, P.I., Clegg, P.D. and Stewart, M.C. (2011). Stem cell-based therapies for bone repair. *The Veterinary Clinics of North America: Equine Practice* **27**(2), 299–314.

Mitchell, J.B., McIntosh, K., Zvonic, S., Garrett, S., Floyd, Z.E., Kloster, A., Halvorsen, Y.D., Storms, R.W., Goh, B., Kilroy, G., Wu, X. and Gimble, J.M. (2006). Immunophenotype of human adipose-derived cells: temporal changes in stromal-associated and stem cell-associated markers. *Stem Cells* **24**, 376–385.

Nixon, A.J., Dahlgren, L.A., Haupt, J.L., Yeager, A.E. and Ward, D.L. (2008). Effect of adipose-derived nucleated cell fractions on tendon repair in horses with collagenase-induced tendinitis. *American Journal of Veterinary Research* **69**(7), 928–937.

Pacini, S., Spinabella, S., Trombi, L., Fazzi, R., Galimberti, S., Dini, F., Carlucci, F. and Petrini, M. (2007). Suspension of bone marrow-derived undifferentiated mesenchymal stromal cells for repair of superficial digital flexor tendon in race horses. *Tissue Engineering* **13**, 2949–2955.

Peroni, J.F. and Borjesson, D.L. (2011). Anti-inflammatory and immunomodulatory activities of stem cells. *The Veterinary Clinics of North America: Equine Practice* **27**(2), 351–362.

Radcliffe, C.H., Flaminio, M.J.B.F. and Fortier, L.A. (2010). Temporal analysis of equine bone marrow aspirate during establishment of putative mesenchymal progenitor cell populations. *Stem Cells and Development* **19**, 269–281.

Radtke, C.L., Nino-Fong, R., Esparza Gonzalez, B.P., Stryhn, H. and McDuffee, L.A. (2013). Characterization and osteogenic potential of equine muscle tissue- and periosteal tissue-derived mesenchymal stem cells in comparison with bone marrow- and adipose tissue-derived mesenchymal stem cells. *American Journal of Veterinary Research* **74**(5), 790–800.

Reggeti, F. and Bienzle, D. (2011). Flow cytometry in veterinary oncology. *Veterinary Pathology* **48**(1), 223–235.

Renzi, S., Ricco, S., Dotti, S., Sesso, L., Grolli, S., Cornali, M., Carlin, S., Patruno, M., Cinotti, S. and Ferrari, M. (2013). Autologous bone marrow mesenchymal stromal cells for regeneration of injured equine ligaments and tendons: a clinical report. *Research in Veterinary Science* **95**, 272–277.

Richardson, L.E., Dudhia, J., Clegg, P.D. and Smith, R.K.W. (2007). Stem cells in veterinary medicine – attempts at regenerating equine tendon after injury. *Trends in Biotechnology* **25**, 409–416.

Rozemuller, H., Prins, H.J., Naaijkens, B., Staal, J., Bühring, H.J. and Martens, A.C. (2010). Prospective isolation of mesenchymal stem cells from multiple mammalian species using cross-reacting anti-human monoclonal antibodies. *Stem Cells and Development* **19**(12), 1911–1921.

Sadan, O., Melamed, E. and Offen, D. (2009). Bone marrow-derived mesenchymal stem cell therapy for neurodegenerative diseases. *Expert Opinion on Biological Therapy* **9**(12), 1487–1497.

Schnabel, L.V., Lynch, M.E., van der Meulen, M.C., Yeager, A.E., Kornatowski, M.A. and Nixon, A.J. (2009). Mesenchymal stem cells and insulin-like growth factor-I gene-enhanced mesenchymal stem cells improve structural aspects of healing in equine flexor digitorum superficialis tendons. *Journal of Orthopaedic Research* **27**(10), 1392–1398.

Schnabel, L.V., Fortier, L.A., McIlwraith, C.W. and Nobert, K.M. (2013). Therapeutic use of stem cells in horses: which type, how, and when? *The Veterinary Journal* **197**(3), 570–577.

Schnabel, L.V., Pezzanite, L.M., Antczak, D.F., Felippe, M.J. and Fortier, L.A. (2014). Equine bone marrow-derived mesenchymal stromal cells are heterogeneous in MHC class II expression and capable of inciting an immune response in vitro. *Stem Cell Research and Therapy* **5**(1), 13.

Sensebé, L. and Bourin, P. (2009). Mesenchymal stem cells for therapeutic purposes. *Transplantation* **87**(9 Suppl), S49–53.

Smith, R.K.W., Korda, M., Blunn, G.W. and Goodship, A.E. (2003). Isolation and implantation of autologous equine mesenchymal stem cells from bone marrow into the superficial digital flexor tendon as a potential novel treatment. *Equine Veterinary Journal* **35**, 99–102.

Smith, R.K.W. (2008). Mesenchymal stem cell therapy for equine tendinopathy. *Disability and Rehabilitation* **30**, 1752–1758.

Smith, R.K.W., Werling, N.J., Dakin, S.G., Alam, R., Goodship, A.E. and Dudhia, J. (2013). Beneficial effects of autologous bone marrow-derived mesenchymal stem cells in naturally occurring tendinopathy. *Plos One* **8**(9), e75697.

Spaas, J.H., Oosterlinck, M., Broeckx, S., Dumoulin, M., Saunders, J., Van Soom, A., Pille, F. and Van de Walle, G.R. (2012). Treatment of equine degenerative joint disease with autologous peripheral blood-derived mesenchymal stem cells: a case report. *Vlaams Diergeneeskundig Tijdschrift* **81**, 11–15.

Spaas, J.H., De Schauwer, C., Cornillie, P., Meyer, E., Van Soom, A. and Van de Walle, G.R. (2013). Culture and characterization of equine peripheral blood mesenchymal stromal cells. *The Veterinary Journal* **195**(1), 107–113.

Stewart, M.C. (2011a). Cell-based therapies: current issues and future directions. *The Veterinary Clinics of North America: Equine Practice* **27**(2), 393–399.

Stewart, M.C. and Stewart, A.A. (2011b). Mesenchymal stem cells: characteristics, sources, mechanisms of action. *The Veterinary Clinics of North America: Equine Practice* **27**(2), 243–261.

Taylor, S.E. and Clegg, P.D. (2011). Collection and propagation methods for mesenchymal stromal cells. *The Veterinary Clinics of North America: Equine Practice* **27**(2), 263–274.

Taylor, S.E., Smith, R.K.W. and Clegg, P.D. (2007). Mesenchymal stem cell therapy in equine musculoskeletal disease: scientific fact or clinical fiction? *Equine Veterinary Journal* **39**, 172–180.

Theoret, C. (2009). Tissue engineering in wound repair: the three "R"s – repair, replace, regenerate. *Veterinary Surgery* **38**(8), 905–913.

Toupadakis, C.A., Wong, A., Genetos, D.C., Cheung, W.K., Borjesson, D.L., Ferraro, G.L., Galuppo, L.D., Leach, K.J., Owens, S.D. and Yellowley, C.E. (2010). Comparison of the osteogenic potential of equine mesenchymal stem cells from bone marrow, adipose tissue, umbilical cord blood, and umbilical cord tissue. *American Journal of Veterinary Research* **71**(10), 1237–1245.

van Buul, G.M., Villafuertes, E., Bos, P.K., Waarsing, J.H., Kops, N., Narcisi, R., Weinans, H., Verhaar, J.A.N., Bernsen, M.R. and van Osch, G.J.V.M. (2012). Mesenchymal stem cells secrete factors that inhibit inflammatory processes in short-term osteoarthritic synovium and cartilage explant culture. *Osteoarthritis and Cartilage* **20**, 1186–1196.

Vandenabeele, S.I.J., White, S.D., Affolter, V.K., Kass, P.H. and Ihrke, P.J. (2004). Pemphigus foliaceus in the horse: a retrospective study of 20 cases. *Veterinary Dermatology* **15**, 381–388.

Verfaillie, C.M., Pera, M.F. and Lansdorp, P.M. (2002). Stem cells: hype and reality. *Hematology* **2002**, 369–391.

Vertenten, G., Lippens, E., Girones, J., Gorski, T., Declercq, H., Saunders, J., Van den Broeck, W., Chiers, K., Duchateau, L., Schacht, E., Cornelissen, M., Gasthuys, F. and Vlaminck, L. (2009). Evaluation of an injectable, photopolymerizable, and three-dimensional scaffold based on methacrylate-endcapped poly(D,L-lactideco-epsilon-caprolactone) combined with autologous mesenchymal stem cells in a goat tibial unicortial defect model. *Tissue Engineering Part A* **15**(7), 1501–1511.

Wilke, M.M., Nydam, D.V. and Nixon, A.J. (2007). Enhanced early chondrogenesis in articular defects following arthroscopic mesenchymal stem cell implantation in an equine model. *Journal of Orthopaedic Research* **25**(7), 913–925.

Zuk, P.A. (2009). The intracellular distribution of the ES cell totipotent markers Oct4 and Sox-2 in adult stem cells differs dramatically according to commercial antibody used. *Journal of Cellular Biochemistry* **106**, 867–877.

32 Hematopoietic Stem Cell Transplantation

M. Julia B. Felippe

32.1 Definition

Hematopoietic stem cell transplantation (HSCT) replaces the hematopoietic cells of a patient with *autologous* (from self), *allogeneic* (from a major histocompatibility complex, MHC-matched related or unrelated donor), or *syngeneic* (from an identical twin) stem cells (Figure 32.1A, B). Non-familial haploidentical HSCT (i.e., using a MHC-matched unrelated donor) has become a resource to patients that require immediate HSCT but a MHC-matching sibling is not available (Huang, 2006). The clinical conditions in which HSCT becomes a treatment option include myeloid and lymphoid malignancies, and acquired or congenital bone marrow failures, such as primary immunodeficiencies and autoimmunity (Copelan, 2006; Or, 2004; Filipovich, 2008). Success in HSCT is associated with MHC matching, pre-transplantation chemotherapy and/or irradiation conditioning for recipient bone marrow ablation, post-transplantation suppression of GvHD, use of antimicrobials, and supportive care. Nevertheless, mortality rates associated with HSCT are still relatively high (approximately 22%).

Incompatible MHC antigens induce severe transplant reactions (graft-versus-host disease, GvHD) and rejections. Even when donor and recipient are MHC-identical siblings, reactions can still occur, due to minor histocompatibility antigens, although such reactions are more likely between non-familial individuals. Nevertheless, changes in protocols throughout the years, using depletion of T cells from donor HSC, transplantation of mega amounts of stem cells, reduced-intensity conditioning, and appropriate antimicrobial therapy, have significantly decreased early transplant-related mortality and GvHD (Koh, 2008).

Fetomaternal tolerance prevents the offspring to build immunity against NIMA (MHC haplotype not inherited from the mother). However, these same individuals are capable of producing anti-non-inherited paternal antigens (NIPA, MHC haplotype not inherited from the father) (Billingham, 1953). Therefore, perinatal exposure to NIMA may affect future development of immunity, which can be clinically useful for increasing HSCT engraftment and decreasing GvHD (Burlingham, 1998).

In transplantation from a sibling donor who is mismatched with the recipient for one MHC haplotype, there is a beneficial effect of tolerance to non-inherited maternal antigens (NIMA) on long-term graft survival, in contrast to non-inherited paternal antigens (NIPA) (i.e., transplantation from a sibling donor expressing maternal MHC-antigens not inherited by the recipient has a greater graft survival than in transplantation from a sibling donor expressing paternal MHC-antigens not inherited by the recipient). Therefore, NIMA-mismatched donors provide an opportunity for patients who would not tolerate GvHD and prolonged immunosuppression.

Non-T cell-depleted NIMA-mismatched haploidentical HSCT can be performed safely by evaluating the reaction of IFN-gamma-producing cells of the donors against NIMA, using mixed-lymphocyte reactions before transplantation (Hirayama, 2012). At the same time, evolving approaches with reduced-intensity and nonmyeloablative conditioning regimens have increased the number of elderly, comorbid and primary immunodeficiency patients eligible for HSCT (Chiesa, 2012).

Outcomes of HSCT include successful engraftment of the donor cells, graft rejection, hematopoietic chimerism (coexistence of donor- and host-derived hematopoiesis), GvHD, engraftment syndrome (ES, granulocyte activation after recovery), thrombotic microangiopathy (small vessel endothelial injury and organ failure), and infections (Jodele, 2014; Spitzer, 2015). Under control, GvHD can be favorable to the patient, as it prevents tumor relapse (known as graft-versus-tumor effect).

32.2 Hematopoietic stem cell sources

Hematopoietic stem cell sources include bone marrow, blood, umbilical cord and amniotic fluid, with different success rates (Chan, 2013). Most HSCT are performed intravenously and, despite comparable success, different engraftment profiles may result from intramarrow versus intravenous routes (Jung, 2007).

Autologous hematopoietic stem cells can be harvested from the patient proactively at birth from umbilical cord and cryopreserved at a cord blood bank, or later in life from blood (using apheresis) or bone marrow (using aspirates), before pretreatment with chemotherapy and radiation. Autologous transplants have a lower risk of infection because recovery of immune function is rapid; however, due to the absence of

Equine Clinical Immunology, First Edition. Edited by M. Julia B. Felippe.
© 2016 John Wiley & Sons, Inc. Published 2016 by John Wiley & Sons, Inc.

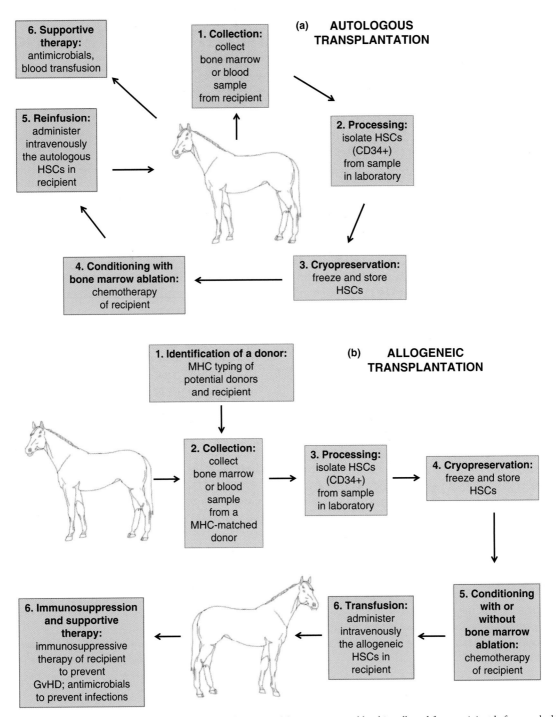

Figure 32.1 (a) Autologous hematopoietic stem cell (HSC) transplantation: **1)** bone marrow or blood is collected from recipient before myeloablative chemotherapy (e.g., for leukemia treatment); **2)** the sample is processed in laboratory for enrichment of HSCs, often using positive selection for the CD34$^+$ marker; **3)** the HSCs are frozen in special medium and preserved in liquid nitrogen until use; **4)** the patient is treated with myeloablative chemotherapy to destroy bone marrow and blood cells; **5)** the patient receives its own HSCs intravenously; **6)** the patient receives supportive therapy with antimicrobials to prevent infections.

(b) Allogeneic hematopoietic stem cell (HSC) transplantation: **1)** A MHC-matched donor is identified using microsatellite typing; **2)** bone marrow or blood is collected from the donor; **3)** the sample is processed in laboratory for enrichment of HSCs, often using positive selection for the CD34$^+$ marker; **4)** the HSCs are frozen in special medium and preserved in liquid nitrogen until use; **5)** the patient is treated with myeloablative (e.g., for the treatment of leukemia) or non-myeloablative (e.g., for the treatment of primary immunodeficiencies) chemotherapy; **6)** the patient receives allogeneic HSCs intravenously; **7)** the patient receives immunosuppressive therapy to prevent graft-versus-host disease (GvHD), and supportive therapy with antimicrobials to prevent infections.

GvHD, some types of cancer are more likely to relapse. Allogeneic transplants also use umbilical cord stem cells despite low cellular yield; yet, still suitable for transplantation to children.

A compatible donor matches the recipient's MHC class I and MHC class II haplotypes. Mismatch of MHC class I increases the risk of graft rejection, and a mismatch of MHC class II increases the risk of GvHD. Mismatches in MHC DNA sequence or in the minor histocompatibility antigens may lead to HSCT failures.

32.3 Pre-transplantation conditioning

In patients with bone marrow tumors, *myeloablative* conditioning regimen with chemotherapy (e.g., melphalan, cyclophosphamide, busulfan, fludarabine) and total body irradiation eliminates the tumoral cells prior to the HSCT. In addition, bone marrow ablation suppresses rejection of allogeneic stem cells (Russell, 2000). In non-malignant hematological diseases, pre-transplant chemotherapy destroys hematopoietic host cells to gain marrow space, while preventing rejection of donor stem cells. Autologous transplants also use a similar approach.

Non-myeloablative regimen uses lower doses of chemotherapy and radiation (or no radiation) that do not cause marked destruction of the bone marrow, and allow recipient-donor chimerism (Toze, 2005). This regimen reduces the risk of lethal infections and allows a graft-versus tumor effect to resist cancer relapse. Immunosuppressive doses are also lower than those used in conventional transplants, in order to allow T cell function in the graft-versus-tumor effect. As expected, clinical signs of GvHD often appear in this regimen, but these signs are used to tailor the immunosuppressive therapy without removing the graft-versus-tumor effect.

The non-myeloablative protocol is also used in non-malignant disorders, such as primary immunodeficiencies, and in the case of haploidentical hematopoietic stem cell transplantation. In the latter, selective T cell allodepletion decreases early transplant-related mortality and GvHD, while enabling robust and prompt engraftment. Nevertheless, the removal of T cells decreases the graft-versus-tumor effect, and cancer relapse is possible. Persistence of natural killer (NK) cell alloreactivity is still possible in leukemia patients using this regimen.

32.4 Post-transplantation immunosuppression

Graft-versus-host disease (GvHD) is associated with high morbidity and mortality in allogeneic post-HSCT (Weisdorf, 1990). Clinically significant GvHD occurs in 34–40% of patients undergoing MHC-matched related donors, 47–52% of patients undergoing MHC-matched unrelated donors, and a higher percentage when lacking MHC-matched donors. In MHC-matched transplantation, GvHD is mediated by donor T cells that recognize minor histocompatibility antigens in the recipient. Therefore, prophylactic immunosuppressive therapy post-transplantation is critical.

Only about 40% of transplanted patients with GvHD will respond to glucocorticoid therapy; therefore, pharmacologic investigations and clinical trials test the efficiency of other immunosuppressive drugs, in single use or in combination (e.g., tacrolimus, methotrexate, cyclophosphamide) (Kanakry, 2014). Proliferating alloreactive T cells are selectively sensitive to cyclophosphamide, which has been a successful prophylactic treatment for GvHD in MHC-matched related and unrelated HSCT, and partially MHC-mismatched HSCT (O'Donnell, 2002; Luznik, 2010).

Antimicrobial therapy (broad-spectrum antibiotics, anti-herpes virus and antifungal medication) and supportive care are also essential. Once engraftment is confirmed, vaccination protocols with primary and secondary immunizations should be followed, in order to develop adaptive immunity against relevant pathogens.

32.5 Hematopoietic stem cell transplantation in the horse

In the horse, single-cell suspensions prepared from liver of equine fetuses were transplanted in 14 foals with severe combined immunodeficiency (SCID), and resulted in no functional engraftment, while three foals developed mild GvHD with hepatic necrosis (Perryman, 1982). It is possible that the thymus of SCID foals could not complete differentiation of HSC or T cell precursors from fetal liver. However, when thymus cells were added to the transplantation protocol, engraftment could be achieved with functional lymphocytes, which were responsive to mitogens and synthesized immunoglobulins, the first successful HSCT in the horse (Perryman, 1979).

HSCT was attempted by the Equine Immunology Laboratory group at Cornell University in a Thoroughbred mare diagnosed with common variable immunodeficiency (CVID). This condition is characterized by late-onset recurrent bacterial infections, due to failure of B cell development in the bone marrow, B cell depletion and inability to produce antibodies, while innate and T cell functions are clinically intact. A healthy female full-sibling was determined transplantation-compatible based on MHC haplotype analyses, using serology (lymphocyte microcytotoxicity assay), reverse-transcription polymerase chain reaction (RT-PCR) of MHC class I, and microsatellite typing. Both donor and recipient were equine leukocyte antigen (ELA) A3/A9, and genome-wide scan panel revealed only four distinct microsatellites.

The recipient mare was treated with a non-myeloablative reduced-intensity conditioning protocol using cyclophosphamide and fludarabine, along with flunixin meglumine, on days minus 4, minus 3 and minus 2 before HSCT. Approximately 135 ml of non-manipulated fresh bone marrow collected from the donor contained approximately 8×10^8 CD34$^+$ cells, which

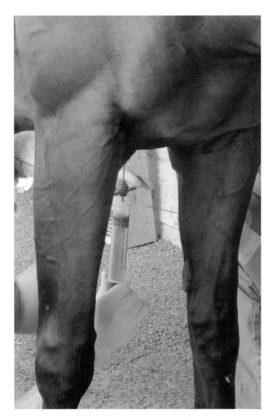

Figure 32.2 Bone marrow aspirate from a horse. Equine bone marrow is collected from the sternebrum after sedation, local anesthesia and aseptic preparation, using a Jamshidi® needle and a collecting syringe containing heparin (Julia Felippe, Cornell University).

were transplanted intravenously (Figures 32.2 and 32.3). Post-transplantation care included: immunosuppression to prevent GvHD (tapering doses of dexamethasone in the first 30 days, then maintenance with prednisolone for 22 days); anti-microbials (valacyclovir for 15 days, fluconazole for 50 days, trimethoprim-sulfadiazine for 115 days); anti-ulcer medication

(omeprazole while on glucocorticoids); daily physical examination; weekly complete blood cell counts and biochemistry.

Overall, the mare tolerated well the conditioning treatment and transplantation, and had mild episodes of colic that were controlled by a daily analgesic dose of flunixin meglumine. Long-term dexamethasone therapy developed increased appetite, muscle waste, and polyuria and polydipsia. Blood work revealed: decreased hematocrit (lowest value 39% on day 3), platelet count (lowest value 110,000 cells/uL on day 9); mild neutropenia (lowest value 4,400 cells/uL on day 24); lymphopenia (lowest value 400 cells/uL on days 3 and 9); increased cellular and cholestatic liver enzymes (gamma-glutamyl transferase, GGT; sorbitol dehydrogenase, SDH; glutamate dehydrogenase, GDH; and aspartate aminotransferase, AST; from day 9 to day 60, with highest values between days 15 and, 20); and hyperglycemia (highest value 195 mg/dL on day 15). With the exception of persistent hypoglobulinemia (average 1.7 g/dL) reflecting hypogammaglobulinemia, all other abnormal blood parameters resolved.

Chimerism (presence of donor genomic DNA) was detected (yet < 1%) in the recipient's blood at 2.5 months after transplantation, using quantitative amplification of microsatellites. Peripheral blood immunophenotyping revealed a transient mild decrease in CD4$^+$ T cell distribution from day 3 to day 9, but sustained high distribution throughout the study period at > 71%; CD8$^+$ T cell distribution did not change. B cell distribution, originally < 1.5%, increased to 3–4% between days 37 and 51, about the same time that chimerism was detected in blood. There was no improvement in serum IgG and IgM concentrations.

The mare was submitted to euthanasia 115 days after HSCT, due to intermittent fevers, malaise and emaciation. No obvious B cell expansion or presence of plasma cells was observed in lymphoid tissues at necropsy. The same level (< 1%) of chimerism detected in blood was measured in the recipient's bone marrow. This is the first report of HSCT in horses that used

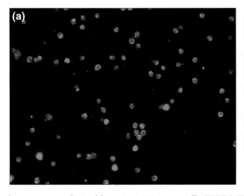
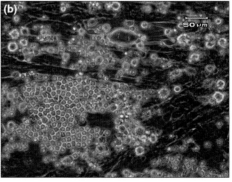

Figure 32.3 Equine bone marrow-derived hematopoietic stem cells (HSCs). The HSC are sorted from the bone marrow cell population, using a monoclonal antibody against the CD34 stem cell marker, and a magnetic bead cell sorting system.
(a) Immunocytofluorescence microscopy shows equine CD34$^+$ HSCs (green fluorescence).
(b) Equine HSC in culture with bone marrow stromal cells that, along with specific cytokines and growth factors, support cell differentiation into specific lineages, in this case B cells (courtesy of Ute Schwab, Cornell University).

a MHC-matching full-sibling as a donor, with conditioning, immunosuppressive, and supportive therapies based on human patient protocols. Maintaining critical equine patients long-term is still a challenge and perhaps cost-prohibitive.

References

Burlingham, W.J., Grailer, A.P., Heisey, D.M., Claas, F.H., Norman, D., Mohanakumar, T., Brennan, D.C., de Fijter, H., van Gelder, T., Pirsch, J.D., Sollinger, H.W. and Bean, M.A. (1998). The effect of tolerance to noninherited maternal HLA antigens on the survival of renal transplants from sibling donors. *New England Journal of Medicine* **339**(23), 1657–1664.

Chan, W.Y., Roberts, R.L., Moore, T.B. and Stiehm, E.R. (2013). Cord blood transplants for SCID: better B-cell engraftment? *Journal of Pediatric Hematology and Oncology* **35**(1), e14–e18.

Chen, X., Hale, G.A., Barfield, R., Benaim, E., Leung, W.H., Knowles, J., Horwitz, E.M., Woodard, P., Kasow, K., Yusuf, U., Behm, F.G., Hayden, R.T., Shurtleff, S.A., Turner, V., Srivastava, D.K. and Handgretinger, R. (2006). Rapid immune reconstitution after a reduced-intensity conditioning regimen and a CD3-depleted haploidentical stem cell graft for paediatric refractory haematological malignancies. *British Journal of Haematology* **135**(4), 524–532.

Chiesa, R. and Veys, P. (2012). Reduced-intensity conditioning for allogeneic stem cell transplant in primary immune deficiencies. *Expert Review of Clinical Immunology* **8**(3), 255–266.

Copelan, E.A. (2006). Hematopoietic stem-cell transplantation. *New England Journal of Medicine* **354**(17), 1813–1826.

Filipovich, A.H. (2008). Hematopoietic cell transplantation for correction of primary immunodeficiencies. *Bone Marrow Transplantation* **42**(Suppl. 1), S49–S52.

Hirayama, M., Azuma, E. and Komada, Y. (2012). Tolerogenic effect of non-inherited maternal antigens in hematopoietic stem cell transplantation. *Frontiers in Immunology* **3**, 135.

Huang, X.J., Liu, D.H., Liu, K.Y., Xu, L.P., Chen, H., Han, W., Chen, Y.H., Wang, J.Z., Gao, Z.Y., Zhang, Y.C., Jiang, Q., Shi, H.X. and Lu, D.P. (2006). Haploidentical hematopoietic stem cell transplantation without *in vitro* T-cell depletion for the treatment of hematological malignancies. *Bone Marrow Transplantation* **38**, 291–297.

Jodele, S., Laskin, B.L., Dandoy, C.E., Myers, K.C., El-Bietar, J., Davies, S.M., Goebel, J. and Dixon, B.P. (2014). A new paradigm: Diagnosis and management of HSCT-associated thrombotic microangiopathy as multi-system endothelial injury. *Blood Review*, Nov 28, 2014 [Epub].

Jung, C.W., Beard, B.C., Morris, J.C., Neff, T., Beebe, K., Storer, B.E. and Kiem, H.P. (2007). Hematopoietic stem cell engraftment: a direct comparison between intramarrow and intravenous injection in nonhuman primates. *Experimental Hematology* **35**(7), 1132–1139.

Kanakry, C.G., O'Donnell, P.V., Furlong, T., de Lima, M.J., Wei, W., Medeot, M., Mielcarek, M., Champlin, R.E., Jones, R.J., Thall, P.F., andersson, B.S. and Luznik, L. (2014). Multi-institutional study of post-transplantation cyclophosphamide as single-agent graft-versus-host disease prophylaxis after allogeneic bone marrow transplantation using myeloablative busulfan and fludarabine conditioning. *Journal of Clinical Oncology* **32**(31), 3497–3505.

Koh, L.P. and Chao, N. (2008). Haploidentical hematopoietic cell transplantation. *Bone Marrow Transplantation* **42**(Suppl. 1), S60–S63.

Luznik, L., Bolaños-Meade, J., Zahurak, M., Chen, A.R., Smith, B.D., Brodsky, R., Huff, C.A., Borrello, I., Matsui, W., Powell, J.D., Kasamon, Y., Goodman, S.N., Hess, A., Levitsky, H.I., Ambinder, R.F., Jones, R.J. and Fuchs, E.J. (2010). High-dose cyclophosphamide as single-agent, short-course prophylaxis of graft-versus-host disease. *Blood* **115**(16), 3224–3230.

O'Donnell, P.V., Luznik, L., Jones, R.J., Vogelsang, G.B., Leffell, M.S., Phelps, M., Rhubart, P., Cowan, K., Piantados, S. and Fuchs, E.J. (2002). Nonmyeloablative bone marrow transplantation from partially HLA-mismatched related donors using posttransplantation cyclophosphamide. *Biology of Blood and Marrow Transplantation* **8**(7), 377–386.

Or, R., Aker, M., Shapira, M.Y., Resnick, I., Bitan, M., Samuel, S. and Slavin, S. (2004). Allogeneic stem cell transplantation for the treatment of diseases associated with a deficiency in bone marrow products. *Springer Seminars in Immunology* **26**(1–2), 133–142.

Perryman, L.E., Buening, G.M., McGuire, T., Torbeck, R.L., Poppie, M.J. and Sales, G.E. (1979). Fetal tissue transplantation for immunotherapy of combined lmmunodeficiency in horses. *Clinical Immunology and Immunopathology* **12**(2), 238–251.

Perryman, L.E., McGuire, T., Torbeck, R.L. and Magnunsn, N. (1982). Evaluation of fetal liver cell transplantation for immunoreconstitution of horses with severe combined immunodeficiency. *Clinical Immunology and Immunopathology* **23**(1), 1–9.

Russell, N., Bessell, E., Stainer, C., Haynes, A., Das-Gupta, E. and Byrne, J. (2000). Allogenic haemopoietic stem cell transplantation for multiple myeloma or plasma cell leukaemia using fractionated total body radiation and high-dose melphalan conditioning. *Acta Oncologica* **39**(7), 837–841.

Spitzer, T.R. (2015). Engraftment syndrome: double-edged sword of hematopoietic cell transplants. *Bone Marrow Transplantation* Jan 12, 2015. [Epub].

Toze, C.L., Galal, A., Barnett, M.J., Shepherd, J.D., Conneally, E.A., Hogge, D.E., Nantel, S.H., Nevill, T.J., Sutherland, H.J., Connors, J.M., Voss, N.J., Messner, H.A., Lavoie, J.C., Forrest, D.L., Song, K.W., Smith, C.A. and Lipton, J. (2005). Myeloablative allografting for chronic lymphocytic leukemia: evidence for a potent graft-versus-leukemia effect associated with graft-versus-host disease. *Bone Marrow Transplatation* **36**(9), 825–830.

Weisdorf, D., Haake, R., Blazar, B., Miller, W., McGlave, P., Ramsay, N., Kersey, J. and Filipovich, A. (1990). Treatment of moderate/severe acute graft-versus-host disease after allogeneic bone marrow transplantation: an analysis of clinical risk features and outcome. *Blood* **75**(4), 1024–1030.

Index

Equine Clinical Immunology, First Edition. Edited by M. Julia B. Felippe.
© 2016 John Wiley & Sons, Inc. Published 2016 by John Wiley & Sons, Inc.